BILLY BUNTER
IN THE LAND OF THE PYRAMIDS

Billy Bunter's Bad Luck
Southward Bound
Harry Wharton & Co., in Egypt
The Lure of the Golden Scarab
Billy Bunter's Bargain
The Shadowed Schoolboy
The Secret of the Scarab
The Eye of Osiris

Vol. XLII Nos. 1277–1284 inclusive

Billy Bunter in the Land of the Pyramids

By

FRANK RICHARDS

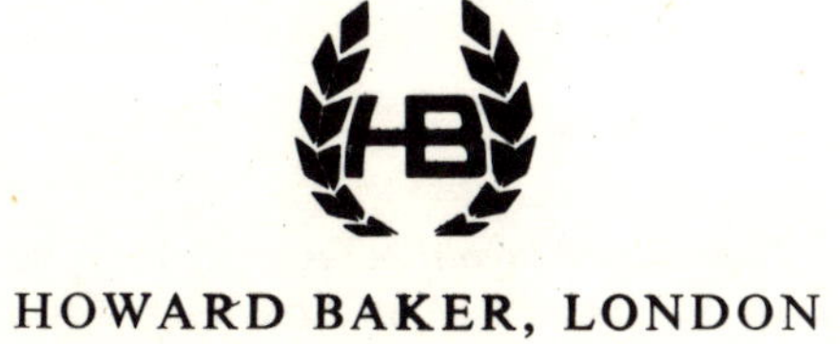

HOWARD BAKER, LONDON

FRANK RICHARDS

Billy Bunter in the Land of the Pyramids (The *Magnet*, 1932)

Originally published in single issues

Howard Baker edition 1969
SBN 09 309890 1

Howard Baker books are published by
Howard Baker Publishers Ltd
47 Museum Street
Bloomsbury, London W.C.1

Printed and bound in Great Britain by
Balding & Mansell Ltd, of London and Wisbech

Few could deny that Charles Hamilton was one of the greatest school story writers of all time — if not *the* greatest.

Writing mainly under the pseudonyms Frank Richards and Martin Clifford his work appeared continuously for over 30 years in those famous Fleetway magazines, the *Magnet* and the *Gem*. Most famous of all, was his immortal character Billy Bunter, the Fat Owl of the Greyfriars Remove: along with those other boyhood heroes Harry Wharton and Co., whose exploits in the *Magnet* delighted generations of readers from 1908 to 1940.

The war unhappily saw the end of the *Magnet*, but the post-war years witnessed the return of the Greyfriars stories in other formats.

However, nothing quite captured the evergreen magic of the original *Magnet*. So here, for the first time, are presented faithful facsimiles of those well-loved papers.

Each volume will contain a complete series. In this, the first volume, we follow the adventures of Billy Bunter and his friends in the land of the Pyramids.

Now read on, gentle reader, and bask in nostalgia for 'the best years of your life'.

"BILLY BUNTER'S BAD LUCK!" This week's grand school story inside.

The MAGNET 2D

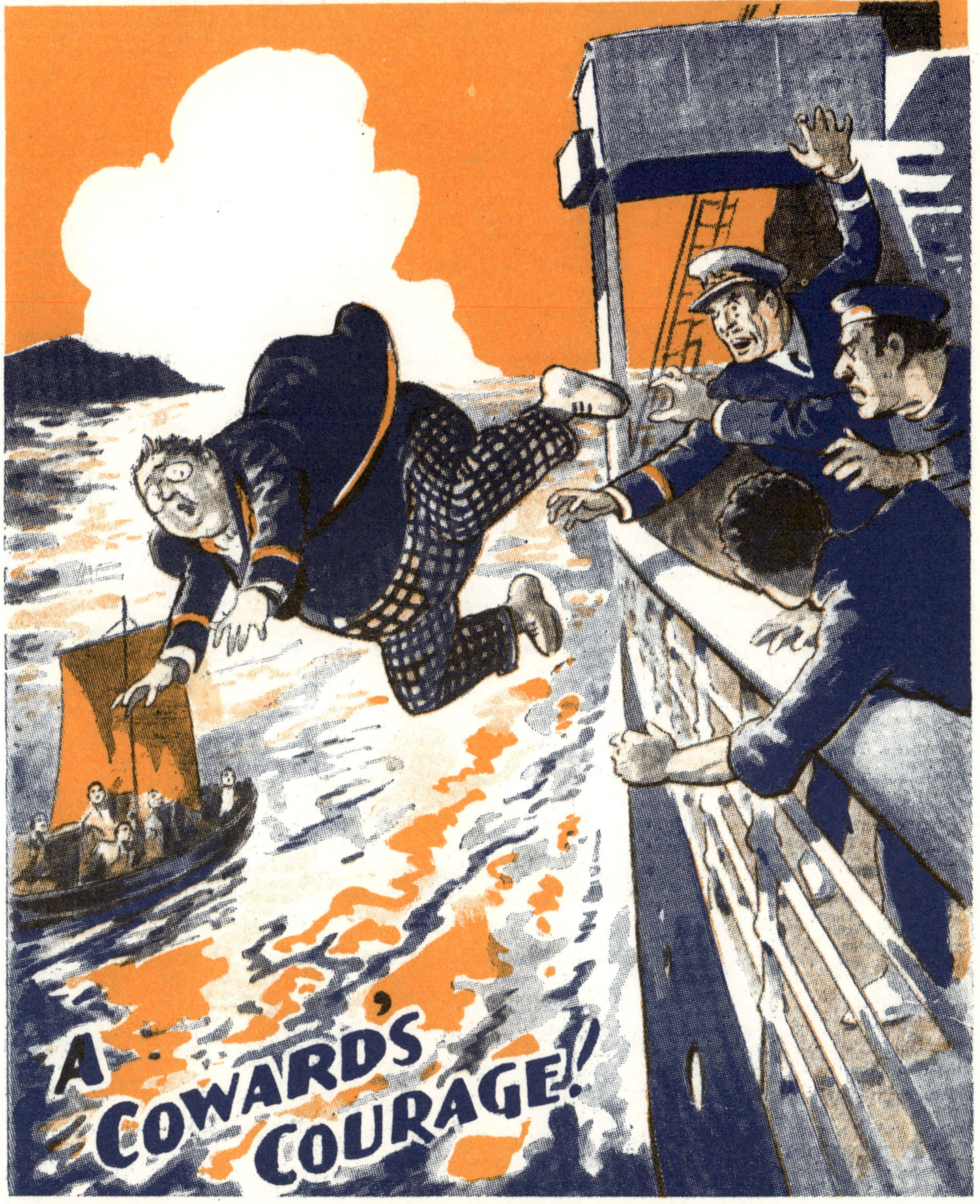

No. 1,277. Vol. XLII EVERY SATURDAY. Week Ending August 6th, 1932.

A CHAT WITH YOUR EDITOR !

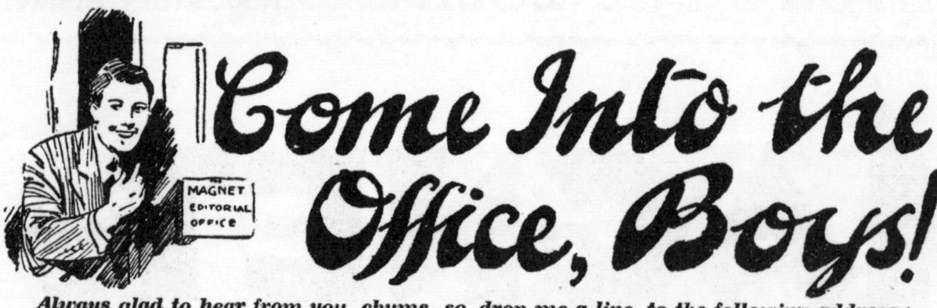

Always glad to hear from you, chums, so drop me a line to the following address: The Editor, The "Magnet" Library, The Amalgamated Press, Ltd., The Fleetway House, Farringdon Street, London, E.C.4.

I HAVE had a large number of letters this week from readers who wish to join the Navy, the Army, the Air Force, and the Mercantile Marine. On many occasions I have given full particulars of how to go about it, and I regret I haven't space to print them again. But boys who wish to join any branch of the fighting forces should apply to their local post office, where they can obtain a free booklet giving full particulars concerning the force in which they are interested.

With regard to the Mercantile Marine, application should be made direct to the shipowners of any particular line. In reply to both F. W. L. (of Chester), and "A Reader," who gives no address, I must warn them that first-class eyesight is an essential for a life at sea, and a stringent eyesight test must be passed before applications can be considered. I am afraid that, even in the steward's department, boys who wear spectacles would not be taken.

* * *

Do you remember the letter I quoted from a Hull reader concerning an alleged mermaid ? Well, here comes a most interesting letter from a Harrow reader, who sends along some information concerning

MERMAID-FAKING AS A BUSINESS !

You will doubtless have noticed that all descriptions of "mermaids" are somewhat similar—and this is the reason why. "Mermaid-faking" is quite a flourishing occupation in many East Indian islands. The natives get hold of the head of a monkey, the arms and body of another animal, and the tail end of a fish. Then these parts are skilfully fixed together in such a manner as to deceive one completely.

The fakers, of course, take great pains over the job, for the more realistic the monster appears, the higher price it commands. The "mermaids" are bought by travellers, and thus find their way to England and other European countries, where they are exhibited.

Apart from these fakes, many of the so-called mermaids which are exhibited in this country are manatees. This is a sea-cow, which has a fish-like body and a finely-wrinkled skin, covered with very delicate hair. The fore limbs form paddles, but they also bear three nails, and have free movement at the shoulder, elbow, and wrist. They have a very mobile upper lip, and eleven teeth.

Manatees never voluntarily leave the water, but if they are caught they are easily tamed.

You can take it for granted that whenever you see a "mermaid" advertised for exhibition, it is either a manatee, or else, as my Harrow reader says, "an impudent (if skilful) fake."

* * *

HERE comes a letter from Bernard Jex (of South Elmsall), who sends along

AN INTERESTING SENTENCE.

Perhaps you know it ? It contains all the letters of the alphabet. Here it is: "The quick brown fox jumps over the lazy dogs." But I can go one better than that. The letter "e," as you all know, occurs most frequently in the English language. It appears three times in the above short sentence. But what about a long sentence (in verse, too !) that contains every letter in the alphabet *except* the ubiquitous "e" ? I don't think it is very well known, and perhaps it might interest you, so I'll print it here :

A jovial swain may rack his brain
And tax his fancy's plight ;
Go quiz in vain,
For 'tis most plain
That what I say is right !

* * *

"A Regular Reader" (of Bristol), writes :

CONCERNING VENTRILOQUISM.

He has been practising this entertaining art for some time, and tells me that he can now speak perfectly without moving his lips. But he can't "throw" his voice, and he asks me to tell him how to do it. Well, I am sorry to tell him that *no one* can actually "throw" their voice. Ventriloquism, as practised even by the greatest exponents, is really an illusion—the voice merely *appears* to be thrown. In other words, my reader must imitate the sound of a voice as it would strike the hearer *if* it came from a certain source. When that is done properly, the hearer really believes that the voice has been thrown. Naturally, when a ventriloquist has dolls with movable mouths to help him, it is much easier to sustain the illusion.

* * *

NOW I am going to award a topping Sheffield steel penknife to Thomas E. Denyer, of 120, Ash Road, Aldershot, Hants, for sending in the following joke :

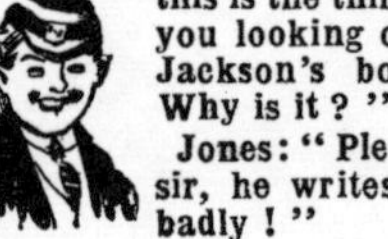
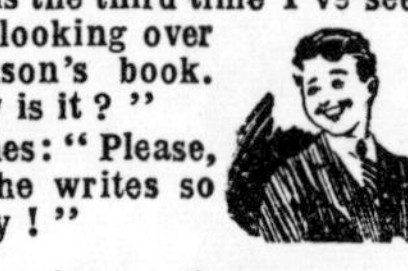

Teacher (during an exam) : "Jones, this is the third time I've seen you looking over Jackson's book. Why is it ?"
Jones : "Please, sir, he writes so badly !"

* * *

Space is running short, so I had better give a few

RAPID-FIRE REPLIES

to various readers who have sent along queries.

Minimum age for Motor-Cycle (and side-car) Driving Licence. ("Regular Reader," of Totton.) At the age of sixteen you can obtain a licence allowing you to drive a motor-cycle, and also a side-car. You must be seventeen to obtain a driving licence for a motor-car.

How to Get Bronzed. (Bristol Inquirer.) Nothing but exposure to the sun and fresh air will give you a real healthy bronze—and you must be very careful not to overdo it. It is against my rules to recommend any chemicals to achieve this result—chemicals are dangerous !

How the "Flying Scotsman" Got it's Name. ("Regular Reader," of Peacehaven.) It was one of the first long-journey trains in this country, and long before the practice of naming trains was adopted the public gave it this nickname because of its speed. "The Flying Scotsman" is the name of the *train*, not the name of the engine. The engine which draws it is one of the "Pacific" type, and the most famous is the "Gladiateur," which holds the world's record for continuous running.

Other Papers in Which the Greyfriars Chums are Featured. (Miss J. R.) You will find other splendid tales of Harry Wharton & Co. in the "Schoolboy's Own Library." I will bear in mind your suggestion to bring in Marjorie Hazeldene and Co., of Cliff House, into the stories. What do other readers think ?

How to Train for a Professional Singer. ("Would-be Singer," of London.) As you live in London, your best plan would be to write to the Guildhall School of Music, John Carpenter Street, E.C.4, and ask them for a prospectus. There are hundreds of first-class musical academies in London.

The Best "Scrapper" in the Remove. (S. Hitchen, of Halifax.) Yes, I think Bob Cherry would top the list of Remove boxers, with Harry Wharton and Mark Linley a close second and third. I will bear in mind your suggestion of publishing a list such as you describe.

* * *

I THINK I have just room for another prizewinner. This time it is: Michael Ward, of Brayestown, Clonee, Co. Meath, I.F.S., who sends in the following Greyfriars limerick and gets a topping prize for it.

Said Coker, as he mounted his bike :
"To do seventy an hour I'd like."
But the foolish young ass
Stepped too hard on the gas
And he stuck in the ground like a pike !

Now a word or two about the treat in store for you in next week's issue of the MAGNET. Frank Richards' long complete story is entitled :

"SOUTHWARD BOUND !"

and it's just the kind of yarn you are bound to appreciate. Wouldn't you give something to accompany the Famous Five on their holiday jaunt to sunny Egypt ? By Jove, it makes my mouth water to think of it ! Brilliant sunshine, blue skies, waving palm trees—and ripping adventures ! Yes, there's certainly a treat in store for you next week !

Although our great adventure serial, "The Island Traders," ends in our next issue, you will have the satisfaction of knowing that I have another special treat to take its place. Watch out for full particulars in next Saturday's MAGNET. Dr. Birchemall, of course, will be well to the fore in another rib-tickling yarn of St. Sam's, entitled :

"HIGH JINKS HIKING !"

Laugh ! Gee, your sides will ache some when you've finished reading it !

Send along your jokes, limericks, and queries, chums ! I'm always pleased to receive them !

YOUR EDITOR.

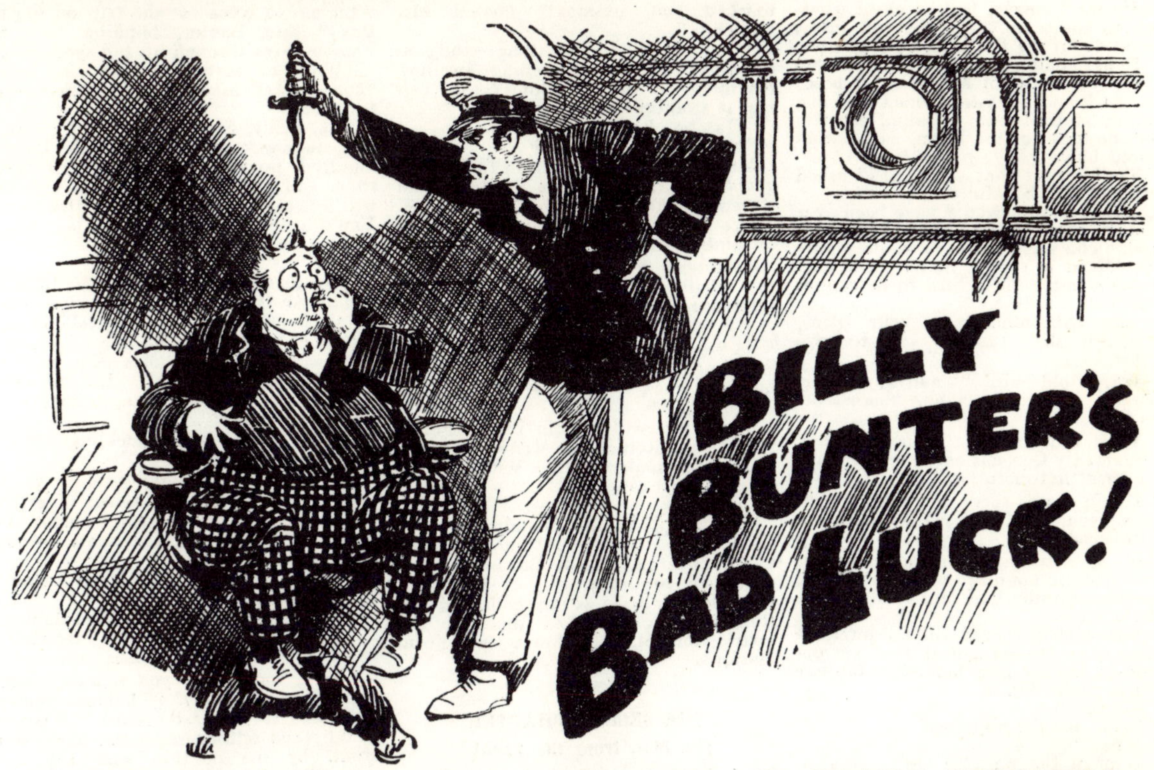

Featuring Harry Wharton & Co. of Greyfriars. By FRANK RICHARDS.

THE FIRST CHAPTER.
Trouble for Bunter!

RAP!

"Whoooop!"

Billy Bunter, sagging over his desk in the Remove Form Room at Greyfriars, was half asleep—until Mr. Quelch's pointer rapped on his fat knuckles. Then he was suddenly awake—very wide-awake indeed.

It was quite a loud rap! But it was not so loud as the yell that followed it. That yell woke every echo in the Form-room, and a good many beyond.

Mr. Quelch, the master of the Remove, was cross that morning. He was suffering from that end-of-the-term feeling—a common complaint among schoolmasters. And it was hot—the hottest day in July. A wasp had sailed in at the open window, and was buzzing about, with an irritating buzz. Twice Mr. Quelch had swiped at that wasp with his pointer, and missed. When he swiped at Bunter he did not miss.

Bunter was sleepy. Even energetic fellows in the Remove felt the drowsy heat a little. Billy Bunter felt it a lot. Never had Latin prose seemed so prosy to Bunter. Quelch's voice, in his fat ears, was merely an irritating buzz—just like that of the wasp. Bunter nodded, and nodded, and his little, round eyes closed behind his big round spectacles, and he was just sliding happily into a delicious dream of ginger-pop and doughnuts, when that rap on his knuckles brought him back, with a jump, to reality.

"Ow, ow! Wow!" gasped Bunter, sucking his fat knuckles frantically.

"You must not go to sleep in the Form-room, Bunter!" said Mr. Quelch.

"I—I wasn't asleep!" gasped Bunter.

"What? Your eyes were shut!"

"I—I listen better with my eyes shut!" gasped Bunter. "I—I heard every word you said, sir! Wow!"

"Oh!" said Mr. Quelch grimly. "In that case, Bunter, repeat my last sentence."

"Oh! I—I—I mean——" stammered the hapless Owl of the Remove.

"You will take fifty lines for untruthfulness, Bunter."

"Oh crikey!"

"And do not utter ridiculous ejaculations in the Form-room!" thundered Mr. Quelch.

"Oh, sir! No, sir! Oh lor'—I—I—I mean, oh, jiminy——"

"Silence!"

Mr. Quelch stalked away from that hopeful pupil, leaving Bunter sucking his knuckles. Remove fellows who had been feeling drowsy, and disinclined for Latin prose on a sultry July morning, sat up and took notice. Evidently Quelch had to be treated with tact that morning. He was in a mood to hand out lickings and detentions. And that afternoon was a half-holiday—the last half-holiday of the term. Nobody wanted detentions.

Billy Bunter's borrowing again! This time he has "borrowed" Lord Mauleverer's title! The result is a string of misfortunes for Bunter and a tip-top story for YOU!

Bob Cherry closed one eye at his chums as the Remove master's back was turned for the moment.

"'Ware beaks!" murmured Bob. "The jolly old bean's got his jolly old back up!"

It was the faintest of whispers, and ought to have been audible only to Harry Wharton, to whom it was addressed. But Henry Samuel Quelch seemed amazingly keen of hearing that morning. He spun round, and fixed his eyes, as penetrating as a pair of gimlets, on Bob Cherry.

"Cherry!"

"Oh crumbs!" gasped Bob, in dismay. "I mean, yes, sir!"

"Were you talking in class, Cherry?"

"I—I—I——"

"Were you talking in class, or were you not talking in class, Cherry?" demanded Mr. Quelch categorically.

"Oh, yes, sir! I—I just whispered to Wharton——"

"You will take a hundred lines, Cherry!"

"Oh! Yes, sir!"

"You will hand them to me before tea," added Mr. Quelch.

"Oh!" gasped Bob.

There was no more whispering in class. Wharton and Nugent, Johnny Bull and Hurree Singh, gave their chum sympathetic glances. The Famous Five had planned an excursion for that afternoon; but lines to be handed in before tea meant that Bob would have to stay within gates till they were done. Mr. Quelch was suffering from the end-of-the-term feeling, and now Bob was going to suffer from it, too!

Latin prose resumed its prosy course. The Remove longed for the end of third school. Perhaps Mr. Quelch was as anxious to be done with his Form, as his Form were to be done with him. But Quelch was a dutiful Form master, and he never slacked, or allowed slacking. On that blazing morning the Remove could have done quite well with a less dutiful master.

Bzzzzzzz!

The wandering wasp was still busy.

Mr. Quelch turned his gimlet eyes on that wasp.

But the gimlet eyes that could almost

petrify the Remove, had no effect whatever on the wasp. The cheerful insect buzzed about the Form-room, regardless of Henry Samuel Quelch. It sailed within two inches of Mr. Quelch's nose, and the Remove master swiped with the pointer, and missed. It sailed cheerily over the heads of the Form, with a continuous buzzing.

"Shall I swat that wasp, sir?" asked Vernon-Smith hopefully.

Chasing a wasp would have been ever so much more entertaining than Latin prose. The whole Remove would gladly have joined in such a chase. But Mr. Quelch was too old a bird to be caught with chaff like that.

"You will remain in your place, Vernon-Smith!" snapped the Remove master.

"Wary old bird!" murmured the Bounder to Tom Redwing, who sat beside him.

"What did you say, Vernon-Smith?" Undoubtedly Quelch's ears were remarkably keen that morning.

"I said I was sorry the wasp should annoy you, sir!" answered Vernon-Smith meekly.

Mr. Quelch gave him a suspicious look. He did not quite believe that that was what Smithy had said to Redwing.

Buzzzzzz!

"Yarooooh!" roared Billy Bunter, as Skinner, on the form near him, surreptitiously tickled him behind a fat ear with a penholder.

"Bunter!"

"Ow! It's the wops——"

"What?"

"I mean the wasp! Ow! It's on me!" yelled Bunter, jumping up. "Ow! I'm stung! Yaroooooh!"

"Sit down, Bunter!" thundered Mr. Quelch. "You are not stung! The wasp is not near you! Take a hundred lines!"

"Oh crikey! I—I thought I was stung!" gasped Bunter. "Something touched my ear! I think it was the wasp, sir——"

"Silence!"

"Oh, really, sir——"

"I shall cane you if you speak again, Bunter."

Billy Bunter did not speak again. He rubbed his fat ear, and grunted. Skinner smiled serenely and winked at Snoop. The wasp sailed to the window, and drummed on the glass with a ceaseless buzz. Billy Bunter blinked round uneasily. He was sure that the wasp had touched him—and he was afraid that the insect might touch him again. Wasp stings were neither grateful nor comforting.

"Bunter," yapped Mr. Quelch, "sit still!"

"Oh dear! I—I'm afraid of that wasp, sir——"

"Silence!"

Billy Bunter sat still, listening with uneasy ears to the buzz. The wasp, discovering that he could not get through glass, left the window, and buzzed over the heads of the juniors once more. The playful Skinner, reaching behind Bunter, tapped the back of his fat neck with the pen-holder.

"Whoooop!"

Bunter fairly bounded.

The form rocked, books went crashing to the floor, and ink spurted from an inkwell. Bunter clasped the back of his neck and roared:

"Ow! I'm stung! Yaroooop! Whooop!"

"Bunter!" shrieked Mr. Quelch.

"I'm stung!" yelled Bunter. "Stung on the back of the neck! Oow! Wow! Yow! I knew that wasp was going to sting me! Yaroooh!"

"I do not believe that the wasp touched you, Bunter!" hooted Mr. Quelch.

"Ow! It did! I'm stung—stung in the neck! My neck's swelling—swelling fearfully——" howled Bunter. "I can feel it swelling——"

"Ha, ha, ha!"

"Silence!"

Mr. Quelch made a stride to Bunter, grabbed him by the fat shoulder, and stared at the back of his podgy neck. There was no sign of a sting—and certainly no swelling.

"Bunter! You are not stung! You are deliberately playing tricks to interrupt the lesson! You are a young rascal, sir!"

"Ow! I—I thought I was stung——"

"Nonsense! You will take three hundred lines, Bunter——"

"Oh lor'!"

"And you will remain in the Form-room this afternoon to write them out. And if you make another sound during class, I shall cane you."

"Ow!"

The wasp, having found the open window at last, sailed out into the quad, and the buzzing ceased. But Mr. Quelch continued to drone, till, at long last, third school came to an end, and the Remove were dismissed—much to the satisfaction of both Form and Form master.

THE SECOND CHAPTER.
The Man from the Yacht!

"I SAY, you fellows!"

"Br-r-r-r-r-r!"

After dinner, Harry Wharton & Co. gathered by the House steps, to consult. It had been the intention of the Famous Five to get out immediately after dinner, and make the most of the last half-holiday of the term. That programme was rather upset by Bob Cherry's detention. Remarks from Billy Bunter were not required while the chums of the Remove discussed the matter. But the plans of the Famous Five were, of course, a trifle light as air, from the point of view of William George Bunter. Billy Bunter had three hundred lines on hand, which meant detention for the afternoon; and that was the most important matter, at the moment, within the wide limits of the universe.

"I say——" recommenced Bunter.

"Shut up, old fat bean," said Harry Wharton. "Look here, Bob, we'd better wait till you get through——"

"The waitfulness for the idiotic Bob is the proper caper," agreed Hurree Jamset Ram Singh.

Bob Cherry shook his head.

"No good you fellows hanging about," he said. "You'd better start, and I'll get after you when I've done those dashed lines. You can get the boat ready——"

"I say, you fellows!"

"Shut up, Bunter! You'll have to arrange about the boat at Pegg," said Bob. "That will take some time. I'll join you as soon as I can, and trot all the way."

"I say, you fellows!" bawled Bunter. "You seem to have forgotten that I've got lines."

"Dry up, old fat bean!"

"But I shan't be able to come with you fellows if I have to stick in the Form-room doing lines!" hooted Bunter.

"We'll try to survive it somehow," said Johnny Bull sarcastically. "We may be able to pull through."

"Oh, really, Bull! I suppose you want me to come for the trip on Pegg Bay!" said Bunter, blinking at the Famous Five through his big spectacles.

"What on earth put that idea into your head?" asked Frank Nugent, in surprise.

"Oh, really, Nugent! Now, look here, you fellows," said Bunter. "Three hundred lines will keep me till tea-time, and that means that you fellows will lose my company for the afternoon. You'd hardly like that, on the last half-holiday of the term."

"Oh, my hat!"

"My idea is to whack out the lines," explained Bunter. "I'll do fifty—I'm no slacker, I hope—and you fellows do fifty each. That will be fair all round. You can make your fists like mine—near enough to pass! Ten to one Quelch won't spot anything. See?"

"Ha, ha, ha!"

"What are you cackling at?" demanded Bunter.

"Your little joke, old bean."

"I'm not joking, you asses! It's the only way—otherwise, I can't come! It means a licking if Quelch spots it—but I'll chance that."

"And we're to chance it, too?" grinned Nugent.

"Exactly! Is it a go?" asked Bunter.

"The go-fulness is not terrific!" chuckled the Nabob of Bhanipur.

"Now, look here, you fellows," said Bunter impressively. "I hope you're not going to be beastly selfish! I never could stand selfishness. Look here, you stand by me in this, and I'll tell you what I'll do—I'll ask the lot of you home to Bunter Court for the holidays. There!"

"Ha, ha, ha!"

"Blessed if I see anything to cackle at! It will be rather a change for you, after your own humble homes, you know!"

"That's settled, then," said Harry Wharton. "We'll trot down to Pegg, and you can trot after us when you're done, Bob."

"What about me?" hooted Bunter.

"Nothing about you, old fat bean."

"I say, you fellows, I mean it!" said Bunter. "I'll have the lot of you at Bunter Court, and it will be a chance for you fellows to mix, for once, in some really decent society, you know. Dash it all, I'll ask the pater to let us have a run in his yacht!" added Bunter recklessly.

"Ha, ha, ha!" roared the Famous Five.

Bunter Court, which was Bunter's magnificent name for his father's detached villa in Surrey, was well known in the Remove. But the Bunter yacht was new.

That day a handsome steam-yacht had been seen to drop anchor in Pegg Bay, a couple of miles from the school. Possibly that had put the idea into Billy Bunter's fat and fatuous brain.

"I mean it," said Bunter. "How'd you fellows like a yachting cruise these hols—dropping in at Continental ports, and all that——"

"Fine!" grinned Bob Cherry.

"Ripping!" chortled Johnny Bull.

"The ripfulness would be terrific!"

"Well, I'll work it!" said Bunter fatuously. "Of course, you fellows aren't really the sort of chaps I should ask——"

"Eh?"

"We generally have members of the nobility. But I'll stretch a point! After all, we're pals, and I never was a snob!"

"Oh crikey!"

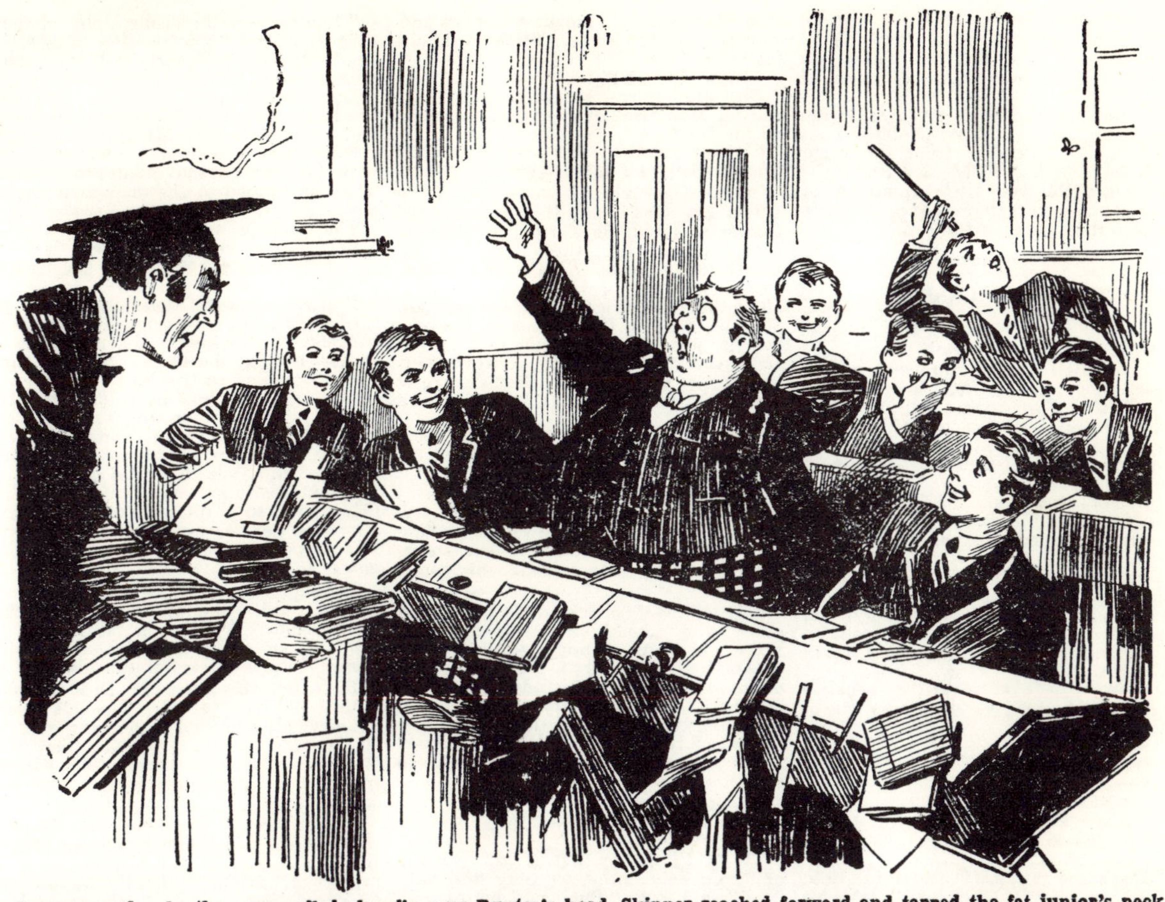

Buzzzzzzzz! As the wasp sailed cheerily over Bunter's head, Skinner reached forward and tapped the fat junior's neck with a pen-holder. "Whooooop!" yelled Bunter, jumping up. "I'm stung! Stung on the back of the neck—ow! Wow!"

"It's a go, then," said Bunter. "You fellows come in and whack out my lines——"

"Bunter!"

"Oh lor'!" gasped Billy Bunter, spinning round like a fat humming-top at the sound of his Form master's voice.

Mr. Quelch was looking out of the doorway of the House. He was going to remind two members of his Form that it was time to turn up for detention. They might possibly have forgotten it, without a reminder.

"Bunter! Were you asking these juniors to write your lines for you?" asked Mr. Quelch, in an awful voice.

"Oh, no, sir!" gasped Bunter. "I—I wouldn't, sir! I—I—I like writing lines——"

"What?"

"Especially for you, sir!" gasped Bunter. "Because—because you're so —so nice, sir!"

"Upon my word, Bunter, go into the Form-room at once! You will write four hundred lines, Bunter."

"Oh jiminy!"

"Cherry, you will go in with Bunter."

Two hapless Removites went into the House, under the gimlet eye of Henry Samuel Quelch. Four members of the Co. walked away to the gates.

"Too bad!" murmured Nugent. "We shan't get that trip in Bunter's yacht now! What a loss!"

"Ha, ha, ha!"

"The lossfulness will be terrific!" chuckled Hurree Jamset Ram Singh.

The four juniors sauntered away cheerfully down the lane, and turned into the footpath through the wood.

Beyond the wood, Pegg Bay and the shining North Sea spread before their eyes.

Brown sails danced on the bay in the bright sunlight, and some distance out, a large steam-yacht was at anchor. The juniors looked at it from the beach, feeling that the owner of that magnificent vessel was a man to be envied.

Having arranged with old Dave Trumper for the hire of a boat, and having packed in it a basket of tuck for tea afloat, the juniors sat down on the rail of the old wooden pier, to wait for Bob Cherry to turn up.

From the yacht's davits, a boat had dropped, and two dark-skinned foreign-looking seamen pulled for the shore. In the stern sat a slim, olive-skinned man, in a yachting cap.

The juniors watched the boat idly as it pulled to the pier, and the seamen hooked on, and the olive-skinned man stepped out. The man, apparently the owner of the yacht, was some sort of a foreigner, though they did not know of what race. He glanced about him, with a pair of eyes that were quick, keen, and intensely black, as he landed, and looked at the four juniors sitting on the rail—and looked again. He seemed to be interested in Harry Wharton & Co. for some reason, why, they could not imagine.

After a long, keen look, he came towards the juniors, and raised his yachting cap in polite salute. Not to be outdone in politeness, the juniors "capped" him in return.

"You will excuse me," said the foreign gentleman, in a very musical voice, "I am a stranger here, and perhaps you can tell me if there is a school called Greyfriars near at hand?"

"Yes, rather, sir!" answered Harry Wharton, with a smile. "We belong to Greyfriars School. It's a couple of miles away."

"Perhaps I can get a conveyance——"

"They'll phone a taxi if you walk up to the inn yonder, sir."

"Thank you." The keen black eyes passed from face to face. "I guessed that perhaps you were Greyfriars boys, seeing you here. Possibly you are acquainted with a boy in the school named Mauleverer—Lord Mauleverer?"

"He's in our Form—the Remove," answered Harry.

The foreign gentleman smiled.

"Perhaps one of you is Lord Mauleverer?" he asked.

Wharton smiled, and shook his head.

"No, he's not with us, sir!"

"Thank you, then I must go to the school," said the foreign gentleman, and, saluting the juniors again, he walked on quickly towards the Anchor.

Harry Wharton & Co. looked after him, rather curiously.

"What the dickens can that foreign johnny want with old Mauly?" asked Johnny Bull.

"Goodness knows!"

The man from the yacht disappeared into the Anchor. He emerged again in a few minutes, and stood waiting by the old porch, till at length a taxicab came grinding up the road. The yachtsman stepped into the taxi, and was driven rapidly away in the direction of Greyfriars.

He disappeared from the eyes of the juniors on the pier. They wondered what business the foreigner from the yacht could have with Lord Mauleverer of the Greyfriars Remove—little dreaming of the strange events that were destined to happen that sunny afternoon.

THE THIRD CHAPTER.
Bunter in a Hurry!

CRASH!

Bob Cherry threw down his pen, and hurled Virgil across the Form-room. P. Vergilius Maro dropped into a corner with a crash, unheeded. The hundred lines were done at last, and Bob was done with the great Mantuan.

"Done!" said Bob. "Thank goodness!"

Billy Bunter blinked up at him dolorously.

Bunter had four hundred lines to write, and while Bob was doing a hundred, Bunter had done only ten. With three hundred and ninety still on hand, the fat Owl was not feeling merry or bright.

"Finished, old chap?" groaned Bunter. "I say, I've done only ten of my lot!"

"Slacker!"

"Oh, really, Cherry! Look here, I'm jolly well not going to finish them," said Bunter. "I'm fed up!"

"Fathead!"

"I'll chance it, and come along with you, old bean!" said Bunter.

"Don't be an ass!" advised Bob. "You can bet that Quelch will have his eyes wide open. It means a licking and detention all the same. Stick to it, old fat bean!"

"Blow Quelch!"

Billy Bunter rose from his desk. There was an expression of deep determination on his fat face.

"Better stick to it," said Bob. "If Quelch spots you going——"

"Bless Quelch!"

The fat Owl's mind was made up. Bunter was not, as a rule, a fellow to take chances. But three hundred and ninety more lines, in a stuffy Form-room on a hot July afternoon, were altogether too thick. Bunter was not, perhaps, keen on the sail across the bay, but he was very keen on getting out of anything in the shape of work, and still keener on taking the lion's share of tea in the boat. Bunter had made up his mind.

"I'm chancing it," he said. "Look here, old chap——"

"Don't be a goat!"

"Beast! You take in your lines to Quelch and keep him busy for a few minutes! See? Keep him from looking out of the window while I cut. Ask him something about deponent verbs, or——"

"Catch me!" chuckled Bob. "If I asked him something about deponent verbs, old bean, he might tell me."

"Oh, really, Cherry! I'll give you a minute to get to his study," said the fat Owl. "Then I'll start, see? Ask him something about your lines—he likes fellows to be interested in that tripe!"

"Better stick where you are, and do your lines!"

"Beast!"

"If you get spotted——"

"Rotter!"

"Well, I'll do my best, if you've made up your silly mind to play the silly goat," said Bob. "But you'd better——"

"You're wasting time, old chap!" said Bunter. "You're like a sheep's head, you know—nearly all jaw. Get a move on!"

Bob Cherry got a move on. He left the Form-room with his lines in his hand, and made his way to Mr. Quelch's study.

Billy Bunter waited a whole minute, with his eye on the Form-room clock. Then he tiptoed to the door and peered out.

The passage was deserted.

Few Greyfriars fellows were indoors on that glorious summer's afternoon. The House was very silent.

Bunter blinked along the passage through his big spectacles, his fat heart beating. Breaking detention was rather a risky business. But by that time, Bob was in the Remove master's study, and there was no doubt that Mr. Quelch would rise to the bait, if Bob asked him to explain something in Virgil. His eyes would not be on his window, and Bunter needed only a very few minutes to get clear. Exertion did not appeal to William George Bunter, but once he was out of the House, he was prepared to put on top speed to the gates.

Taking his courage in both hands, as it were, Billy Bunter crept out of the Form-room. A minute later he was blinking out of the open doorway of the House, into the blaze of sunshine.

To reach the gates, he had to pass within full view of Mr. Quelch's study window. But he had no doubt that Bob Cherry was playing up, and that the Remove master was expounding Virgil, in which case his eyes could not be on the quad.

It was neck or nothing, and Bunter chanced it. He rolled down the House steps, and started for the gates at a rapid run. Seldom did Billy Bunter put on speed, but now he fairly flew. His feet seemed scarcely to touch the ground as he went.

But it was, as so often happens, a case of more haste and less speed. At that terrific burst, Bunter ought to have reached the gates in a minute or so. Naturally, he had not calculated on Mr. Prout, the master of the Fifth Form, stepping into the path from under the elms, as Bunter came hurtling by like a charging rhinoceros. Naturally, he had forgotten the existence of Mr. Prout, just as Mr. Prout had forgotten the existence of William George Bunter. They were suddenly reminded of one another's existence, as they established contact.

Bunter crashed, and Prout flew.

"Oooooh!" spluttered Prout, as he staggered and sat down.

"Yowp!" gurgled Bunter, as he reeled back from the shock.

Prout sat up, gasping.

"I—I—you—you—oooogh—what—oh—ow!" Prout's first remarks were incoherent. "Upon my word! Bless my soul! Bunter——"

"Oh! Ow! Ooooooogh!"

"You—you—how dare you?" gasped Prout. He heaved up his portly form and grasped the fat junior by the collar. "Bunter! I repeat, how dare you rush along the path like—like—like a wild Indian, and—and—ooooch? I shall take you to your Form master, Bunter! Wooooh! I shall insist upon—ooch!—the most exemplary—wooogh—punishment, for this—ugh—gug—gug—this outrageous conduct! Wooooogh!"

"I—I—I say——" gasped Bunter. "I—I—I'm in a—a—a hurry——"

"Come with me!" boomed Prout.

"Oh crikey!"

In the lowest of spirits, Billy Bunter was led back to the House, with

Prout's plump hand on his collar. Prout gasped as he went. Billy Bunter groaned. He was marched into the House, still with the plump hand on his collar; and his spirits were down to zero when they arrived at Mr. Quelch's study door. Prout tapped and opened the door.

" . . . per noctem plurima volvens." Mr. Quelch was speaking in the study in his kindliest tone.

Seldom—very seldom—did a fellow bringing in lines to Mr. Quelch display any personal interest in those lines. Quelch was not in the best of tempers that day, but this naturally had an ameliorating effect on him.

"By night revolving many things, Cherry, you will see—why—what—Mr. Prout—what——"

Mr. Quelch broke off, staring at Prout and Bunter. Bob Cherry stared at them, too. Evidently Bunter had made his dash for freedom—and, equally evidently, he had had no luck. Bob had done his best; he had kept Quelch's eyes off the window, but in vain.

"Mr. Quelch," boomed Prout, "I have brought this boy to you——"

"Bunter, what are you doing out of detention?" thundered Mr. Quelch. "What have you to say, Bunter?"

"Oh crikey!"

That, apparently, was all Bunter had to say!

"Detention!" repeated Mr. Prout. "Ah, no doubt that was the reason why this boy—this reckless young rascal—was racing down the path like—like a wild Hottentot! I have been knocked over, Mr. Quelch; I have been felled—felled to the earth by this boy——"

"This boy will be punished most severely, Mr. Prout. You may leave him in my hands!"

And Prout rolled away, leaving the unhappy Owl in Mr. Quelch's hands.

Mr. Quelch eyed him like a basilisk.

"So you have broken detention, Bunter?"

"Oh, no, sir! I—I—I——"

"You will bend over that chair, Bunter."

"Oh lor'!"

Whack, whack, whack!

"Yow ow-ow!"

"Silence! As I cannot trust you to remain in the Form-room, Bunter, you will remain in this study and write your lines under my own eyes."

"Ow!"

"You may sit at the table, Bunter. And now, Cherry," said Mr. Quelch with a change of manner, "per noctem plurima volvens——"

Really, it was unnecessary for Mr. Quelch to go on expounding Virgil; it was no longer any use, in the circumstances. But Mr. Quelch, being happily unaware why he was expounding Virgil, went on with it; and Bob Cherry listened with as much interest as he could muster for five long minutes. Then he was very kindly dismissed.

He gave the fat Owl a commiserating look as he went—receiving in return a doleful and dismal blink. There was no more breaking detention for Bunter! Under his Form master's gimlet eye he was safe!

The hapless Owl settled down to lines; and Bob Cherry left the House, went down to the gates, and started on his way to Pegg.

THE FOURTH CHAPTER.

Lord Mauleverer is Wanted!

TAP!

Mr. Quelch gave a slight grunt, apparently not pleased by the tap on his door.

Billy Bunter, on the other hand, looked up hopefully.

Mr. Quelch was engaged on a pile of papers, and he did not want an interruption. Billy Bunter was engaged on a pile of lines, and he did want an interruption.

The Remove master was working busily on one side of the study table. Billy Bunter was working busily on the other. If his pen slacked down, a lift of Quelch's eyebrows across the table was sufficient to set it going again. Under Quelch's gimlet eye, even the champion slacker of Greyfriars could not slack.

Bunter could have groaned. He had turned out a hundred lines. The remaining three hundred seemed to stretch in an endless vista before him. Really, it was more than flesh and blood could stand—Billy Bunter's flesh and blood, at all events. Almost was Bunter tempted to make a sudden, reckless dash from the study, regardless of consequences. But not quite. Such a proceeding required more nerve than dwelt within the extensive circumference of William George Bunter.

But a tap on the door was welcome to Bunter's fat ears. Even a minute's interruption was worth something. And if Quelch, by some stroke of fortune, was called away from the study, there was no doubt about what Billy Bunter was going to do. He was going to bolt!

It was Trotter, the House page, who entered, and he brought in a card for Mr. Quelch. Bunter blinked hopefully at the Remove master as he glanced at it. If this meant a visitor for Quelch, it meant a chance for the Owl of the Remove.

"Kalizelos!" Mr. Quelch read the name on the card aloud, evidently surprised to read a Greek name there. Mr. Quelch had an extensive acquaintance among the ancient Greeks, but he was not acquainted with any modern Greeks.

"I've showed the gentleman into the visitors' room, sir," said Trotter.

"Very good," said Mr. Quelch. "But why have you brought this card to me, Trotter, instead of taking it to the headmaster?"

"The gentleman asked to see Lord Mauleverer's master, sir," answered Trotter, "and his lordship being in your Form, sir——"

"Oh, quite so!" said Mr. Quelch, evidently puzzled, however. "Very well, Trotter, tell Mr. Kalizelos I will be with him in a few minutes."

"Yessir!"

Trotter retired.

Mr. Quelch laid the card on the table and proceeded to finish the paper on which he had been engaged when the interruption came. Mr. Kalizelos, whoever he was, had to wait a few minutes.

Billy Bunter blinked inquisitively at the card.

He had never heard of Mr. Kalizelos before, as obviously Mr. Quelch never had; and that gentleman's visit did not concern the Owl of the Remove in the very least, but Bunter was always inquisitive.

K. KALIZELOS.
Dealer in Antiques.

That was the inscription on the card.

What on earth a dealer in antiques could want with Lord Mauleverer, of the Greyfriars Remove, was rather a mystery; but it was clear that his business must be with Mauly, as he had asked for Mauly's Form master.

Mr. Quelch rose from the table at last and picked up the card again. He turned to the door and then turned back to Bunter. The fat Owl scribbled industriously, wondering whether the beast guessed his secret thoughts.

"Bunter!"

"Oh, yes, sir!"

"You will not leave this study during my absence, Bunter."

"Oh, no, sir!"

"I shall be absent a very short time, Bunter. I shall expect you to have made due progress with your lines when I return."

"Oh, certainly, sir!"

Mr. Quelch gave him a rather grim look and left the study. He walked away to the visitors' room. In that apartment he found his unexpected visitor awaiting him.

A slim, olive-skinned man was seated by the big window that looked on the quadrangle. His dark face was handsome in its own foreign way; his eyes, of an intense black, fixed keenly on the Form master. He was a total stranger to the Remove master and to Greyfriars, though, as it happened, there were four Greyfriars juniors who had seen him. It was the man who had landed from the yacht in Pegg Bay, and spoken to Harry Wharton & Co. on the old pier.

"Mr. Kalizelos?" asked Mr. Quelch, with a glance at the card in his hand and another at the olive-skinned yachtsman.

"Precisely, my dear sir!" said the man from the yacht. He spoke in excellent English, in a low and melodious voice. "I beg a thousand pardons for this intrusion——"

"Not at all, sir," said Mr. Quelch. "If you will kindly state your business I——"

"I desire to see Lord Mauleverer, who, I understand, is one of your pupils, sir," said Mr. Kalizelos.

"I am Mauleverer's Form master," answered Mr. Quelch; "but I must inquire what business you may have with a Greyfriars boy, sir, as you are a stranger to me."

Mr. Kalizelos smiled, showing a gleam of dazzling white teeth under his little black moustache.

"Perfectly, sir! I quite understand that! My card tells you that I am a dealer in antiques. I am chiefly interested in Egyptian antiquities."

"No doubt. But——"

"The late Lord Mauleverer, sir, your estimable pupil's father, was, as perhaps you are aware, a distinguished Egyptologist, and made many explorations, years ago, in the tombs of the ancient kings of Egypt."

"I have heard so. But——"

"His late lordship's collection of Egyptian relics is now at Mauleverer Towers," continued Mr. Kalizelos. "By the kindness of Sir Reginald Brooke, Lord Mauleverer's guardian, I have been enabled to see them—a very great pleasure to me, sir."

"Quite, but——"

"It was my desire, sir, to take photographs of certain articles in the collection," explained Mr Kalizelos. "Sir Reginald Brooke had no objection, but he considered, very properly indeed, that Lord Mauleverer's permission should be given."

"Oh!" said Mr. Quelch.

"I can scarcely doubt, sir, that his lordship will give me this permission," said Mr. Kalizelos. "If I may speak a few words to him, I am sure that he will have no objection to make. Sir Reginald Brooke, indeed, has assured me that making the request is merely a matter of form, and that his ward will give me permission at once for the photographs to be taken of the articles at his magnificent home, sir."

Mr. Quelch smiled.

"I have no doubt of it," he answered.

"You are very kind," said Mr. Kalizelos. "I apologise a hundred times, sir, for taking up your valuable time."

"Not at all, Mr. Kalizelos," said the Remove master. "But as to-day is a half-holiday, it is possible that Lord Mauleverer is not within gates. If you will wait, I will ascertain whether the boy is in the House, and, if so, you may certainly see him."

"I can only thank you, sir!" said Mr. Kalizelos, in his musical voice, and Mr. Quelch left the visitors' room, leaving Mr. Kalizelos with a smile of polite satisfaction on his olive face.

But as soon as the door closed behind the Greyfriars master the expression on Mr. Kalizelos' face changed very much.

The smile disappeared, as if wiped away by a duster; the lines of the olive face hardened, and a glitter came into the deep black eyes. The Greek breathed hard and deep.

"At last!" he muttered, half-aloud, a remark that certainly would have astonished Mr. Quelch had he heard it, and might have caused him to suspect that the handsome Greek was something else as well as a dealer in antiques—and that he had business with Lord Mauleverer that he had not stated to Lord Mauleverer's Form master.

The Greek did not sit down again.

He stood with his eyes on the door, watching it for the expected schoolboy to enter—and the look on his face was that of a watching tiger.

THE FIFTH CHAPTER.

Bunter the Nobleman!

BILLY BUNTER put a bullet head out of Mr. Quelch's study doorway, and blinked along the corridor through his big spectacles.

Like Moses of old, he looked this way and that way—and there was no man!

For the second time that afternoon Bunter was going to "chance" it. He hoped for better luck at the second attempt.

With that beast, Quelch, jawing to somebody in the visitors' room, it seemed probable that the coast would be clear. Billy Bunter waited in the doorway, watching and listening, with his fat heart thumping. But he screwed up his courage at last and rolled out.

This time he did not go at a rush. He almost tiptoed his way down the long corridor. Neither did he intend to leave by the door on the quad. The fat Owl's idea was to scuttle up to the Remove passage, and leave by the box-room window at the back of the House. Hoping that Quelch was still safe with his unexpected visitor, Bunter reached the stairs and started up.

Then he halted.

On the next flight of stairs above he sighted a familiar form. It was that of Mr. Quelch, going upstairs. Fortunately, his back was to Bunter, and he did not think of glancing round. Billy

Bunter gave one horrified blink at his Form master's back, and gasped, and turned, and fairly flew.

"Oh crikey!" gasped Bunter.

He had supposed that Mr. Quelch was still in the visitors' room. Apparently, however, the Remove master had already got through with Mr. Kalizelos, and Bunter concluded that that gentleman was gone.

But for the fact that Quelch, for some reason, was going up to the Remove studies, Bunter might have met him face to face!

He shuddered at the thought.

The fat junior blinked at the open doorway of the House. In the quad, only a short distance from the steps, the portly figure of Mr. Prout was in sight, in conversation with Mr. Wiggins.

Bunter backed hastily away from the door.

Prout knew that he was detained—and he did not want to catch Prout's eye again.

"Oh lor'!" murmured Bunter.

Quelch, above, cut him off from the Remove passage; Prout, outside, cut him off from the quad. And any minute Quelch might come down, or Prout might come in. Moments were precious.

In sheer desperation, the fat junior crossed to the door of the visitors' room.

That apartment had windows on the quad, and it would be easy to watch for an opportunity, when the coast was clear, and drop from one of the windows, as the room was on the ground floor. And if Quelch missed him from his study, he would not be likely to look for him in the visitors' room—at least, Bunter hoped so.

It was a case of any port in a storm. Bunter hesitated, with his fat paw on the door-handle. A portly shadow fell across the sunlight from the quad—Mr. Prout was coming in.

That decided Bunter. A few moments more, and Prout would see him—and the game would be up! Swiftly he turned the door handle, opened the door of the visitors' room, stepped inside, and closed the door after him.

"Lord Mauleverer!" said a musical voice.

Bunter jumped.

As he had seen Quelch going up to the junior studies, he had taken it for granted that Quelch's caller was gone. It had not occurred to his fat brain that Mr. Kalizelos might be waiting alone in the visitors' room for any reason. He had had no doubt that the room was empty.

But it was not empty.

A slim, lithe, olive-skinned man stood looking at Bunter, bowing, with a smile on his face. The tiger's look with which Mr. Kalizelos had watched the door vanished as the door opened, and he was instantly the polite, smiling antique dealer again.

Bunter blinked at him.

He was too startled to speak for a moment.

Mr. Kalizelos bowed with foreign grace, his black eyes on the fat junior.

"I thank your lordship for giving me a few minutes of your lordship's time," he said.

Bunter blinked.

His fat brain was not quick on the uptake; but he remembered, from what had been said in Mr. Quelch's study, that Mr. Kalizelos had called in reference to Lord Mauleverer.

It dawned on him that the foreign gentleman was waiting for Mr. Quelch to send Mauleverer to him, or bring him to the visitors' room.

The Greek's mistake was natural.

He was waiting there for Lord Mauleverer, and when a schoolboy entered he naturally supposed that it was Mauleverer. The room obviously was not one that was used by junior schoolboys, except to see visitors in.

Bowing and smiling, the Greek came nearer to Bunter.

His keen black eyes scanned the fat face, as if with the intention of memorising his supposed lordship's features.

"Oh!" ejaculated Bunter. "You—you're waiting to—to see——"

"I am waiting to see you, my lord!" said Mr. Kalizelos, with another bow. "I have not had the pleasure of seeing you before, but—you are Lord Mauleverer, my lord?"

Billy Bunter opened his fat lips—and closed them again. He was about to tell the foreign gentleman that he was not Mauleverer; but second thoughts—not always the best—supervened.

Bunter's fat brain was working at full pressure. He had to keep in cover—Prout was in the Hall outside the door. Bunter could not possibly walk out of the visitors' room, with Prout outside. He had to stay where he was, and certainly he could not confide to this foreign gentleman that he was a young rascal under detention, dodging the masters.

Truthfulness had never appealed to William George Bunter. He had no use for it. Indeed, Remove fellows declared that Bunter never told the truth if he thought that a "whopper" would do. That might be an exaggeration; but undoubtedly Billy Bunter, in moments of difficulty, was prepared to roll out whoppers to any number and any extent. If this merchant thought he was Lord Mauleverer, at least he could stay in the room till the coast was clear. That was enough for Bunter.

"I——" began Bunter. "Yes! Of—of course! I—I suppose you're Mr. Kalizelos!"

The fat junior's confused manner caused the Greek to eye him sharply. But if he had any doubt, it was removed at once by Bunter mentioning his name. Lord Mauleverer, certainly, had never heard of Mr. Kalizelos, and he could only have heard the name from his Form master, who had gone to find him. It was scarcely likely that any other boy at Greyfriars had heard it. Mr. Kalizelos knew nothing, of course, of the fat Owl having been in Mr. Quelch's study when his card was taken in.

"I—I'm glad to see you, Mr. Kalizelos," hurried on Bunter. "N-n-nice afternoon, isn't it?"

The Greek, whose face had hardened and sharpened for a moment as he eyed the fat schoolboy, was all smiles again.

"Oh, quite, my lord!" he said. "We have very warm weather—almost as warm as in my own country."

"What's that?" asked Bunter, not so much from his usual inquisitiveness as from the necessity of saying something.

"Egypt, my lord."

"Egypt!" repeated Bunter, blinking at him. Bunter had a hazy belief that all the inhabitants of Africa were black. "But you're not a darkey."

Mr. Kalizelos stared for a moment. Then he smiled.

"I am a Greek, my lord—an Egyptian Greek. There are many Greeks in Egypt."

"Are there?" said Bunter.

"Descended from the Grecian colony planted in that country by Alexander of Macedon, my lord."

"Oh!" said Bunter. Bunter had heard of Alexander the Great; though the less he learned about that ancient monarch, or any other, the better Bunter liked it.

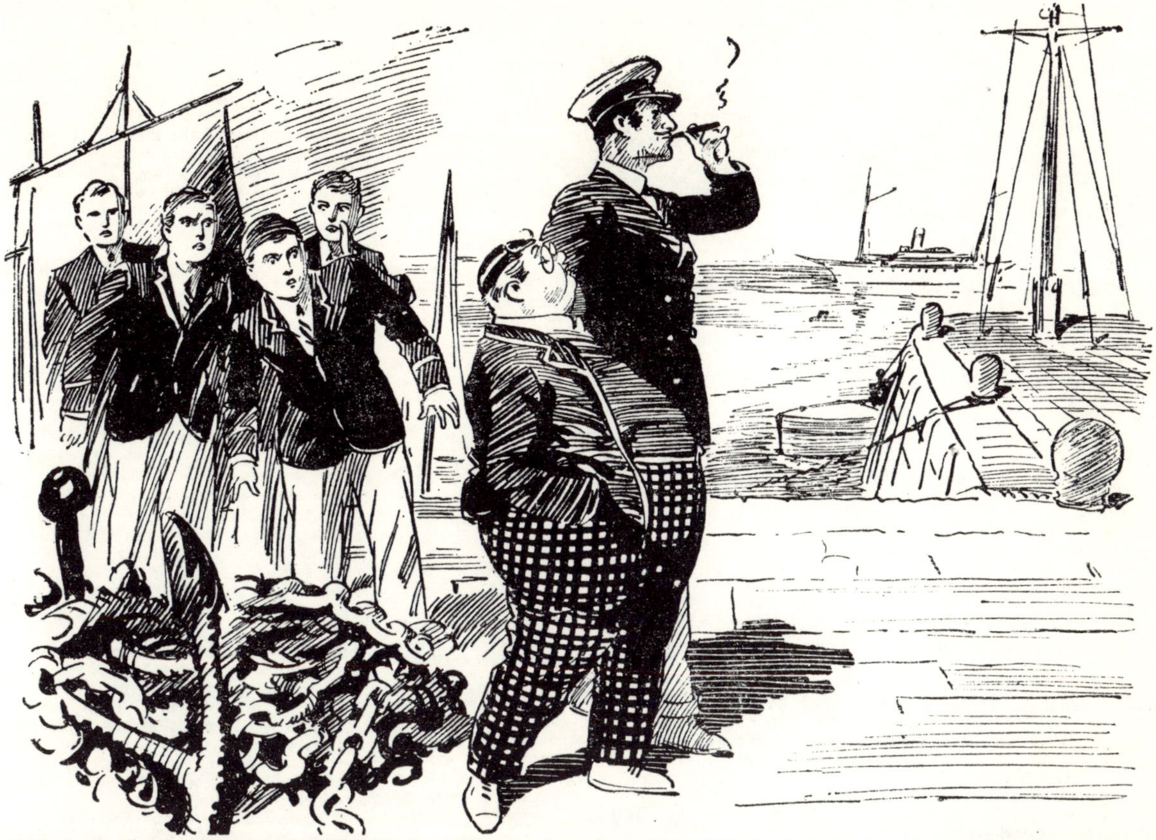

"Oh, here you are, Bunter!" said Wharton. "You've turned up at last!" Instead of acknowledging his school-fellows, the Owl of the Remove turned up his fat nose and walked on with Mr. Kalizelos. It was the cut direct!

"But to come to business, my lord——"

"Oh! Ah! Yes," said Bunter.

He moved across to the window. It was open, and near at hand the quad looked deserted. In the distance Bunter could hear shouting on the cricket ground; but close at hand the coast was clear.

"I took the liberty of calling," said Mr. Kalizelos, following his supposed lordship to the window.

"Oh, yes!" Bunter was in terror every moment of the door opening to reveal Mr. Quelch or Lord Mauleverer. "But the fact is I'm sorry, and all that, but I've got to speak to a chap——"

"But, my lord——"

"He's just gone out of gates!" gasped Bunter. "I—I shall have to cut after him, or—or I shall lose him. Sorry, you know—awfully sorry—can't stop a single moment——"

With that the fat junior plunged out of the open window and dropped into the quad, under the astonished eyes of the Greek.

Mr. Kalizelos made a swift stride to the window, and watched the fat figure scudding across to the gates.

His black eyes glittered

What Mr. Kalizelos might think of his peculiar conduct Bunter had no time to consider. The coast was clear, and it was a chance to escape, and that was all that mattered to Bunter.

Only for a moment Mr. Kalizelos stood watching him.

Then he crossed to the door, quitted the room, and walked quickly out of the House.

The taxi in which he had arrived stood on the drive. The Greek spoke a sharp word to the driver.

"You see that fat boy? I wish to speak to him. Follow him!"

"Yessir!"

The Greek stepped into the taxi, and the chauffeur put it in motion at once. Billy Bunter reached the gates and scudded into the road. A moment later the taxi turned out of the gates after him. The Greek's black eyes scintillated with triumph as he looked from the window at the fat figure plugging along the sunny road.

———

THE SIXTH CHAPTER.

Amazing!

LORD MAULEVERER yawned.

"Don't come in, fathead!" he called out.

It was a tap at his study door that drew that remark from his lordship.

Lord Mauleverer's elegant form was stretched on his study sofa. Mauly was lazy at the best of times, and on a blazing afternoon in July he was at his laziest.

Strenuous fellows like Harry Wharton & Co. might sail on the bay, or knock the ball about on the cricket field. But Herbert Mauleverer preferred his study sofa.

Stretched at full length, with his hands clasped behind his noble head, Mauleverer was taking it easy.

The only fly in the ointment was the possibility that some fellow might butt in and disturb his comfortable repose.

Hence his remark as the tap came at his door.

The door opened.

"What?" ejaculated a voice that seemed to have an edge on it.

"Oh, begad!" gasped Lord Mauleverer in dismay.

He leaped from the sofa.

A moment before Lord Mauleverer had looked as if he could hardly move if the alarm-bell rang to announce that the House was on fire. But at the voice of Mr. Quelch he moved like a Jack-in-the-box.

"Oh, sir!" gasped Mauleverer, his cheeks crimson as he blinked in dismay at his Form master. "I—I—I didn't know it was you, sir."

"I presume not!" barked Mr. Quelch.

"I—I'm aw'fly sorry, sir——" stammered the schoolboy earl.

"You should not be idling in your study in this glorious weather, Mauleverer," said Mr. Quelch severely.

"Oh, n-no, sir!" stammered Mauly, "I—I wasn't exactly idlin', sir; I—I was thinkin' out a—a problem, sir."

"Indeed," said Mr. Quelch, his brow clearing. "I am glad to hear that, Mauleverer. I have heard from Mr. Lascelles that your mathematics are far—very far—from satisfactory."

"I—I mean——"

"If you are in a difficulty, my boy, I will find time to help you with the problem to which you refer," said Mr. Quelch kindly.

"Oh! Ah! I—I mean, it was the problem of the hols, sir!" gasped the unfortunate slacker of the Remove.

"The what?"

"The holidays, sir. I—I haven't decided about the holidays, and as we break up in a few days I was thinkin'——"

"You are a foolish and absurd boy, Mauleverer!" snapped Mr. Quelch.

"Oh! Yes, sir!"

"You should not be idling indoors. However, it is fortunate, in a way, as someone has called to see you, that I have found you in the House," said Mr. Quelch.

"Is it nunky, sir? I—I mean Sir Reginald Brooke?" asked Mauleverer.

"No; it is a Greek gentleman, named Kalizelos," answered Mr. Quelch.

"Never heard of him, sir."

"Very probably. It appears, Mauleverer, that this gentleman has been allowed to see your late father's collection of Egyptian antiquities at Mauleverer Towers, and he desires your permission to take photographs of some of them."

"He's very welcome, sir," answered Lord Mauleverer.

"You may see him, Mauleverer. The man appears to be a respectable antique merchant, but as he is a total stranger here it will be best for you to see him in your Form master's presence."

"Very well, sir!"

"You may follow me to the visitors' room, Mauleverer."

"Yes, sir."

Mr. Quelch walked out of the study, and Mauleverer, casting what the poet describes as a "longing, lingering look behind" at his sofa, followed. Lord Mauleverer was more than willing to oblige the Greek gentleman, or any other gentleman, but he was not willing to leave his study sofa for the purpose. But there was no help for that, and he followed the Remove master down the stairs.

They arrived at the visitors' room, and Mr. Quelch opened the door and walked in, followed by Mauleverer.

"Here is Lord Mauleverer, Mr. Kalizelos!" he said. "Why—what—where—— Goodness gracious!"

Mr. Quelch stared round the room as if he could hardly believe his own gimlet-eyes—as indeed he hardly could.

The room was empty.

He had left the Greek gentleman waiting there. He had not been gone more than six or seven minutes. But during that short space of time, the Greek gentleman had vanished.

It was amazing, indeed, inexplicable. Mr. Quelch was both astonished and annoyed. Mr. Kalizelos had seemed to him a gentleman with very courtly manners. But this abrupt and inexplicable departure was really shocking bad manners.

"Extraordinary!" said Mr. Quelch.

He stared round the room, as if he half-expected to see the Greek gentleman emerge from some corner.

"Is—is he gone, sir?" asked Mauleverer, as astonished as his Form master.

"He certainly appears to be gone, Mauleverer! I cannot understand this at all!" snapped Mr. Quelch.

He whisked out of the room, very much annoyed indeed. Prout was in the offing, and the Remove master called to him.

"Prout! Have you seen anything of a gentleman—a foreign-looking man—who was waiting here?"

Mr. Prout glanced round.

"Certainly, Quelch! He left the visitors' room a few minutes ago—and went out to his taxi."

Mr. Quelch stepped to the open door of the House. The taxi was gone. He turned back, frowning.

"This is very remarkable," he said. "The man called, stating that he had a reason for speaking to Mauleverer; and he seems to have left while I was fetching the boy. It is extremely odd."

"Very odd, indeed, sir!" said Mr. Prout in surprise. "If you are not acquainted with the person——"

"Not in the least; he was quite a stranger."

"Then it would be as well to ascertain that nothing is missing—such as the umbrellas——"

Mr. Quelch shook his head, and Mauleverer grinned. The Remove master could not suspect a man of Mr. Kalizelos' wealthy appearance of nefarious designs on the umbrellas! But he was very puzzled, and very perturbed.

However, there was nothing to be done, and Mr. Quelch was anxious to get back to his study and his pile of papers.

"As the man appears to have left, Mauleverer, you may go," he said.

"Yes, sir!"

Lord Mauleverer travelled slowly and laboriously back to the Remove passage, and sank down on his study sofa with a sigh of relief—no doubt turning his noble mind once more to the problem of the holidays.

Mr. Quelch, with his lips set, returned to his own study.

There another surprise awaited him.

He fully expected to find that Bunter had been slacking, and had done nothing while he was out of the study. He was prepared, in that case, to give Bunter the keenest edge of his tongue. But Bunter's chair was vacant, and his pen lay in a sea of blots on his unfinished lines. Bunter was gone!

"Upon my word!" gasped Mr. Quelch.

His face set grimly.

He made a step to the door—and stopped! He realised that the fat truant was likely to be far enough away by that time. Having taken the risk of breaking detention, he was not likely to linger.

Mr. Quelch sat down to his pile of papers again, with an expression on his face that might have curdled the fat Owl's blood if he could have seen it. Fortunately, William George Bunter could not see it.

THE SEVENTH CHAPTER.

The Spider and the Fly!

"MY lord!"

Billy Bunter blinked round in surprise.

Once safe out of the school gates, Bunter had started down Friardale Lane as fast as his fat little legs could carry him. He heard the buzz of a motor behind him and drew to the side of the lane to let the vehicle pass. But it did not pass; it slowed down, and a musical voice from the window addressed the panting fat junior.

"Oh!" gasped Bunter, as his big spectacles turned on Mr. Kalizelos at the window of the taxi.

For a second, he wondered why the foreigner had followed him. He was at the school to see Mauleverer; and he had not yet seen Mauleverer. But Kalizelos, of course, supposed that Bunter was Mauleverer, as the fat Owl remembered at once. Apparently his business with the schoolboy earl was so urgent that he had followed on from the school.

The olive face of the Greek was smiling. There was no doubt that he was surprised and puzzled by the extraordinary behaviour of the supposed Mauleverer; but he had his own reasons for being pleased by the turn of events. He smiled and bowed from the taxi window.

"I—I say, I—I'm in a hurry," gasped Bunter, with an anxious blink back towards the school gates. "I—I've got to speak to a—a chap——"

"May I offer your lordship a lift?" asked the Greek.

At that stage in the proceedings, Bunter would have told the Greek that he was not Lord Mauleverer, simply to get rid of the man.

But the offer of a lift banished that thought from his fat mind.

A lift was exactly what Bunter wanted.

Whether Mr. Quelch would look for him when he missed him, he did not know; but it was quite possible that he would, or that he would request a Sixth Form prefect to do so. Bunter was anxious to put a safe distance between his fat person and the school. Later, he had to face the music for breaking detention and getting away. That was bad enough. But it would be altogether too bad, if he was hooked back with a hand on his collar, to face the music without having got away at all. The offer of a lift was a windfall to the podgy truant.

"Oh! I say, that's jolly decent of you," gasped Bunter.

"Your lordship would like a lift?"

"I'd jolly well like it no end," said Bunter, with great sincerity. "Just what I'd like! I—I'm in a fearful hurry."

"Pray step in, my lord."

Kalizelos opened the taxi door.

Bunter stepped in; hardly able to believe in his good luck! The door closed, and the taxi rolled on again.

"You are looking for a friend, I understand, my lord?" asked the Greek, his keen, black eyes on Bunter's flushed, podgy face.

"Oh! Ah! Yes!" Bunter had almost forgotten that "whopper" already. "Yes! Quite! But—I—I think I've lost him—the fact is, I want to get to Pegg—if you're going that way——"

The black eyes glistened.

Even Bunter, obtuse and unobservant as he was, could see that the Greek was glad to hear that he wanted a lift to Pegg. Why, it was a mystery; unless the antique merchant was glad of a chance to oblige a nobleman.

"I am now returning to Pegg, to my yacht there, my lord!" said Kalizelos. "It will be a great pleasure to have your lordship's company."

"Oh, good!" said Bunter.

His assumption of Lord Mauleverer's identity was turning out a better speculation than he had dreamed.

Obviously, this foreign gentleman, polite as he was, would never have offered a lift to a young rascal dodging out of detention. He was happy to offer it to Lord Mauleverer! Bunter sagely resolved to continue to be a peer of the realm, at least, until the seaside village was reached. In the taxi, he was likely to arrive there before Bob Cherry, who was walking. He would be in ample time for the trip in the Remove boat—and what was more important, for the tea in the Remove boat! Billy Bunter was feeling quite elated.

The taxi sped down Friardale Lane towards the village. At the stile on the footpath, a sturdy schoolboy was about to clamber over, to take the path through the wood, a short cut to Pegg. Billy Bunter grinned as he saw Bob Cherry. He had twice as far to go, by road, but he had no doubt of arriving first in the taxi.

"Hallo, hallo, hallo!" Bob Cherry glanced round and stared at the sight of the fat face in the taxi, "Bunter!"

Bob stared blankly at the fat junior as the taxi came up. He had left Billy Bunter safe under Mr. Quelch's gimlet-eye, and he was amazed to see him careering along Friardale Lane in a taxi. Bunter grinned at him.

Mr. Kalizelos frowned, for a moment. For reasons of his own, as yet unimagined by Bunter, the Greek did not want Lord Mauleverer to pick up a friend en route. To his relief, Bunter did not ask him to stop. He waved a fat hand to Bob, and the taxi whizzed on.

Bob stared. He turned from the stile and shouted to the fat Owl.

"Hold on! If you're going to Pegg, give a fellow a lift, old fat man."

Bunter did not seem to hear.

The taxi whizzed on.

If Bob Cherry had entered the taxi, it would not have been many minutes before Kalizelos discovered that "Lord Mauleverer" was not Lord Mauleverer at all; and the lift to Pegg would have been a thing of the past.

So Bunter judiciously turned a deaf ear to Bob Cherry.

"Hold on, you fat sweep!" roared Bob.

Bunter grinned. The taxi swept on towards Friardale.

"My hat! The fat worm!" growled Bob Cherry, in disgust. And he turned back to the stile, clambered over it, and proceeded by the short cut through the wood at a rapid trot.

Kalizelos glanced curiously at his "lordship."

"That was a schoolfellow of your lordship's?" he remarked.

"Oh! Yes," said Bunter. "Not the man I was—was looking for! Never mind him—he can walk."

Billy Bunter leaned back, glad of the rest after his exertions, and taking his fat ease. He was safe from pursuit now, and safely booked for a free ride to Pegg.

Nothing could have happened better, from Billy Bunter's point of view, at least. And now that his fat mind was at ease, Billy Bunter's inquisitive curiosity was awakened.

The olive-skinned Kalizelos was rather an unusual sort of visitor for a Greyfriars fellow, and his business with Lord Mauleverer must be rather important and pressing, as he had hurried after his supposed lordship from the school.

Everybody's business but his own had a deep interest for Billy Bunter, and as the Greek believed him to be Mauly, he had only to ask to learn all about it. Never had a Paul Pry, in fact, had a better opportunity for satisfying his curiosity.

He blinked at the handsome olive face of the Greek, finding that the black eyes were watching his stealthily.

"Let's see, what was it you came to see me for, Mr. Kalizelos?" asked Bunter breezily. "We can talk now."

"Oh, quite, your lordship!" said Mr. Kalizelos. He was watching the fat, obtuse face with a calculating eye. "But we shall be at Pegg in a few minutes. My yacht is there——"

"That yacht yours?" asked Bunter, with interest. "I've heard the fellows talking about it. Mauly says it's a ripping yacht."

"Mauly!" repeated Mr. Kalizelos.

Bunter caught his breath.

Billy Bunter lived and moved and had his being in spoof; but although he belonged to the class of persons who should proverbially have good memories, Bunter had a bad one—and he was liable to give himself away at any moment.

"A—a—a pal of mine!" he stammered, thankful that he had said Mauly and not Mauleverer. "Chap named—named Maulson—we call him Mauly for short. I say, you must do jolly well out of the secondhand business if you keep a yacht on it!"

Kalizelos looked at him.

This sort of fatuous impertinence was part and parcel of Billy Bunter's fascinating character; but it was not what was to be expected from a peer of the realm.

But it was not the Greek's cue to be offended by bad manners. Only for a second the smile faded from his olive face.

"We make our small profits, my lord," he said smoothly.

"Jolly big profits, I should think, to keep a yacht!" said Bunter. "Shouldn't have thought there was so much in secondhand furniture."

The Greek's black eyes gleamed for a moment.

"I am an antique dealer, my lord," he said. "In Cairo I have a large establishment. That is why I am interested in your lordship's collection of Egyptian relics. Your lordship's late father brought back many curious things from Egypt."

"Oh! Yes! Rather!" agreed Bunter, remembering that he was Lord Mauleverer. "Lots and lots!"

"Among other things, a very interesting scarab," said Mr. Kalizelos, his eyes on Bunter's fat face.

"Dozens of them," answered Bunter, inwardly wondering what on earth a scarab was.

Kalizelos smiled.

"No doubt, no doubt," he said. "Egyptian scarabs are by no means uncommon. But the one to which I refer is of very special interest. I speak of the Golden Scarabaeus."

"Oh!" gasped Bunter. "The—the Golden Scarabaeus! Exactly!"

"Your lordship is well acquainted with it, of course?"

"Oh! Yes! Know it like a book!" said Bunter.

"No doubt it is still in the collection left to your lordship by your lordship's late father?"

"Oh! Quite! Wouldn't part with it for worlds!" said Bunter. "We—we keep it in a special room at Bunter Court."

"Indeed! Your lordship does not keep it with the rest at Mauleverer Towers?" exclaimed the Greek.

Once more Bunter had stumbled!

"Oh! Yes! No!" he stammered. "We—we keep some of the things at—at Bunter Court—one of my country houses, you know. Hallo, there's the sea."

Bunter was rather glad to be in sight of his destination. Twice he had nearly given himself away, and he did not want to enlighten the Greek till he was safely landed at Pegg. After that he did not care how soon the man from Cairo discovered that his leg had been pulled.

"That is my yacht, my lord," said Kalizelos, with a gesture towards the handsome vessel riding at anchor in the distance. "If your lordship is at leisure, might I venture to beg your lordship to pay a visit to my poor vessel? It would be an honour and a distinction."

"Oh!" said Bunter.

With all his wily cunning the Greek could not keep a shade of anxiety out of his face. He was angling warily for this fat fish; and, so far, the supposed Mauleverer had played into his hands. But at this stage of the proceedings Kalizelos hardly hoped that fortune would continue to smile on him so benignly.

But he need have had no doubts.

It was very doubtful indeed whether Lord Mauleverer would have accepted the invitation from a total stranger. But there was no doubt that William George Bunter would.

"Well, the fact is, I was going to tea with some friends," said Bunter, blinking at the Greek. "I can't very well miss my tea."

"If your lordship would deign to accept some refreshment on my poor yacht——" said Kalizelos, his black eyes glinting.

Billy Bunter blinked at the well-dressed Greek and then at the handsome and, evidently, very expensive yacht. A lordly guest on the yacht was undoubtedly likely to fare better than whacking out a basket of tuck with five fellows in a boat. And Bunter was not quite certain yet that he would be able to wedge into the Remove boat at all. That had been his intention, certainly; and he had great skill in wedging in at other fellows' spreads. Still, there was a doubt. A bird in hand was worth two in the bush!

"Done!" said Bunter.

"I thank your lordship!" said Kalizelos. "Believe me, I appreciate the honour your lordship does me!"

"Yes, I don't suppose you often get a lord on your yacht!" agreed Bunter fatuously.

"Oh! Ah! Quite!" gasped Kalizelos.

The taxi ran on into the cobbly street of Pegg, and stopped at the wooden pier, where the yacht's boat was waiting. Kalizelos paid off the taxi, and walked on the pier, with Billy Bunter rolling by his side. It was settled now, in Bunter's fat mind, that he was going to be Lord Mauleverer till after tea on the yacht!

THE EIGHTH CHAPTER.

Cut!

HARRY WHARTON & CO. rose from the rail where they were seated. In the distance they spotted Bob Cherry, emerging at a rapid trot from the wood into Pegg Lane. Bob was still at a distance when the taxi came whizzing up from the direction of Friardale, and, to their astonishment, Billy Bunter stepped out and came on the pier, with the olive-skinned man they had seen land from the yacht.

"That fat chump!" said Johnny Bull.

"The fathead must have broken detention," said Harry Wharton. "Asking for trouble, as usual!"

"That yachting sportsman must have given him a lift," said Frank Nugent. "Bunter's in luck—and we're not!"

"He said he was going to Greyfriars to see Mauleverer," remarked Wharton. "He must have got through pretty quick to be back so soon. Trust Bunter to stick him for a lift, if cheek would do it!"

"Now we're landed with the fat frog, I suppose!" grunted Johnny Bull. "Are we letting him come in the boat, or kicking him across the beach?"

Harry Wharton laughed.

"It's the last half-holiday of the term," he said. "Let the fat bounder wedge in."

"In the esteemed circumstances the kickfulness is not the proper caper," agreed Hurree Jamset Ram Singh.

"Better get in some more grub, then!" grunted Johnny Bull. "We've only enough for five. We shall want enough for ten now!"

The chums of the Remove made up their minds to it. Evidently Bunter had broken detention, and booked himself for a licking, to join the boating party; and it was, after all, the last half-holiday of the term, and there was the happy prospect before them of not seeing William George Bunter again till next term. So, though the addition of the fat Owl to the party did not exactly have an exhilarating effect on them, they resolved to grin and bear it with fortitude.

They were quite unaware, so far, that Bunter's plans had changed since he had scooted out of Greyfriars.

The picnic-basket in the boat had no temptation for a fellow who was going as a wealthy man's guest on a magnificent yacht. Billy Bunter was prepared to turn up his fat little nose at that picnic-basket in his new and peculiar circumstances.

So far from being pleased to see the juniors waiting on the pier, not yet started on their trip, Bunter was annoyed and alarmed.

Tea on the yacht depended on Kalizelos continuing to believe that he was Lord Mauleverer. One careless word from these fellows would knock the whole thing on the head.

Bunter would have been glad had the chums of the Remove given him the "marble eye" as he passed them on the pier. But having nobly made up their minds to give him as cordial a welcome as possible, the juniors gave him quite pleasant looks.

"Oh, here you are!" said Harry. "You've turned up, after all."

Bunter trembled inwardly. Another word might spoil the whole thing. These irritating beasts had to be got rid of.

Instead, therefore, of answering, Bunter turned up his fat nose, and walked on with Mr. Kalizelos, little dreaming how relieved the Greek was that he showed no desire to join up with them.

The four juniors stared after him blankly. It was the cut direct.

The yacht's boat was waiting farther along the pier, and Bunter was anxious to get into it and push off. He hastened his steps.

"What on earth——" ejaculated Johnny Bull.

"Hasn't the fat idiot come here to land himself on us, after all?" exclaimed Nugent, in astonishment.

"Making out he doesn't know us!" exclaimed Johnny Bull, in deep wrath. "Turning up his silly nose. Why, I'll go after him, and rub his nose on the pier!"

"Fancy being cut—by Bunter!" gasped Wharton. "What is the fat chump's game? Cut—by Bunter! My hat!"

"The cutfulness was terrific and preposterous," grinned Hurree Jamset Ram Singh.

The juniors stared blankly after Bunter. It was a relief, so far as that went, to find that the fat Owl did not want to join the boating party, after all. But what Bunter's new and remarkable manners and customs might mean was a deep mystery. He had walked past them with his nose in the air as if they were obstreperous fellows whom he did not care to know. It really was astounding.

"Let's go and bump him on the pier!" growled Johnny Bull, deeply incensed.

"Oh, let him rip!" said Harry. "We'll kick him later. He seems to have landed himself on that yachting man somehow—goodness knows how! Let him rip, and a good riddance!"

"The goodfulness of the riddance is great, but the cheekfulness of the idiotic Bunter is preposterous!"

Billy Bunter blinked back rather uneasily when he reached the yacht's boat. He was relieved to see the Greyfriars fellows remaining where they were. Mr. Kalizelos gave him a hand into the boat, and Bunter plumped down in the stern.

"Let's get off," he said. "I don't want to have anything to do with that crowd—cheeky lot of rotters, you know. They think they can glue on to a chap, just because they belong to the same school. I get a lot of that sort of thing."

"No doubt, my lord," said Kalizelos.

"Oh, exactly! Being a lord, you know——" said Bunter.

The boat pushed off. Mr. Kalizelos had his own excellent reasons for desiring to get afloat as soon as possible. The two foreign-looking seamen bent to the oars, and the boat shot away across the bay towards the anchored yacht.

Billy Bunter, safe now from awkward revelations, grinned back at the juniors on the pier, and waved a fat hand. He had no doubt that they were envying him.

"Well, my hat!" said Harry Wharton. "The fat chump's going out to the yacht! How on earth has he wangled it?"

"Beats me hollow!" said Johnny Bull.

"The hollowfulness is terrific!"

Surprised and a little curious, the juniors watched the boat pulling for the yacht. Billy Bunter's fat face was looking round at them, growing smaller and smaller in the distance, his spectacles flashing back the rays of the sun. Somehow or other—how was a mystery—the fat Owl seemed to have "wangled" an invitation to the yacht. They watched the boat reach the anchored vessel, and saw the accommodation ladder let down, and watched Bunter heaving his weight up it. His spectacles gleamed at them from the yacht's deck, and they saw a fat hand waved. Then Bunter disappeared from sight, and the boat was swung up to the davits, which looked as if Bunter was not leaving again soon.

"Hallo, hallo, hallo!"

Bob Cherry came trotting on the pier, breathing hard.

"Oh, here you are!" said Harry. "All ready!"

"Isn't Bunter here?" asked Bob.

Wharton pointed to the yacht.

"Bunter's there!" he answered.

"What on earth is he doing there?" exclaimed Bob.

"Goodness knows!"

"Well, my hat! He passed me in Friardale Lane in a taxi with a foreign-looking chap," said Bob. "The fat villain refused to give me a lift. I've run all the way!"

"And he cut us when he got here," grinned Nugent. "Cut us dead!"

"I'm going to kick him when we get in!" growled Johnny Bull.

"He's palled on to that yachting chap somehow, and given us the go-by," said Harry Wharton, laughing. "More power to his giddy elbow! Let's get the boat out now you're here, Bob."

And dismissing Billy Bunter and his mysterious proceedings from their minds, the Famous Five stepped the mast in Trumper's boat, and ran cheerily out of the bay before the wind.

THE NINTH CHAPTER.
In Deadly Peril!

KONSTANTINOS KALIZELOS smiled as he trod the deck of the yacht Zeus. The Egyptian Greek was full of satisfaction. He looked, indeed, like a man who could hardly believe in his own good luck. Billy Bunter could not help observing how pleased the Greek seemed to be, and he attributed it partly to his own engaging manners, and partly to the fact that Kalizelos believed him to be a lord. He was soon to discover that the Greek had other reasons.

Bunter blinked round at the yacht with interest, and several dark-skinned seamen looked at him curiously, and an officer, to whom Kalizelos spoke in his own tongue, grinned openly as if entertained.

Bowing and smiling, Kalizelos requested the fat junior to accompany him below, and Bunter, in a state of fat satisfaction, rolled down into a handsome saloon. There were evidences of wealth on every hand, and Bunter wondered how a Greek dealer of Cairo made it all. He could have no doubt that the "grub" on such a vessel would be superb, and he felt that he was in great luck. This was rather better than a whack in the picnic-basket among a lot of hungry schoolboys in a dashed old fisherman's boat. At all events, it seemed better—as yet.

In the saloon Kalizelos waved Bunter to a seat, and closed the door by which they had entered. The smile on his dark, handsome face had developed into an ironical grin. From the porthole near at hand Bunter had a glimpse of the Remove boat dancing out from the pier. But he gave it only a careless glance. Bunter was feeling very superior to a mob of schoolboys in a hired boat. By this time, indeed, the fat Owl almost believed that he really was a lord.

"Not a bad little turn out," said Bunter patronisingly, blinking at the grinning Greek. Lofty patronage was Bunter's idea of a nobleman's manners and customs. "Not at all bad." He blinked at the door, wondering why Kalizelos had closed it so carefully. The next item on the programme, from Bunter's point of view, should have been the steward with tea—a large and substantial tea. "I say, if you don't mind my mentioning it, I'm a trifle peckish. What about tea?"

"I will give orders, my lord," said Kalizelos. "But first let us have a few

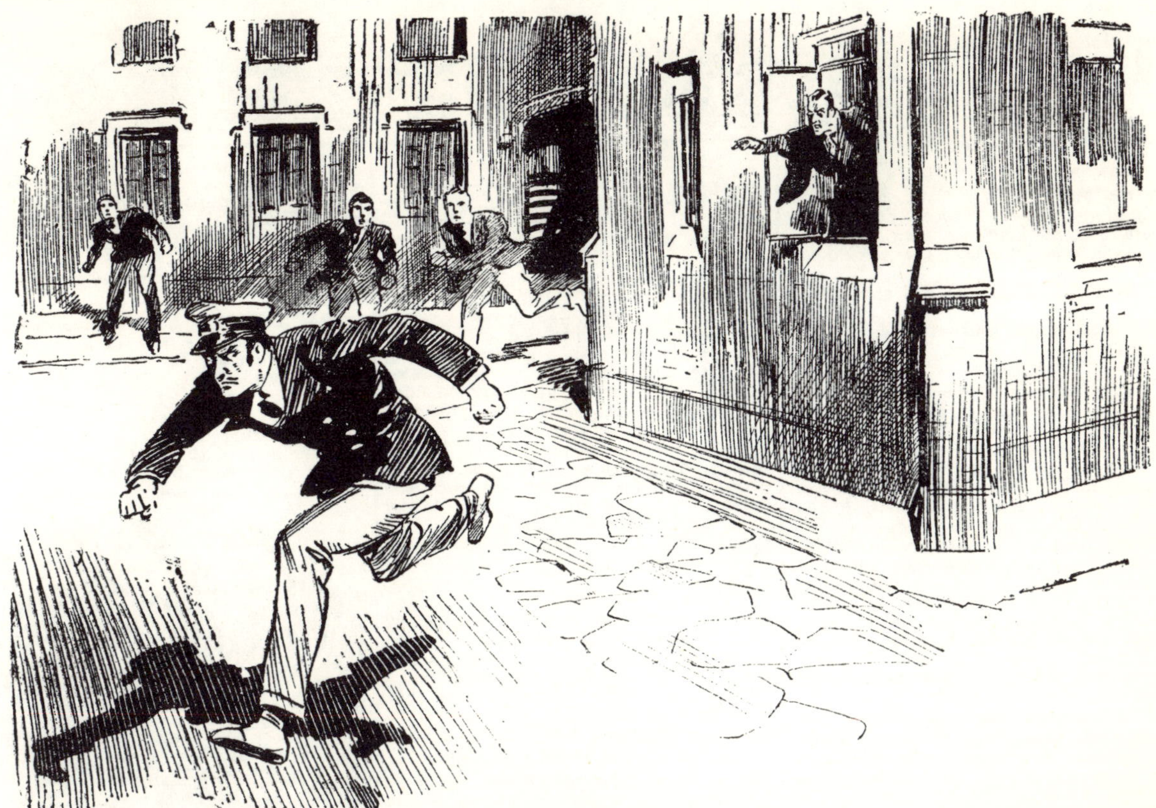

With the swiftness of a deer, Kalizelos raced across the quadrangle in the direction of the gates. "Stop him!" shouted Mr. Quelch from the window. "Wingate—Coker—Price—stop that man at once!" The seniors rushed after the fleeing Greek.

minutes of conversation. We may talk more at our ease here than at the school, I think."

"Oh, all right!" said Bunter, feeling for the first time a faint feeling of uneasiness as the black eyes scintillated at him.

He wondered what the Greek was looking at him so queerly for, and whether he was suspecting that his leg had been pulled.

"Your lordship is the present owner of the Golden Scarabaeus," said the Greek. "It is only lately that I have learned that this precious scarab was taken from the tomb of A-Menah by the late Lord Mauleverer, and brought by him to England. It is for that reason, Lord Mauleverer, that I left Cairo, and came to this country in my yacht."

"W-w-was it?" asked Bunter.

He would rather have discussed tea than scarabs, especially as he did not know what a scarab was. He felt that he was on delicate ground. If old Mauly had inherited that scarab, whatever a scarab was, from the late Lord Mauleverer, no doubt Mauly knew what it was; but Bunter didn't, and he was rather afraid of giving himself away.

"I desire to possess the scarab of A-Menah," explained Kalizelos, "and I have already seen your guardian, Sir Reginald Brooke, on the subject."

"Oh!" said Bunter.

"But your guardian has no power to part with it, and he explained that until your lordship comes of age, neither have you the power to sell it."

"Oh! Yes! Exactly," agreed Bunter. "No good talking about it, is it?"

"I think so, my lord," said Kalizelos smoothly. "I have not made so long a journey for nothing; and I do not intend to return to Egypt without the Golden Beetle."

"The—the what?" ejaculated Bunter.

"I think you understand me, my lord."

"Nunno! You were speaking about scarabs or something—what's that got to do with beetles?"

The Greek stared at him.

"Come, my lord," he said, "you are very well aware that the Golden Scarab, now in your possession represents the sacred beetle of ancient Egypt."

"Oh!" gasped Bunter. "Does it? I—I didn't know a scarab was a beetle! What the thump do you want a beetle for?"

"I see that you are getting on your guard, my lord, though hitherto you have played into my hands like a child," said the Greek. "But it is too late—you are now on board my yacht—in my hands and at my mercy."

Billy Bunter jumped.

"Wha-a-t?" he ejaculated.

"Be assured, my lord," said Kalizelos, "I have no desire to harm you, if you accede to my wishes. I must have the golden scarab and I would not allow a hundred lives to stand in my way."

"Oh lor'!" gasped Bunter.

He blinked at the Greek in terror through his big spectacles. There was no smile on Kalizelos' face now. It was as hard as if carved in bronze, and the black eyes had a glitter that sent a cold chill down Bunter's spine, warm as the July day was.

"Your guardian, the old man Brooke, may have had some suspicion of me," went on Kalizelos. "At all events, he would not allow me to see the precious scarab, and would not reveal where it was kept. He may have had, from your father, some hint of its value. Once the scarab was in my hands, I should have kept it, even if I had had to drive a knife to his heart to do so. But he gave me no chance."

"Oh!" gurgled Bunter.

Evidently there were drawbacks to being a peer of the realm, a millionaire, and possessor of a unique collection of Egyptian antiquities. Billy Bunter began to wish that he was back in Quelch's study writing lines! The Greek's glittering black eyes almost froze his blood.

"I came to your school, my lord," resumed Kalizelos, "to see you—merely in order to know you by sight. That was all I hoped to accomplish by my visit, and I had a tale ready to tell to account for desiring to see you. Once I knew you, I should have taken measures for you to be seized, and sooner or later you would have fallen into my hands. By a singular chance, you have walked into the trap of your own accord—I never hoped for such good fortune."

"Oh!"

"Now you are here," said Kalizelos, "on this ship, every man is at my orders and devoted to me. Your life is in my hands, my lord."

"Oh crikey!"

Bunter was not thinking of tea now.

He blinked at the Greek in terror. It dawned upon his podgy brain that he was like a fat fly in a spider's web. His only consolation was that he was not, after all, Lord Mauleverer, as the Greek believed. But he was fearfully dubious how Kalizelos might receive that information, when he imparted it.

(*Continued on page* 16.)

BIRCHEMALL'S B

By DICKY

I.

TINGER-LINGER-TING!

The sharp wring of the telly-fone-bell echoed throughout St. Sam's, and Dr. Birchemall, the revered and majestick headmaster, flung aside his birch with an eggs-clamation of annoyance.

"Bust the blinking tellyfone!" he said in his refined way. "It's always the blinking same—no sooner do I kom-mense a blinking birching than the blinking fone interrupts me! What are you blinking at me for, Jolly?"

"W-was I blinking, sir?" asked Jack Jolly, who was one of the four juniors who had just fourgathered in the Head's study to be birched black and blew. "I'm awfully sorry!"

"I'll make you sorrier still in a minnit!" growled the Head, picking up the receever. "I'll bash you with this birch till you howl and squeal for the mercy you'll never get! At the same time, of corse, I shall treat you with strikt and imparshal justiss. Hello! Who's speaking?"

Jack Jolly & Co. natcherally couldn't hear the answer to that question. But, whatever it was, it had a startling effect on the Head. His neeze started nocking together, beads of perspiration stood out on his forrid, and, although he seemed almost deprived of the power of speech, his teeth chattered incess-antly.

"Oh, crikey!" the juniors herd him mutter to himself in dismay. Aloud, he said: "I suppose you're wringing up about those overdew instalments on my bike? Sorry and all that, but I'm afraid I can't do anything this week. Can't you let it stand over for another year or so?"

Jack Jolly & Co. nudged each other and grinned.

"The old, old, story," said Frank Fearless, sotto vocey. "I wonder if the Head has ever settled a dett in his life, yet?"

"Never!" declared Bright. "Or, at least, hardly ever!"

A series of strange noises came from the earpeace of the fone while Fearless and Bright were speaking. It sounded rather like an earthquake going on at the other end of the wires, and the juniors notissed the Head's face turn garstly white as he lissened.

"What!" he eggsclaimed, when the noises came to an end. "You mean you're threttening to send a dett-collector along to the skool to booly me into paying it? Impossibul! Think of my position! Surely you'd never be such rotters as to——"

There was a sudden crash from the earpeace, indikating that the jentleman at the other end had wrung off.

Dr. Birchemall replaced the receever and turned to the juniors, uttering a deep, deep groan as he did so. It was serprizing to see the change that had come over him. His skollerly dial, which only five minnits before had been smiling and happy at the prospect of wacking Jack Jolly & Co., was now the picture of misery.

"Woe is me!" he cried. "A lass and a lack! I am undone!"

"Yes, I notissed that, sir," nodded Jack Jolly, with a glarnse at the Head's weskit which had several buttons miss-ing. "Can we help you, sir? Perhaps the House dame can sew on some new buttons for you."

"Fathead!" snorted the Head. "I was speaking metafiggeratively, not literally. Still, Jolly, now that you make the sujjestion, there is just a charnse that you can help me."

"Delited to do so, sir!" grinned Jack Jolly, who began to see a way of escape from their prommised flogging. "These chaps will help me, won't you, chaps?"

"Yes, rather!" corussed Fearless, Merry, and Bright.

Dr. Birchemall nodded.

"Thank you kindly, boys. Under the sercumstances, of corse, I shall cansel the walloping I intended giving you and let you off with a sollum warning never to pull faces at your headmaster again! And now to give you an idea of what I want doing. As you will have gathered from my remarks on the fone, I am in rather a tight corner. Messrs. Mugleigh's, of Muggleton, are pressing me for the settlement of the balance owing on my old jigger. They have just had the awful cheek to thretten me with a big burleigh booly of a dett-collector!"

"Shame!"

"'Shame' hardly describes it. It's utterly disgraceful. I really don't know what commerse is coming to these days," said Dr. Birchemall, with a sad shake of his head. "However, that's by the way. The main thing is that this wacking grate booly is coming to see me. What am I to do?"

"Can't you let them have the bike back?" sujjested Jack Jolly.

"I wish I could, Jolly!" was the Head's reply. "Unforchunitly, how-ever, I raffled it a short time ago, and it is not now in my possession. No; my idea is to give this beastly dett-collector such a hot welcome that he'll never want to come near St. Sam's again. That's where you come in!"

"Oh crikey!"

"If you want to help me in this emerjency—and it will pay you to do so," said the Head, with a sideways glarnse at his birch, "I sujjest that you all go down to the gates, wait for this dett-collector to turn up, and give him a real ruff-house. Think you can mannidge that?"

Jack Jolly & Co. grinned.

"Rely on us, sir!" said Jack Jolly. "This is a task that's after our own harts, isn't it, you fellows?"

"Yes, rather!" corussed Jack Jolly's loyle followers.

The Head got out his fountin-pen and drew a deep breth of releef.

"Thanks awfully for offering to help me, boys," he said gratefully. "If you do the job well, I'll stand you a free feed afterwards. Keep an eye out for anyone who looks like a dett-collector, and, as soon as you see him, go for him like tigers! Now you can buzz off—or, as the vulgar would put it, you may go!"

"Thanks, sir!" grinned Jack Jolly & Co.

And they quitted the study, determined to do all they could to help Dr. Birchemall out of his awkward predicament.

II.

JACK JOLLY & Co. waited down at the gates for half an hour on the look-out for Dr. Birchemall's eggs-pected visitor. During that time there were plenty of callers, including the milkman, the baker, a newspaper-boy delivering a pink sporting jernal for Bounder of the Sixth, and a lorry-driver delivering a ton of birches for the Head. But nobody resembling a

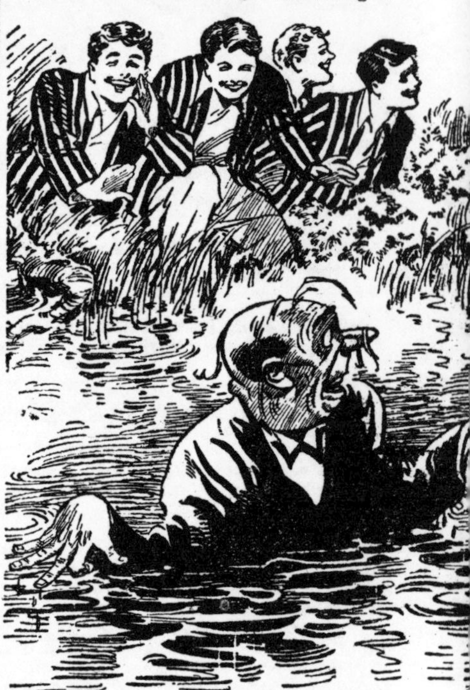

dett-collector turned up, and the juniors were just beginning to get restiv when a sudden eggsclamation from Frank Fearless raised their hoaps again.

"Here he is!" said Fearless, pointing down the road.

The rest of the Co. looked. One glarnse was sufficient to tell them that this was their eggspected visitor, for he had beetling eyebrows and a low, cunning eggspression on his fizz.

WOULD YOU BELIEVE IT?

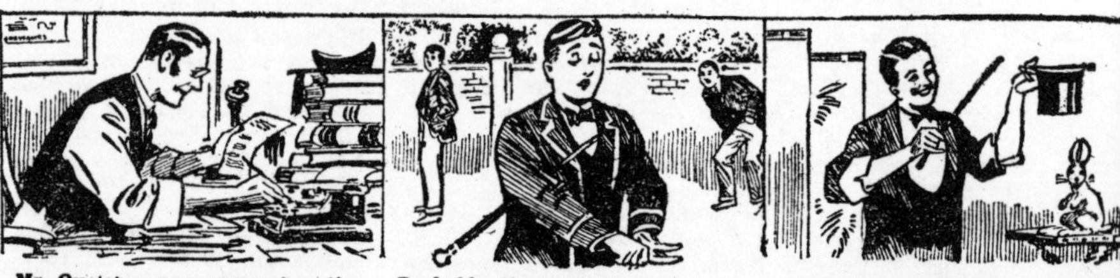

Mr. Quelch is now engaged on the tenth volume of his famous History of Greyfriars. He claims this will be the most exhaustive school history yet written.

Probably the best-dressed fellow at Greyfriars is Cecil Reginald Temple, the dandified captain of the Upper Fourth.

Oliver Kipps is a clever amateur conjuror and hopes for a stage career. He can produce almost anything out of a top hat.

[...]G BLUNDER!

[...]UGENT.

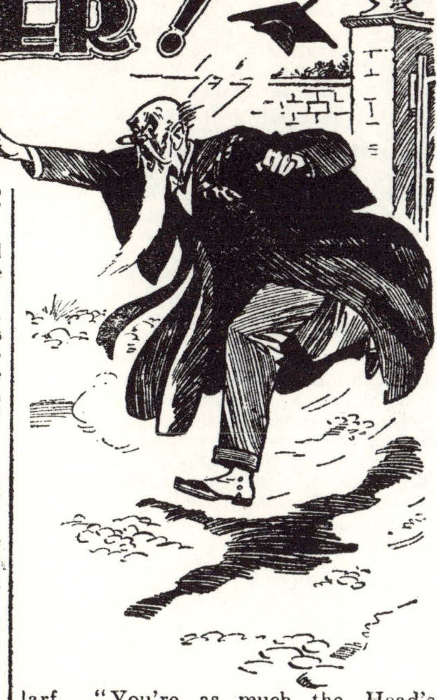

"What an ugly-looking villan!" grinned Merry. "He reminds me somewhat of the Head."

"It's our man all right, though," said Jack Jolly. "Leave it to me and wade in when I give the werd!"

"All sereen, old chap!"

A moment later the visitor arrived at the gates and pawsed in front of the Fourth-Formers.

"Good-mourning!" he remarked, regarding the juniors from under his black eyebrows. "Trot me along to your headmaster, Dr. Birchemall, one of you, will you? I want to see him privitly, and I particularly don't want to be annownced."

That was enuff for Jack Jolly.

"Wade in, you fellows!" he cride, and hurled himself on the newcomer with terriffick force.

The others were not long in following his eggsample. Frank Fearless grabbed the man by the ears, Merry seezed his hair, and Bright dived for his feet.

"Yarooooo!" roared the suspected dett-collector, as he collapsed in the road with four determined juniors on top of him. "Mersy!"

"'Mersy,' indeed!" cride Jack Jolly skornfully. "A fat lot of mersy you'd have shown our Head once you got him in your klutches! Have you got him, you fellows?"

"Yes, rather!"

"Then carry him over to the pond and throw him in!"

"Help!" cride the visitor, struggling fewriously. "You're making a garstly mistake—there's nothing fishy about me!"

"Throw him as far as you can, you fellows," ordered Jack Jolly, leading the struggling group across to the pond. "Here we are! One—two—three—go!"

The juniors hurled their burden with all their mite, and the suspected dett-collector shot through the air like a boolet from a gun.

Bang!

With a deffening eggsplosion he collided with the surfiss of the water and disappeared in the pond.

When he came up again some seconds later, his sholders were covered with green slime, while his face was purple with rage. The langwidge he used was the most highly-cullered the juniors had ever herd.

"You young villans!" he howled, as he started wading for the shore. "I'll have you flogged and eggspelled for this! How dare you attack your Headmaster's cuzzin!"

"Headmaster's cuzzin, ratts!" retorted Jack Jolly, with a skeptical larf. "You're as much the Head's cuzzin as I'm your aunt!"

"Ha, ha, ha!"

"You—you——"

Before the visitor could say more, there was a sound of hurried footprints from the direction of the skool gates, and Dr. Birchemall himself arrived on the seen.

The Head gave one look at the juniors, then his eyes turned to the specter in the pond. And then, to the serprize of the juniors, he gave a yell.

"Cuzzin Herbert!"

III.

"M-M-MY hat!" gasped Jack Jolly. "Then it's true! He's not the dett-collector, after all, but the Head's cuzzin!"

"Oh crums!"

It was a startling discovery, and the juniors looked awfully nervuss as they went to the side of the pond to help Cuzzin Herbert on to terrer-firmer. They were wondering how the Head would take it.

They didn't wonder for long. As soon as Cuzzin Herbert was landed, Dr. Birchemall turned on them with fury in his fizz.

"You dastardly young villans!" he cried. "You have chucked your own Headmaster's cuzzin in the pond! This is the last thing I wished, for he happens to be very welthy—I mean, he happens to be an awfully nice jentleman! How dare you!"

"We're awfully sorry, sir!" said Frank Fearless. "We thought he was the dett-collector."

The Head glared.

"I haven't the phoggiest notion what you're talking about, Fearless! What should I know about dett-collectors?"

"Oh crikey!"

Cuzzin Herbert snorted.

"The young villans just did it for a lark, I fansy!" he remarked.

"I can hardly swallow that, my dear cuzzin!" said the Head, with a frown. "In any case, they won't crow for long, for I intend to give them the bird with a vengenz when I get them in my study!"

"But it was quite a mistake, sir!" pointed out Jack Jolly. "When this jentleman came on the seen, we thought he was just a common loafer and not a bit well-bread; but now, of corse, it's obvious that he's dripping."

"Ratts!" said the Head crustily. "You boys will follow me up to my study; and you, Cuzzin Herbert, shall have the plezzure of seeing me lay it on thick and hevvy!"

"Jolly good idea!" said Cuzzin Herbert, looking a little Molly-fied.

And with that, he joined the Head and squelched his way up to the Skool House.

It was ruff luck on the juniors and no mistake. But there was nothing else for it, but to bear their punishment with fortitude.

This, of corse, they did, and when the Head laid it on with all the vigger of his strong right arm, Jack Jolly & Co. just gritted their teeth and yelled and howled with stoical indifference.

• • • • •

At tea-time that day, Jack Jolly & Co. were once more summoned to the Head's study.

Dr. Birchemall was grinning all over his dial by this time, and the chums of the Fourth rightly guessed that Cuzzin Herbert had left some of his welth behind him when he shook the dust of St. Sam's from off his feet.

"Trot in, my boys!" said the Head jenially, as they entered. "I'm sorry about this morning; but you will realise, or corse, that by chucking my cuzzin in the pond you placed me in rather a dellicate predicament."

"Eggsactly, sir!" said Jack Jolly, with a slite smile. "Of corse, you acted like a rotter and a beast to us. But we forgive you, don't we, you fellows?"

"Yes, rather!" said the Co.

Dr. Birchemall smiled.

"That is very jennerous of you, my boys, I must say. I mite add that, since my cuzzin's visit, my financial position has improved a little with the result that I have been able to pay Mugleigh's another instalment on that bike. So you need worry no more about that dett-collector. And now, what about tea with me?"

"Thanks awfully, sir!"

"Squatty-voo, my dear boys, and I will order a repast that will live in your memory for years!" said the Head. "I will ring for the House dame."

Dr. Birchemall did so, and, true to his werd, ordered a meal that the Co. remembered for a long, long time.

What they cheefly remembered about it, though, was the remarkable speed with which the Head grabbed everything on the table and ate it before they had a chance to begin.

THE END.

(Next week's story of Jack Jolly & Co.: "HIGH JINKS HIKING!" is absolutely spiffing, chums, so prepare yourself for another hearty laugh!)

GREYFRIARS FACTS WHILE YOU WAIT!

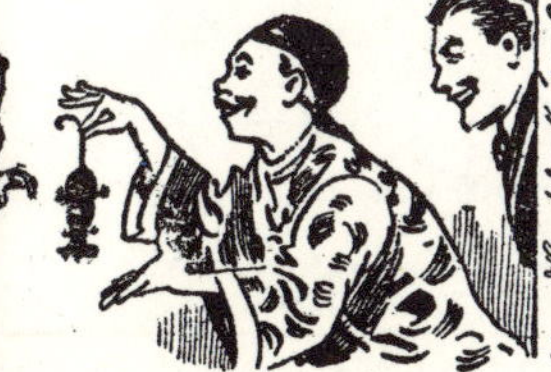

[...]u never know what's in a pie [...]at Wun Lung has made. He [...]s a weakness for cats and [...]ice and other "impossible" [...]gredients!

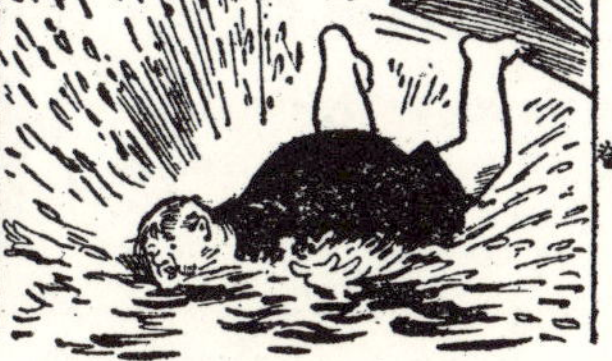

Sammy Bunter makes almost as big a splash as his major when he goes in swimming—which isn't very often. Pity the poor fishes when he does!

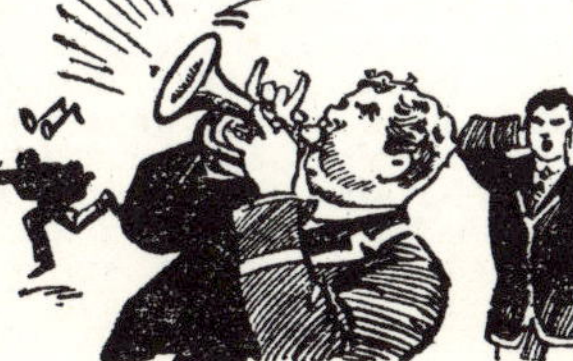

Johnny Bull is the only cornet player at Greyfriars. And when he's practising there's a great demand for cotton-wool at the local chemist's.

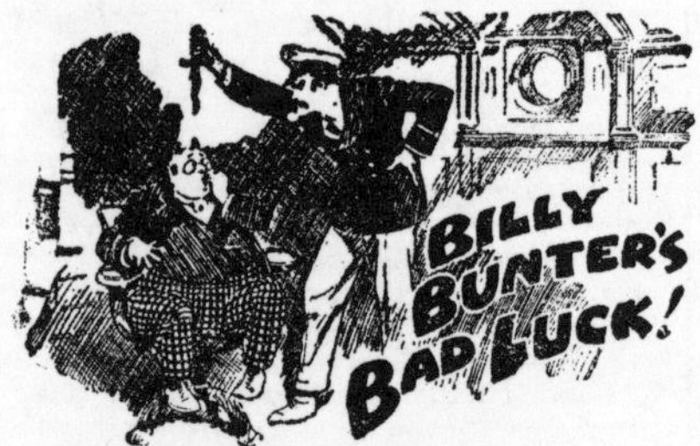

(*Continued from page 13.*)

The man did not look the kind of man to be trifled with, with impunity.

The terror in his fat face evidently afforded the Greek satisfaction. Had Bunter really been the Earl of Mauleverer, that nobleman would have been, in the Greek's hands, like clay in the hands of the potter.

Bunter staggered from his seat.

"I—I—I—I want to go ashore," he stuttered. "My—my friends will be waiting for me——"

"Sit down, my lord."

"I—I'd rather go ashore now!" mumbled Bunter.

"Sit down!" rapped the Greek, in a tone that made Bunter jump. The fat junior fell rather than sat.

"Now let us talk business," said Kalizelos. "I am here to obtain the scarab; you understand that. You, my lord, know where it is kept—you will give me the most precise information, to enable me to lay my hands on it. Once it is in my possession, you will be released, unharmed. But do not seek to deceive me—your life depends on it."

"Oh crikey!"

"Until I lay hands on the Golden Scarab of A-Menah, you remain a prisoner on my yacht at sea. Yet I will deal with you fairly," went on Kalizelos. "The intrinsic value of the scarab, as a piece of gold, is little—perhaps twenty—thirty pounds in your English money. I know not, as I have not yet handled it. But I will pay one thousand pounds for the scarab, my lord, willingly. Is it a bargain?"

"Oh crumbs!"

"Is not that a good offer?" asked Kalizelos. "The scarab has a value to me—that is my own secret. To your lordship, it is only one of the many curios that the late Lord Mauleverer brought from the land of Egypt many years ago. To you it has no special value. But there are those in Egypt, my lord, who would wade in blood to possess it."

"B-b-but——" stammered Bunter.

"You will give the scarab into my hands," said the Greek. "Sell it if you wish, at the price I have named. Hand it to me, and take a thousand pounds in English money as compensation. But the scarab I must and will have—and if money does not tempt you, my lord, —I have heard that you are very rich—I offer you your life in exchange for the Golden Beetle."

"I—I—I say——"

"Is it a bargain, my lord?"

Bunter's teeth chattered.

Had he been Lord Mauleverer, or had he even known where the mysterious scarab was to be found, no doubt it would have been a bargain. Billy Bunter was not of the stuff that heroes are made of.

But it was not in Bunter's power to make it a bargain, as he knew nothing about the scarab, and had never even heard of it till Kalizelos spoke of it.

"Your answer, my lord?"

"I—I can't!" stammered Bunter. "You—you see——"

"Think again, my lord," said the Greek, in a low tone of deadly menace. "If you refuse to part with the sacred scarab of A-Menah, the next heir to the Mauleverer estates may part with it. Think again!"

Kalizelos stepped to the wall and took down a curved Oriental dagger that hung there as a decoration. Bunter's heart thumped. It seemed almost incredible to the fat junior, but there was no doubting it. Had Lord Mauleverer fallen into the Greek's hands, his life would have been in dire peril at that moment. And now it was Bunter's life that was in peril—unless the revelation that he was not Mauleverer would save him. His teeth chattered, and his little round eyes goggled at the Greek through his big round spectacles.

The bright Damascus steel flashed before his eyes, and Bunter gave a squeal of terror.

"Your answer, my lord!" said Kalizelos, with a snarl that showed his gleaming white teeth. "Life or death depend on your word. The scarab—or you will not live to see the sun set."

"I—I can't!" gasped Bunter. "You see, I—I—— Oh lor'! I—I say, I ain't Lord Mauleverer! I'm Bunter! Oh lor'!"

THE TENTH CHAPTER.

Desperate Courage!

THE man from Cairo stared blankly at the terrified fat junior. The curved dagger, catching the sunlight, flashed in his hand, and his jetty eyes flashed over it. Whatever he had expected from the fat schoolboy certainly he had not expected that announcement. And, for the moment at least, it was plain that he did not believe it. His dark face grew more savage and threatening.

"Oh dear!" groaned Bunter. "I wish I hadn't bunked out of Quelch's study! I wish I was back at Greyfriars! Oh crikey! I say, I ain't Lord Mauleverer—I—I ain't anything like him! Oh crumbs!"

"It is useless to lie to me, my lord!" said the Greek. His well-cut lip curled in a sneer. "I did not expect a nobleman to lie to save his skin."

"I—I ain't a nobleman!" groaned Bunter. "Any Greyfriars man could tell you that I ain't Lord Mauleverer. I don't know anything about his beastly scarab! I don't even know what it is. Oh crikey!"

The Greek eyed him doubtingly now.

It was Billy Bunter's fond belief that any stranger might have taken him for a nobleman on account of his aristocratic looks. But, as a matter of fact, the Greek had been rather surprised to find that Lord Mauleverer was this podgy fellow, evidently a fool, and obviously a funk. Billy Bunter's denial that he was Mauleverer began to carry conviction to his mind.

A flash of rage came into his black eyes that made Bunter squeak with fear.

"You are not Lord Mauleverer!" exclaimed the Greek, at last, in a hissing voice. "You have deluded me!"

"I—I was only pulling your leg!" groaned Bunter. "You see, I was detained this afternoon, and I was dodging out, and—and it was really only a—a—a joke, you know. Oh dear! I was getting away from old Quelch, and—— Oh lor'!"

"If you are not Lord Mauleverer, who are you?"

"Oh dear! I'm Bunter!"

Kalizelos gritted his white teeth.

The rage in his dark face made Billy Bunter quake.

"Then where is Lord Mauleverer now?" he snarled.

"I—I suppose he's at the school. Slacking in his study, most likely. He's jolly lazy——"

"Then if I had waited I should have seen him! And you deceived me, deluded me. Fool! I Konstantinos Kalizelos, have been deluded, deceived, by a fool of a schoolboy—an ass—a dolt! But it is not too late!"

The Greek replaced the dagger on the wall, much to Bunter's relief. He stood for some minutes, with his dark brows puckered in thought.

Billy Bunter watched him in terror.

The Greek believed him now; he could see that. The plotting rascal realised that, while he had supposed that he was trapping Lord Mauleverer, he had only been helping a fatuous, unreflecting duffer to escape detention. It was a bitter pill for the wily Greek, who prided himself upon his keenness and cunning, to swallow; but he could see that the terrified junior was telling the truth, and he was quick to grasp how matters stood.

After the first few moments of savage rage and disappointment, he was cool again, thinking the matter out.

It was not too late.

His sudden departure from Greyfriars, without seeing the boy he had called to see, must have seemed strange and unaccountable to the master he had interviewed there. But he could invent some plausible explanation. The cunning Greek was at no loss for trickery. The fat fool was safe on the yacht, and could give no warning. It was easy to return to the school and see Lord Mauleverer, as he had originally planned. Once he knew the boy by sight, he could lay plans for his kidnapping; and this fatuous trickster could be taken care of, and could not betray him.

He turned to Bunter again, with one of his swift, tigerish movements.

"It is not too late," he said. "You will remain here, fool! You have made my task more difficult, but it is not too late. You know too much now, you fat fool! You will remain a prisoner here until Lord Mauleverer is in my hands."

"I—I say——" stammered Bunter.

"Siopesate! Hold your tongue! If we were not in English waters I would secure your silence by dropping you into the sea, with a weight at your heels!" snarled the Greek.

"Oh lor'!"

"As soon as I have seen Mauleverer I shall return here and put to sea, and you will sail with me!" snarled Kalizelos. "You will remain a prisoner here until——" He broke off.

Billy Bunter shuddered.

Now that he knew the plans of the man from Egypt, and a word from him would put the schoolboy earl on his guard, it was obvious that the Greek could not afford to let him go. He was to remain a prisoner until Mauleverer was in the hands of his enemy. But it seemed to him that he could read a more terrible intention in the gleaming black eyes of the Egyptian Greek.

"Remain here, fool!" said Kalizelos, between his teeth. "I shall order my men to throw you into the sea if you quit this room."

"Oh crikey! I—I want to stay here! I—I like being here!" gasped Bunter.

"Fool!"

The Greek hurried from the saloon.

"Oh crikey!" groaned Bunter.

He heard the boat lowered, and the plash of oars.

Kalizelos was gone.

Bunter knew where he was gone. He was bound for Greyfriars to see Lord Mauleverer there. He could have no hope that Mauleverer would fall into his hands as Bunter had done. That would come later, once he knew the schoolboy earl by sight. Sooner or later he would succeed, there could be no doubt about that, as Mauleverer was totally unconscious of danger. Probably the Greek's chance would come when the school broke up for the holidays, and Mauly was on his way home. In the meantime——

In the meantime, obviously, Bunter had to be kept from putting the schoolboy earl on his guard. The yacht would put to sea immediately Kalizelos returned, and then——

Once out of sight of English land on the wide waters, with no eyes to see, was the man from Egypt likely to keep the fat junior a prisoner on the yacht, or to make sure of his silence by a more deadly method? It seemed to Bunter that he had read a fearful intention in the black eyes of the Greek, and he shuddered with terror at the thought that it was not his liberty, but his life, that would be in danger, once the yacht was out of sight of land.

But there was no escape for Bunter.

It was clear that the crew of the yacht were men picked for the Greek's service. He had nothing to hope from them. He had not the slightest doubt that they had orders to deal with him drastically if he ventured to go on deck, and that they would carry out the orders.

The yacht was anchored half a mile out. When he blinked from the porthole the shore was merely a blur to him. There was no hope of help from the shore.

Harry Wharton & Co. knew that he was on the yacht, and if he did not return to school they would say so; but long before calling-over at Greyfriars the yacht would be far out to sea.

Bunter groaned dismally.

He blinked from the porthole. The yacht's boat, with Kalizelos in it, was already out of sight. The Greek had landed. and was on his way to the school.

"Oh lor'!" groaned Bunter.

From the bottom of his fat heart he wished that he was back in Mr. Quelch's study, writing lines. But it was rather too late to wish that. Alternatively, as the lawyers say, he wished that he had joined the Famous Five, after all, in the sailing-boat. He wished, in fact, that he was anywhere but where he was at the present moment. Billy Bunter had often had cause to repent of his trickery, but never had he repented so deeply and sincerely as he did now.

A brown, patched sail glancing on the sunny waters caught his eyes as he stood blinking dismally shoreward.

Five figures could be seen in the boat.

Billy Bunter's heart gave a jump.

Harry Wharton & Co., unconscious of the eyes—and the spectacles—that watched them from the yacht in the distance, were sailing merrily on the bay. The Greek had given no thought to the schoolboys he had seen on the pier. Bunter had given them no thought till now. Now his fat heart thumped at the sight of them. If they came near enough for a yell to be heard——

But they did not look like passing within hail of the yacht. And Bunter realised, too, that a yell from the porthole, whether it was heard by the Removites or not, would certainly be heard by the crew on deck, and they would take instant care that it was not repeated. His fat mouth opened and closed again.

He watched the sailing-boat with haggard eyes behind his big spectacles. It was passing within easy view, and he saw several of the juniors glancing towards the yacht, doubtless remembering that the fat Owl was on board her, though little dreaming in what circumstances.

The boat was drawing nearer; but it would not pass close, and in a few more minutes it would be gone! Bunter opened his mouth once more, and once more he closed it. But he was making up his fat mind to a desperate resolve now.

Whatever courage Billy Bunter might have possessed had oozed out at his fat finger-tips. He was in a state of palpitating, shuddering funk. But from the extremity of fear he drew a kind of desperate courage. Once the Greek came back and the yacht put to sea he was lost! That most peaceful of animals, the sheep, is the most desperate of animals once in a state of desperation. So it was with Billy Bunter. He was so frightened that he dared not be afraid. There was one chance for him, and he knew it; the Remove boat was all that stood between him and the merciless plotter from Egypt. From sheer terror Billy Bunter acted as a courageous fellow would have done.

He did not stop to think; he dared not think! He tore open the door and tore on deck.

Four or five dark-skinned men were close at hand, and they ran at him at once. Had Bunter intended to wave or call to the passing boat he would have had no chance. But that was not his intention. Before a hand could be laid on him the fat junior bounded to the rail and flung himself into the sea.

THE ELEVENTH CHAPTER.

Removites to the Rescue!

"HALLO, hallo, hallo!"

Bob Cherry stared.

He stared in amazement, his eyes almost bulging from his head at what he saw.

"Great pip!" gasped Harry Wharton.

"Bunter——"

"What——"

"Good heavens!"

The juniors in the boat stared at the yacht blankly. Harry Wharton was at the tiller, and even as he stared in utter amazement at the sight of Billy Bunter pitching over the rail into the sea, he gave the tiller a twist, and the sailing-boat shot towards the yacht.

"Bunter!" gasped Johnny Bull. "Is he mad? He didn't fall—he jumped from——"

Bob Cherry grabbed a boathook. Nugent dragged at the sheet. The boat shot like an arrow towards the yacht's side.

The rail was lined with dark faces, staring down. Some of the yacht's crew were already rushing to lower a boat.

But the Famous Five were first in the field.

Billy Bunter was swimming desperately. Bunter was about the worst swimmer at Greyfriars, but he had reason to be glad just then that "ducker" was compulsory at the school. Had Bunter been able to dodge learning swimming, undoubtedly he would have dodged it. His swimming, according to Bob Cherry, was enough to make the fishes sit up on their tails and laugh. Still, he could swim after a fashion. After the the first plunge he came up, spluttering wildly, and swam, and was at least able to keep himself afloat, in calm waters, for a few minutes. A few minutes were not needed, however; in considerably less than one minute the Remove boat was rushing down on him and Bob was hooking at him with the boathook.

"Grooooogh! Ooooch!" spluttered Bunter.

"Got him!" gasped Bob.

"Get him in!"

Frank Nugent leaned over as the boathook hauled Bunter to the gunwale, and grasped the fat junior by the collar. Hurree Jamset Ram Singh lent a prompt hand, and Bunter was dragged, dripping and spluttering, into the boat.

There was shouting from the yacht; excited, dark faces staring at the schoolboys. Bunter sat up streaming with water.

"Ow! Help! I say, you fellows——"

"What's this game, you potty ass?" yelled Bob Cherry. "What do you think you are up to? Trying to commit suicide, or what?"

"Help! Keep them off! Quick!" yelled Bunter frantically. "They'll be after us! Help! Murder——"

"Mad!" gasped Johnny Bull.

"Quick!" shrieked Bunter. "Get away before they can get after you. They'll murder the lot of you——"

"What the thump——"

Harry Wharton & Co. stared at Bunter and stared at the yacht. That the fat junior could have been in any danger on board that vessel was amazing to them. But there was no mistaking the frantic terror in his face, or his desperate act in leaping into the sea.

A boat dropped from the yacht's davits, and half a dozen dark-skinned men were in it, and already it was pulling swiftly towards the Remove boat.

Wharton gave a twist to the tiller and the sailing-boat shot away before the wind. Amazing as it was, well-nigh incredible, the juniors could see that the foreign seamen were coming as enemies; that they were after Bunter! Why, was an utter mystery; but there was no mistaking the fact. Only in time the sailing-boat shot away, and as the sail filled with wind the yacht's boat was dropped astern. But the seamen, with set, dark faces, pulled hard in pursuit.

"They're after us!" almost babbled Bob Cherry. "They're after us, and Bunter! What the jolly old thump——"

"What the dickens——"

"Keep her before the wind," said Harry Wharton quietly. "They won't get near us with oars! You're all right now, Bunter."

"Oh crikey!"

"But what the thump——" gasped Nugent.

"Oh dear! G-get ashore, you fellows!" stuttered Bunter. "I say, you fellows, run ashore as fast as you can, and—— Oh dear!"

"They won't get near us, old fat bean! We're sailing three or four lengths to their one," said Harry reassuringly.

"Get to the shore, you beast!" howled Bunter. "I'm not to be murdered to please you!"

"Wha-a-at?"

"I say, you fellows—— Oh crikey!"

Harry Wharton glanced back. The yacht's boat was pulling in pursuit, but it had no chance against the sailing-craft. The Remove boat danced away from it. Even Billy Bunter was a little reassured as he blinked back and saw how fast the distance was widening.

"Well, if this doesn't beat the band!" said Bob Cherry blankly. "If Bunter's not mad, and they're not mad, what does it mean, you men?"

"Ask me another!" said Harry.

"I say, you fellows, they're after Mauly!" groaned Bunter.

"Mauly!" repeated Wharton.

"Oh dear! You—you see, I—I got a lift from that beast by pretending that I was Mauly——"

"You spoofing sweep!"

"How was I to know that he was after Mauly and looking for a chance to kidnap him!" groaned Bunter. "I—I thought I was going to have a jolly good tea on that yacht. Oh dear!"

"Kidnapping Mauly!" repeated Wharton. "What on earth——"

"He's gone back to Greyfriars after Mauly now——"

"Who has?" yelled Wharton.

"That Greek beast—Kalizelos, he calls himself! He's after some beastly Egyptian rubbish that Mauly's pater brought home from Egypt. Oh dear! I say, you fellows, get ashore. If they get steam up on the yacht they'll run us down!"

"Oh, my hat!"

"They've chucked it!" said Johnny Bull, looking back at the pursuers. "But if they up anchor and follow us by steam we're done! Better run ashore, you men."

"Yes, rather!"

The yacht's boat was swinging up to the davits again in the far distance. There was no doubt that if the steam-yacht got under way it would not take long to run down the sailing-craft, and the juniors headed for the shore. The Famous Five handled a sailing-boat well, and they ran close to the wind, heading for the beach at its nearest point.

Minute followed minute as the boat raced through the water. Billy Bunter blinked back at the yacht with scared eyes through his spectacles. But the sailing-boat ran on swiftly and bumped on the sandy beach a mile along the circling bay from the pier. Billy Bunter rolled out in hot haste, heedless of water up to his fat knees, and plugged up the sand, gasping and spluttering. Harry Wharton & Co. stayed only to drag the boat above high-water mark and then followed him.

"Now, you fat duffer, let's know what it's all about," said Bob Cherry.

Billy Bunter did not answer. He needed all his breath for running. He plugged desperately on till he reached Pegg Lane and the beach was left behind. There at last he halted, and staggered against a tree, gasping for breath. He was feeling safe at last. Even Bunter realised that the crew on the yacht could not venture to land and pursue the schoolboys inland.

"Oh! Ow! Wow!" gasped Bunter. "I say, you fellows, I—I'm winded! Oh dear! I wish I'd stayed in Quelch's study! Oh crikey!"

"Tell us what's happened, you fat chump!" exclaimed Wharton. "If old Mauly's in any danger——"

"He jolly well is!" gasped Bunter. "That Greek beast thought I was him, you know, and he bagged me! Oh dear!"

"Cough it up, fathead!"

Billy Bunter spluttered out his story, the chums of the Remove listening in amazed silence. But for the fact that they had seen, with their own eyes, Bunter's desperate escape from the yacht, it would have been incredible to them. Now they could not doubt.

"So that scoundrel—Kalizelos, as you call him—has gone back to the school after Mauly!" exclaimed Wharton. "He must be there by this time, or very nearly, in a taxi——"

"We've got to get after him!" exclaimed Bob Cherry.

Wharton shook his head.

"No time! But we can get Quelch on the phone from the Anchor, at Pegg. That will be in time to put a spoke in his wheel. I'll cut off and get Quelch on the phone."

And without wasting another moment the captain of the Remove started at a run for Pegg, covering the ground at a speed he had never exceeded on the cinder-path.

THE TWELFTH CHAPTER.

A Timely Warning!

BUZZZZZ!

Mr. Quelch uttered a sound which—if Form masters could be supposed to snort—would certainly have been taken, by any hearer, for a snort.

He was annoyed.

Already, that afternoon, there had been interruptions and annoyances. There had been Bunter's bolt from the Form-room, and Prout's complaint of the fat junior barging him over in the quad; then the visit of the antique merchant from Cairo, and his mysterious and inexplicable departure after wasting Mr. Quelch's time; then the vanishing of Bunter from the study.

It had been quite an annoying afternoon, and Mr. Quelch was feeling that end-of-the-term feeling more than ever. Now, as he laboured through his pile of papers, the buzz of the telephone bell came as the last straw.

Buzzzzz!

The Remove master laid down his pen, and crossed over to the telephone, and jerked the receiver from the hooks. He barked into the transmitter rather like a ferocious mastiff.

"Well?"

"Is that Mr. Quelch? Wharton speaking."

"Wharton!" Quelch growled this time instead of barking. "Really! Why have you rung me up, Wharton? Are you not aware that you should not interrupt your Form master and waste his time? I see no reason why——"

"It's important, sir—awfully important!" came the breathless voice of the captain of the Remove. "Mauleverer is in danger, sir!"

"What? What?"

"Mauleverer, sir—danger——"

"Nonsense!"

"I assure you, sir——"

"Rubbish!"

"Please listen, sir! Has a man—a Greek—named Kalizelos, called to see Mauleverer?"

"That is the case, Wharton, though I fail to see how you can be aware of it!" snapped Mr. Quelch.

"Is he at the school now, sir?"

"No! He is not! I fail to see how it concerns you, Wharton, but the man left without waiting to see Lord Mauleverer."

"Then he hasn't come back yet, sir?"

"Come back?" repeated Mr. Quelch acidly. "I do not suppose that it is his intention to come back. Certainly I shall speak to him very plainly if he does so. What do you mean, Wharton?"

"He is Lord Mauleverer's enemy, sir, and looking for a chance to kidnap him——"

"Do not be absurd, Wharton!"

"He came off a yacht now anchored in Pegg Bay, sir. Bunter somehow made him believe that he was Lord Mauleverer, and he got hold of Bunter."

"Bunter has broken detention—have you seen Bunter?"

"Yes, sir. The Greek took him on the yacht, thinking that he was Lord Mauleverer, and Bunter jumped into the sea to escape, and we picked him up in our boat."

"Goodness gracious!"

"According to what Bunter says, the man left him on the yacht to keep him from giving warning, while he went back to the school to have another try for Mauleverer. If he has not reached Greyfriars yet, he is on his way. I've rung you up to warn you, sir! For goodness' sake, sir, don't let him get at Mauleverer."

"This is a most extraordinary story, Wharton!"

"I know, sir! But Mauleverer is in danger. The man is a desperate villain from what Bunter says happened on the yacht——"

"Bunter is a foolish, untruthful, exaggerative boy, Wharton. Have you any reason, from your own knowledge——"

"We saw Bunter jump into the sea to escape, sir, and a boat from the yacht chased us after we picked him up."

"Bless my soul! I can hardly believe that the man will return here, Wharton, but I shall certainly take measures——"

Tap!

The study door opened. Mr. Quelch looked round at Trotter.

"The foreign gentleman, sir," said Trotter. "He wishes to see you again, sir. I've showed him into the visitors' room, sir."

"Upon my word! Mr. Kalizelos?"

"Yessir!"

Mr. Quelch's jaw set grimly.

"Tell Mr. Kalizelos that I will be with him in a few moments, Trotter."

"Yessir."

The page departed and closed the door.

"Wharton!" Mr. Quelch spoke into the transmitter again. "Are you there, Wharton?"

"Here, sir!"

"The man, Kalizelos, has just arrived, and I am about to see him," said Mr. Quelch. "So far Bunter's statements appear to be borne out. Return to the school at once, Wharton, and bring Bunter with you."

"Very well, sir."

Mr. Quelch put up the receiver and left the study. His face was grim as he made his way to the visitors' room. In that apartment the Greek was waiting, and he rose from a chair and bowed with lithe grace to the Remove master.

The Greyfriars master eyed him grimly. Obviously, Kalizelos was unaware of Bunter's escape from the yacht, and did not dream that the Form master had been warned. There was a surprise in store for Konstantinos Kalizelos. He addressed Mr. Quelch smoothly, in his musical voice, with a deprecating smile.

"I have to beg a thousand pardons, my dear sir," he said. "No doubt you

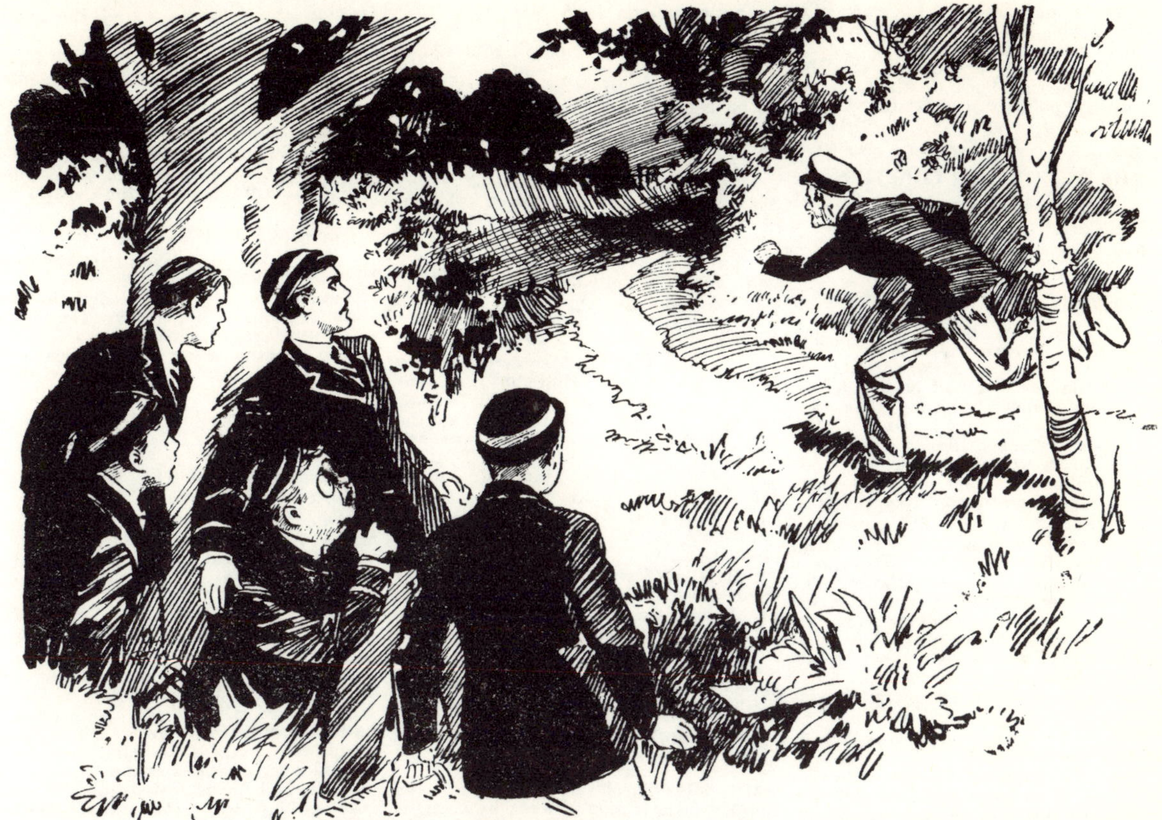

"Hallo, hallo, hallo!" exclaimed Bob Cherry suddenly, as there came the sound of swiftly running feet on the footpath, and a dark-skinned man, running hard, burst into view. Bunter gave a squeal of terror at the sight of the Greek, and dodged behind Bob Cherry. "Ow! Help!" he howled. "Keep him off!"

were surprised by my leaving so abruptly, without having seen——"

"I was!" interrupted Mr. Quelch curtly.

"You will, I feel sure, excuse my apparent discourtesy, when I explain the matter," said Kalizelos.

"I shall be very glad to hear your explanation, sir, of so very singular an action!" said Mr. Quelch.

"I was deceived, sir, by a foolish schoolboy's prank. The boy entered this room while I was waiting, made me believe that he was Lord Mauleverer, and asked for a lift in my car."

"Indeed!"

"Later he confessed to this foolish prank, sir, and so I lost no time in returning here—with a thousand apologies for taking up your so valuable time——"

"What has become of the boy you mention?"

"I left him at the village of Pegg, my dear sir, which we had already reached before I discovered the facts——"

"You did not take him on your yacht?"

Kalizelos started violently.

His black eyes narrowed, gleaming with suspicion and alarm.

"My yacht?" he repeated mechanically.

"I understand that you landed from a yacht in Pegg Bay, Mr. Kalizelos."

"I did not know that you were aware of that circumstance, sir. But it is the case, certainly."

"Did you take the boy on the yacht?"

"Certainly not!"

"You did not do so, still under the belief that he was Lord Mauleverer?"

"No!" muttered the Greek. "Why should you suppose——"

"You did not, still believing him to be Lord Mauleverer, threaten him on board your vessel, and put him in a state of fear?"

The Greek breathed hard. Unless this dry-looking, stern-featured schoolmaster was a magician, Kalizelos could not guess how he knew all this. But he scented danger now.

"You did not leave him on your yacht, and return here to make another attempt to see the real Lord Mauleverer, with the object of attempting to kidnap him?"

"My dear sir——"

Kalizelos broke off. With all his coolness and nerve, he was utterly confounded. He cast a hunted look towards the door. But Mr. Quelch was standing between him and the door, and evidently had no intention of moving.

"It may interest you to hear," said Mr. Quelch, in a grinding voice, "that the boy Bunter escaped from the yacht after you left——"

"What?"

"That he was helped by some schoolfellows, and that I have been apprised, sir, by telephone, of all that has happened."

Kalizelos almost staggered.

"You have chosen to come here, sir," said Mr. Quelch. "You will remain until you have been questioned by the police. You spoke falsely, sir, in stating your reason for desiring to see Lord Mauleverer—and most certainly you will not be allowed to see him. I shall take every care, sir, that the boy does not come into your presence. Whether you can be charged with kidnapping for your action with regard to the boy Bunter I do not know—but this I know, sir, that you will be detained here until you have explained yourself to the police."

The Greek made a stride forward, his hand slipping under his coat. The Remove master eyed him, with icy contempt.

"There is ample help at hand, sir, to secure you!" he snapped. "Attempt to leave this room, and you shall be detained by force."

The Greek's eyes blazed. His dusky hand came out from under his coat without the weapon he had obviously thought of producing. He stood facing the Remove master, panting.

"You will remain here till the boy, Bunter, reaches the school, and you will be questioned by a police-inspector in the boy's presence!" rapped Mr. Quelch. "I have no doubt that I shall be able to give you into custody, and I shall certainly do so, Mr. Kalizelos."

Kalizelos gave him a black, bitter look. Then, with a sudden swiftness like the spring of a tiger in the jungle, he reached the open window and leaped out into the quadrangle.

"Goodness gracious!" gasped Mr. Quelch.

He rushed to the window.

Kalizelos, with the swiftness of a deer, was running for the gates. The taxi was waiting on the drive, but the Greek did not attempt to reach it. He had not a second to lose.

"Stop him!" Mr. Quelch shouted from the window. "Stop that man! Wingate—Coker—Price! Stop that man!"

There were a dozen fellows in sight in the quad, and they stared round in amazement. Mr. Quelch pointed after the fleeing Greek.

"Stop that man! Seize him!" he shouted.

There was a rush after the Greek. But Kalizelos had too good a start, and his feet seemed scarcely to touch the ground as he fled. He darted out of the open gates and vanished.

"Bless my soul!" gasped Mr. Quelch.

And he hurried back to his study to ring up the police station at Courtfield.

THE THIRTEENTH CHAPTER.

The Last of the Greek!

"I SAY, you fellows——"

"Come on, fathead!"

"But, I say——"

"Get a move on!"

"Shan't!" roared Billy Bunter.

Harry Wharton had rejoined his chums after leaving the Anchor. The sail on the bay that afternoon was a thing of the past; it had been briefer, though much more exciting, than the Famous Five had anticipated. Mr. Quelch had instructed the captain of the Remove to return to the school and bring Bunter—and that was the next item on the programme. But William George Bunter had quite other ideas.

Now that the danger was over, Billy Bunter was himself again. No man had landed from the yacht; the foreign crew evidently did not venture to carry the pursuit ashore. Bunter was at leisure now to remember that he was hungry—and to remember what awaited him when he found himself under his Form master's gimlet eyes again.

"Now, look here, you fellows," said Bunter, blinking at the chums of the Remove, "I'm not going back till call-over, see? I've cut detention, and old Quelch will lick me. You know that."

"Serve you jolly well right!" grunted Johnny Bull.

"Beast! I'm hungry!"

"Get a move on!"

"You've got a basket of grub," said Bunter. "Well, let's have a picnic in the wood, see? We shall be safe from those foreign beasts there! I'm fearfully hungry——"

"Are you coming?"

"No!" roared Bunter. "I'm not coming! I've got a licking coming for breaking detention. Think I'm going to have the licking and detention, too? Don't be a silly ass!"

"You fat Owl! Quelch told me to bring you back——"

"That's all right," said Bunter. "You can tell Quelch you lost sight of me, and were looking for me till call-over——"

"Oh, my hat!"

"Now, what about the picnic?"

"Nothing about the picnic, old fat man! Come on! You walk behind him, Bob, and help him."

"Yarooooh! Leave off kicking me, you beast!" yelled Bunter. "I'm coming, ain't I? I—I want to come! If you kick me again, you beast, I'll——Yarooop!"

And Billy Bunter started—quite in a hurry! Johnny Bull carried the basket of tuck—still unopened. Wharton had left word at the Anchor for Mr. Trumper, and the boat was left where the juniors had dragged it up the beach for the old fisherman to collect. The Famous Five were anxious to get back to the school to learn what had happened since Wharton had telephoned.

Billy Bunter was by no means anxious about that. What Bunter was anxious about was the contents of the picnic basket. Likewise, he was anxious to postpone seeing Mr. Quelch until the latest possible moment. But there was no help for William George Bunter. With Bob Cherry walking behind him, ready to give his assistance at any moment, Billy Bunter rolled on to the school and did not even dare to lag.

His only consolation was to tell the chums of the Remove what he thought of them as he went. What he thought of them was not at all complimentary; but the cheery juniors did not seem unduly perturbed.

With an occasional lift from Bob Cherry's foot to keep him going, the fat Owl rolled along the path through Friardale Wood—every now and then casting a longing blink at the picnic basket.

"Hallo, hallo, hallo!" exclaimed Bob suddenly.

The juniors halted.

There was a sound of swiftly running feet on the footpath under the shady branches.

A dark-skinned man, running hard, burst into view. His olive face streamed with perspiration as he ran.

Billy Bunter gave a squeal of terror.

"Ow! Help! Keep him off!"

The fat junior dodged behind Bob Cherry, his eyes almost bulging through his spectacles at the sight of the Greek.

Kalizelos halted, panting.

"It's the man from the yacht!" shouted Bob. "Collar him!"

But it was only for a second that the juniors glimpsed the Greek. He turned from the footpath and plunged into the wood, dashing away among trees and thickets and brambles with the swiftness of a wild animal. He was gone almost in the twinkling of an eye.

"I say, you fellows, keep him off!" howled Bunter.

"You fat chump! He's gone!" snapped Wharton.

"Oh crikey!" gasped Bunter. "I—I say, you fellows, let's get back to Greyfriars! Oh dear! Hurry up, for goodness' sake! Oh crumbs! If that beast comes back—— Oh lor'!"

Billy Bunter started again, without waiting for assistance from Bob. The juniors resumed their way. For once they had to hurry to keep pace with Billy Bunter. The sight of the Greek had revived all the fat Owl's terrors, and he was yearning to find himself safe within the walls of Greyfriars—even if Mr. Quelch's cane awaited him there! He plugged on as fast as his fat little legs could whisk, panting for breath.

"Looks as if that sportsman has been to the school and left in rather a hurry!" grinned Bob. "I suppose he's making for his yacht before the police can get hold of him."

"I say, you fellows, hurry up——"

"Fathead! The man's on the run," said Harry. "He wants to get out to sea before he can be stopped."

"Hurry up, you beast!"

The juniors chuckled, and hurried on after Bunter. They had no doubt that Kalizelos was making for his yacht, to get to sea at the earliest possible moment. But to Billy Bunter, it seemed that the Greek's fierce black eyes were gleaming from every shadow in the trees and thickets; and he plunged on desperately, panting and gasping—without even a blink at the lunch-basket. The fat Owl did not slacken speed till the wood was left behind, and they came out into Friardale Lane. Even then he kept on at a gasping trot till the school gates were reached. He rolled in, gurgling for breath.

There was an excited crowd in the quadrangle when the juniors came in. Fellows were discussing the escape of the man who had leaped from the window of the visitors' room in great excitement. Harry Wharton & Co. learned what had happened by the time they reached the House.

"I say, you fellows." Bunter came to a halt at last. "I say—grooogh—I'm winded—I say, I'm not going to see Quelch! If he asks about me, tell him you couldn't find me, see? If you're going to see the beast, I'll mind that basket for you while you're gone, see?"

"Come on, fathead!"

"Look here, you beast—leggo my ear—wow! I'm coming."

The Famous Five proceeded to their Form master's study. Billy Bunter rolled in reluctantly with them. To his surprise and to his great relief, Mr. Quelch took no particular notice of him. Billy Bunter did not, as he supposed, fill his Form master's thoughts to the exclusion of all other matters. Mr. Quelch gave his attention to Wharton.

"Please tell me exactly what occurred, Wharton," he said.

He listened quietly, while the captain of the Remove told him of the rescue of Bunter and the flight from the yacht's boat. Then he turned to the fat Owl. Bunter quaked. But the Remove master did not refer to his "bolt" from the study. He told Bunter to give him a succinct account of what had happened while he was with the Greek. He made no comment till the fat junior had finished. Then he came to the subject which was uppermost in Bunter's mind, if not in everybody else's.

"You have broken detention this afternoon, Bunter, taking advantage of my absence from the study——"

"I—I didn't——"

"What?"

"I—I mean, I—I wasn't——"

"Be silent, Bunter! I shall not punish you, as it has turned out so very fortunately," said Mr. Quelch. "Your disrespectful, unthinking, foolish and absurd conduct has had the unexpected result of giving us warning that another boy in the Remove is in danger; and that danger can now be guarded against. For this reason, I shall pardon you."

"Oh!" gasped Bunter. "Good! I—I mean——"

"You may leave the study."

Bunter was only too glad to leave the study. He had feared that he would have to remain there to complete that unfinished imposition. He rolled away with fat satisfaction in his face.

"You have acted very well and very sensibly, Wharton," said Mr. Quelch graciously. "But for the warning you gave me by telephone, Kalizelos would certainly have seen Mauleverer, and the boy's safety might have been endangered. The police will now be looking for the rascal. You may go, my boys."

The Famous Five followed Bunter from the study.

"I fancy the bobbies will be looking for that Greek Johnny rather too late," remarked Bob Cherry, as they went down the passage. "He wasn't losing any time getting back to his yacht. He's got the anchor up before this."

"Let's go up and see!" suggested Nugent; and the juniors went up to the Remove dormitory, from which there was a clear view of Pegg Bay, far away across the tree-tops.

There was no longer an anchored yacht to be seen in the bay. But far away seaward a black trail of smoke lay against the sky, and under it a speck on the sea was vanishing into the east. Even as the juniors watched, the speck disappeared from sight; and only a blur of smoke, dispersing in the wind, remained. Konstantinos Kalizelos was gone!

THE FOURTEENTH CHAPTER.

Up to Bunter!

LORD MAULEVERER, of the Remove, the following day, was the cynosure of all eyes at Greyfriars School.

His lordship, earl and millionaire as he was, was so modest a youth by nature, that he seldom filled much space in the public eye. But that was all changed now—rather to his lazy lordship's discomfort. Mauly did not like the limelight.

But there was no help for Mauly! He had the limelight now, whether he liked it or not.

Fellows who hardly knew him stopped him in the quad or the passages to ask him about the mysterious scarab, and the mysterious Greek who had, apparently, come all the way from Egypt after it.

Great men of the Sixth Form, even prefects, were interested in the matter: and Mauly was even asked to tea in a Sixth Form study that day.

In the Remove, of course, there was only one topic—Kalizelos the Greek, and his quest of Mauleverer's mysterious scarab.

Most of the fellows, probably, had never heard of a scarabaeus before; but they all heard about it now.

Billy Bunter had told his tale of adventure fifty times at least; and it grew more and more wonderful every time he told it—Billy Bunter not being trammelled by any special regard for facts.

Second thoughts are said to be best; and on second thoughts, Bunter had hit on a much better version of the story than the one he had related to Mr. Quelch in his study.

It appeared now—since Bunter had had time for second thoughts—that it was not merely to dodge out of detention that he had played his weird pranks the previous day. It was—on second thoughts—with the object of saving old Mauly from danger, that Bunter had, as it were, rushed into the breach. So far from being scared, or frightened, or anything of that sort, Bunter had gone into the thing with cool courage and presence of mind, regardless of peril, and entirely for Mauly's sake. And Bunter seemed quite pained when this version of the story, which really was ever so much better, evoked nothing but laughter in the Remove.

Probably a hundred times, that day, Lord Mauleverer was called upon to tell fellows about that mysterious scarab.

But Mauly had little to tell.

Like many fellows born to great possessions, Mauly was rather indifferent to those possessions. Certainly he had never given much attention, if any, to the collection of Egyptian antiquities which the late earl had brought home to Mauleverer Towers.

"Yaas, there's a scarab," Lord Mauleverer admitted. "In fact, there's a lot of jolly old scarabs. As far as I can make out, Egypt used to be stacked with scarabs, which seems to be some sort of a grasshopper——"

"Beetle, ass!" said Harry Wharton.

"Is it a beetle?" asked Mauly innocently. "Yaas, now I come to think of it, it's a beetle or something of the sort. I don't like beetles myself—loathe 'em, in fact—but the jolly old Gippies seem to have been frightfully gone on beetles."

"They had sacred beetles, fathead—sort of superstitious stuff like mascots," said Bob Cherry. "They wore them as amulets."

"Did they?" yawned Mauly. "Queer taste, what? Well, there's lots of them in the Egyptian Room at Mauleverer Towers—lots and lots."

"But it's one special one that Kalizelos was after," said Nugent. "According to Bunter, he called it the Golden Scarab—the sacred beetle of A-Menah which——"

"Yaas, I believe I sort of remember it," said Mauly. "An ugly little beast of a thing, made of gold, though, with queer marks on it. Worth a few quid, very likely—and that Greek johnny must be off his rocker if he's really willing to give a thousand pounds for it, as he told Bunter."

"It must be worth more than a few quid, fathead," said Bob, "if that sportsman is trying to kidnap you to get hold of it."

"Yaas; but I don't see it! Anyhow, he won't get hold of it now, or of me, either!" chuckled his lordship. "Wasn't it jolly lucky that the Greek sportsman got hold of Bunter yesterday by mistake? Fancy Bunter comin' in useful, you know."

"Is that all you know about your own scarab, Mauly?"

"That's the lot, dear men."

"Then what the thump does Kalizelos want it for?"

"Goodness knows."

Evidently, Lord Mauleverer knew little enough about the mysterious scarab that had brought the lawless Greek from Cairo. But what little he knew he had to repeat over and over again to curious fellows; till he was inexpressibly bored with the subject; and wished from the bottom of his heart that the Scarabaeus of A-Menah had never been in his possession at all.

Of the Greek, nothing more was heard. The yacht Zeus had steamed promptly out of Pegg Bay, and vanished into the North Sea; and it looked as if Kalizelos was gone for good. It was rather doubtful exactly how far he had rendered himself amenable to the law. He could scarcely be charged with kidnapping, as the fatuous Owl of the Remove had gone on board the yacht of his own accord, though there could be no doubt as to his intentions. And though Bunter had been threatened, he had not, after all, been harmed.

But the Greek evidently did not want to put the matter to the test. He had fled in his yacht, and so far as could be learned by the police, the Zeus was no longer in English waters.

He had failed, and his failure had put Mauleverer on his guard! It was certain that, as Mauly remarked, Billy Bunter had come in useful for once.

Mauly's opinion was that the Greek had gone back to his own country—aware that the game was up, and going while the going was good.

That seemed probable to the other fellows, with one exception. The exception was Billy Bunter.

Billy Bunter dropped into Mauleverer's study that evening, with a very serious expression on his fat face, after prep.

Mauly suppressed a groan. Billy Bunter had, howsoever, unintentionally and inadvertently, done his lordship a great service, and Billy Bunter was not the man to let it be forgotten. Mauly felt that it was up to him to give Bunter his head, in the circumstances. So instead of groaning at the sight of the fat Owl, his lordship contrived to smile.

"Take a pew, old bean," he said.

Bunter sat down, blinking at him through his big spectacles with alarming seriousness.

"I've been thinking this over, Mauly," he said.

"Yaas."

HERE'S ANOTHER GREYFRIARS LIMERICK!

Burly Bolsover, with muscles all bursting,
To eclipse every record was thirsting.
With a bar-bell he toyed,
But got very annoyed
When it broke, and he said: "How disgusting!"

A POCKET WALLET has been awarded to Leslie Webb, of "Santoy," Stafford Road, Bloxwich, Staffs, author of the above winning effort.

"I've saved you from fearful danger, old chap——"

"You've mentioned that before!" murmured Lord Mauleverer.

"If you're going to be an ungrateful beast, Mauly——"

"Oh dear!"

"There's not a lot of fellows," said Bunter severely, "who would let themselves be collared by a desperate, ferocious kidnapper, to save another fellow from danger, Mauly. There's precious few."

"Oh, quite," said Mauly, "and you're not one of the few, old bean!"

"Oh, really, Mauly——"

"Is that Toddy calling you in the passage, Bunter?"

"No, it isn't! I've been thinking this over, Mauly! I've saved you from one fearful danger, as you know. But you're still in danger, old chap! You fancy that Greek blighter has gone——"

"Looks like it, old fat man."

"Well, my idea is this," said Bunter. "He's cleared off, to keep away from the peelers, but he's going to hang on somewhere, on the quiet, and have another try at the scarab, see?"

"Shouldn't wonder," yawned Mauly. "He seems a determined sort of bloke. Is that Bob Cherry callin' you?"

"No, it isn't! As you're still in fearful danger, Mauly, and as I've saved you once, I'm going to keep on looking after you."

"Awf'ly good of you, Bunter!" groaned Mauly. "I say, did I hear Wharton shoutin' to you?"

"No, you didn't! Now, while you're here at school, you're fairly safe," pursued Bunter. "I can keep an eye on you, see?"

"Oh! Yaas! Thanks!"

"But we break up for the hols. in a day or two, old chap! Once out of my sight, what will you feel like?"

"No end bucked!" said Mauly.

"What?"

"I—I mean, it's all right," said Mauleverer hastily. "Don't you worry, Bunter!"

"You see, I can't help worrying," said Bunter, shaking his head. "When a pal's in danger, I'm not likely to think of myself—not that I'm one of those fellows who think much about themselves, anyhow. I'm going to see you through, Mauly. I've had a lot of invitations for the holidays, but I'm turning them all down on your account, old chap. I've come here to tell you that you can rely on me!"

"Oh gad!" groaned Lord Mauleverer.

"Rely on me, old fellow," said Bunter. "I'm coming home with you for the holidays, and keeping an eye on you all the time. You'll be in danger—fearful danger—but with me there, you——"

"Oh dear!"

"With me there, you will be all right. It's up to me, and I'm going to do it," said Bunter. "I've already written to a lot of people who are keen to have me for the vac, telling them it can't be done. I'm sticking to you, Mauly."

"Don't!" groaned his lordship.

"Eh?"

"Stick to somebody else, old fellow—there's a good chap."

"Oh, really, Mauly! If that's what you call gratitude——"

"Oh dear!"

"I'm used to ingratitude," said Bunter. "But, really, this is rather thick, Mauly, after I've saved your life and——"

"Groan!"

"If you don't want me to come home with you for the holidays, Mauleverer, after I've saved your life——"

"Groan!"

"I say, Mauly, what's the matter with you?"

"You!"

"Beast!" roared Bunter. "I—I—I mean, you will have your little joke, old chap! It's all right—I'll come! I'm not the man to let a pal down when he's in danger! Is it settled, old fellow?"

"I'm afraid so!" groaned Mauly dismally.

"He, he, he!" Bunter decided to take that answer as a joke. "All right, then—it's a go, Mauly! Rely on me to stick to you at Mauleverer Towers all through the vac. It's up to me." Bunter rose from the chair. "I'll cut along now and tell Smithy, and Temple of the Fourth, and Hilton of the Fifth, and Sykes of the Sixth, that I shan't be able to accept their invitations. We're going to have a jolly time together these hols, Mauly, what?"

Bunter rolled out of the study, leaving Lord Mauleverer blinking after him dismally—not looking like a fellow who was expecting a jolly time at all!

THE FIFTEENTH CHAPTER.

Who's for Egypt?

"EGYPT!"

"Yaas!"

It was the last evening of the term. The Famous Five of the Remove were gathered in Study No. 1. There was no prep that evening, and they were discussing the hols instead of prep, a much more agreeable occupation, till it was time for supper in the Hall. Welcoming glances were turned on Lord Mauleverer when he ambled in; his amiable lordship was a welcome visitor in any study. Wharton pulled out the armchair, and Mauly sank into it, crossed one elegantly-trousered leg over the other, smiled cheerfully at the Five, and propounded the query whether they knew anything about Egypt.

The Famous Five grinned. Mauly in search of knowledge was rather a new Mauly. He had not, perhaps, quite so rooted an objection to acquiring knowledge as Billy Bunter had. But he did not like the process.

"You want to know about Egypt?" asked Harry.

"Yaas."

"Well, we've had some Egypt in geography class. It's a country in Africa, old bean, chiefly composed of the banks of the River Nile."

"I know that much," admitted Lord Mauleverer, "and I know that some jolly old beans named Pharaoh used to reign there, and one of them came a mucker in the Red Sea with all his giddy chariots and horses. It was colonised by—by—was it Christopher Columbus?"

"Ha, ha, ha!" yelled the Famous Five.

"Wrong?" asked Mauly.

"Just a few!" chuckled Nugent. "Egypt was conquered, and partly colonised by Alexander the Great—if that's what you mean—a jolly old Greek."

"Yaas, that's it. I knew it was somebody," assented Mauly. "I'm not bad at history, you know. Not a whale on it—but not bad!"

"Later, it was a Roman province——" declared Bob Cherry.

"And the Arabs mopped it up——" said Johnny Bull.

"And the Turks——" said Wharton. "Lots of people took a turn. And the French, in Napoleon's time. Then there were the Mamelukes, and the giddy Turkish pashas, and after them Tommy Atkins dropped in and set the place to rights."

"Oh! Yaas! Frightfully interestin', isn't it?" said Mauly, yawning. "But what I chiefly want to know is, is it fearfully hot in the summer?"

"Terrifically, my esteemed Mauly!" said Hurree Jamset Ram Singh.

"Like a furnace, what?" asked Mauly.

"More or lessfully."

"Dangerous animals—lions and tigers and things?" asked Mauly. "Poisonous serpents, and ferocious brigands, and things like that?"

"Not exactly," said Wharton, staring. "What the dickens—— Plenty of scorpions, I believe."

"Well, scorpions are dangerous, ain't they?"

"They're not nice! But what——"

"Frightfully hot, and reeking with scorpions!" said Lord Mauleverer thoughtfully. "I think I'll go."

The Famous Five gazed at Lord Mauleverer. That fortunate youth was able to spend his holidays in any country he chose to name, expense being no object. But why he should select a country because it was frightfully hot, and had scorpions in it, was rather a mystery.

"You see, my uncle, old Brooke, is going out to Egypt," explained Lord Mauleverer. "He's got a lot of land in a sort of fruity part of the country, called the What's-its-name——"

"We haven't had that with Quelch," remarked Bob gravely.

"I—I mean the what-do-you-call-it——"

"Ah! That makes it quite clear!"

"Ha, ha, ha!"

"The—the—the——" Mauly made a mental effort. "The—the Fayyum! Goodness knows what the Fayyum is—I don't, and don't want to a lot. But nunky's got a big estate there, and there's some question of cutting a canal, or something, and he's goin' to see about it, and it occurred to him that I might like to go. Far as I know, people go to Egypt for the winter, and it's not what you'd call a summer resort. Still, a lot of people must live there all the year round—so I suppose it will be all right. After all, the hotter it is the better, in a way—if you're sure of the scorpions."

"What the thump——"

"What I mean is, Bunter's comin' home with me for the hols," said Lord Mauleverer. "He says I'm under a fearful obligation to him, an' I suppose he knows. Think Bunter would like a fearfully hot country, stacked with scorpions?"

"Ha, ha, ha!" roared the Famous Five.

"I hardly think he would," said Mauleverer hopefully. "And if he wouldn't care to go, it makes Egypt seem rather attractive, doesn't it?"

"Ha, ha, ha!"

"If Bunter asks you anythin' about Egypt, don't forget to mention the scorpions, will you?" asked Mauly. "You might pile 'em on a bit, perhaps! Think you find scorpions in the beds at the hotels?"

"Hardly!" grinned Bob. "Chiefly in the jolly old tombs, I think."

"Isn't there a desert, or somethin' in Egypt?"

"Bags of it!"

"That's where you perish miserably of thirst, isn't it?" asked Mauly. "Well, if Bunter asks you anythin' about Egypt, put it on a bit about the desert—and fearful sufferings from thirst. Hunger, too—that will make Bunter think!"

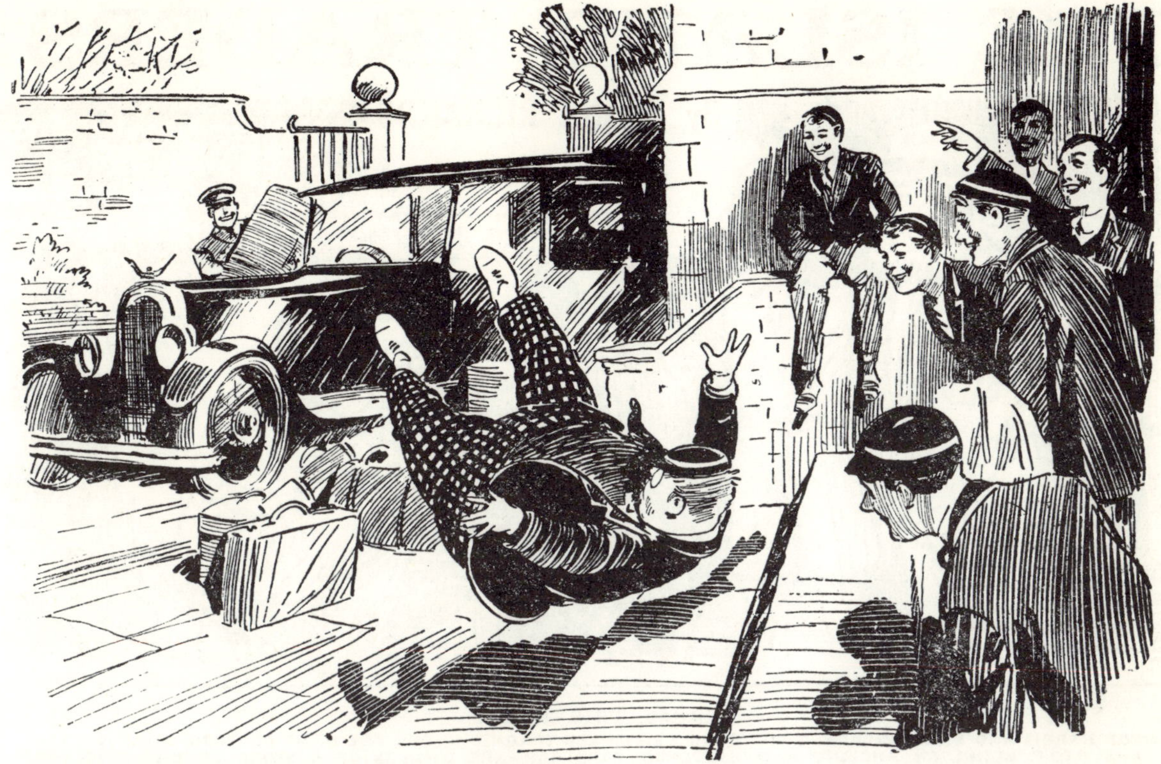

"For goodness' sake, cut off, you fellows!" snapped Bunter. "If you fancy you're sticking on to Mauly and I, all I can say is—yarooooop!" Bunter made that final remark, as Bull gave him a shove that sent him bumping down the steps.

"Ha, ha, ha!"

"And don't forget the fearful heat—like a furnace in summer—and the scorpions—awful scorpions, and—and I think you might put in a lion or a tiger, or so. What?"

"Ha, ha, ha!" yelled the Famous Five.

"And plague," said Mauly. "Bunter's bound to hate plague—plagues are awfully dangerous."

"But there isn't any plague, fathead!"

"Oh, draw it mild!" said Mauly. "I may not be a whale on history, but I've heard about the plagues of Egypt."

"You frabjous ass! The plagues of Egypt were more than six or seven thousand years ago."

"There might be one left over," said Mauly. "You never know—in the East, you know. If you mention them to Bunter you can pass lightly over the date——"

"Ha, ha, ha!"

"But we shan't be seeing Bunter, fathead," said Harry. "We break up to-morrow, and we're all looking forward to not seeing Bunter again till next term."

"But he's coming home with me, so he says, at least," said Mauly, "and I'm afraid he means it. Ain't you fellows coming to Egypt with me?"

The Famous Five stared.

"Are we?" gasped Bob Cherry.

"I hope so! Jolly country, you know," said Mauleverer persuasively. "Lots of tombs—for fellows who like 'em—fellow who pegged out all of a sudden would find one handy——"

"Oh, my hat!"

"And — and sunshine," said Mauleverer. "No end of sunshine. And—and camels! And—and dates—they grow on palms, you know—are you fellows fond of dates? Succulent fruit, I believe. You'd better come."

"But, you ass——"

"Now look here, why can't you fellows come with me for the hols?" demanded Lord Mauleverer.

"You haven't asked us yet, fathead!" roared Bob Cherry.

Lord Mauleverer started.

"Haven't I really?" he ejaculated.

"Ha, ha, ha!"

"I knew there was somethin' I was goin' to say to you fellows the other day, only I forgot——"

"Ha, ha, ha!"

"Sure I didn't ask you?" inquired Mauly. "Well, I'm askin' you now. We'll put in a week at Mauleverer Towers, if you'll come; and I'll show you that jolly old scarab that the Greek sportsman was after, what? If there's some jolly old secret about it, you may be able to spot it. Then we'll fix it up for Egypt. Nunky rather wants me to go, and he says I can bring any friends I like. You fellows are friends of mine, aren't you?"

"Bosom pals, if you're standing a holiday in Egypt, old bean."

"Ha, ha, ha!"

"The only drawback is that Bunter's comin'—but you men can stand him for a week, can't you? And he will want to give Egypt a miss, if you pile it on about the fearful heat, and the awful scorpions——"

"The pilefulness will be terrific."

"Is it a go, then?" asked Mauly, detaching himself from the armchair.

"We shall have to ask our people first—but I think you can call it a go, old bean," said Harry Wharton smiling.

"Good egg! Jolly glad you're comin', old things—if we don't drop Bunter, you can help me stand him. But if you tell him a lot about the plagues and things——"

"Ha, ha, ha!"

Lord Mauleverer nodded amiably, and ambled out of the study. A moment later he put his head back into the doorway.

"Wasn't there a famine in Egypt once?" he asked. "I seem to have heard somethin' of the sort."

"Ha, ha! Yes!"

"Well, look here, if you could give Bunter a sort of idea that it was still on, you know——"

"Ha, ha, ha!"

"And don't forget the scorpions!"

And Lord Mauleverer ambled away, leaving the Famous Five chortling.

THE SIXTEENTH CHAPTER.
Off for the Holidays!

"I SAY, you fellows——"

"Hallo, hallo, hallo, old fat frump!"

"You're not gone yet?" said Billy Bunter, blinking at the chums of the Remove.

"Do we look as if we're gone?" asked Bob.

"The gonefulness is not terrific, my esteemed fat Bunter," smiled the Nabob of Bhanipur.

"Well, most of the fellows are gone," said Bunter. "Time you started. You'll lose your train."

The Famous Five chuckled. Greyfriars School was breaking up for the summer holidays, and, as Bunter said, a lot of the fellows were gone already. Billy Bunter was not gone—he was not going till Lord Mauleverer went, and Lord Mauleverer was not going till the big car arrived to take him away. That tremendous car was even now turning in at the gates of Greyfriars, and gliding up to the House, and the Famous Five, standing on the steps, watched it coming.

Billy Bunter was not yet aware that

(*Continued on page 28.*)

OUR THRILL-PACKED STORY OF SOUTHERN SEAS ADVENTURE!

THE ISLAND TRADERS!

By FRANK RICHARDS

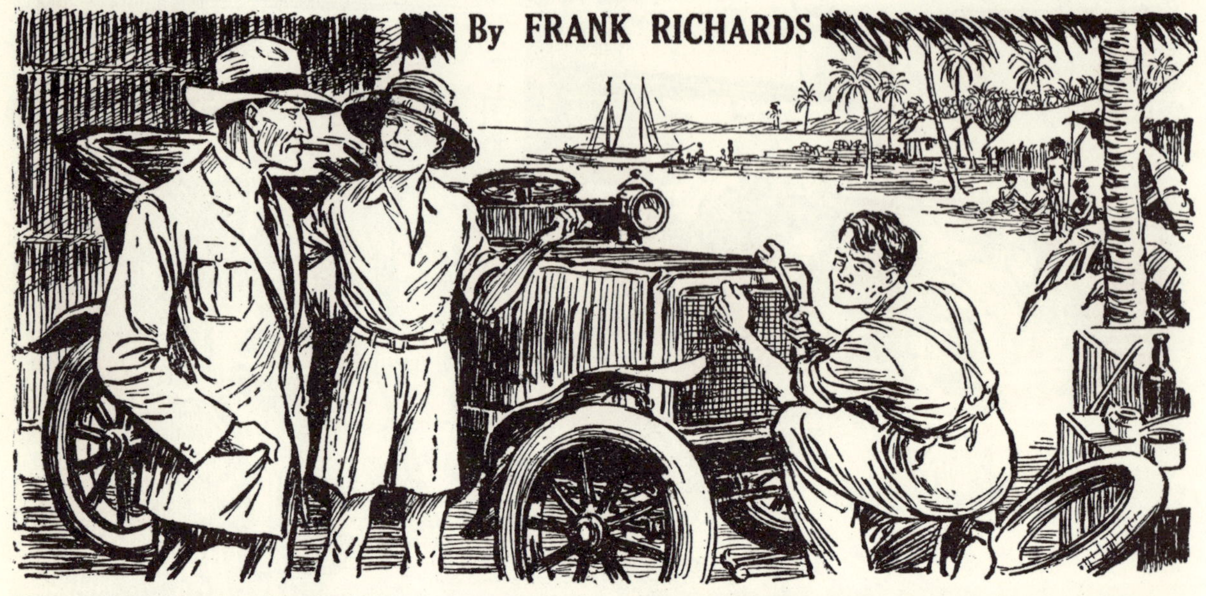

READ THIS FIRST.

BOB HARRIS AND BILLY McCANN, TWO YOUNG BRITISHERS TRADING UNDER THE NAME OF "BOB, BILLY & CO."—THE "CO." BEING AN ANCIENT AND BATTERED FORD CAR—ARE OWNERS OF A STORE ON KALUA ISLAND. KNOWING THAT A VAST TREASURE LIES HIDDEN ON THE SITE, DAVID BONE, A RASCALLY AMERICAN TRADER, OFFERS TO BUY THE STORE, BUT THE ISLAND TRADERS REFUSE TO SELL. AFTER SEVERAL FRUITLESS ATTEMPTS TO DRIVE THE PARTNERS OFF THE ISLAND, BONE BRIBES PURKISS, A BEACH-COMBER, TO FIRE THE STORE. BOB AND BILLY ARE SETTING OUT IN SEARCH OF PURKISS, WHEN BOB'S SUSPICIONS ARE AROUSED BY THE ARRIVAL OF JACKY, THE HOUSE-BOY, HOLDING SOMETHING TIGHTLY CLENCHED IN HIS HAND. "DON'T WORRY ABOUT HIM," SAYS BILLY, "IT'S PURKISS WE WANT!"

The Two Crimson Specks!

"HOLD on a minute I tell you!" cried Bob. Then, turning to the house-boy, he asked:

"What feller thing you keep along hand belong you?"

"Feller pill, sar, plenty magic pill, makee along Soo-oo, sar," said Jacky. He opened his hand, with visible reluctance, and showed a small pill-box, such as were used for the quinine pills often taken by all the white inhabitants of Kalua. "Big witch-doctor Soo'oo makee pill, sar, makee this feller Jacky plenty strong."

Bob burst into a laugh. Soo'oo, the cunning old devil-doctor, did a great business among the natives with magic pills. It came into Bob's mind that that was why Kolulo-ululo had been at the hut that morning. No doubt he had fetched the magic pill from the devil-doctor for Jacky.

"Are you coming?" snapped Billy.

"Right-ho!"

Bob followed his chum towards the coral rock on the beach.

Jacky, breathing hard, hurried on towards the hut. He carried the pill-box with great care, and once, when he stumbled on a point of rock cropping up in the sand, and almost dropped the box, he gave a cry, and his brown face blanched with terror.

He reached the hut and passed into its dusky interior. There was a scratch, a flicker of light, and a candle glimmered. Jacky stared from door and window, a shiver running through his brown limbs. Then, taking a knife, he pricked off the lid of the pill-box, first laying it carefully on the table.

The glimmer of the candle showed his brown face wet with perspiration. It shone on the contents of the box—something that stirred, something that glowed a bright crimson in the candle-glimmer. There were two crimson specks in the pill-box.

Jacky, with a careful hand, inserted the tip of a palm-leaf into the box. A red speck was lifted out, and Jacky bent for a moment over Bob Harris' bunk. The red speck disappeared in the blankets. Then the second crimson speck was lifted out with equal care, on the tip of the palm-leaf, and dropped into Billy McCann's bunk.

Jacky blew out the candle, and then stepped out of the hut. The starlight, shining on his face, showed it almost grey and streaming with sweat.

. . . . .

Billy McCann gave a snort of anger and dropped the lawyer cane.

"Suffering cats!" he growled.

Pete Purkiss, the beach-comber, lay at his feet. The starlight glimmered on a pallid, sick face.

Bob Harris whistled softly. They had found the beach-comber, the wretched degenerate who had burned down the store for a bribe from David Bone. But even the incensed Billy, as he looked at him, did not feel disposed to handle the lawyer-cane.

The man, stretched in the sand, was half-conscious. He was muttering to himself indistinctly. He was clad only in thin cotton shirt and shorts, ample for the hot day on Kalua, but little protection against the cold of night. And night on Kalua was sometimes very cold. It was cold now, after the sun had gone, and the barely clad wretch was shivering.

His eyes, burning with a strange light, looked up at the partners. But he did not seem to recognise them.

"Poor wretch!" muttered Bob.

Billy snorted.

"He's got out of the thrashing! I can't lay a hand on him now."

"You can't!" agreed Bob.

A mumble came from the wretch at their feet. Evidently Purkiss had spent David Bone's bribe in Tu'uka's village, not wisely but too well. Native "kava" and unlimited square-face had done their work. The strength of the miserable beach-comber, sapped by long years of intoxication, had given out entirely after that last prolonged "drunk." It was a man deadly sick who lay sprawling in the starlit sand; a man who would be dead in the morning if he was left there for the night. And there were few on Kalua who were likely to give a thought to a white man who had "gone native" and fallen so low that even the natives abandoned him.

"Let him lie!" growled Billy, and he turned away.

Bob hesitated.

The man was a rascal; a disgrace to his race, a shame to his colour. He had ruined the island traders at the order of David Bone. But there was pity in Bob's face; he could not leave the wretch to die.

"Billy, old bean——" Bob hesitated.

Billy McCann uttered a sound like a snarl.

"You soft ass! Don't I know what's in your silly head?" he growled. "That brute's ruined us for a handful of dollars from David Bone. And now you want to play the Good Samaritan and look after him."

"So do you, Billy," said Bob, with a smile.

Billy was scowling blackly. But his black scowl melted into a grin. He was no more impervious to compassion than his partner.

"I suppose we can't leave him here," he grunted. "You're a fool, Bob, and I'm another! The biggest pair of silly idiots on Kalua! Take one end of the brute. This means having him in the hut to-night; nobody else on Kalua is fool enough to take him in. Is he going to have your bunk or mine?"

"Mine!" said Bob.

"Rats! He can have mine!" snorted Billy. "I can take a blanket on the floor."

"Rot!" said Bob. "We'll shove the poor wretch in my bunk, and I'll take a blanket on the floor. It's my idea to stand by him."

"It's my idea as much as yours, Mr. Harris. I'm as big a fool as you, if you come to that!" snapped Billy.

They lifted the shivering, mumbling wretch from the sand. His staring eyes were on them unseeingly.

"This way, Purkiss," said Bob. "Pull yourself together a bit."

His voice seemed to strike some chord of memory in the wretched man, for Purkiss eyed him, snarling.

"Let a man alone!" came in a thick mutter from his lips. "Who says I fired the store?"

"Never mind that now. Come on!"

Purkiss resisted feebly. Some dim realisation seemed to be working through the fog of his brain.

"I know you!" he muttered. "Let me be—let me be! Look for David Bone; it was his doing! Look for that nigger Loo. Let me be!"

"We're helping you, you fool!" growled Billy. "We're taking you to a shelter for the night. Shut up!"

Purkiss stared at him with bleared, uncomprehending eyes. But he made no further resistance, and the partners half-led, half-carried him up the beach.

"Here, you Jacky!" called out Bob.

The house-boy was leaning on the palm outside the hut. He started forward, a shadow in the gloom.

"Yes, sar."

"You light feller candle along hut."

Jacky stared curiously at the sagging figure between the two partners. He went into the hut and lighted a candle. Purkiss was helped into the little building.

"My bunk, Billy," said Bob.

"Mine!" growled Billy.

"Look here——"

"Rats! This way!" Billy McCann heaved the sagging form towards his own bunk, and Bob gave in.

"You feller boy, turn back the blankets," said Bob.

Jacky did not stir, his dilated eyes staring at the partners of Kalua.

"Do you hear?" snapped Billy.

"Yes, sar!" gasped Jacky. "You no go put that feller Purkiss along bed belong you, sar?"

"Turn back the blankets, you fool!" roared Billy.

Jacky approached the bunk, but in a very gingerly way. There was terror in his face, terror and consternation.

"Oh, sar!" he gasped. "You no put that feller along bunk belong you, sar! Where you sleep, sar?"

"Mind your own business and do as you're told. Plenty quick!"

"Jacky's never heard of the Good Samaritan, Billy!" chuckled Bob.

"Turn those blankets back, you swab!" roared Billy. "You want me knock seven bells out of you?"

Jacky, with trembling hands and watchful eyes, turned back the blankets in Billy's bunk at last. It was as if he feared to touch the bunk or anything that lay on it.

"What's the matter with the nigger?" growled Billy.

"Blessed if I know," said Bob, staring at the house-boy. "Shove him in!"

Purkiss was laid in the bunk and the blankets drawn over him. Jacky backed across the room, staring with dilated eyes. Then he made a sidling movement towards the door. Billy stared round at him.

"Where you go?" he snapped. "You stop along this place. Get a blanket off the other bunk and hand it here."

Jacky moved towards Bob's bunk. He stretched out a hand to take a blanket from it, and then drew it back suddenly. Bob and Billy stared at him in amazement. What was the matter with the house-boy was a mystery to them.

"Plenty quick, you swab!" snapped Billy.

Jacky stretched his dusky hand to the bunk again. Then, suddenly turning, he made a spring towards the open doorway.

Billy stared at him in stupefaction. But Bob Harris acted promptly. His grasp fell on the house-boy as he leaped, and Jacky was dragged back and jammed against the wall of the hut. Suspicion—a fearful suspicion—was in Bob's mind now, and the look in his eyes made Jacky cringe with terror.

"Now, what's this game?" said Bob, between his set teeth.

"You let this Kanaka go, sar!" panted Jacky. "Me no stop along this place. Me no stop along you, sar."

"Won't you!" said Bob grimly. His grasp tightened on the wriggling house-boy. "What name you 'fraid touch feller bunk?"

Jacky, instead of answering, struggled to free himself. Bob knocked his head on the wall with a resounding crack, and there was a dismal howl from the house-boy.

"You speak, mouth belong you!" hissed Bob. "What name you too much plenty fright touch feller bunk?"

"What the suffering cats——" began Billy.

"Get Purkiss out of that bunk!" gasped Bob.

"What the——"

"Get him out!" roared Bob. "Do you want to murder him?"

"In Heaven's name——"

"Get him out!" shrieked Bob. "No—hold this nigger while I get him out!"

He flung the house-boy at the amazed Billy and leaped to the bunk where Purkiss lay.

Back into Bob's mind had come the memory of the pill-box Jacky had held hidden in his hand. Back into his mind came the picture of Kolulo-ululo, searching the distant beach with a palm-leaf in his hand for something that he dared not let his fingers touch.

He knew now why David Bone had let Soo-oo lift the taboo so that the house-boy might come back. In a flash of hideous revelation he knew.

"Keep that nigger safe!" he panted. "Don't touch the bunk! On your life don't touch the bunk!"

Jacky struggled wildly. But he crumpled up in Billy's sinewy grip.

Billy watched his partner, open-eyed. Bob had warned him not to touch the other bunk. But he had himself to touch the one where Purkiss lay to save the beach-comber's life, if his hideous suspicion was true. With careful hands that trembled a little in spite of himself he turned back the blankets and lifted the beach-comber out on to the floor. There he laid him down and bent over him, searching him with straining eyes.

"Thank Heaven!" he breathed.

"What——" gasped Billy.

"Can't you see?" hissed Bob. "There's death in the bunks, and that infernal nigger—— Hold him!"

The house-boy made a desperate effort to tear away, but Billy McCann's grasp on him was like iron.

"Bring him here!" said Bob. "Pitch him into the bunk!"

A scream of terror came from the house-boy.

"No, sar! No touch feller bunk!" he screamed. "You no put this feller along bunk, sar!"

He shrieked and writhed in Billy's grasp.

"Pitch him in!" said Bob grimly.

"What's in the bunk, Bob?" asked Billy McCann very quietly.

"Something that that nigger's put ready for us, I fancy! Something that the pig-hunter dug out of the beach, and that Jacky brought back in a pill-box. Something that would clear us off Kalua for ever if it touched us!" hissed Bob. "Something that would leave the ground clear for David Bone! Pitch him in and let him have it!"

Jacky shrieked.

"This feller die along bunk, sar! This feller no stop any more altogether, s'pose go along bunk, sar!" He struggled frantically. "Little red one stop along bunk, sar!"

"I thought so!" said Bob grimly.

Billy McCann's ruddy face became as pale as death.

"The little red one!" he breathed.

Well he knew the "little red one" of the Kanakas; the tiny crimson spider whose sting was sudden death. The sweat ran down Billy's face. Death he knew how to face, and had faced many times. But a shudder of horror ran through him as he thought of the sting of the death-spider.

His grasp closed on the house-boy till the native's bones seemed almost to crack under it.

"So that's it?" breathed Billy.

"That's it!"

"Me plenty solly, sar!" moaned Jacky. "Old big devil-doctor Soo-oo he tellee this Kanaka, sar, put little red one along bunk, sar; me plenty 'fraid along Soo-oo, sar! He terrible big devil-doctor, sar!"

Bob looked at him. He was almost tempted to throw the Kanaka into the bunk to meet the fate he had planned for his masters.

"Suffering cats!" muttered Billy McCann.

Bob picked up a pair of pliers and searched the bunk. Deep in the blankets a tiny crimson speck glowed in the candle-light. A grip of the pliers put an end to it. He crossed to the other bunk and searched again. The search was long, but the crimson speck came to light at last and again the pliers gripped, and the death-spider ceased to be.

"Is that all?" he asked, his eyes on the house-boy.

"Yes, sar! Two little red ones, sar!"

"You shall sleep in a bunk to-night."

"Yes, sar!" mumbled Jacky.

Obviously there had been only two of the death-spiders. The house-boy's terror was gone now. His terror of the little red ones.

"All clear now, Billy," said Bob. "Take him away!"

Billy McCann picked up a thick stick and led the house-boy out of the hut. For the next five minutes there was wild howling and yelling to the sound of heavy lashes. When Billy came back into the hut the house-boy crawled away into the bush, with an ache in every bone in his brown-skinned body.

In the candle-light the partners of Kalua looked at one another across the unconscious beach-comber on the floor.

Bob wiped his forehead.

"If we hadn't taken Purkiss in, Billy——"

Billy McCann grinned faintly.

"Good Samaritans, and their jolly old reward!" he said. "We've saved Purkiss' life, and he's saved ours. Suffering cats! When I get a chance at David Bone——"

"We've got to get at him—after this!" said Bob grimly. "We've got to find a chance."

And that chance was coming!

What the Beach-comber Knew!

"THE Osprey!"

"David Bone's cutter."

Bob and Billy spoke simultaneously.

Bob Harris had come out of the hut, where he had been giving a drink to Purkiss, the beach-comber, lying in one of the bunks, a wreck of a man. Billy McCann had come out of the lean-to where the old Ford was garaged. And their eyes fell at the same moment on the graceful cutter that was threading its way through the reef passage into the lagoon.

Bob's eyes flashed. Billy McCann took a harder grip on the spanner in his oily hand.

"That rotter's come back!" said Bob.

"That swab!" muttered Billy. "The hound! To dare to come back to Kalua after——"

"It's because he thinks his rotten work is done that he's come back," said Bob quietly. "He doesn't expect to see us alive, Billy."

"He will find out that we're alive," said Billy McCann grimly.

The partners of Kalua watched the cutter glide into the lagoon. Among the native crew that moved on the deck they made out the figure of David Bone, the 'Frisco trader, in white ducks and panama hat. Bone, with a black Borneo cheroot between his yellow teeth, was staring at the beach as the Osprey glided on to her anchorage.

He did not see the two island traders standing in the shadow of the palm before the hut. But his sharp eyes, under his leathery, puckered brows, were turned in that direction. It seemed to the partners that they could discern a sardonic grin on the leathery face of the American trader. He was staring at the black mass which marked where the store had stood—the ruins of the island traders' property, burned out by an incendiary. No doubt that sight of the blackened ruin was a welcome one to the eyes of David Bone.

"If we had proof," muttered Bob, "every white man on Kalua would lend a hand to string him up, if we could prove——"

"Isn't his coming back here proof enough?" growled Billy McCann. "We know he set the nigger to put the death-spiders in our bunks through that Santa Cruz boy, Loo. He's come back because he thinks it's done. That's proof enough for me."

"And for me," said Bob. "But——"

Billy gave a snort.

"I know it's not enough for the High Commissioner of Fiji, but it's enough for me to crack his rascally head!"

Bob Harris smiled.

"He's come back," repeated Billy, glaring at the cutter. "He tried to buy the store under threats. He put up the devil-doctor to lay a taboo on us to ruin our trade. It didn't work. And he set Purkiss to fire the store. That didn't beat us. And he fixed it up for us to be stung by death-spiders. Now he's come to bag the prize."

"It's no good telling Kalua that, Billy. Nobody would believe that David Bone was so set on getting hold of the site of our store. We can't even guess ourselves why he wants it."

"We know he wants it bad, from what he's done."

"I know. But I can't imagine why, and you can't. And I fancy we shall never find out."

"He may tell us himself, if I get a grip on the back of his skinny neck," said Billy.

A faint voice called from the interior of the hut, and Billy snorted.

The partners of Kalua had taken in Purkiss, the beach-comber, returning good for evil, and saved the wretched man's life. For three days now he had lain a sick man in the hut, tended by the partners in turn. But Billy, at least, was more than fed-up with him.

But they looked into the hut. Purkiss was sitting up in his bunk, a startled expression on his bearded face. He had heard the talk of the young traders outside, and it had evidently disturbed him. The beach-comber was looking better; he was on the mend, but he was still a sick man.

"What do you want, Purkiss?" asked Bob, kindly enough.

Bitterly as the man had injured him and his partner, he could not feel anything but pity for the human wreck that lay before him.

"I heard what you said. Is that David Bone's cutter?"

"Yes; the Osprey."

"Then he's coming back to Kalua?"

"Looks like it."

"Look here, Purkiss," said Billy McCann gruffly. "We know you fired our store, and that Mr. Bone put you up to it. You know we know it. Tell the truth to all the island, and we may be able to get at that swab with the law."

"The law will never touch David Bone," said the beach-comber. "S'pose I owned up—what then? I never saw Bone. His nigger, Loo, gave me the order, and the dollars for doing it. Who's to prove that Bone knew anything about it? That Santa Cruz nigger will deny the whole thing. If I talk myself black in the face, it leaves you where you were."

"That's so," said Bob, with a sigh. "Bone covers up his tracks too jolly well, Billy. He's too deep for us."

Purkiss eyed them curiously.

"You boys have been decent to me," he said. "You picked me up, as good as dying on the beach, and brought me here. After what I'd done"—the wretched man's face worked for a moment—"I ain't going to thank you. Talk won't do you any good. But after the way you've helped me, I'm going to help you."

Bob smiled faintly.

"How can you help us?" he asked.

"More than you think," grunted Purkiss. "I've been weeks in Tu'uka's village, before I came back to the beach. You know I've lived among the natives, and know their lingo. I've heard a lot of talk. That Santa Cruz nigger, Loo. I—I dare say you reckoned it was his first sight of Kalua when David Bone brought him here."

"Hadn't thought about it," said Bob. "But I suppose so. Kalua is a long step from Santa Cruz."

"Well, he's been here before, and knows the island like a book," said Purkiss. "He was a prisoner here in the old days—before white men came to Kalua, when old Mokatoo was king of the island. He made himself useful to the old chief, and they didn't eat him, as they did most of their prisoners. He was a slave in Mokatoo's grass palace for years. Plenty of niggers in Tu'uka's village knew him. Tu'uka himself remembered him. He escaped from Kalua in a canoe in those old days. I reckon he wouldn't have gone among them, even now, only he's got David Bone behind him, and that sees him safe."

He panted for breath.

"He's been the go-between between Bone and the niggers here, fixing things up for you. He fixed it with me to burn down the store. He fixed it with your house-boy to put the death-spiders in your bunks. He's got a reason, and David Bone's got a reason. And when I learned, from the talk of the niggers, that Loo had been on Kalua for years in old Mokatoo's time, and had been kept in Mokatoo's house, I knew the reason."

Bob and Billy exchanged a quick glance.

The deadly enmity of David Bone had been plain enough, but the cause of it had utterly baffled them. They wondered now whether the beach-comber could let in light on that strange mystery.

"And the reason?" asked Bob.

"Old Mokatoo's treasure."

"Wha-a-t?"

Bob almost laughed. Ever since they had been on Kalua the partners had heard, again and again, the talk of the treasure of the old King of Kalua, but they had never believed the story.

"You know the yarn," said Purkiss. "Before white men settled here old Mokatoo traded with the schooners that called at Kalua for years—forty years and more. He sold them copra, pearl-shell, pearls, slaves, too, in the old days. Like all the island chiefs he would never touch paper money—never trusted it. Traders had to pay him in golden Australian sovereigns, as they do all through the Pacific. Old Mokatoo hoarded his treasure. He may have had ten thousand—twenty thousand sovereigns—by the time Tu'uka's spear made an end of him. It's no secret that Tu'uka killed him for his treasure, though he never found it afterwards. The old villain had hidden it somewhere safe out of sight."

"But—what——"

"The village was burned down in the fighting, and when white men came here, Tu'uka and his crew went back of the bush. Your store was built on the spot where old Mokatoo's palace once stood, as you know. White men have

Printed and published every Saturday by the Proprietors, The Amalgamated Press, Ltd., The Fleetway House, Farringdon Street, London, E.C.4. Advertisement offices: The Fleetway House, Farringdon Street, London, E.C.4. Registered for transmission by Canadian Magazine Post. Subscription rates: Inland and Abroad, 11s. per annum; 5s. 6d. for six months. Sole Agents for Australia and New Zealand: Messrs. Gordon & Gotch, Ltd., and for South Africa: Central News Agency, Ltd.—Saturday, August 6th, 1932.

hunted for the treasure. I hunted for it for years while I was combing the beach here. The niggers hunt for it in the bush to this day. It's never been found."

"But what's this got to do with Loo, or David Bone, or us?" grunted Billy McCann.

"This much — that they're after Mokatoo's treasure."

"Suffering cats!" said Billy McCann, staring blankly at the man in the bunk.

"You don't believe me?" grunted Purkiss. "Well, that's that! Loo hasn't let on a word to the niggers. It's as much as his life's worth, I reckon. They'd cut him to pieces for the secret. But as soon as I knew he'd been years in old Mokatoo's palace I knew what he was after. Old Mokatoo had help in hiding the treasure, I reckon. Not a Kalua boy; no native here knows anything about it. He trusted his slave, because only he stood between Loo and the cooking-pots. When Loo escaped from Kalua he knew where the treasure was hidden."

"My hat!" repeated Bob.

"Loo's kept his secret for years, hoping to get a chance. He's let David Bone into it. He could do nothing alone; with the American at the back of him he had the power in his hands. He's sharing the secret with Bone to get hold of the treasure. That's what he's on Kalua for; that's what David Bone is after. Take it from me."

The beach-comber sank back in the bunk.

"But—but," Bob almost stuttered, "if there's anything in that—I own up it looks like it—what's that got to do with us? David Bone could come here and hunt for the treasure if he liked. We couldn't stop him if we wanted to."

"Suffering cats!" yelled Billy McCann.

Purkiss grinned sourly.

"Your partner's tumbled, Mr. Harris," he said.

Bob stared at his partner.

"Billy! What the thump——"

"Got any eyes?" yelled Billy in great excitement. "The store stood on the site of old Mokatoo's palace. Got any optics? Can't you see, feller eye belong you?"

"Blessed if I can!" said Bob, bewildered. "What——"

"Where would Mokatoo be likely to bury his stack of quids?"

"In the bush——"

"Bush be blowed! What about the floor of his jolly old palace?" yelled Billy.

Bob Harris jumped.

"His sleeping-room most likely, where he could sleep over it," chuckled Billy. "Right on the spot, Bob! What?"

Billy McCann rubbed his plump hands.

"That's why David Bone wanted to buy the store! That's why he wanted to buy the site! That's why—everything! Can't you see, you old codger, now it's as plain as daylight?"

"My only hat!" said Bob, realising the truth at last.

A Shock for David Bone!

DAVID BONE stepped ashore from the cutter's whaleboat. The boat pulled back to the Osprey, and the American trader walked up the beach.

Many eyes were turned curiously upon him.

Bob and Billy had made no secret of their belief that the trader from 'Frisco had been at the bottom of all their long series of disasters, which had brought them to the verge of ruin—if not over the verge. All Kalua wondered whether there was anything in it—doubting; for so far as all Kalua could see, the 'Frisco trader had no motive for that deadly and implacable vendetta.

If he had a motive it was in accordance with his known character, that was certain. So the traders and planters wondered. But they did not think of telling David Bone what they wondered or surmised. Mr. Bone was too powerful a man in the islands for any planter on Kalua to offend him if he could help it. Even old Mackay, a good friend to the island firm, was careful to keep out of any personal trouble with David Bone.

Mr. Bone walked up the beach as if it belonged to him. So it might have if he had liked, for he was rich enough to ever, and clicked his yellow teeth hard together, biting clean through his cheroot, as two boyish figures emerged from the shadow of a bungalow.

David Bone stopped dead.

The American trader had plenty of nerve. He needed it for his methods of business. But for once his nerve was shaken.

What colour there was in his leathery face faded out of it, and his flinty eyes dilated under his puckered brows as he stared at Bob Harris and Billy McCann.

For a long moment he stared at the two young traders whom he had believed dead, his eyes almost starting from their sockets. Then his hand flew to his hip.

But he realised more than ever, to his amazement, that he did not need to draw a weapon. There was no hostility in the looks of the island traders.

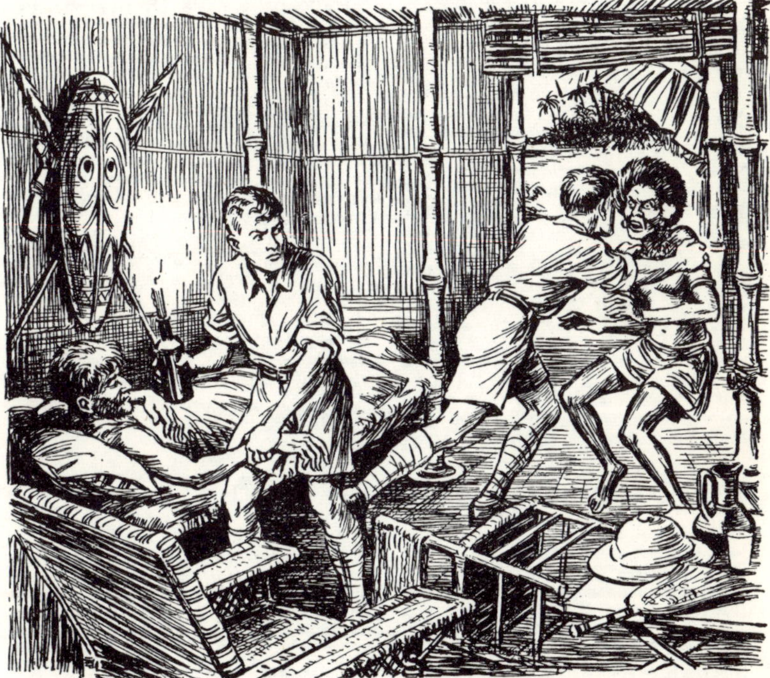

Bob Harris grasped the house-boy and jammed him against the wall of the hut. "What name you 'fraid touch fellow bunk?" "This feller die!" shrieked Jacky. "Little red one stop along bunk, sar!"

buy Kalua—all except the island store. All the money in the Pacific would not have bought out Bob, Billy & Co. at the behest of the American trader.

But Mr. Bone was under the impression now that the island traders had paid dear for their obstinacy. He had offered to buy them out, and they had refused. David Bone was not the man to take a refusal. The Santa Cruz boy had been left on the island with ample funds and a free hand. David Bone had no doubt that the partners of Kalua had ceased from troubling.

There was a sour smile on his leathery face as he walked up the beach, nodding here and there to an acquaintance.

Mr. Bone, as a business man, preferred peaceful methods. The island traders had refused to sell, and had refused to clear off Kalua. But they had had to take what was coming to them. Mr. Bone was going to cast a regretful glance at their graves before he took possession of the abandoned site of the burned-out store.

With that pleasant impression in his mind Mr. Bone walked up the sunny beach. He gave a violent start, how-

Bob Harris raised his grass hat politely to Mr. Bone. Billy McCann, who had once broken a stout lawyer-cane on Mr. Bone's lean back, grinned at him cheerily and followed Bob's example.

"On Kalua again, Mr. Bone?" said Bob.

"Eh! I—I guess so!" stammered David Bone. He was utterly taken aback, and out of his depth.

"This island is looking up when a man of your size makes special trips to it," said Billy McCann gravely. "This is your second visit, sir! Not buying a store this time?"

Mr. Bone recovered himself. He registered a mental vow to make Loo pay for his failure when he had counted on the Santa Cruz boy's success as a certainty.

"Why, yep!" he answered easily. "I've heard your store was burned down. But I guess the site will suit me for building a new store on, and I'm open to make a fair offer."

(Don't fail to read the concluding chapters of this adventure story in next week's MAGNET.)

BILLY BUNTER'S BAD LUCK!

(*Continued from page 23.*)

the Famous Five were booked for Mauleverer Towers. The holiday in Egypt could not be definitely settled till they had communicated with home—though the chums of the Remove had no doubt about it—but, anyhow, they were going home with Mauly for a week at the Towers. Nobody, however, had taken the trouble to mention that circumstance to the fat Owl.

"Here comes Mauly's car," said Bunter. "Well, I shall have to say good-bye to you fellows. Sorry I can't take you with me."

"Eh?"

"But it would hardly do," explained Bunter. "A fellow can be pally with all sorts of fellows at school, but when he s staying with a titled friend, he has to be a bit particular, you know."

"Oh!"

"I hope you'll have a good time in your humble homes, old chaps," said Bunter generously.

"Thanks awfully!" said Harry Wharton gravely.

"The thankfulness is terrific, my esteemed and idiotic Bunter."

"Well, you'd better be off," said Bunter. "Where's that ass Mauly—slacking about somewhere I suppose? Topping car, isn't it—not like my pater's Rolls, of course—still, a good car. Look here, you fellows if you're hanging about to see Mauly——"

"Just that!" said Bob cheerily.

"Oh, you own up, do you?" sneered Bunter. "Well, I can tell you there's nothing doing. If you'd treated me a bit more decently this term, I'd have put in a word for you—in fact, asked Mauly to ask you. But have you treated me decently? Only yesterday you refused to cash a postal order for me, Wharton——"

"I'll refuse again to-day, if you like, fatty."

"You kicked me the day before yesterday, Bull——"

"Like another?" asked Johnny Bull.

"Taking you all round, you're an ungrateful lot," said Bunter. "Now, look here, cut off! Fishing for invitations for the holidays is rather rotten, you know."

"You ought to know!" agreed Nugent.

"Ha, ha, ha!"

"It's rather thick, hanging on to see Mauly, like this," said Bunter scornfully. "I must say I despise fellows who grease up to a wealthy chap, and fish for invitations, and all that. Not the sort of thing that I could do myself."

"Ha, ha, ha!"

"Blessed if I see anything to cackle at. Look here, here comes Mauly—now, the sooner you fellows clear off the better. If you fancy you're going to stick on to Mauly, you can wash it right out. I'm looking after my pal Mauly, and I can jolly well tell you that I'm not going to let a blessed Bank Holiday crowd glue on to him——"

"Hallo, hallo, hallo! Here's the jolly old car, Mauly!" roared Bob Cherry.

"Yaas, old bean!"

Lord Mauleverer came out of the House.

"For goodness' sake, cut off, you fellows!" snapped Bunter. "Go and catch your train—and take your third-class tickets—he, he, he! Leave old Mauly alone. If you fancy you're sticking on to us, I can only say——Yarooooooooooop!"

Billy Bunter made that final remark unintentionally, as Johnny Bull gave gave him a gentle push, which tipped him off the steps.

Bump, bump, bump, bump!

Billy Bunter negotiated the House steps rather like a barrel, roaring as he rolled, and he landed in the quad spluttering.

"Ha, ha, ha!"

"Yoooop!"

Billy Bunter sat up.

"Ready, you men?" asked Lord Mauleverer cheerfully. "Baggage on, what? Get the baggage on, Watson!"

Bunter scrambled to his feet. He set his spectacles straight on his fat little nose, and gave the Famous Five a devastating blink, as they came down to the big car.

"I say, Mauly——" howled Bunter.

"Yaas, old fat bean."

"If you've asked these fellows——"

"Yaas."

"Well, look here, I see enough of them in the term—too much, in fact, and I don't want to see anything of them in the hols, see?" hooted Bunter.

"Yaas."

"And if they're coming I'm jolly well not!"

"You don't mean that, old chap?" asked Mauly.

"I do!" said Bunter firmly. "Leave them out, or leave me out. I mean it, Mauly!"

"Good! You fellows can't possibly desert me now," said Mauleverer. "Tumble in! Good-bye, Bunter!"

"Wha-a-t?"

"Good-bye! Pleasant hols, old man! See you next term."

"Ha, ha, ha!"

Lord Mauleverer and the Famous Five packed themselves into the car. Billy Bunter glared at them, with a glare that almost cracked his spectacles.

"Why, you—you beast!" he gasped. "I—I—I mean, my dear old chap, I wouldn't let you down for worlds! I say, you fellows, make room for a chap!"

"Ha, ha, ha!"

"Comin' after all?" asked Mauly.

"Yes, old fellow, I'm not the man to let you down," said Billy Bunter affectionately. "Is it likely?"

"'Fraid not," agreed Lord Mauleverer.

And William George Bunter was in the car as it rolled away from Greyfriars; though had William George been able to foresee the wild adventures that were in store for him, it is probable that he would have let his pal Mauly down, with a bump!

THE END.

(*Harry Wharton & Co. are booked for the most thrilling holiday adventures of their lives. On no account, therefore, should you miss the next yarn in this grand new series. It's entitled: "SOUTHWARD BOUND!"*)

“SOUTHWARD BOUND!” Thrilling Holiday Yarn of Schoolboy Adventure—Inside.

The MAGNET 2D

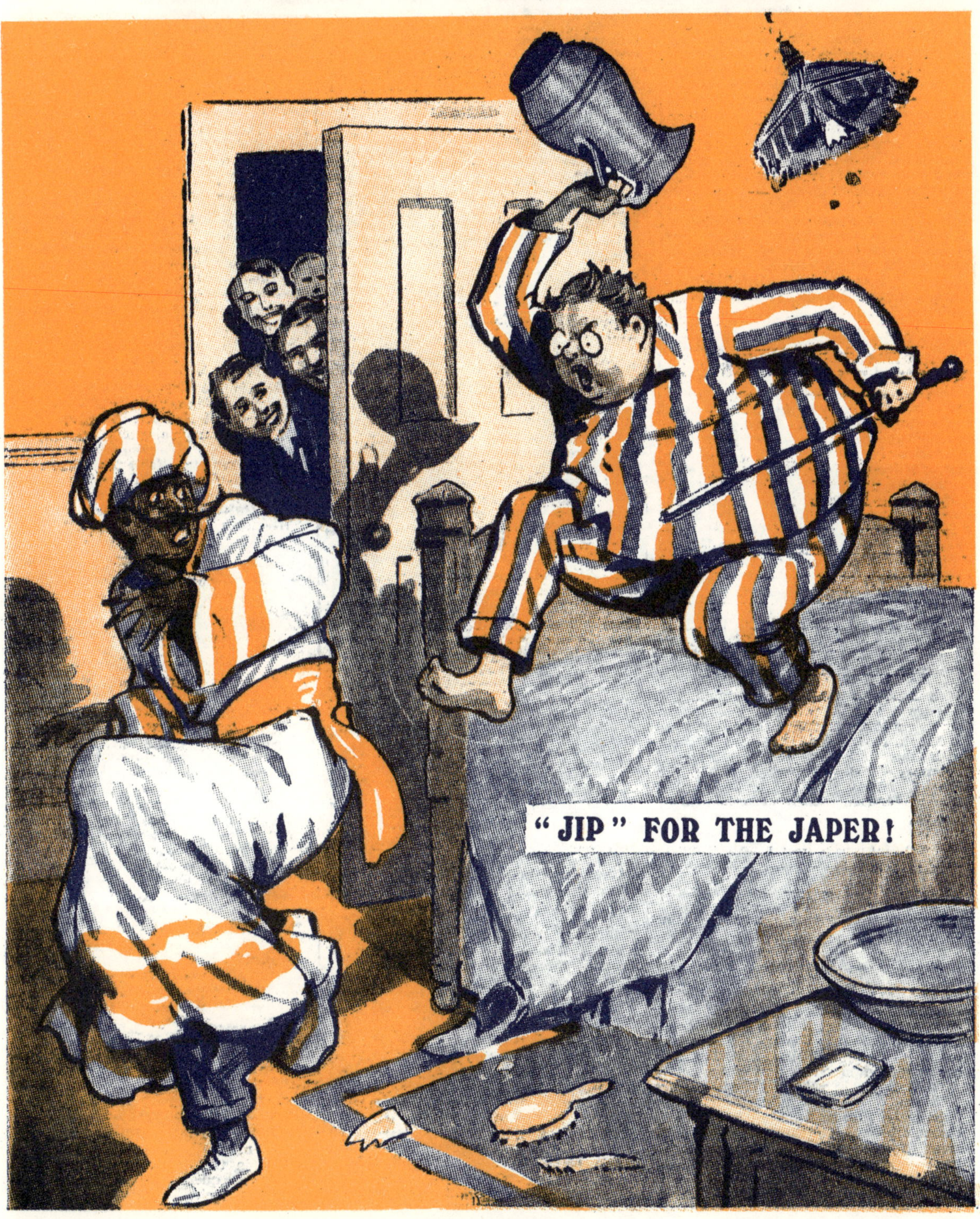

No. 1,278. Vol. XLII. EVERY SATURDAY. Week Ending August 13th, 1932.

NEWS AND VIEWS FROM ALL QUARTERS.

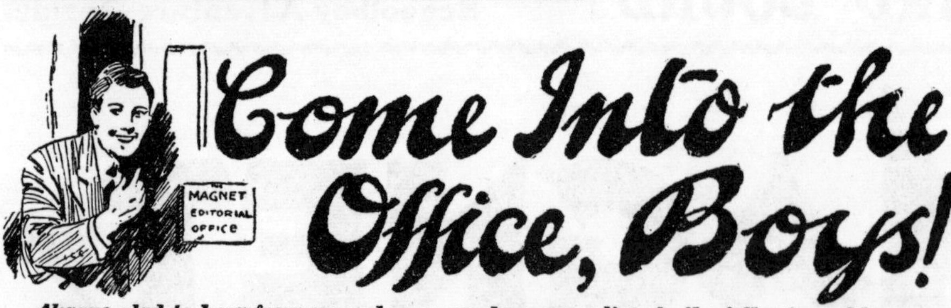

Always glad to hear from you, chums, so drop me a line to the following address: The Editor, The "Magnet" Library, The Amalgamated Press, Ltd., The Fleetway House, Farringdon Street, London, E.C.4.

I HAVE received quite a number of letters this week asking for information regarding the chums of Greyfriars. For instance, Joe Henderson, of South Bank, asks me if Frank Richards was the originator of Harry Wharton & Co. The answer is "Yes." Frank Richards wrote his first story of Harry Wharton in 1908—and has been going strong ever since! A Rainworth reader, who signs himself "China," asks me if it is possible to obtain a copy of the first issue of the MAGNET. I am afraid it is not possible to buy one now—unless some old reader still has one in his possession, and is willing to part with it.

However, it is possible to *read* the first issue! Any reader who is on a visit to London will find

THE "MAGNET" IN THE BRITISH MUSEUM.

It will be necessary to apply for a reader's-ticket, but once that is obtained all back numbers of the MAGNET can be consulted. Full information as to how to obtain permission to consult back issues for reference purposes can be obtained from the Museum Reading Room authorities.

Answers to other queries which this same reader asks are: (2) Harry Wharton is fifteen years of age, and (3) the other members of the now "Famous Five" were already at Greyfriars when Harry Wharton first went to the school.

ANOTHER query from A. John Ashmore, of Hull, asks which characters were first in the field—Harry Wharton & Co., or Tom Merry & Co.? This distinction belongs to Tom Merry & Co. The "Gem," our splendid companion paper, commenced in March, 1907. The MAGNET commenced with the first story of Greyfriars in February, 1908. Nipper & Co., of St. Franks, and Jimmy Silver & Co., of Rookwood, came along at a later date. The very first of all these famous characters who are "still going strong" were Jack Blake and Figgins, who were already at St. Jim's before Tom Merry went there.

Now comes another query regarding our stories.

IS GREYFRIARS A REAL SCHOOL?

Several readers have asked me that, including William Hale (no address given), and William Stewart, of Birkenhead. Well, although there is no actual school called "Greyfriars," Mr. Frank Richards has modelled his stories upon an actual school. The characters, of course, are fictitious, but this popular author draws upon real life for his descriptions of various characters—which is why they actually seem to live. So, although you cannot hope to go to Greyfriars, you will find the counterparts of Harry Wharton & Co. in hundreds of schools in Great Britain.

Get ready for a chuckle, chums! This funny yarn comes from Reginald Lowis, of Girsby, Hainton, Lincoln, who gets a splendid Sheffield steel penknife for it.

Teacher: "Tell me the longest word you know."

Bobby: "Elastic, teacher."

Teacher: "Oh, but that's not a long word."

Bobby: "No; but you can stretch it, teacher!"

Send along your yarns and limericks, chums. I assure you our prizes are worth having!

NOW for a few

RAPID-FIRE REPLIES.

Average Weight of a Boy of $15\frac{1}{2}$ (J. H., of Yorkshire): The average weight of boys is as follows: 13 years, 6 stone; 14 years, 6 stone 8 lbs.; 15 years, 7 stone 5 lbs. Boys of $15\frac{1}{2}$, therefore, should average about 7 stone 12 lbs. The average height cannot be calculated, as some boys grow more quickly than others. Scots boys are generally the tallest, then come Irish, English and Welsh, in the order indicated.

Cost of Printing a Magazine (A. J. A., of Hull): The cost of printing varies all over the country. Any local printer will be pleased to give you a quotation, but I am afraid you will find it very expensive for such a magazine as you describe. I am afraid I don't know the address for which you ask.

Why Do Onions Make One "Weep"? (D. R. F., of Croydon): Because the onions give off fumes which irritate the eyes. Fluid sacs in the eyes exude the fluid they secrete in order to wash away the irritating fumes.

The First Stories of Harry Wharton & Co. ("Interested Reader," of Heswall): I am afraid that both the first issues of the MAGNET and of "The Schoolboys' Own Library" are now out of print, and cannot be obtained.

The Second Largest Film Producing Country in the World ("Film Fan," of Ealing): America, of course, produces the largest number of films per year—but you are wrong when you think that Britain produces the second largest. This distinction—you would hardly believe it—belongs to Japan! Japan produces 300 more films a year than we do!

Lights That Penetrate Fog (G. G. H., of Penarth): Infra-red rays penetrate fog—which is why torch flares are more use in a fog than electric lights. By means of infra-red rays letters can actually be photographed *without even opening the envelopes!*

The Most Famous Cricketer (Norman Lemon, of North Shields): Opinions differ, of course. Admirers of Jack Hobbs generally claim the distinction for him—and he certainly seems to have earned it! But other cricketers have their admirers, too! The record individual score is held by Don Bradman, who scored 452 not out, in a match between New South Wales and Queensland.

Did Columbus First Discover America? (O. H., of Leith): No! America was discovered by Vikings in the 10th century, some considerable time before Columbus made his voyage.

The Record Football Score (W. Reay, of South Shields): This happened in a Scottish Cup-tie, on September 12th, 1885, when Arbroath beat Bon Accord (Aberdeen) by 36 goals to nil!

THE last-mentioned reader also sends along some interesting information regarding

A RECORD FAST,

which has just been completed in his home town. Harry Rennie lived without food in a glass coffin for 72 days. He drank only water and smoked cigarettes—and his average daily consumption of cigarettes was 150! There was no room in the glass coffin in which to stand. This period constitutes a new world's fasting record.

There is just room to squeeze in a prize-winning limerick which earns a magnificent pocket wallet for W. Turner, of Ivy Cottage, Pyllmeynic, near Chepstow, Mon.

Said Coker to Potter and Greene:
"My bike is the fastest you've seen,
For when I get going
There's never no knowing
Whenever again I'll be seen."

LOOK out for next week's issue, chums. The long story of Greyfriars is entitled:

"HARRY WHARTON & CO. IN EGYPT!"

By Frank Richards,

and it continues the adventures of Harry Wharton & Co. on their holiday trip to Egypt. It is packed with thrills—and fun!

As you are already aware the curtain rings down this week on "The Island Traders." But why worry? As in the past, so in the future, the MAGNET will always take the lead where serial stories are concerned. Next week you will be able to enjoy the opening chapters of one of the most thrilling adventure tales of the "good old days" ever published. In

"THE RED FALCON!"

By Arthur Steffens

you will meet Hal Lovett and his staunch pal, Jerry McLean, both of whom, as the result of strange circumstances, become Knights of the Road. Thrills and perils galore loom ahead for Hal and Jerry, but they face them all unflinchingly. Be sure and read this stirring story, chums. It will hold you spellbound from the first chapter.

This bumper issue will also contain another highly amusing St. Sam's yarn, "The Inn of Mystery," while, of course, I will be in the office, as usual, ready to answer your queries, and to give any advice you may require.

YOUR EDITOR.

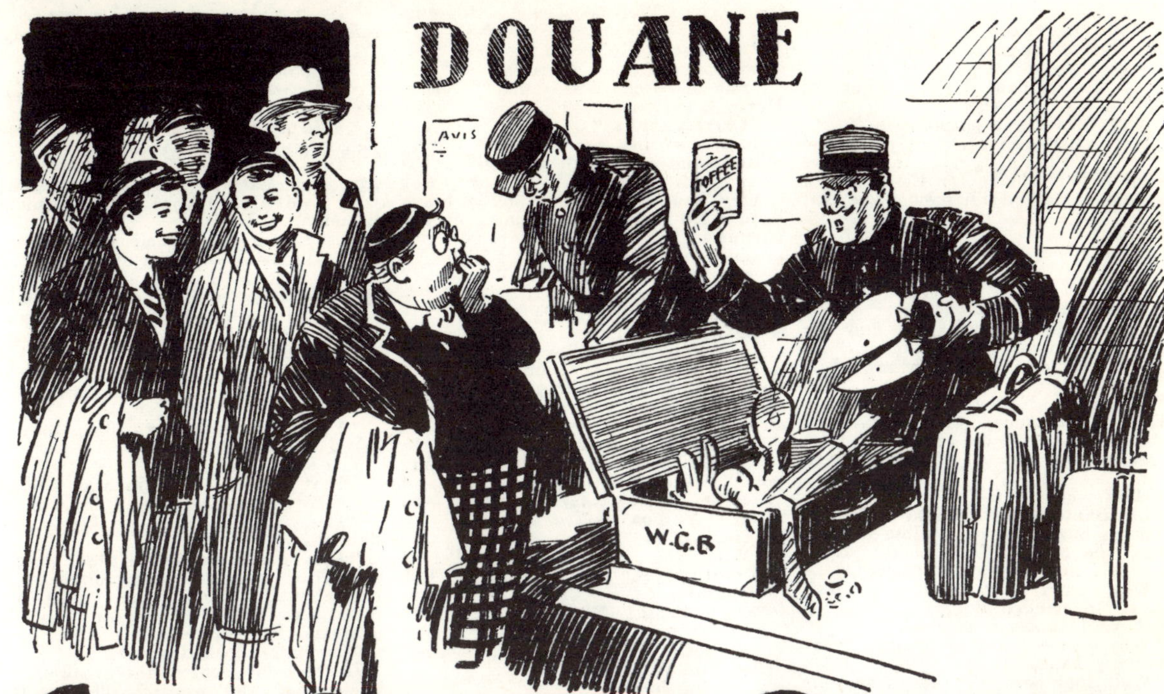

SOUTHWARD BOUND.

By FRANK RICHARDS.

THE FIRST CHAPTER.
On the Road!

"WHERE'S my toffee?"

Billy Bunter woke up.

Bunter had been asleep for a couple of hours, and his reverberating snore mingled more or less musically with the hum of the big car.

It was a hot day. The summer sun blazed down on the long, white roads. The drowsy heat, and the hum of the engine, lulled Billy Bunter to slumber. Fields and meadows, green pastures and dusky woodlands flashed past the car, without interesting William George Bunter. He was interested in a large packet of toffee till he went to sleep; and when he awoke, his thoughts naturally reverted to the toffee. He had dropped off with a sticky chunk in his fat hand; but when his eyes opened behind his big spectacles, his fat paw was empty. And he blinked suspiciously at the other fellows in the car.

It was a big car—but it was well filled. Lord Mauleverer, of the Greyfriars Remove, sat in the corner farthest from Bunter. The farther he was from Bunter, the more comfortable Mauly felt. That feeling was shared by Harry Wharton & Co.; but somebody had to sit next to Bunter, and Bob Cherry nobly made the sacrifice.

The Famous Five of Greyfriars were going home with Mauly for the holidays, in happy anticipation of a jolly good time, and there was only one fly in the ointment, so to speak, but it was a very fat fly, and its name was Billy Bunter. But on break-up day, free from lessons and masters, for weeks and weeks to come, the Famous Five felt that they could stand even Billy Bunter with equanimity.

Five faces wore very cheerful looks; and Lord Mauleverer smiled with placid contentment. Still, it was a relief when Billy Bunter went to sleep. His snore started, but his conversation stopped. And of the two inflictions, the snore was rather preferable.

Now he had woke up, his snore stopped and his conversation started. All the juniors in the car felt that it was a change for the worse.

"I say, you fellows——"

"Go to sleep again, old fat man!" said Frank Nugent persuasively.

Somewhere in Egypt lies a hidden treasure worth a quarter of a million pounds—and the only clue to its whereabouts is to be found from a golden scarab which is now in the hands of Harry Wharton & Co.

"Something woke me up!" said Bunter accusingly. "The car jolted, or something. It woke me up."

He blinked at Lord Mauleverer.

"You've got a rotten chauffeur, Mauly."

"Yaas."

"Not like my pater's chauffeur at Bunter Court."

"Yaas."

"Shut up, old fat man, and go to sleep!" said Johnny Bull. "You're much nicer asleep."

"The noisefulness is great, but the nicefulness is terrific," agreed Hurree Jamset Ram Singh.

"Yah! Where's my toffee?"

Billy Bunter sat up and blinked round him through his big spectacles. He knew that that toffee had been in his fat fingers when he went to sleep. It was no longer in his fat fingers. Bunter wanted to know where it was; and he wanted to know at once. Evidently he suspected the other fellows of having had felonious designs on that chunk of toffee.

"Look here, Cherry, if you've scoffed my toffee——"

Bob Cherry chuckled.

"Have you had it, Wharton?"

"Not guilty," said Harry Wharton, laughing.

"Look here, Nugent——"

"Fathead!"

"Well, somebody's had that toffee!" roared Bunter. "Have you got my toffee, Mauly?"

Lord Mauleverer shuddered.

"Good gad! No!" he gasped. "Wouldn't touch it with a barge-pole, old bean."

"If it was you, Bull——"

"Ass!"

Nobody in the car was likely to have "scoffed" the sticky chunk of toffee, that had been sticking to Bunter's fingers. Really, it was not appetising or attractive—except to Bunter.

"If you've got my toffee, Inky——"

"The gotfulness is not terrific, my esteemed idiotic Bunter," chuckled Hurree Jamset Ram Singh. "Perhaps it has dropped on the floor while you were sleeping snorefully."

Billy Bunter blinked down among innumerable feet.

"For goodness' sake give a fellow room," he grunted. "Hardly room to move in this car. Not like my pater's Rolls, at Bunter Court, Mauly."

"Yaas!" said Mauly.

"Well, you want room for two or three, fatty!" remarked Bob Cherry.

"I wish you'd hang one of your feet out of the window, Cherry. Lots of room in the car, then!"

"You cheeky fat porpoise——"

"Well, where's that toffee?" demanded Bunter. "I'm hungry! If I were taking a party home for the holidays, I should put a lunch-basket in the car, Mauly."

"Yaas."

"I think you fellows might look for that toffee! You know I'm short-sighted! Beastly selfishness all round. I jolly well think——"

"For goodness' sake, let's find the toffee!" exclaimed Frank Nugent. "He will shut up for a minute or two while he's wolfing it."

"Oh, really, Nugent——"

Bob Cherry stooped, and disinterred a sticky chunk from the rug on the floor. A considerable amount of dust adhered to it.

"Here you are, fatty."

Billy Bunter grunted as he took it.

"Some beast's been treading on this toffee," he said. "Look at it! Lend me your hanky to wipe it, Cherry."

"Why can't you use your own hanky?" demanded Bob.

"It would make it all sticky."

"Why, you—you fat frump, what about my hanky?"

"Well, look here, I'll wipe it on your sleeve—keep still——"

Bob Cherry did not keep still. He jerked his arm away as suddenly as if it had been electrified.

"Keep that sticky muck away from me!" he bawled.

"Oh, really, Cherry——"

"Mauly, old man, do you mind if we open the door and spill Bunter along the road?" asked Harry Wharton.

Lord Mauleverer grinned. Probably he would not have minded very much. But Billy Bunter was his guest for the summer holidays; so his lordship refrained from stating what he thought on the subject of Bunter.

The fat Owl of the Remove wiped the toffee on his own handkerchief—nobody else's being available. Really, it did not matter very much; nothing could have made Bunter's handkerchief much stickier, or much more in need of a wash. Then he transferred the delightful object to his mouth. Billy Bunter had a large mouth; but the chunk of toffee was large, and filled it almost to capacity. The fat junior leaned back in his seat, looking a little more good-humoured. One fat cheek bulged out like a ripe red apple, and there was a gurgling sound of satisfaction from the Owl of the Remove.

And then the car jolted again, over a rough rut of dried mud on the country road. It was quite a severe jolt, and all the passengers jerked in their seats. Billy Bunter bounced like a punchball, and Bob Cherry grabbed him and dragged him back into his seat. From the fat Owl came a wild, weird, guggling gurgle.

"Groooooooogh!"

"What the thump——"

"Grrrrrrrggh!"

"What——"

"Yurrrrggggghh!"

Billy Bunter's fat face was crimson, his eyes almost popped through his big spectacles, and he gasped and gurgled, and gurgled and gasped, frantically. The Famous Five stared at him in amazement, wondering what on earth was the matter. Then they guessed! The toffee was going down the wrong way—in bulk!

"Urrrrrrgh Wurrrgh! Ooooch! Grooooch! Woooooooooch! Gug gug-gug!"

"My hat! He's choking——"

"The chokefulness is terrific——"

"Pat his back, Bob—quick!" gasped Harry Wharton.

"Urrrrrggggghh!"

Smack, smack, smack! Bob Cherry patted Bunter on the back with vigour and rapidity—especially vigour. Bob Cherry had a hefty arm and a heavy hand. No doubt Billy Bunter needed patting on the back. But it was barely possible that Bob overdid it a little.

"Ooooogh! Grooogh! Woooooh!" gurgled Bunter.

Smack, smack, smack!

"Urrrrrggggghh!"

The troublesome toffee shot floorward again. Billy Bunter found himself suddenly relieved of that impediment to his speech. But Bob Cherry was still going strong.

Smack, smack, smack, smack!

"Yaroooh! Stoppit!" shrieked Bunter. "Leave off hitting me, you beast! Wharrer you hitting me for, you rotter? Yarooooop!"

"Ha, ha, ha!"

"Why, you thankless fat porker, I was patting your back!" exclaimed Bob indignantly.

"Ow! Beast! Wow!"

"Better have a few more——"

"Yaroooh! Keep off, you beast!" yelled Bunter.

"Ha, ha, ha!"

Billy Bunter sat back in his seat, glaring at the Famous Five with a glare that almost cracked his spectacles.

"Beasts!" he roared. "Now, that toffee's gone again! Look here, find that toffee—see?"

"Here, old bean," said Lord Mauleverer, and he handed a box of chocolates across to the fat Owl, "try these!"

"Oh!" said Bunter. His fat brow cleared. "Right you are!" He lost no time in trying the chocolates. "I say, Mauly, these are good! I'll finish the box, if you like."

"Do, old fat man!"

"And look here, Mauly," said Bunter generously, "you can have the toffee, old chap!"

"Oh gad!" gasped Lord Mauleverer. "I—I—I don't think I care very much for toffee, thanks, old top!"

"Ha, ha, ha!"

And the toffee remained where it was.

THE SECOND CHAPTER.
Pursued!

HURREE JAMSET RAM SINGH looked back from the rear window in the big car, with a serious and thoughtful shade on his dusky face. His chums looked at him rather curiously. It was the tenth time, at least, that the Nabob of Bhanipur had looked back, scanning the long, white road behind the car with searching eyes.

Billy Bunter, having finished the chocolates, was composing himself in his corner to snore again. Lord Mauleverer was on the point of nodding.

But the drowsy summer heat and the purring hum of the car did not have a soporific effect on the Famous Five. Those energetic youths were merry and bright and wide awake, and most alert of all was the dusky junior from India's coral strand.

After a long, long look at the winding road behind the car, the nabob turned to his comrades, and the serious expression on his face arrested their attention.

"Hallo, hallo, hallo! What's up, Inky?" asked Bob.

"The upfulness, I think, is terrific!" said Hurree Jamset Ram Singh gravely. "This esteemed and ridiculous car is being followed."

"Followed?" repeated Harry Wharton.

"Lots of cars on the road, Inky," said Nugent.

"The lotfulness is preposterous!" agreed the nabob. "But look back with your own absurd eyes, my ridiculous friends."

The Co. crowded their faces at the little window in the back of the car and looked. Some distance behind, in a cloud of dust, a big, powerful Austin was humming in their wake. It was closed, and whether there were passengers inside they could not see; but they could see the chauffeur plainly, and make out that he had a dark face under the peak of his cap.

"You've seen that car before, Inky?" asked Johnny Bull.

The nabob nodded.

"That esteemed Austin was behind us when we left the school," he said.

"The same car?" asked Bob dubiously.

"I have seen it a dozen times since," said Hurree Jamset Ram Singh. "It has fallen out of sight many times, but it always turns up again like an estimable bad penny."

The juniors looked grave.

In the excitement of the break-up, of packing-up and getting off for the summer holidays, they had almost forgotten the peril that had threatened Lord Mauleverer; but not quite.

They remembered Kalizelos, the Greek from Egypt, who had come from far-off Cairo, in quest of the mysterious scarab that was in the schoolboy earl's possession. But for the trick played by Billy Bunter, which had led the Greek to believe that the fat Owl was Lord Mauleverer, there was little doubt that Mauly would have fallen into the hands of the man from Egypt.

Mauly gave very little thought—if any—to his peril; but his friends were very keenly on the alert for another attempt to be made on him.

The juniors were miles from Greyfriars now, and it was odd, at least, if the high-powered Austin had hung behind them all the time. In ordinary circumstances they would have taken no heed of it. But if the man from Egypt was still in England, the circumstances were not ordinary.

"That chap at the wheel looks foreign, so far as one can make out his chivvy under that cap," said Johnny Bull. "It's not Kalizelos; but it might be one of his gang. He had a lot of his own sort with him on his yacht."

"I say, you fellows——"

"Shut up, Bunter!"

"Beast! What are you blinking at?" asked Bunter irritably. "Some beast trod on my foot!"

"Mauly, old man," said Harry.

"Yaas." Lord Mauleverer opened his half-closed eyes. "I'm not goin' to sleep! I heard all you fellows were sayin'. You were talkin' cricket, weren't you?"

"Fathead! It looks as if this car has been followed from the school," said Harry. "If that's so, it shows that Kalizelos never cleared off when his yacht put to sea, and he's after you again."

Lord Mauleverer yawned.

"All serene! Let him rip!"

"Ass! We've got to make sure! Tell the chauffeur to slow down and see if that car passes us."

"Oh, all right, dear man!"

Lord Mauleverer spoke to the chauffeur, and Watson slowed down from forty to twenty. The Austin came swiftly on, drawing nearer and nearer. It had been doing forty on the wide country road, and could easily have passed the schoolboys' car now. But before it came close, the dark-skinned chauffeur slowed down the Austin keeping behind.

"He's not passing us, then," said Nugent, after a long pause.

"I say, you fellows——"

"Go to sleep, Bunter!"

"Beast!"

"Tell Watson to let her out, Mauly," said Harry.

"Yaas."

The Rolls leaped into speed again. Watson let her out to fifty. The Austin dropped away for a minute, then picked up speed, and came roaring on at fifty. for the holidays to protect you? Haven't I turned down a host of invitations, and put up with this Bank Holiday crowd you've brought along for the hols, simply to look after you and protect you?" demanded Bunter.

"Oh, gad! Have you?"

"Yes, I jolly well have!" said Bunter warmly. "My idea is that that Greek blighter will be after you again, some time or other, and I'm bound to stand by you as a pal. I say, you fellows, let me have a look."

Bunter rose to his feet, barged the juniors aside, and blinked back along the road through his big spectacles. The next moment he gave a squeak of alarm.

"Ow! I say, you fellows, tell the chauffeur to let the car out! Oh dear! I say, it's that beast again!"

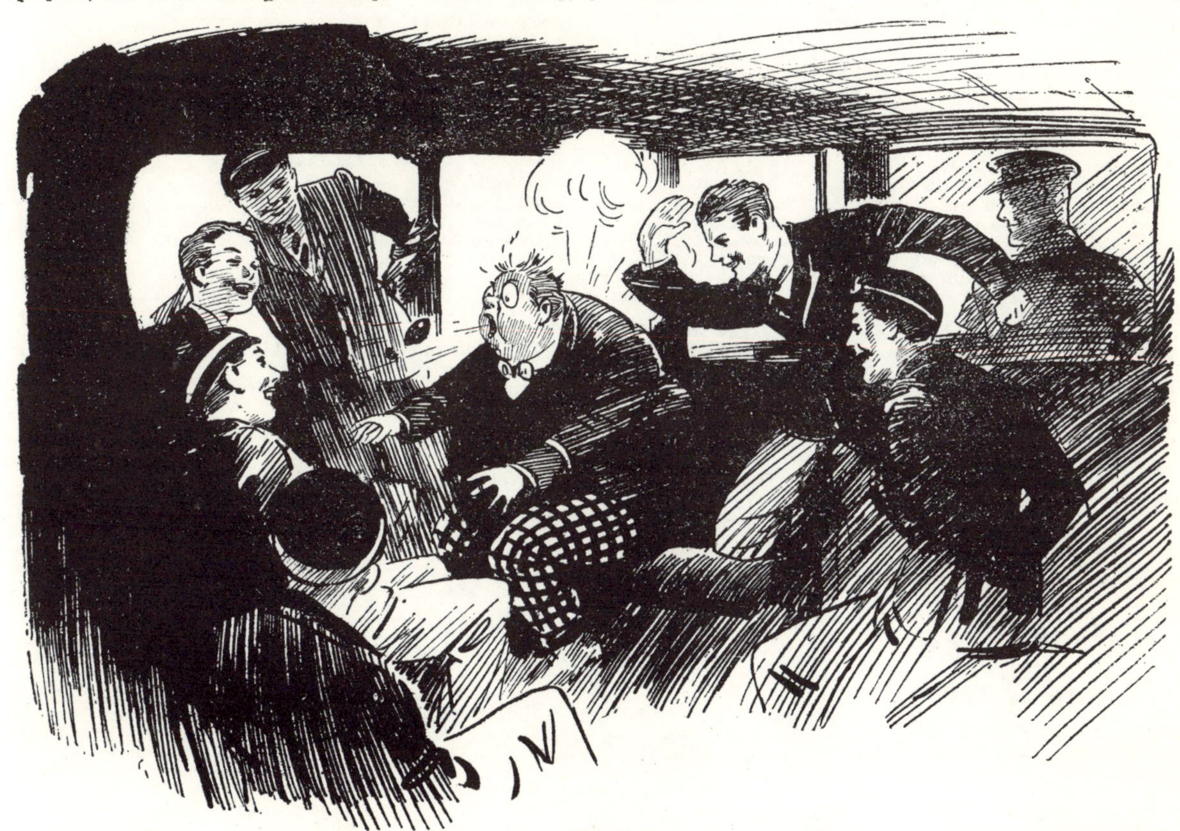

"Yurrrrrrgggghh! Urrrrrrrrggh!" Bunter was gurgling and gasping frantically. "My hat!" cried Wharton. "Bunter's choking! Pat him on the back, Bob—quick!" Bob Cherry patted Bunter on the back with vigour and rapidity, and the troublesome toffee was brought to light.

"We can't see anybody in the car!" said Harry.

"I've seen that man who's driving, before—he was on the yacht when that beast Kalizelos got me there!" gasped Bunter. "I saw him there!"

"Sure?" asked Harry.

"Yes, you beast! Make the chauffeur go faster!" yelled Bunter. "I tell you they're after us, and there may be a gang of them packed in that car. If they catch us on a lonely road——"

"Chance for you to protect Mauly!" grinned Bob Cherry.

"Beast!" howled Bunter.

Now that it was certain that the enemy were in pursuit, Billy Bunter did not seem so keen on protecting his pal, Mauly. He seemed considerably alarmed for his own podgy self.

Watson let out the Rolls again, at an almost terrific burst of speed. Trees and hedges flashed by. But the high-powered car behind was let out, too, and it kept pace. Billy Bunter plumped into his seat with a gasp. He was not looking sleepy now. His little, round eyes were very wide open behind his big, round spectacles.

There was no doubt that Bunter had—inadvertently—saved Mauly from the clutches of the man from Egypt, and it was on that account that his good-natured lordship had allowed the fat Owl to hook on for the summer holidays. Possibly Bunter, who had a fertile imagination, and who feared no foe when the foe was out of sight, really believed that he was going with Mauly to protect him. If so, he woke up, as it were, when he found that the enemy were in sight. Obviously Bunter, at that moment, wished that he was anywhere but in the magnificent Rolls which was bearing the Greyfriars fellows towards Mauleverer Towers.

There could hardly be a doubt now. The Austin was following the schoolboys' car, keeping it in sight, letting the Rolls make the pace.

Again the Rolls dropped to twenty. Again the Austin dropped to twenty behind.

"That settles it!" said Harry. "They're after us!"

"The settlefulness is terrific!"

"I say, you fellows, don't be nervy," said Billy Bunter. "I'm with you, you know!"

"Fathead!"

"I don't suppose there's anybody after us," said Bunter. "Only your nerves, old chaps. If that Greek shows up again, Mauly, don't you be afraid. I'm here to look after you! What are you grinning at, Mauly?"

"Was I grinning, old bean?"

"I've saved your life once!" said Bunter, with dignity. "They'd have had you if I hadn't let them think I was you, and faced the danger for you, and pulled you through. You know that! Ain't I coming home with you

"I—I say, you fellows——" he stuttered.

"Shut up, fatty!" said Bob. "No good funking now. Look here, you men, it's plain enough that they're after us. But what's their game?"

"Kalizelos, if he's in that car, doesn't know Mauly by sight," said Harry Wharton. "That was how Bunter spoofed him. But he may have found out that this car came from Mauleverer Towers—may have had some spy watching the place and picking up information. If he knows that it's Mauly's car, he knows that Mauly's in it."

"Yaas, that's it," said Lord Mauleverer placidly. "Easy enough for him to pick that up. And as he's seen all you fellows before, an' knows that you're not me, he won't be long in pickin' me out, what? Lucky Bunter's here to protect me. If there's any shootin' I shall keep behind Bunter——"

"Yaroooh!"

"Luckily, Bunter's wide enough to give a chap plenty of cover——"

"Beast!" roared Bunter.

"Ha, ha, ha!"

"Blessed if I see anything to cackle at!" howled Bunter. "I can tell you that Greek is a desperate beast. Look here! All he wants is that silly Egyptian scarab that Mauly's got at home. I think Mauly had better let him have it, and then the beast will go back to Egypt and let us alone, see? It's not worth much, Mauly—and, anyhow, I'll pay for it if you like."

"Who's going to lend Bunter the money to pay Mauly for his scarab?" asked Bob Cherry. "Or is he going to pay for it with that bad sixpence he couldn't pass at the tuckshop yesterday?"

"Ha, ha, ha!"

"I don't know whether that jolly old scarab is worth anythin'," said Lord Mauleverer, "but I know that scoundrel isn't goin' to get his thievin' hands on it!"

"No fear!" said Harry. "And it must be worth something for that rascal to run such risks to get hold of it. Kalizelos hasn't come all the way from Egypt for nothing, and he's risking prison. Look here, you fellows! If Kalizelos is in that Austin, we can have his car stopped at the next police station, and give him into custody. The police have been looking for him since he bagged Bunter on his yacht near Greyfriars. Let him follow us into the next town——"

"Good egg!"

"I say, you fellows, they're going to catch us in some lonely place!" gasped Billy Bunter. "I say——"

"That's their game, I suppose," said Bob. "But we can jolly well put paid to it. We shall be in Maidstone soon, and we'll stop at the police station, and put the jolly old peelers on to him."

The juniors continued to watch, bunched at the window while the car ran swiftly on towards the ancient city on the Medway. Once or twice they caught the glitter of the black eyes of the foreigner who was driving the Austin, and they wondered whether he had spotted them looking back. They could have little doubt that the enemy had planned to overhaul them on some long, lonely stretch of road—of which there were a good many on the hundred-mile run to Mauleverer Towers.

Had not Hurree Singh spotted the pursuit, such a plan would have been easy to carry out. Now, however, it seemed to the Greyfriars party that "paid" could be put to it. There was a charge against the Greek, on which he could be handed over to the police, and if he was in the Austin that was the most effective way of dealing with him.

"Hallo, hallo, hallo!" exclaimed Bob Cherry suddenly. "They're chucking it!"

"My hat!"

Maidstone was in sight ahead, when the Austin suddenly turned from the road, and vanished round a corner. The juniors stared. The pursuer had disappeared from sight.

"Gone!" said Bob.

"The gonefulness is terrific!"

Bob chuckled.

"They spotted us watching them," he said, "and I dare say they guessed what we should do. Anyhow, they've chucked it."

Billy Bunter blinked back along the road. Plenty of cars were humming along in the sunlight; but the Austin was gone.

The Owl of the Remove recovered his courage on the spot.

"I say, you fellows, it's all right," he said. "Don't be funky, you know. Blessed if I ever saw such a nervy lot!"

"Kill him, somebody," said Bob.

"Beast!"

Billy Bunter settled down to sleep again, and snored. Maidstone was left behind, and the Rolls purred on, on its long journey westward, the juniors glancing back every now and then to watch the road. But there was no sign of the Austin again, and it seemed clear that the Greek had given up the game. Which was rather a relief to the Greyfriars party, though now they knew, beyond the shadow of a doubt, that Lord Mauleverer's peril was not over, and that the man from Egypt was still in quest of the mysterious scarab of A-Menah.

———

THE THIRD CHAPTER.

Desperate Measures!

"PENNY for 'em, Inky!" grinned Bob Cherry.

Hurree Jamset Ram Singh sat silent, a thoughtful shade on his dusky face, while his comrades chatted, and Bunter snored, and the car ate up the miles. The nabob was thinking, and he smiled faintly as Bob offered him a penny for the result.

"My esteemed chums," said Hurree Singh, "I have been thinkfully reflecting. What are we doing in this car now?"

"About thirty, old bean," said Lord Mauleverer.

"But the esteemed car could do sixty."

"Easily. Want to go faster?" asked Mauly.

"Not at all, my absurd Mauly. But the execrable Austin that was following us could do as much as this car."

"What about it, Inky?" asked Harry Wharton, looking attentively at the nabob's thoughtful face. "What have you got in your head now?"

"Cough it up!" said Bob. "I can see that he's got something in his jolly old black noddle."

"I was thinkfully reflecting, my worthy and idiotic chums, that while we are doing thirty, perhapsfully the ridiculous Austin is doing sixty."

"That won't hurt us, will it?"

"My absurd meaning is that, by taking another road, they may have passed us, out of our esteemed sight, and got ahead of us on this road," said Hurree Jamset Ram Singh. "In which case, my ludicrous friends, they can pick us up wherever they like, before we reach our idiotic destination."

"Oh, my hat!"

"Oh gad!" said Lord Mauleverer.

Harry Wharton nodded slowly. The Rolls was keeping up an average of thirty, and it was easy enough for the pursuers to get ahead if they liked. They had been dropped near Maidstone, and the Austin had not been seen since. But if Kalizelos had let the car out he might be twenty miles ahead now.

It was a startling thought that perhaps the pursuers, who had been dropped behind, might now be waiting for the Greyfriars party ahead. But obviously it was possible, indeed probable, now that the nabob suggested it.

"Oh gad!" yawned Lord Mauleverer. "I'll tell you what, you men—that giddy Greek is beginnin' to be a bore! Ten to one old Inky's got it right."

"The possibility is terrific," remarked Hurree Jamset Ram Singh, "and if I may make a suggestive remark——"

"You can make a suggestion, if you like, or a remark," chuckled Bob Cherry. "Get it off your chest!"

"The esteemed enemy is probably watching for us ahead, as his knowfulness of our route is terrific. But if we go roundfully, and arrive at Mauly's absurd home from the other side——"

"Good egg!" said Bob. "That will bunker the old bean! He can watch this road till the cows come home, if he likes, if we're on another. We can go fifty or sixty miles round, and come back through Winchester to Mauleverer Towers. What, Mauly?"

"Yaas, but"—Lord Mauleverer hesitated—"I don't like the idea of dodgin' the rascal! I'd rather punch his face."

"Fathead!" said Harry Wharton. "If we get held up on a lonely stretch by a gang of them, we shan't have much chance of putting in punches."

"Yaas, but, dash it all, I can't be kept in a jolly old bandbox, you know! Still, perhaps you're right. Rather a lark to leave the jolly old Grecian watchin' the road we shan't travel by." His lordship chuckled. "I'll tell Watson."

The car turned from the road.

Dodging the enemy did not appeal to Lord Mauleverer, or to his friends, but evidently it was the wisest course. There was no doubt that Kalizelos was a desperate man, and that he would hesitate at little or nothing to get the schoolboy earl into his hands. The schoolboys had no chance in a scrap with an armed gang, and on some long, lonely stretch of road they would be at the mercy of the man from Egypt. All the party realised that Hurree Singh's foresight had probably saved them from running into a trap from which there would have been no escape.

They settled down to a long run, making a wide detour far from the road that led direct into Hampshire. Whether Kalizelos was watching that road or not, he could not watch all the roads, and they had no doubt of eluding him now. Now the car was let out, and the miles raced by under the wheels, the route lying through Sussex instead of Surrey. Mauleverer Towers was some miles on the London side of Winchester; but the car, after a long run, came to the ancient cathedral city from the western side.

Billy Bunter ceased to snore when Winchester was passed, and opened his eyes behind his spectacles.

"I say, you fellows——"

"Sleep, baby, sleep!" chanted Bob Cherry.

"Oh, really, Cherry, ain't we nearly there?" asked Bunter. "I say, I'm getting jolly hungry! Time we got in, I think! This is a pretty slow car, Mauly! If I'd thought of it I'd have phoned for my pater's Rolls to take us to your place. I've often done seventy in it."

The juniors grinned. The fat Owl was unaware that sixty miles or more had been added to the journey.

"Wake me up when we get in!" yawned Bunter; and, to the relief of the rest of the party, he closed his eyes again and once more a deep snore drowned the hum of the car.

Far in the distance the ancient turrets of Mauleverer Towers came into sight over the tree-tops.

"Hallo, hallo, hallo!" yelled Bob Cherry suddenly.

He pointed from the window.

"The Austin!" exclaimed Wharton.

From a side road the car had passed, a big Austin shot out into view behind them. It was the car they had dropped in Kent.

"Here we are again!" grinned Bob. "They're after us, Mauly."

"Yaas!" yawned Mauly. "Let her out, Watson."

The juniors looked back as the Rolls tore on. Behind them the big Austin roared. A man could be seen beside the driver now—a supple, olive-skinned man with eyes black as jet.

"That's Kalizelos!" said Bob.

"Is that the sportsman?" asked Mauly, watching the handsome, dark face of the Greek. "He won't catch us now; we're nearly home."

The Rolls raced on towards the great gates of Mauleverer Towers, now only half a mile ahead. The Austin, going all out, kept pace, but did not gain.

The juniors grinned as they looked back. They could guess what had happened. There could be no doubt now that Hurree Singh had been right, and that Kalizelos had got ahead to waylay the party on the road. But when they failed to appear the Greek had doubtless guessed that they had taken the alarm and changed their route. That left the man from Egypt no recourse but to scour the roads round Mauleverer Towers in the hope of catching sight of the big Rolls again. Fortune had favoured him to this extent; he had sighted them. But they were almost in now, and, so far as the juniors could see, he had no chance.

Bang!

"Great pip!" gasped Johnny Bull.

Bang! Bang!

The pistol-shots rang from the man beside the dark-faced driver. For a moment the schoolboys supposed that the Greek was firing on them. Then they realised that he was shooting at the tyres. The bullets spattered on the road under the Rolls as it shot round a bend in the road. Watson gave a jump in his seat, but did not look round; the car was going at a breakneck pace. He kept it going. The juniors felt a thrill at their hearts. A burst tyre at that speed——

"I say, you fellows!" Bunter yawned. "What's that row? Is it thunder?"

Bang! Bang!

"The villain!" breathed Wharton.

Had it been a matter of minutes the Greek would no doubt have stopped the Rolls by that desperate method; perhaps at a cost of life or limb to the occupants. But it was only a matter of seconds.

"I say, you fellows——"

"Here we are!"

Bang!

The park gates were open. The Rolls rocked on two wheels as Watson turned in at the wide gateway. The big oaks and beeches on the drive flashed by, merged into one another at the speed. Watson slowed down up to the house. The juniors stared back breathlessly, wondering whether the Greek was desperate enough to follow them in at the park gates. But Kalizelos stopped short of that. The Austin shot past the gateway and vanished.

Bob Cherry gasped.

"My hat! We're well out of that!"

"Lucky we didn't fall in with them on a lonely road!" said Nugent. "That scoundrel wouldn't stop at much!"

"I say, you fellows——" Billy Bunter blinked round peevishly. "Are we in at last? Frightful long time we've been on the road! This isn't much of a car, Mauly."

"Yaas."

"I say, what was that row?" asked Bunter. "It wasn't thunder? Somebody letting off fireworks?"

"Ha, ha, ha!"

"Yes; jolly dangerous fireworks, old fat bean," grinned Bob Cherry, as the Rolls came to a stop at the entrance of Lord Mauleverer's mansion, and the great door opened, revealing the portly figure of Porson, his lordship's butler. "It was the jolly old Greek potting at us, my fat tulip."

"Yarooooh!"

"All serene now, Bunter," said Harry Wharton.

"Beast! Lemme gerrout!" yelled Bunter.

"Ha, ha, ha!"

"Lemme gerrout!" shrieked the fat Owl.

He plunged for the door. Watson had dismounted and opened it, and Billy Bunter came out like a bullet from a rifle.

He tore up the steps at frantic speed. Porson, portly and majestic, was in the doorway. Bunter did not even see him. He crashed.

"Ooooough!" gasped the butler of Mauleverer Towers, as the fat Owl established sudden contact with his well-packed waistcoat.

He sat down with startling suddenness.

"Ow!" gurgled Bunter, as he sprawled over Porson. "Ow! Beast! Gerrout! Leggo! Rotter! Oooogh!"

"Ha, ha, ha!"

Billy Bunter scrambled up and vanished into the house.

Porson sat up and gasped.

The juniors came grinning in. Porson was a dignified butler, worthy, in his natural state, of the highest traditions of Mauleverer Towers. But for once Porson received his lordship at his lordship's door in an utterly undignified manner.

Had Porson been told that he would ever receive Lord Mauleverer, sitting down in the doorway and clasping both hands to his waistcoat, Porson would have repudiated the suggestion with scorn.

But that was exactly what he did on this occasion.

"Oooogh!" gasped Porson. "Oooop! Wooooooh-hoooooop! My lord—— Grooogh! My—— Oooooch! Lord! Warrrroooop!"

Three or four footmen rushed to help Porson up. Supported on one side by James, and on the other by John, Porson endeavoured to collect his accustomed dignity, and to speak with his usual calm aplomb. But all he could say was:

"Woooooh! Goooooh! Goooooch!"

And the footmen led him away, still gurgling.

THE FOURTH CHAPTER.

Bunter Declines!

"SCORPIONS——"

"And lions——"

"And plagues—you fellows have heard about the plagues of Egypt——"

"And the famines——"

"Then there's the sand-storms——"

"And the burning sun—hot as a furnace——"

"Hotter!"

"The hotfulness is terrific!"

"Better not tell Bunter. He will find it out soon enough for himself when he gets there."

"Beasts!" murmured Billy Bunter.

Bunter was seated in a deep armchair in the old armoury that Lord Mauleverer used as a "den." With his podgy figure filling the big chair, and his fat little legs stretched across another chair, his fat thumbs stuck in the armholes of his waistcoat, Billy Bunter presented a picture of comfort, if not of elegance or beauty. Several lunches were packed away inside Bunter, and he had retired to that comfortable chair for a nap.

Harry Wharton & Co. came into the room, apparently unaware that he was there. They stood in a group by the window, their backs to Bunter, while they discussed Egypt and the attractions of that famous land.

Billy Bunter blinked inimically at their backs, through his big spectacles. He did not make his presence known. If the fellows were discussing matters not intended for his fat ears, Billy Bunter was not the fellow to let them know that he was there.

"No, keep it dark from Bunter," said Harry Wharton gravely. "He will know what it's like when he finds a scorpion in his bed in Egypt."

"Let him be happy as long as he can," said Bob Cherry. "No need to tell him he may be gobbled up by a lion in the Libyan Desert."

"Bunter won't last long enough to be gobbled by a lion," said Johnny Bull, shaking his head. "He will melt away like tallow when he gets under the Egyptian sun."

"Poor old Bunter!"

"Might give him the tip what to expect," said Nugent.

"No, no! He might chuck us, if he knew. And what should we do without Bunter?"

"True!"

"But if he's bitten by a scorpion——"

"Well, that will save him from being gobbled by a lion——"

Billy Bunter could keep silent no longer.

"Beasts!" he roared.

The Famous Five spun round from the window, with surprised looks worthy of members of the Remove Dramatic Society.

"Hallo, hallo, hallo! He's here!" exclaimed Bob.

"Oh, my hat! Did you hear what we were saying, Bunter?"

"Yes, I jolly well did!" snorted Bunter. "Keeping it dark, were you, you rotters? You'd like me to be bitten by scorpions!"

The fat junior rose from the armchair. His very spectacles gleamed with wrath and indignation.

"Now, look here, you fellows, what's this rot?" he demanded. "I knew there was something on—I've spotted that. Is Mauly going to Egypt for the holidays?"

"That's it, old bean," assented Bob. "We're going with him. And as you're staying with Mauly for the hols, you're coming, too, of course."

"Well, I can tell you I'm jolly well not!" declared Billy Bunter. "I'll stay here with Mauly, or I'll go with him if he likes to make it Margate. But I'm not going to Egypt, and that's flat."

"Ripping country, old bean!" said Bob Cherry solemnly. "No end of a catch to get a holiday in Egypt."

"That's a bit different from what you were saying just now, when you thought I didn't hear you!" sneered Bunter.

"Oh! Ah! Yes! But——"

"Lots of things to see, Bunter," said Frank Nugent. "There's the jolly old Sphinx——"

"Blow the Sphinx!"

"And frightfully interesting tombs," said Johnny Bull. "You'd need a tomb, you know, if a scorpion bit you."

"Beast!"

"As for the plagues of Egypt——" said Bob. "I—I don't think there are really any plagues there now!"

"Yah! I'm jolly well not going to be bitten by scorpions, and catch plagues, to please you, I know that!" said Billy Bunter. "And I'm jolly well going to tell Mauly so. I'm going to tell him so plainly."

"My esteemed Bunter——"

"Yah!"

Billy Bunter rolled towards the door—apparently to seek Lord Mauleverer at once, and talk plainly to him.

The chums of the Remove exchanged joyous grins.

"It's worked!" murmured Bob.

Really, it seemed to have worked like a charm.

The Greyfriars fellows had now been some days at Mauleverer Towers, and it was time to get ready for the journey to Egypt with Mauly's uncle, Sir Reginald Brooke.

Bunter was landed on Mauly for the holidays; he had done Mauly a service, and for that reason his long-suffering lordship felt bound to stand the fat and fatuous Owl. If Bunter decided to accompany the party to Egypt, Mauly felt that he could not say him nay.

For which reason his friends were coming to the rescue, as it were. That happy description of the famous land of Egypt, which Bunter supposed that he had overheard by chance, seemed to have worked the oracle.

Billy Bunter, evidently, was not attracted by a prospect of scorpions, lions, plagues, and burning heat like a furnace.

Bunter rolled away, leaving the juniors grinning. But as he reached the door Lord Mauleverer came into the armoury.

"Oh, here you are, you men," said Mauly. "Like to come along to the Egyptian Room and have a look at that jolly old scarab—the one that the Greek johnny is after, what?"

"Yes, rather, old bean," said Bob.

"I say, Mauly——" Billy Bunter planted himself in front of Lord Mauleverer, and fixed his eyes, and his spectacles, on the schoolboy earl's surprised face. "I've got a bone to pick with you. Never mind the scarab now—just listen to me."

"Yaas," sighed Lord Mauleverer.

"I hear that you're going to Egypt for the hols."

"Yaas."

"Well, I think it's rot!"

"Yaas."

"I came here," said Bunter accusingly, "expecting to pass the vacation here. It's not quite up to the style of Bunter Court; but I could be comfortable here. Still, if you want a change, I suggest Margate."

"Yaas."

"I dare say you don't know much about Egypt, Mauly, but it's frightfully hot, packed with scorpions, and there are plagues and famines, and all sorts of things. Well, give it a miss, old chap, see?"

"Yaas—I mean, no!" said Lord Mauleverer. "You see, my uncle's going to Egypt, while my aunt's in Switzerland, to look after an estate he's got in the—the—the—the what's-its-name——"

"The Fayyum!" grinned Bob Cherry.

"Yaas, that's it! Well, I'm goin' with him, and my friends are comin' with me, and if you'd like to come, Bunter——"

"Well, I wouldn't!" said Bunter emphatically.

Lord Mauleverer brightened up.

"Begad! Mean that, Bunter?" he asked.

"Yes, I jolly well do! You'd better give it a miss," said Bunter. "I tell you plainly that if you go to Egypt for the hols you lose my company."

"Oh gad!" ejaculated Lord Mauleverer.

"I mean it!" said Bunter emphatically. "So there you are, Mauly! I'll stay here with you, or I'll come to Margate, or Blackpool. But I jolly well won't go to Egypt, and that's flat!"

"Look here, Bunter, you can't let us down, old man!" said Bob Cherry, shaking his head.

"Rats to you!" said Bunter. "Now, then, Mauly, yes, or no? Are you going?"

"Yaas."

"In that case," said Bunter, with dignity, "I consider that you've let me down, and I'm done with you. I shall go to Margate. You can lend me a car to get to Margate, I suppose?"

"Why not phone home for your pater's Rolls?" asked Bob.

"You shut up, Cherry! Look here, Mauly——"

"My dear chap, I'll lend you a car with pleasure," said Lord Mauleverer, with alacrity. "I'll tell Watson to land you right on the pier at Margate."

"Well, that's all right," agreed Bunter. "But there's one more thing. Owing to coming away with you to look after you, you know, I haven't been home, and I'm short of tin. I think you might lend me a fiver—I mean a tenner—till I get a remittance from Bunter Court."

"Any old thing," said Lord Mauleverer.

"Thanks!" said Bunter carelessly, as his lordship opened a remarkably well-filled notecase, and a banknote changed hands. "I'll settle this later, Mauly."

"The latefulness will probably be terrific," murmured Hurree Jamset Ram Singh.

"You shut up, Inky! No good my sending this back by post, if you're going to Egypt," said Bunter thoughtfully. "I'll leave it over till next term at Greyfriars, Mauly."

"Yaas."

"And I hope you'll enjoy the plagues and scorpions," added Bunter sarcastically, as he rolled back to the armchair.

"Yaas."

Lord Mauleverer left the armoury with the Famous Five. The Greyfriars fellows might have been looking forward to enjoying the plagues and scorpions, judging by their smiling faces. Lord Mauleverer seemed quite bucked. His lordship glanced rather curiously at the Co. as they went along to the Egyptian Room.

"You men been pilin' it on about the jolly old scorpions and things?" he asked.

"Just a few," grinned Bob.

Lord Mauleverer chuckled.

"Bunter's goin' to make this trip to Egypt a jolly old success," he remarked.

"Eh—how?"

"By goin' to Margate."

"Ha, ha, ha!"

The ancient and mysterious land of Egypt had many attractions for the Greyfriars fellows. But there was no doubt that it seemed more than ever attractive, now that it was settled that Billy Bunter was going to Margate.

THE FIFTH CHAPTER.

The Face at the Window!

HARRY WHARTON & CO. looked round with keen interest in the Egyptian Room at Mauleverer Towers. They had seen the room before on previous visits to Mauly's home without much

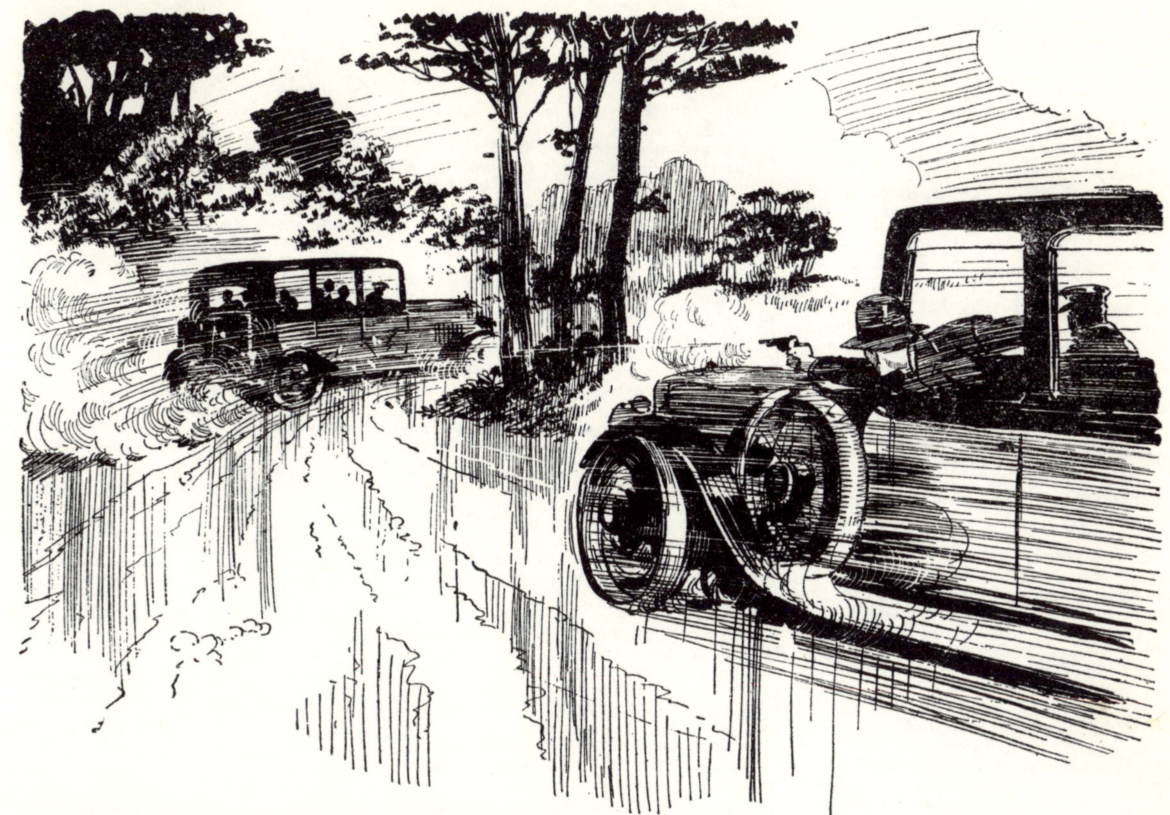

As the Rolls containing the Greyfriars juniors shot round the bend, the Greek, in the pursuing car, aimed for the tyres. Bang, bang, bang ! " The villain ! " breathed Wharton, as bullets spattered on the road under the Rolls as it tore on.

interest; but now that they were going to Egypt everything connected with that mysterious land had an attraction for them.

The late Lord Mauleverer, whom Mauly hardly remembered, had spent many years in the land of the Pharaohs, exploring ancient tombs and ruins, and he had brought home a great collection of Egyptian antiquities. There was a huge stone sarcophagus with a lid the juniors could hardly lift. There were swathed mummies which seemed rather creepy. There were rolls of papyrus covered with strange characters they could not read. There were old weapons and jewels and strange garments, and there were many specimens of the sacred scarab of the old Egyptians.

Mauly's uncle, Sir Reginald Brooke, was in the room when they came in, and the old baronet showed the chums of the Remove about the room, and explained many of the curios and antiquities to them, while Lord Mauleverer sat on the old sarcophagus and nobly forbore to yawn. His lordship had too many possessions to value them very highly. And probably he had given hardly a thought to the wonderful collection in the Egyptian Room.

But it was the Golden Scarab, the sacred scarabaeus of A-Menah, that chained the attention of the juniors. This scarab was kept in a special glass-topped case by itself, and the juniors gathered round to look at it rather eagerly. It was for the sake of that scarab that Konstantinos Kalizelos had travelled from Cairo. It was for that scarab that the Greek had attempted to kidnap Lord Mauleverer, for which attempt he was now being hunted by the police. It was obvious that some unknown value was attached to the golden beetle, though the juniors could not begin to guess what it was.

That it had an intrinsic value was clear, for it was formed of gold, and its eyes were two tiny diamonds. But the value of the metal and the stores could hardly have been more than thirty or forty pounds, and certainly did not account for the Greek's desire to possess it.

So far as the juniors could see, it was simply a beetle formed of solid gold, such as the ancient Egyptians wore as amulets to protect them, as they fancied, from evil fortune and the evil eye.

Strange hieroglyphics were engraved on the shining surface of the beetle's body, but what they meant, if they meant anything, the schoolboys had not the faintest idea. Egyptian lore had been left out of the curriculum at Greyfriars.

"So that's it," said Bob Cherry.

"That is it, my boy," said Sir Reginald Brooke, with a smile. "It is thousands of years old, like most of the things in this room. But why the man Kalizelos desires to possess it, is a mystery to me, unless"—he smiled again and shook his head—"unless he is a believer in an ancient and rather vague tradition, or perhaps I should say superstition, that the possessor of the scarab of A-Menah holds in his hand the key to a wonderful treasure."

"Oh, my hat! A clue to a treasure!" exclaimed Bob. "Are those queer marks on it the jolly old clue?"

Sir Reginald smiled again.

"No. Those queer marks, as you call them, are simply an inscription stating that the scarab belongs to A-Menah, who appears to have been a great man in Egypt in ancient days. I cannot read them myself, but I have a translation."

"Sort of name and address of the owner?" said Johnny Bull.

"Yes; nothing more."

"Then where's the jolly old clue?" asked Bob.

Sir Reginald laughed.

"There is no clue. It is simply, as I have said, an ancient superstition. I cannot believe that a keen and wily man like Kalizelos believes in such nonsense. Ignorant Egyptian fellaheen might believe that the scarab possesses some magic properties, but a Greek dealer of Cairo could hardly share such a belief. So his motive for seeking to get hold of the scarab is quite a mystery."

The baronet unlocked the case and lifted the scarab out.

It passed from hand to hand, the juniors examining it curiously.

The golden beetle was heavy, though hardly so heavy as they would have expected if the gold was solid. A fragment of a golden chain was still fastened to it, which had once passed round the dusky neck of an Egyptian tens of centuries ago. Except for the hieroglyphics which indicated the name and title of its ancient possessor there was nothing marked on it. How it could possibly furnish a clue to a treasure was unimaginable, unless, indeed, it was invested with some ancient magic which the Greyfriars fellows were not likely to believe. Yet it was certain that Kalizelos had spent money like water, and risked the prison gates closing upon him, to obtain possession of it. But they could hardly suppose that the wily Greek believed in magic.

"Anyhow, that sportsman is after it, like a jolly old dog after a bone," said Bob Cherry. "If he found out where it was kept he might drop in and borrow it, Mauly."

"This room is safely protected from burglars," said Sir Reginald. "There are many valuables here. But——"

"Hallo, hallo, hallo!" ejaculated Bob Cherry. "Look!" He pointed to the window into which the August sun was blazing.

A face was pressed to the glass.

The juniors stared almost spellbound at the dusky, olive face with the gleaming eyes of jetty black, that was pressed to the window-pane.

"The Greek!" shouted Wharton.

"Oh, my hat! Kalizelos!" exclaimed Lord Mauleverer, jumping up from the stone lid of the sarcophagus.

The juniors rushed to the window.

For an instant the Greek's black, scintillating eyes glittered at them through the glass, but before they reached the window the head outside disappeared.

Kalizelos was gone.

Sir Reginald Brooke quickly unlocked the window and opened it, and the juniors stared down. Beneath the window was thick, old ivy, which was swaying and rustling as the supple Greek slithered down. Even as they looked, he dropped to the ground and ran, and vanished round a corner of the building.

"After him!" shouted Bob.

The juniors dashed pell-mell out of the Egyptian Room and down the stairs. They tore out of the house, and rushed in the direction where the Greek had disappeared.

But Kalizelos had not lost a second, and he had vanished. Up and down the shrubberies the juniors hunted, but there was no sign of the man from Cairo.

The juniors' faces were grave as they returned to the house at last. Sir Reginald Brooke met them in the hall, and his face was also grave. The police were hunting for the Greek, yet it was certain that he was still at hand, haunting the vicinity of Mauleverer Towers, in the desperate hope of laying lawless hands on the scarab. There was no doubt that he had seen it in the hands of the schoolboys when his dark face was pressed to the window of the Egyptian Room. He was gone—but the thought was in every mind that he would return—that he was not done with yet—and it seemed to the chums of the Remove that a shadow of dark mystery and peril lay in the house—a shadow that fell from the mysterious East.

THE SIXTH CHAPTER.

Bunter, Too!

BILLY BUNTER grinned.

Sprawling in Mauly's most comfortable armchair, in Mauly's den, the fat Owl of Greyfriars was reading

Bunter was not much of a reading man, and when he did read, his taste ran, as a rule, to yellow-covered novels which described the weird adventures of amazing crooks and still more amazing detectives who popped up in the most unexpected way, in a different disguise every time. But on this occasion, Billy Bunter was reading a volume that contained information—which was not at all in his line. And he was grinning over it, as over a good joke, which was still more surprising.

The volume had an attractive coloured cover, showing a picture of the Sphinx, with an Arab mounted on a fiery steed in the foreground, and a pyramid in the background. It was entitled, "Why Not Egypt?"

That valuable volume was issued by a tourist firm in London, and it was crammed with information of the most attractive kind. "Chuck's Tours," it appeared, enabled you to see Egypt from the Delta to Wady Halfa without any trouble and almost without any expense, and the whole trip was a sheer delight from beginning to end. There was no mention of scorpions, lions, plagues, or famines. Even the heat was not mentioned. And Billy Bunter grinned as he blinked at attractive page after page. According to Messrs. Chuck, Egypt was more attractive than even Margate!

Since the trip to Egypt had been decided on, the chums of Greyfriars had been looking up the subject, and this was one of the volumes they had consulted. Now Billy Bunter was consulting it—with the result that he was making another change in his plans. It dawned on Billy Bunter's fat brain that his fat leg had been pulled—and he was no longer thinking of making the trip to Egypt a happy success by standing out of it!

There were voices and footsteps in the doorway, and Bunter hurriedly shoved the volume out of sight under the cushions on the chair. He blinked round as the Famous Five came in with Mauly.

"I say, you fellows!" grinned Bunter.

"Hallo, hallo, hallo! Off to Margate, old bean?" asked Bob.

"He, he, he!" Bunter rose from the chair, and blinked at the juniors. "I say, you fellows, I've changed my mind! Don't you worry, Mauly, old man—I'm coming with you, after all!"

"Oh, gad!"

"I've been thinking it over, you see," explained Bunter. "I saved your life at Greyfriars, Mauly——"

"Oh dear!"

"And I came home with you for the hols, to keep an eye on you, old chap, and watch over your safety, as you know——"

"Give us a rest, old chap!"

"And I'm not going to desert you," said Bunter, shaking his head. "I never was the man to let a pal down. Rely on me to see you through in Egypt, Mauly."

Lord Mauleverer suppressed a sigh. Harry Wharton & Co. gazed at the fat and grinning Owl.

"Don't forget the scorpions, old fat man," said Bob.

"I rather like scorpions," said Bunter.

"Oh, my hat! And the mosquitoes, and——"

"No worse for me than for you fellows!" grinned Bunter.

"And the lions——"

"It's chiefly the lions that have made me decide to come," explained Bunter calmly. "You fellows will be in danger. Well, you'll get funky. You'll need a fellow with some pluck to see you through. That's where I come in."

"Oh crikey!"

"There was a terrific famine in Egypt once," said Bob. "If there should be another——"

"That's all right. I shall set you fellows an example by keeping a stiff upper lip, you know."

"Better think again, old fat bean," said Johnny Bull.

"I've thought it out," said Bunter. "If there's danger, well—I like danger; you know my pluck! If there's hardships, I'm the fellow to rough it, without grousing, and keep your courage up for you by my example. I don't expect a lot of pleasure from this trip—feeling responsible for the lot of you, and all that! But I feel it my duty to stick to you. Duty comes first, you know—I always was a whale on duty! Selfish fellows like you would hardly understand—but that's how it is! You can rely on me, Mauly! I'm sticking to you like glue, old chap!"

"Yaas," groaned Lord Mauleverer. "I was afraid it was rather too good to be true——"

"What?"

"I—I mean, it's all right!"

"Look here, Mauly——"

"Is that nunky callin' me?" asked Mauly, and he walked out of the armoury and disappeared.

Billy Bunter grinned at the Famous Five. Even Bunter could not suppose that the Greyfriars fellows were bucked by the news that he was sticking to them, after all. But that was a trifle light as air to William George Bunter. Bunter was not going to be left out, and so far as the fat Owl could see, that was all that mattered.

"So you're not going to Margate, after all?" said Bob.

"He, he, he! No!"

"You feel safe here?" asked Bob.

"Eh?"

"That Greek blighter is hanging about——"

"He, he, he!"

"Shouldn't wonder if he came butting in some dark night after the scarab," said Johnny Bull.

"He, he, he! If he does, leave him to me!" said Bunter. "He scares you fellows stiff, but I'll handle him all right. The fact is, I shouldn't feel that you fellows would be safe if I went. In the circumstances, I feel bound to protect you. Rely on me!"

"You fat idiot!"

"Yah!"

Billy Bunter rolled out of the room and shut the door after him. The Famous Five looked at one another.

"The fat villain's tumbled to it, somehow, that we were pulling his leg!" growled Johnny Bull. "If he really believed there was any danger, he would be off to Margate like a shot."

"It's too bad!" grunted Bob Cherry. "Mauly's rather an ass to stand it. We ought to think of some way of rescuing him from Bunter."

"My esteemed and idiotic chums," murmured Hurree Jamset Ram Singh, with a glimmer in his dusky eyes, "the dangerfulness is not terrific, but the estimable Bunter is a preposterous funk. Suppose——"

"Go it, Inky!" said Bob hopefully.

"Suppose a fierce and ferocious desperado should break into the idiotic Bunter's room in the deadliness of night——"

"What the thump!" said Harry Wharton. "If Kalizelos came here, he would make for the Egyptian Room, after the scarab. He wouldn't bother about Bunter."

"But if the excellent Bob were to borrow some of the Egyptian costumes from Mauly's idiotic collection, and black his face with some absurd blacking——"

"Ha, ha, ha!" yelled Bob.

"And enter the absurd Bunter's room with a scimitar or a yataghan, in his ridiculous hand——"

"Ha, ha, ha!"

"Good egg!"

"I'm on!" chuckled Bob Cherry. "We'll try it on this evening. If that fat villain fancied there was any danger, he would be off to Margate as fast as petrol could carry him. And if a ferocious Egyptian barges into his room, and——"

"Ha, ha, ha!"

With grinning faces, the chums of the Remove proceeded to discuss the details of the plot.

Outside the door of the armoury another fellow was grinning.

It was Billy Bunter!

His fat ear was glued to the keyhole.

Bunter had been rather interested to hear what the fellows might be saying after he was gone. He found what they were saying unexpectedly interesting!

There was a fat grin on his face as he rolled away.

THE SEVENTH CHAPTER.

Bold Bunter!

"I SAY, you fellows——"

"Hallo, hallo, hallo!"

"I'm going up to my room to write some letters."

"Oh!"

"Don't disturb me," said Bunter.

"Oh!"

The Famous Five exchanged glances as the fat Owl departed.

It was evening, and Billy Bunter had been resting for some time in an arm-chair; he needed a rest after the dinner he had packed away. Now, with the announcement that he had letters to write, he rolled off to his room.

Bob Cherry chuckled.

"Couldn't be better!" he murmured.

Really Billy Bunter seemed to be playing into the hands of the plotters, as if to afford them an opportunity of carrying out the "wheeze" that had been evolved by the active brain of the Nabob of Bhanipur.

That wheeze was the last chance of making Bunter come "unstuck," which was a consummation devoutly to be wished.

For Mauly's sake, if not for their own, the Famous Five felt that it was up to them.

Garments borrowed from the Egyptian collection, and a bottle of liquid blacking, were already in Bob Cherry's room. Only an opportunity was needed, and Bunter was providing it!

There was no doubt, in the minds of the juniors, that if a fearful-looking black man established contact with Billy Bunter, the fat Owl would be convinced that one of Kalizelos' gang was after him; and if Bunter believed that, there was not the slightest doubt that he would make for the safety of Merry Margate at the earliest possible moment. Now was the time!

Lord Mauleverer was in the library with his uncle, discussing details of the trip to Egypt. His lordship had been told nothing of the little scheme; the Famous Five were doing good by stealth, as it were.

"Come on!" said Bob, when Bunter was gone. "Fairly asking for it, isn't he? Thoughtful of him to give us a chance like this, what?"

"Ha, ha, ha!"

The Famous Five ascended the stairs and entered the corridor on which all the rooms of the juniors opened.

They tiptoed past Bunter's door.

Light glimmered from under that door, and they could hear the fat Owl moving within.

Silently they reached Bob Cherry's room and lost no time in getting to business.

Four grinning juniors helped to make Bob up. The result was undoubtedly startling.

In a long djibbah, sandals, and a turban, and with his face blacked, Bob did not perhaps look much like a genuine Egyptian; but he certainly looked a fearful and dangerous character, whom no one would have wanted to meet alone on a dark night.

He surveyed his reflection in the glass and chuckled.

"My hat! Blessed if I should like to meet myself, got up like this, in a lonely place!" he remarked.

"Ha, ha, ha!"

"Bunter will alarm the whole house when he sees you!" grinned Nugent. "Never mind, if he starts for Margate in the morning."

"The startfulness for esteemed and merry Margate is the sine qua non," remarked the Nabob of Bhanipur.

"Well, we're ready," said Harry Wharton. "Come on!"

He opened the door quietly and glanced into the corridor. Suppressing sounds of mirth, the Famous Five crept along on tiptoe to Bunter's door.

From within came a familiar sound to which the juniors were accustomed in the Remove dormitory at Greyfriars.

Snore!

Bunter, apparently, had fallen asleep over his letters—if he really had gone to his room to write letters.

Snorrrrrre!

"Quiet!" murmured Bob, and he opened the door and looked in.

Billy Bunter was seated in an arm-chair, with his eyes shut and his mouth open, snoring peacefully. The juniors grinned as they looked at him.

There was no sign of letter-writing! Apparently Bunter had gone to sleep instead. As a matter of fact, little as the juniors guessed it, the sly Owl had been deliberately giving them an opportunity to "get on with it," and he had fallen asleep while waiting for them to butt in.

Bob stepped into the room.

In the bright electric light he looked a fearsome figure. Four juniors clustered outside the door, which was left ajar.

Snore!

A sudden, fearful yell, close to his fat ear, awakened Billy Bunter. The snore ceased, and his little round eyes opened behind his big round spectacles.

He blinked at the fearsome black man, and for a moment his eyes bulged. But it was only for a moment.

Instead of leaping up, with a howl of terror, Bunter sat where he was, blinking at the fearful apparition.

He was quite calm.

"Ha! Dog of a Faringhee!" exclaimed the black man in a deep, throaty voice. "I have found thee!"

Billy Bunter groped behind him in the chair.

The next moment the black man had the surprise of his life.

According to programme, the fat Owl ought to have been scared out of his podgy wits, and the juniors expected him to bolt from the room in a state of frantic funk.

But somehow the plot did not go according to programme.

Bunter's fat hand came swiftly from behind him, and there was a large, fat, juicy orange in it.

Whiz!

Crash!

Bunter was not a good marksman, but the range was too short for even Bunter to miss.

The orange crashed in Bob Cherry's eye, and he staggered back, taken quite by surprise, and sat down with a bump.

"Oh!" he gasped.

The next instant Bunter sprang from the chair.

But he did not bolt for the door yelling with terror. He jumped at the fearsome black man.

Thump, thump!

A fat fist crashed on Bob Cherry's blackened nose and another on his chin. The hapless japer went over on his back.

Thump, thump, thump, thump!

"Ow! Oh, my hat!" yelled Bob, forgetting that he was a black man. "Oh crumbs! You potty porpoise! Yarooooh!"

Billy Bunter's fat fists were crashing on him with terrific vim. Right and left the fat Owl thumped and thumped, and Bob rolled and roared.

He scrambled away and leaped to his feet. As he did so, Bunter seized a poker from the fireplace and a water-jug from the washstand; then, leaping on his bed, he faced Bob again.

"Oh crikey!" gasped Bob. "Keep off, you potty idiot!"

Bunter swiped again with the poker, and Bob leaped away just in time. Evidently something had gone wrong with the plot. So far from being in a funk, Billy Bunter was handling the situation in a really masterly way. Apparently he was not afraid of a black man.

He followed Bob up as he retreated, still swiping with the poker. Bob Cherry jumped and dodged like a kangaroo.

"Oh, my hat!" gasped Harry Wharton in amazement.

"Yaroooh!" roared Bob, as the poker landed. "Keep off, you fat villain! Keep that poker away, you podgy maniac! Yoooop!"

Swipe!

Harry Wharton threw the door open, and Bob dodged out into the passage. Bunter followed on.

A swipe of the poker, perhaps by accident, caught Harry Wharton, and he roared. Another swipe elicited a frantic howl from Johnny Bull.

"Look out, you silly owl!" gasped Nugent.

"I say, you fellows, collar him!"

shouted Bunter. "Hold him while I brain him with this poker——"

"Oh crikey!"

"It's one of that gang, you know—Kalizelos' gang!" yelled Bunter. "Don't let him get away!"

"Oh crumbs!"

"Look here, you fat chump——"

"Come on!" roared Bunter, charging down the passage after Bob Cherry, brandishing the poker.

"Keep off!" shrieked Bob. "You silly owl—— Oh, my hat! Oh crumbs! Oh, Jehosophat!"

Spipe, swipe!

A poker, at close quarters, was quite unpleasant. Bob Cherry dodged frantically, and fairly bolted down the passage. After him rushed Bunter, still swiping, leaving the rest of the Co. staring after him, almost babbling with amazement.

"Will you keep off?" shrieked Bob. "You silly Owl, you'll be braining me next! I tell you—— Yaroooop!"

He jumped away from the poker again on the landing, missed his footing, and rolled down the stairs.

"I say, you fellows, back up!" yelled Bunter, and he plunged down the staircase after the hapless Bob.

Bob Cherry did the stairs in record time. At the foot of the stairs he sat up, gasping for breath. Porson and James and John came up, staring in amazement at the black man in a tangled djibbah, with his turban hanging down over one ear and disclosing a mop of flaxen hair such as no black man had ever been known to possess. The library door opened, and Sir Reginald Brooke and Lord Mauleverer came out in haste.

"What——" ejaculated the old baronet in astonishment.

"A black man!" gasped Porson.

"A jolly old nigger!" gasped Lord Mauleverer. "Here, collar him!"

Bunter came hurtling down the stairs, poker in hand.

"Leave him to me!" roared Bunter. "I can handle him! Leave him to me, Mauly! I'll brain him——"

"Yarooooh!"

Bob Cherry squirmed frantically away. The poker crashed on the floor a foot from him as he squirmed.

"Good gad!" exclaimed Sir Reginald. "What——"

"Collar him!" panted Mauleverer.

James and John hurled themselves on the black man. They grasped him by either arm. Bunter aimed with the poker, and the black man yelled wildly:

"Keep that fat maniac off! I'm not a nigger, you silly asses, I'm Bob Cherry! Keep him off!"

"Oh gad!" gasped Lord Mauleverer. He pushed Bunter back. "Go easy with that poker, old fat man!"

"I'm going to brain him——"

"Keep him off, will you?" yelled Bob.

The Co. came running down the stairs, amazed, dismayed, and disconcerted. Harry Wharton jerked the poker away from Bunter. That poker had done damage enough—in fact, a little too much. Sir Reginald Brooke surveyed the discomfited juniors rather sternly.

"You may release that boy," he said to James and John. "He is quite unrecognisable, but I know his voice. Cherry, what does this mean?"

"Oh crikey!" gasped Bob. "I've got a dozen bumps——"

"It—it—it was a lark!" gasped Wharton. "It's only Bob, got up as a darkey to scare Bunter——"

"Not so jolly easy to scare me," said Billy Bunter disdainfully.

"Absurd!" said Sir Reginald, and he went back to the library.

"So it's you, is it, Bob, old chap?" said Bunter. "Of course, I never knew it was you! Did you think you could scare me? He, he, he!"

"You fat villain!" roared Bob. "You jolly well knew it was me, or you'd have been scared stiff——"

"Oh, really, Cherry——"

"And I'll jolly well——"

Bob Cherry made a stride towards the grinning fat Owl. A good many swipes from the poker had reached him, and he was feeling hurt.

Lord Mauleverer pushed him back, grinning.

"Hold on, old bean," he grinned. "You asked for it, you know!"

Billy Bunter curled a fat lip.

"So it was a trick, was it?" he said, with lofty scorn. "You fancied you could frighten me—as if I'm a fellow to be frightened! You've known me long enough to know that pluck's my long suit! Of course, I never knew it was Cherry—I never heard the fellows talking it over in the armoury, and hadn't the faintest idea that they were playing tricks. You fellows will have to think of something better than this, if you want to frighten me! He, he, he!"

Billy Bunter rolled away, with his fat little nose in the air. The Famous Five looked at one another with sickly looks. It was a ghastly frost, and the fat Owl had scored all along the line!

Harry Wharton & Co. retreated up the stairs, leaving Porson and James and John grinning, and Lord Mauleverer chuckling. And Billy Bunter grinned after them, as they went, with a fat and triumphant grin.

THE EIGHTH CHAPTER.

In Merciless Hands!

LORD MAULEVERER came into his room, after saying good-night to his friends in the corridor.

There was a thoughtful expression on Mauly's face. That evening, while the Famous Five amused themselves by knocking the balls about in the billiards-room, and Billy Bunter snoozed in an armchair while he waited for bed-time, Mauly had been occupied in a way rather unusual for his lazy lordship.

His father had been, in his younger days, a famous explorer in the strange land of Egypt, and an enthusiastic Egyptologist, as the collection in the Egyptian Room at the Towers showed. Many of the late earl's notes and journals were still in existence, kept in a cabinet in the Egyptian Room, and Mauly had often intended to go through them, though, as a matter of fact, he had never done so. But this evening he had sorted out the old papers, and looked out the references to the Golden Scarab of A-Menah.

Until Kalizelos came on the scene, Lord Mauleverer had given little thought to the sacred scarabaeus, but of late his thoughts had rather concentrated on it. And he had read with great keenness all that the late earl had written in his notes about it, and he had found the subject unexpectedly interesting. He was thinking of it when he came up to bed, and the Golden Scarab was in his pocket.

The August day had been hot, and the night was warm. Mauly crossed to the open window, which looked on the balcony that ran under the windows of all the rooms occupied by the Greyfriars party. The other fellows had gone to bed, and as Mauly stood looking out into the summer night, spangled with stars, the lights went out in the adjoining windows one by one.

From one of the rooms came the sound of a deep snore, showing that Billy Bunter was asleep, and Mauly smiled faintly. But the grave and thoughtful look returned to his face. He turned from the window at last, but he did not go to bed. He was not inclined for sleep. He took the Golden Scarab from his pocket, and laid it on the table, where the golden surface glimmered and gleamed in the electric light. He threw himself into a chair, his eyes on the metallic beetle.

What he had been reading on the subject was running in his mind, and in the silence of the night he seemed to feel the strange and mysterious spell of Egypt upon him.

The golden beetle that lay gleaming under his eyes, bright and undimmed, could have told many strange tales. It had belonged to A-Menah, a great soldier of the reign of Rameses the Second, who was Pharaoh in Egypt thirteen centuries before the beginning of the Christian era.

A-Menah, in those ancient days, had gone forth to war with his Lord Rameses, and fought against the Hittites in Asia Minor, with sharp sword and twanging bow in a charging chariot, drawn by two fiery steeds, with the charioteer by his side.

More than three thousand years had passed since A-Menah, under the banner of the Pharaoh, had darted his arrows at the fierce Hittites on the plains of Syria, in the forgotten battles of Kadesh. Yet, when he stood in his war-chariot, shooting fiery arrows over the plumed heads of his plunging horses, laying the Hittites low, he had worn the Golden Scarab as an amulet, to keep off evil fortune—and it had looked the same in the eyes of that fierce old Egyptian, as it looked to Lord Mauleverer now. All things else were changed, but the glimmering golden beetle was unchanged.

And A-Menah, as Lord Mauleverer had learned from his father's papers, had brought home a treasure from the war—a wonderful diamond that was called the Eye of Osiris, from its size and brilliance and immense value.

And the tradition existed, traced out in the picture-writing on ancient papyrus, that whoever possessed the Golden Scarab of A-Menah, should surely possess that great treasure, the Eye of Osiris.

Was it that tradition that caused the wily Greek of Cairo to seek the sacred scarab? Thinking it over in the quiet of the night with his mind full of Egyptian lore, it did not seem so improbable to Mauleverer now. Was there some strange secret in that glimmering golden object under the electric light that would guide the one who possessed it to the discovery of the Eye of Osiris—the wonderful diamond which had been lost to human knowledge when the mummy of A-Menah was swathed in fine linen and laid in a sarcophagus in the heart of a towering pyramid?

Mauleverer wondered.

He could not read the pictured inscription engraved on the scarab; but he had the translation, which told nothing but that the sacred beetle had belonged to A-Menah, great and glorious in war, servant of the thrice-glorious Rameses, Pharaoh of Egypt and Lord of Syria, slayer of the Hittites.

In those strange hieroglyphics there was no clue. Then in what way could the golden beetle guide its possessor to the discovery of the Eye of Osiris? Unless, indeed there was truth in ancient tales of Egyptian magic?

Somehow, as Mauleverer sat gazing at the gleaming beetle, he did not smile at the thought. His thoughts were back in dim past ages—before the Christian era—before the Roman Empire had been thought of—before Alexander marched out of Macedon—the dim, dim past,

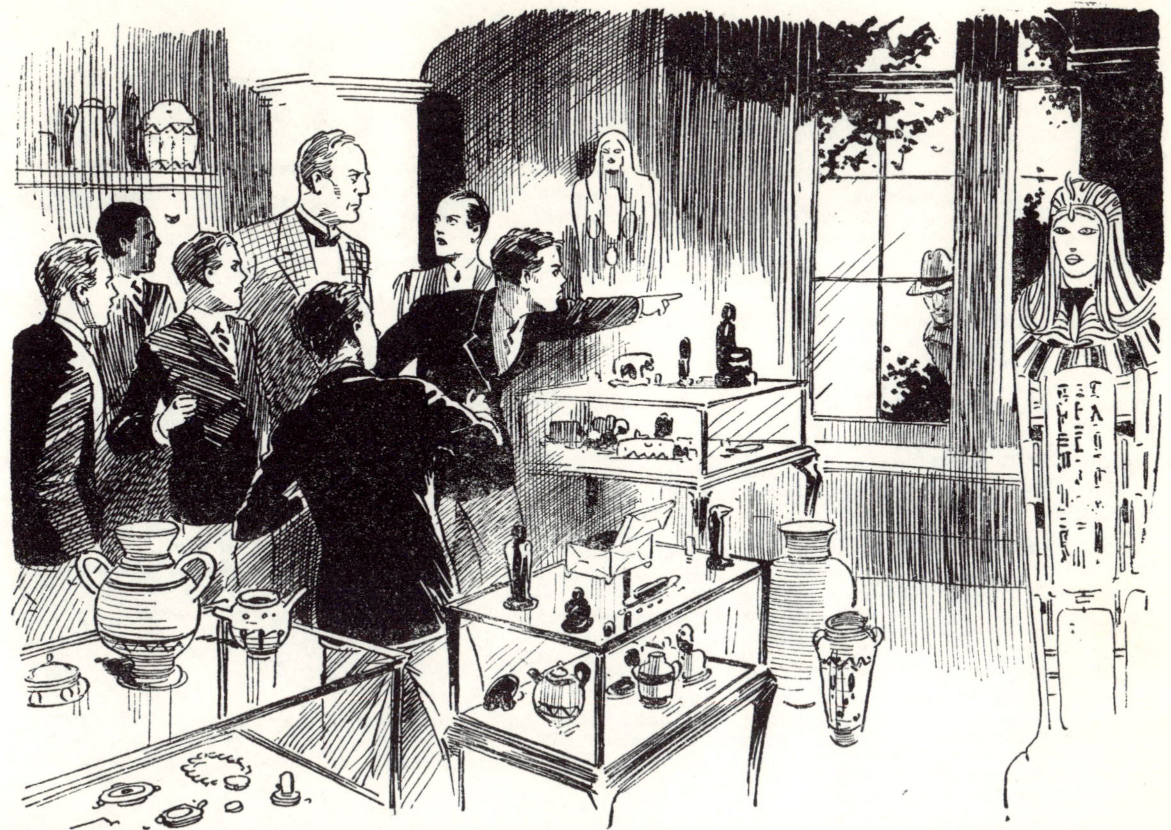

" Hallo, hallo, hallo ! " ejaculated Bob Cherry, suddenly pointing to the window. " Look ! " Sir Reginald Brooke and the Greyfriars juniors stared, spellbound, at the dusky, olive face pressed to the window-pane. " The Greek ! " shouted Harry Wharton.

when England had been a savage island, and Egypt a great and powerful kingdom—when the Sphinx first looked out over the sands of the desert, and the great Pyramids were a-building. Strange things had happened in those strange old days.

There was a faint sound in the silent room.

Mauleverer did not heed it.

From a screen that stood by the bed a dark, olive-skinned face looked out and two jetty black eyes glittered at the schoolboy earl.

Mauleverer did not turn his head.

With the stealthy tread of a cat, the supple Greek crossed to the door, behind the half-dreaming schoolboy, and turned the key in the lock.

The faint click of the key caught Mauleverer's attention, and he started. He glanced round, and sprang to his feet, as he saw the olive face and glittering eyes of the Greek.

For a second his heart leaped. Then he was calm again. His hand closed over the golden scarab on the table as he faced the man from Egypt.

The Greek smiled—a smile that was tigerish.

"Silence, my lord!" he said, in his low, musical voice. "I have locked the door and help cannot come. It is death to call!"

Lord Mauleverer breathed hard.

He had been half-dreaming, dreaming of old Egypt. Now he came back at a bound to reality. He knew that he was in danger—deadly danger. But he was cool as ice as he watched the man from Cairo.

The soft summer breeze played in at the open window from the balcony. Mauleverer realised, only too clearly, that he had been careless. Evidently the Greek had climbed to the balcony and concealed himself in the room, to wait for Mauleverer—to deal with him alone where his friends could not help him.

Mauleverer did not call out. The Greek was within reach of a spring, and he was ready to spring like a tiger, and there was no chance of help coming in time.

The black eyes blazed with triumph at the cool, steady face of the schoolboy earl.

"What do you want here?"

Lord Mauleverer spoke calmly.

Kalizelos showed his gleaming white teeth.

"You can guess, my lord! I have waited and watched! I hid myself here—for you—to force you at the point of my dagger, to lead me to the golden scarab and place it in my hands. But I have been more fortunate than I hoped. The scarab is here. You need not cover it with your hand, my lord—I have seen it. I know that it is the scarab of A-Menah. Give it to me!"

Lord Mauleverer's hand tightened on the golden beetle.

The Greek came a step nearer.

"I have learned many things, my lord, while I have watched and waited, and I have spies in my service," he said. "I know of your lordship's intended visit to Egypt. Fool! Did you think that, with the scarab in your hand, you might find the treasure that has been hidden from all eyes since Rameses was on the throne of Egypt?"

Mauleverer started.

That thought had not been in his mind; but it was a natural suspicion on the part of the Egyptian Greek.

"That wasn't the idea, Mr. Kalizelos!" answered Mauleverer. "My friends and I are goin' to Egypt just for a holiday."

"You think you can deceive me so easily?" sneered the Greek.

Mauleverer shrugged his shoulders.

"Honest Injun, dear man," he answered. "But now you've put the idea in my head, by Jove, I'll take the jolly old scarab along with me, and put in for the treasure. Thanks for the tip!"

The Greek stared at him searchingly.

"You had not thought of it?" he asked.

"Not till now!" smiled Mauleverer.

"And now——"

"Now I'm takin' the tip, as I've said."

Kalizelos laughed mockingly.

"Even if you could escape me now, my lord, and keep the scarab, do you dream that it would guide you to the treasure?"

"Why not, as well as another?" asked Mauly. "It's a sportin' chance, anyhow."

The Greek laughed again.

"From your words, my lord, it is plain that you do not dream of the secret of the scarab—that it is hidden from your eyes," he said. "Here or in Egypt, the scarab will tell you nothing."

"But you fancy it might tell you somethin'?" asked Lord Mauleverer, watching the man curiously.

"I know the secret, my lord," said Kalizelos coolly. "In my antique shop in Cairo, many thousands of old papyri have passed through my hands—and I am skilled in reading the pictured writing of the old Egyptians. There came into my hands a papyrus, written by a scribe at the order of the soldier

(*Continued on page* 16.)

HIGH JINKS I

By DICKY NUGENT.

I.

MR. I. JOLLIWELL LICKHAM, the Fourth Form master at St. Sam's, rushed into Dr. Birchemall's study with a startled eggspression on his dial.

"Sir," he gasped, boughing respectively before the Head's desk, "a most eggstraordinary thing is happening in the quad. A four-horse break has just rolled up the carriage-drive, and is now standing in front of the Skool House. The driver says you ordered it, which, as Euclid remarked, is abserd!"

"Shakespeare, you mean, Lickham, not Euclid. I'm serprized at your ignorance!" said Dr. Birchemall, the stately and skollerly Head of St. Sam's. "Anyway, my dear fellow, the driver is right. I did order it. Have you forgotten that to-day is the day when we start our summer hollerdays?"

"But we don't need a break for our summer hollerdays, do we?" asked Mr. Lickham, in serprize.

The Head larfed.

"Of corse we do, idjut!" he said in his most refined manner. "This is the day when we break up, so, natcherally, I have ordered a break up. See?"

Mr. Lickham grinned.

"I see, sir! Well, let's hoap now you've got the break up that it won't break down. By the way, sir, if I mite be so personal, where are you spending the vack this year?"

Dr. Birchemall coffed and eyed the master of the Fourth with a somewhat fishy eye.

"I'm glad you mentioned that, Lickham," he said. "I had forgotten to tell you before. I've decided to axxept your invitation and stay with you."

Mr. Lickham recoiled, as from a blow.

"Look here, sir——" he eggsclaimed.

Dr. Bichemall smiled.

"Say no more, Lickham! I know how you feel about it. You are overwhelmed with gratitude—nacherally."

"But I'm not!" said Mr. Lickham. "That's just it, sir. What I was going to say was that I don't remember inviting you to stay with me."

Dr. Birchemall cullered furiously.

"Are you sujjesting that I made it up, then, Lickham?" he asked sharply.

"I dare say you did, sir," answered Mr. Lickham bluntly. "It's rather a habit of yours to axxept invitations that were never given when you've nowhere to go. But, anyway, you won't want to come with me. You see, sir, I'm spending my hollerday working on a fishing trawler."

"On a fishing trawler?" repeated Dr. Birchemall, agarst. "Surely you must be codding?"

"No, sir. We're catching mackerel, as it happens!" grinned Mr. Lickham. "I'm sure it's not the kind of hollerday you'd care for, sir."

"It certainly isn't!" snorted the Head. "I'm jolly glad the scales have fallen from my eyes in time. Under the sercumstances, I wouldn't spend the vack with you if you went down on your hands and neeze and begged me. Why, I'd rather go hiking with Jolly and his friends of the Fourth!"

"Why not, sir?" asked Mr. Lickham. "I gather that they're well supplied with dough."

The Head frowned.

"I wish you wouldn't be so slangy, Lickham. What you mean is not 'dough,' but 'oof.' That, of course, makes no difference to me. But it occurs to me that if they are rather flush with munny they ought to have some one of orthority to look after them. Perhaps, now I come to think about it, it is my duty to go with them."

"You'll have to walk, sir," pointed out Mr. Lickham.

"I'll have to do nothing of the kind!" retorted the Head. "What hiking there is to be done will be done by Jolly and his friends. Personally, I shall ride in a sedan chair. They can have the plezzure of carrying me."

"M-m-my hat!" gasped Mr. Lickham. "And where do you think you're going to obtain a sedan chair, sir?"

Dr. Birchemall larfed.

"As it happens, there is one very close at hand—in the skool museum, to be precise. Kindly trot along and get the porter to bring it out in front of the House, will you, Lickham? I must change into hiking clobber now. My mind is made up.

"'A-hiking I shall go,
Along with Jolly & Co.'

"I can foursee a really ripping hollerday for me now. Hurrah!"

And Dr. Birchemall, in his eggsuberence of spirits, performed a series of handsprings round the study while Mr. Lickham hurried off to the skool museum.

II.

"READY, you men?" asked Jack Jolly of the Fourth.

"Ready, I, ready!" replied Merry and Bright and Fearless, in corus.

"Then we'll make a start. Goodbuy, you fellows!" called out the leader of the Fourth to the crowd in the dormitory. "Hoap you all have a jolly good hollerday!"

"Same to you, old chap!"

Jack Jolly & Co. then quitted the dormitory, grinning all over their dials. They were going on a hiking toor for the first part of their holler-

WOULD YOU BELIEVE IT?

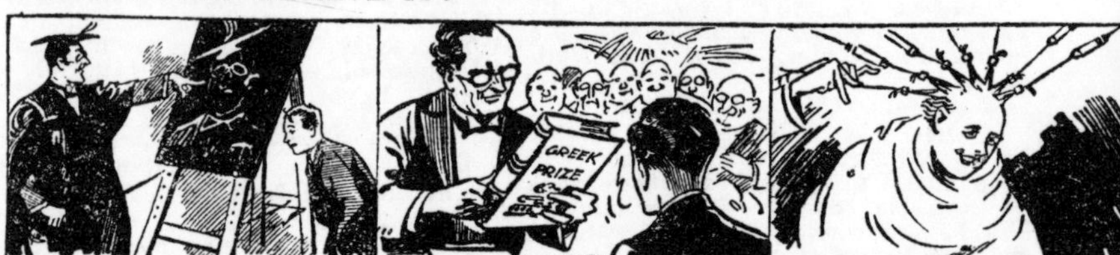

Harold Skinner is a clever caricaturist, and has often been in trouble through caricaturing Mr. Quelch on the blackboard!

Mark Linley, a giant at sport, is also a giant at Latin and Greek. He was admitted to Greyfriars as a Scholarship boy.

Anthony Treluce has been convicted of having a "permanent wave" in secret at a Courtfield hairdresser's.

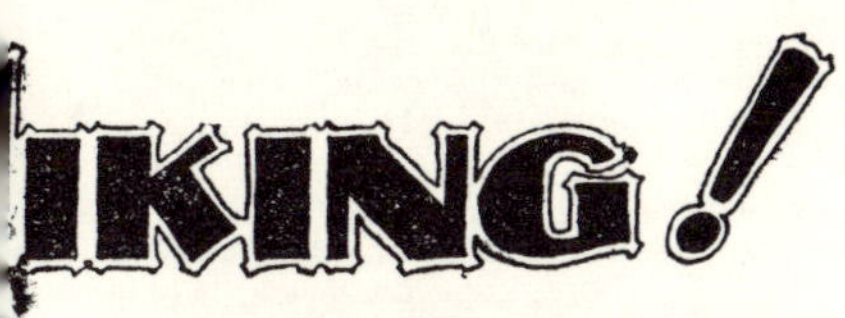

days, and they were keenly looking forward to it.

They were dressed in hiking shorts and open-necked shirts. And a fine, hansom quartet they looked as they tramped down the stairs on their way out of the Skool House, wissling as they went.

They stopped wissling and stared instead when they got outside the door of the Skool House.

The site that greeted their astonished eyes was enuff to make anybody stare. Drawn up at the bottom of the steps was a sedan chair that looked as if it dated back to the year dot. Seated in that sedan chair, dressed in hiking shorts, jersey, and the inevvitable mortar-board, and smirking at the passers-by, was no less a person than Dr. Birchemall!

"What the merry dickens——" gasped Jack Jolly & Co.

At that moment the Head spotted them.

"Hikers ahoy!" he bawled in his cultured voice. "Just making a start, boys?"

"Yes, rather, sir!" grinned Jack Jolly, as he and his pals crowded round the old-fashuned contrivance. "But what's the meaning of this? Are you preparing to take the part of Punch in a Punch and Judy show? If so, you ought to be a grate suxxess, for you're the most villainous-looking Punch I've ever seen!"

"Ha, ha, ha!"

"Silence!" bawled the Head, glaring indignantly at the historical Fourth-Formers. "Your wild guess is very wide of the mark, Jolly. You ought to know better than to suppose I should ever dessend to running a common Punch and Judy show. Selling peanuts or ice-cream—yes. But running a Punch and Judy show—never! The fact is, I am going hiking."

"Going hiking, with this portable drawing-room to carry about with you?" cride Jack Jolly. "Why, sir, you must be potty!"

Dr. Birchemall larfed—a somewhat sinnister larf.

"You are making a slite mistake, my dear Jolly. I don't intend to carry it myself. My intention is to be carried in it!"

"Did you say you were going hiking, or miking?" inquired Frank Fearless; and there was another yell from the Co.

"Ha, ha, ha!"

"Dashed if I see anything to larf at!" eggsclaimed the Head warmly. "I consider it's a jolly good wheeze to go hiking in a sedan chair. It cuts out that tiresome bizziness of walking!"

"Well, it may be a good wheeze from your point of view, sir," grinned Jack Jolly, "but the fellows who're going to carry you must be silly asses!"

Dr. Birchemall chuckled.

"You're quite right, Jolly, they are. Their names, as a matter of interest to you, are Jolly, Merry, Bright, and Fearless."

"Wha-a-at?"

It was a yell from the Co.—a yell of amazement and dismay.

"You are serprized," grinned the Head. "I had an idea, somehow, that you hadn't tumbled. Once you get over the first shock of serprize, of corse, you will be delited at the prospect of having me with you for your hiking toor."

But Jack Jolly & Co. didn't look a bit delited. All sorts of emotions were depicted in their dials, but the emotion of delite was conspikuous only by its absence.

"Suppose we refuse?" asked Jack Jolly rebelliously.

"In that case," answered the Head, stroking his beard reflectively, "I shall write your parents, informing them that, owing to mewtinous conduct on your part, I have been compelled to cansel your hollerdays and keep you swotting at St. Sam's."

"You—you——"

"Well, boys, if you're ready, we'll make a start!" said the Head briskly. "I sujjest you take one pole each. Keep your packs on your sholders—they will keep your backs straight! Squad, 'shun! Quick march!"

There was no help for it. Weather they wanted to do so or not, Jack Jolly & Co. simply had to take Dr. Birchemall with them now; even a hiking hollerday with the Head was better than a swotting hollerday at St. Sam's.

Muttering to themselves, the Fourth-Formers seezed their respective poles and heaved the sedan-chair off the ground. Two minnits later, accompanied by roars of larfter from the fellows in the quad, they were tramping through the gates on the first stage of their hiking toor!

III.

TRAMP-TRAMP! Tramp-tramp!

"Few!"

Jack Jolly & Co. were tired. They were also very hungry, despite the fact that they were fed-up to the teeth. The shades of nite were falling fast, a slite drizzle of rain had begun to drop, and the juniors were almost collapsing.

The only member of the party who remained cheerful was Dr. Birchemall. Inside his sheltered nook, he was humming blithely.

"'I'm happy when I'm hiking,
Trah-lah-lah-lah-lah——'"

All of a sudden, Dr. Birchemall poked his head out of the winder.

"Got any toffy, any of you?" he inquired. "If so, pass it to me immejately. If there's one thing I do hate, it's greediness. Give me the lot at once!"

Jack Jolly's eyes gleemed, as he drew a sticky mess out of his pocket.

"Here you are, sir!" he said, suddenly jamming it all over the Head's face. "I do hoap you'll like it, sir!"

"Ha, ha, ha!" yelled Fearless and Merry and Bright; while the Head gasped and spluttered furiously as he endevvered to scrape the sticky compound off his fizz.

"Bust you!" roared Dr. Birchemall, when he had recovered his powers of speech. "I wanted it to skoff, fathead, not to decorate my dial with! Any more nonsense like that, Jolly, and I shall make you rue the day you came out hiking with me! I'm tired of hiking for to-day, by the way. Stop at the most eggspensive hotel you can find, and we'll put up there for the nite!"

"Who's going to pay, sir?" inquired Frank Fearless.

Dr. Birchemall coffed.

"I'm afraid you'll have to, for the time being. I left my wad of tenners on the grand piano before I came out. You'll get it back after the hollerdays, my boys! Carry on!"

"Grate pip!"

"Well, if this isn't the giddy limmit!" said Frank Fearless, as they staggered forward once more. "Not content with foisting himself on us for the toor, the old buffer eggspects us to pay as well!"

(*Continued on page 27.*)

GREYFRIARS FACTS WHILE YOU WAIT

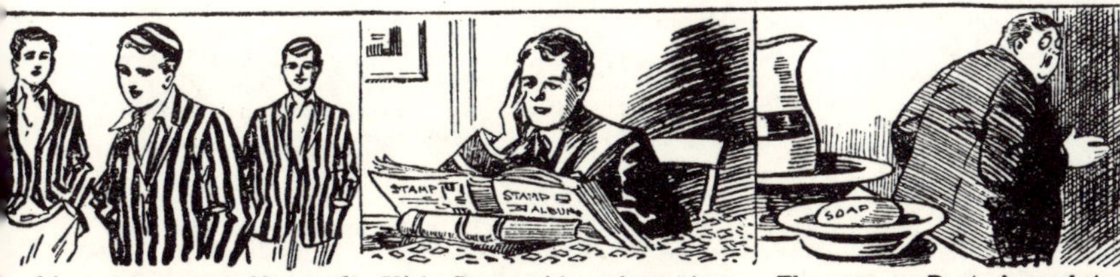

reyfriars colours are blue and hite. They were adopted at e foundation of the school in 1716.

Micky Desmond has a large stamp collection, and hopes some day to make a real "find."

The soap on Bunter's washstand in dorm. lasts six times as long as any other fellow's.

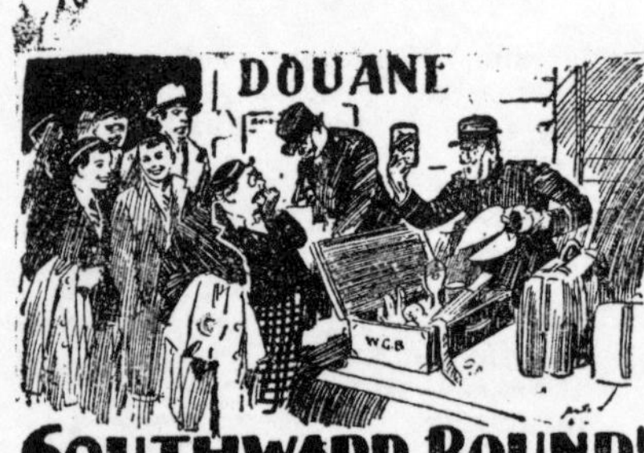

(*Continued from page* 13.)

A-Menah, to be given to his son Menarsis after his death. Whether it was placed in the hands of Menarsis or not I cannot say—but in that ancient scroll is written the secret of the scarab."

"Oh!" murmured Lord Mauleverer.

He understood now why the olive-skinned man had come from Cairo in search of the scarab.

"Tradition says that the possessor of the golden scarab will surely possess the Eye of Osiris, the diamond that was worth more than the fortune of a king in the days of the Pharaohs—that is worth a quarter of a million pounds in modern English money. And tradition says true, my lord, as I have learned from the scroll of the scribe employed by A-Menah three thousand years ago. When this knowledge came to me, I began at once to search for the scarab of A-Menah; I learned that it had fallen into the hands of your lordship's father, and that he had taken it out of the land of Egypt into his own country. That is why I am here."

"I see."

"Without the knowledge that I possess the scarab is valueless to you—it will tell you nothing. To me, knowing what I do, it is worth a quarter of a million pounds."

"And to me—if I hit on the secret!" said Lord Mauleverer.

"You will never find the secret, my lord, even if you keep the scarab. I should not have dreamed of it had I not read what was written in the papyrus. Give it me!"

The Greek came a step nearer.

"Your life, my lord, or a hundred lives, will not stand between me and riches beyond the dreams of avarice. Give me the scarab, and I go—leaving you unharmed. Sell it to me, and I will give you, as I told the fool Bunter, a thousand pounds in English money. But the scarab I will and must have!"

Lord Mauleverer smiled contemptuously.

He picked up the golden beetle and slipped it into his pocket. He faced the Greek, quietly, coolly, with steady eyes and clenched hands.

"Will you lose your life for that bauble, my lord?" said the Greek, between his teeth. "It has little value to you."

"If it had no value whatever it would make no difference," answered Lord Mauleverer coolly. "Do you think you can bully and frighten me, you rotter? If the scarab leads to a treasure, it may or may not lead me—but you won't get your thieving hands on it, at any rate."

The Greek's black eyes flashed.

"For the last time, Lord Mauleverer, I——"

"Chuck it!" said Mauleverer.

"Death, then!" hissed the man from Cairo, and with the spring of a tiger he leaped on the schoolboy earl.

Lord Mauleverer would have shouted for help as he grappled with the Greek. But the tigerish swiftness of the man from Egypt gave him no chance.

Sinuous fingers were on his throat, choking back the cry he would have uttered, and the schoolboy earl went to the floor, the Greek above him.

Mauly was strong and sturdy, and he struggled desperately, but he seemed like an infant in the hands of the wiry, muscular Greek.

The cruel fingers gripped his throat, silencing him; the black eyes blazed down at him, merciless as the glaring orbs of a lion of the Libyan Desert; and in those terrible moments the schoolboy earl of Greyfriars felt himself passing into the valley of the shadow of death!

THE NINTH CHAPTER.
In the Nick of Time!

BOB CHERRY turned his head on his pillow, grunted, and turned again, and sat up in bed.

Generally, Bob slept like a top. But he was not feeling as usual now. Swipes from a poker in a reckless hand were not trifles to be disregarded. Billy Bunter had wielded the poker not wisely, but too well. There were about a dozen bruises distributed over Bob; and he had more aches and pains than he was inclined to count.

Hurree Jamset Ram Singh's "wheeze" had been a frost, and the only outcome was to keep Bob from balmy slumber. And at last Bob gave up the attempt to sleep, and turned out of bed.

He wondered whether any of the other fellows were still awake. The hour was late, and the house was silent and still.

He threw a coat on over his pyjamas, slipped on a pair of slippers and opened his window. Then he looked out on the balcony.

Bob was a gregarious fellow, and he did not like staying up alone in the silent watches of the night. If the other fellows were asleep, however, he had no idea of awakening them; but he hoped that a walk up and down the balcony, under the summer stars, might make him more disposed to sleep.

He stepped from the french window of his room, and immediately became aware that one, at least, of his friends was still up. All the other windows were dark, but light streamed from Lord Mauleverer's window.

"Oh, good!" murmured Bob, relieved.

If old Mauly was sleepless, too, he would probably like a "jaw." Bob strolled along the balcony to Lord Mauleverer's room, and looked in through the open window.

As the light was burning he expected to see Lord Mauleverer out of bed, or perhaps sitting up in bed to read. But what he actually did see made him jump almost clear of the balcony.

For an instant he stared blankly, unable to believe his eyes which almost started from his head.

Lord Mauleverer was on his back on the carpet, and bending over him, gripping his throat with cruel, choking fingers, was the olive-skinned man from Egypt, Konstantinos Kalizelos, the Greek.

For one instant Bob was spellbound.

Then he woke to sudden action. Not a sound came from Mauleverer, the slim sinuous fingers choked him into silence. No sound came from the Greek as he bent to his murderous work. His black eyes blazed down ruthlessly. Not for a moment did the assassin dream that an interruption would come; and Mauleverer had no hope of it. But it came, and it came suddenly.

Bob Cherry came through the open window with a bound, and, before either the Greek or his victim knew that he was there, his clenched fist struck.

The blow, with all Bob Cherry's beef behind it, crashed into the handsome, olive face, and Kalizelos, with a startled cry, reeled sideways, and rolled on the floor.

Lord Mauleverer was released. The cruel grip was gone from his throat, and he gasped spasmodically for breath.

"Mauly!" panted Bob.

The Greek, taken by surprise as he was, and dazed by that terrific blow, was on his feet in an instant with the activity of a cat. His dark face was distorted with rage, and his dusky hand groped for a weapon. But Bob Cherry was on him in a twinkling. He drove his fist again into the Greek's face, sending him spinning, and Kalizelos crashed over, a dagger flying from his hand as he drew it out.

Lord Mauleverer scrambled breathlessly up.

"Oh, good man!" he gasped.

Bob's grasp was on the Greek, holding him down.

"Back up, Mauly!" he panted.

"Yaas, begad!" gasped Mauleverer.

Kalizelos struggled to his feet with Bob Cherry clinging to him. Lord Mauleverer had hold of him the next moment. The Greek's black eyes burned; the olive face was convulsed with fury. With a strength that few would have suspected to dwell in his slim, supple body he dragged himself to the window, the two juniors clinging to him and seeking to drag him down again. Bob Cherry shouted to his comrades as he struggled with the Greek. His powerful voice rang far and wide, and there was an answering shout along the balcony.

Help was coming!

But the Greek, with a frantic effort, tore himself loose from the grasping hands, and made a desperate spring from the window. He stumbled on the balcony and fell as Harry Wharton came speeding along from his window. He was up again in a second, and Wharton staggered back from a fierce blow. The next moment the Greek was scrambling over the rail of the balcony, and as Bob Cherry rushed at him he let go, and dropped into the shrubberies below.

"Bob," gasped Wharton, "what—who—what——"

"My esteemed Bob——"

Hurree Singh came racing up, followed by Nugent and Johnny Bull. All the Co. were awake now.

"It's the Greek!" panted Bob. "Kalizelos——"

There was a crashing in the shrubberies under the balcony. The fall was a long one. It seemed almost impossible that the falling man could have escaped without injury. The juniors rushed to the balustrade and peered over in the starlight.

"Look! There he is!"

"He's running!"

The Greek, hurt or not, was on his feet, and running. His lithe figure was visible for a moment in the starlight, and then it was gone. A faint sound of fleeing footsteps died away in the night.

THE TENTH CHAPTER.

Off to Egypt!

"MAULY, old man——"

"You're hurt!"

The chums of the Remove gathered anxiously about Lord Mauleverer. The schoolboy earl was rubbing his throat tenderly. The marks of the Greek's wiry fingers were only too plainly to be seen there. Mauly had had a narrow escape. And there was little doubt that Bob Cherry had saved his life.

His lordship smiled faintly.

"All serene, old beans!" he said. "Right as rain! I've had rather a jolt. That blighter meant business, by gad!"

"We'd better rouse the house, and get after him!"

Mauly shook his head.

"No good makin' a fuss now; he's gone. I fancy he's doin' about sixty in a car by this time."

Harry Wharton nodded. It was useless to pursue the Greek, now that he had escaped from their hands. Certainly he was not likely to linger.

"Besides, we shan't see him again—in this country," added Mauleverer. "I rather think we may see him on his own jolly old heath when we get to Egypt. Not here, I imagine."

"Why?"

"I've told him I'm taking the giddy scarab to Egypt with me," explained Mauleverer.

"Well, you were rather an ass to let him know that, old chap," said Nugent. "He will be climbing the pyramids after us."

"My dear man, he had guessed it," grinned Mauleverer. "He had the idea that we were goin' out to Egypt on account of the giddy scarab, and lookin' for jolly old A-Menah's treasure—see? So he would have been on our track in any case. He let out that he's come across an old papyrus, and learned from it the secret of the scarab—that's why he's after it."

Mauleverer took the golden scarab from his pocket, and held it up to the light, gleaming and glistening.

"He jolly nearly had it," he said. "He would have had it, but for you, Bob, old bean! And me, too! Determined beggar, you know! He says that the treasure is worth a quarter of a million pounds, in the shape of a diamond called the Eye of Osiris—wonderful old diamond that hasn't been seen for three thousand years, but was fearfully famous at one time. I've been readin' it up in my pater's papers. We're going to take the scarab with us, and put in for the treasure—what? That will make the trip a bit more excitin'."

"Yes, rather," agreed Bob. "But I'm blessed if I see how that beetle is going to show the way to the treasure, Mauly! It can't be anything but a superstition."

"Kalizelos doesn't think so—and he's a wily bird. Perhaps it's a jolly old magic beetle—sort of 'Open sesame.' stunt—what?" grinned his lordship. "The Greek's got it from a giddy ancient document, so he says—chapter and verse. He's willin' to risk his neck for the scarab. Looks as if there's somethin' in it."

The juniors looked curiously at the golden beetle. That there could be magical powers in the ancient amulet they did not, of course, believe. But, otherwise, it was unimaginable how the sacred scarab could possibly afford a clue to the vanished treasure of the days of Rameses II. But there was no doubt that they were keenly interested, and that the idea of a treasure-hunt among the pyramids and tombs of old Egypt attracted them.

"But there's one thing," added Lord Mauleverer gravely, "I'm up against that blighter Kalizelos, and I wouldn't let him have the scarab for love or money, if only to show him that a fellow can't be bullied. But he's a tough customer, and it means danger—not the jolly old tourist holiday that we were thinkin' of—but real danger. If you fellows don't like the idea——"

"Fathead!"

"I don't know whether I ought to let you men in for it," said Lord Mauleverer. "I'm rather keen on takin' the scarab along and puttin' in for the treasure. But if you'd rather not, I'll chuck the idea, and leave it stacked in the bank when we go—what?"

"I don't fancy any bank in England would keep it safe from Kalizelos," said Harry Wharton. "Banks can be burgled, Mauly, and ten to one the Greek would get hold of it sooner or later."

"Yaas, that's so. The only safe place for it is in a fellow's pocket," agreed Lord Mauleverer. "But you fellows can——"

"Fathead! We'll handle Kalizelos all right if he bothers us in Egypt!" said the captain of the Remove. "I fancy it's all bunkum about the treasure. Still, if there's a diamond worth a quarter of a million pounds knocking about, we'll pick it up——"

"Ha, ha, ha!"

"I'll rig a ribbon or somethin' on the thing, and wear it round my neck, like jolly old A-Menah used to, three thousand years ago," said Lord Mauleverer. "Might drop it out of my pocket."

"That's a good idea!"

"My esteemed and ridiculous chums," said Hurree Jamset Ram Singh. "A wheezy good idea has occurred to my ridiculous and debilitated brain——"

"Cough it up, Inky!"

"The absurd Kalizelos will be after the esteemed Mauly for the ludicrous scarab," said the nabob, "and if he should get his disgusting hands on him the scarab will be a goner! Suppose that the absurd article should be entrusted to the keeping of one of Mauly's execrable friends——"

"Inky, old man, you're a giddy jewel!" said Lord Mauleverer. "That's the bright idea! It would be rather a lark if the Greek johnny got hold of me, and when he got there the cupboard was bare—what?"

"Jolly good wheeze!" said Bob Cherry. "Even if the brute guesses that one of us is minding it, he couldn't guess which one. If you'll trust it out of your hands, Mauly——"

"Glad to!" answered Mauleverer. "Likely as not I should lose it—I'm always losin' things. Might lose anythin' knockin' about in Egypt—except Bunter! What offers?"

He held up the golden scarab.

It was decided that Wharton should take charge of the golden scarab. There was no doubt that it was safer in his hands, than in the careless hands of his lordship.

Wharton proceeded to tie a black silk ribbon to the golden beetle, where a chain had once been fastened to it, and he put the ribbon round his neck.

"This doesn't leave me, night or day," he said, "until we get back to England!"

"And if it leads to the giddy treasure, all we've got to do is follow in our father's footsteps!" chuckled Bob Cherry.

"Ha, ha, ha!"

The juniors went back to bed, but Bob Cherry remained in Lord Mauleverer's room for the rest of the night. Danger made little impression on Mauly's noble mind; but his friends decided for him that he was not to be left alone again at night, and his lordship submitted with his usual easy-going tolerance. And Bob looked very carefully to the fastenings of the window before he turned in.

But there was no fresh alarm. Indeed, the juniors had little doubt that Lord Mauleverer was right, and that now that the Greek was assured that the scarab would accompany them to Egypt, he would keep clear of Mauleverer Towers. But they were fully expecting to see the Greek again in the land of the Pharaohs; and they wondered, too, whether the lawless rascal would dog their steps on the journey.

But the chums of Greyfriars were quite confident that they could take care of themselves; and there was no doubt that the idea of hunting for the "Eye of Osiris" gave an added zest to the trip to the Nile.

A few more days and the Greyfriars party were ready to start, and the big car came round to carry them on the first stage of their journey.

Billy Bunter had a very thoughtful look that morning. For the last time the fat junior was debating in his mind the rival claims of Margate and Egypt. He decided in favour of Egypt—for a good reason. Mauly's tenner would not last long at Margate; but in Egypt Mauly would be a horn of plenty that would not run dry till the end of the holidays. So, though Bunter, as a matter of taste, preferred Margate, he settled on Egypt, and his fat person was packed into the car.

THE ELEVENTH CHAPTER.

Bunter Speaks French!

"VOUS n'avez rien à déclarer, messieurs?"

"Leave it to me," said Billy Bunter.

"Fathead!"

"You'd better leave speaking French to me, you fellows——"

"Ass!"

"Beast!"

The Channel had been crossed.

Innumerable porters in baggy trousers had seized upon the baggage of the Greyfriars party, and carried it from the steamer into the Douane, where it was ranged on the long counters for the Customs officials to deal with it.

Sir Reginald Brooke was no doubt capable of seeing to the matter; but Billy Bunter had to wedge in.

At Greyfriars School, Bunter's French made Monsieur Charpentier, the French master, almost weep.

But that, according to Bunter, was because Monsieur Charpentier was rather an ass, and did not understand what a dab Bunter really was at French.

Anyhow, Bunter was going to air his knowledge, and he proceeded to give it an airing.

The polite Customs official asked them whether they had anything to "declare," and, as Sir Reginald was farther along the counter, dealing with another official, it was a chance for Bunter.

"Rong!" said Bunter cheerfully.

The Custom's man blinked at him.

"Plait-il?" he ejaculated.

"Rong!" repeated Bunter.

The Frenchman smiled and shook his head.

"Je ne comprends pas l'anglais, monsieur!" he said.

"Eh! What is he saying, you fellows?" asked Bunter.

"Ha, ha! He's saying that he doesn't understand English!" roared Bob Cherry.

"I wasn't speaking English, you ass, I was speaking French——"

"Ha, ha, ha!"

"Blessed if I see anything to cackle at! It's pretty thick to put a man in charge here who doesn't understand his own language!"

"Oh, my hat!"

"Mais, messieurs, repondez, si'l vous plait," said the Customs man. "Vous avez quelque-chose a declarer?"

"Rein?" answered Harry Wharton; and the man understood this as French, though Bunter's "rong" had been foreign to his ears.

"C'est ca," said the Frenchman, and he chalked Wharton's suit-case.

"Silly ass!" said Bunter. "He seems to understand you, Wharton. I suppose he's some provincial dummy, and doesn't catch on to the Parisian accent. That must be it."

"Ha, ha, ha!"

"Et vous, monsieur?" asked the Frenchman, addressing Bunter.

"Moi, rong!" said Bunter. "Rong? Savee? Don't you comprong your own blinking lingo, you ass? J'ai rong to declare in my bag, no quelque-chose at all!"

The most finished French scholar would hardly have understood French of that variety. The man stared at Bunter, and, instead of chalking his bag, to pass the customs, he proceeded to open it. As it was locked, he asked Bunter for the key, pointing to the lock. Bunter understood the gesture, if not the French, and grunted angrily.

"Look here! What do you want to ouvrez my bag for, when you haven't jolly well ouvreyed the others?" he demanded.

"Ouvrez, si'l vous plait!" rapped the official. "Ouvrez, monsieur!"

"You silly ass, open the bag!" exclaimed Wharton. "You've made him think you've got something to declare, with your silly babble!"

"Oh, really, Wharton——"

"Ouvrez!" yapped the Customs man, losing some of his politeness. "Je vous dis, monsieur, ouvrez, et toute de suite."

"There's no sweets in my bag," explained Bunter. "I ate them all on the boat."

"You frabjous owl!" roared Johnny Bull. "Toute de suite means at once."

"He means you're to open the bag at once, you fat owl!" said Nugent. "Get going, or we shall lose the train!"

"Don't be an ass, Nugent! He was asking me if there are any sweets in the bag. I suppose sweets are contraband here. Silly lot, the French! Well, there ain't any sweets——"

"Ouvrez toute de suite, monsieur!"

"Pas de sweets," said Bunter, in French—Bunter's French. "Non pas any sweets, pas de toot."

"Open that bag, you fat Owl, or I'll jolly well biff you!" exclaimed Bob Cherry.

"I can't find the key, you see."

"Oh, you benighted bandersnatch!"

"Ouvrez!" yapped the Customs man angrily now. He had a suspicious eye on Bunter. Evidently he suspected the fat Owl of having smuggled goods in his suitcase, and of being unwilling to let them be seen.

Porters gathered round the juniors on one side of the long counter, Customs officials and clerks gathered round the Frenchman on the other side. There was a babble of tongues. The Greyfriars party were getting most of the attention of the Douane. Billy Bunter went through one pocket after another in search of his key. Six or seven Frenchmen were speaking all at once now, and a gendarme drew near, with watchful eyes, evidently to prevent the supposed smuggler from bolting all of a sudden.

Sir Reginald Brooke, having got the larger baggage through, came back to the juniors and turned his eyeglass in surprise on the scene.

"What is the matter here?" he asked.

"Only Bunter speakin' French, nunky," answered Lord Mauleverer. "It seems to worry them somehow."

"The silly chumps don't understand good French!" hooted Bunter. "They think I've got sweets in my bag——"

"Open the bag at once, you foolish boy!"

"Oh, really, sir——"

"Lose no more time!" exclaimed Sir Reginald sharply. "The train for Paris will be starting soon."

"I can't find the key! I know I put it somewhere! Oh, here it is!" The key came out at last, with a couple of bullseyes sticking to it. "Now the silly owls can jolly well see that there's no sweets in the bag!"

The bag was opened.

All the rest of the baggage had been passed after a very cursory examination, but the Customs man went through Bunter's bag with meticulous care, obviously in a very suspicious frame of mind.

Fortunately, there was nothing there of a contraband nature, and the official, still looking suspicious, chalked the bag, and it was transferred to a porter's shoulder again.

"Thank goodness," said Nugent. "If you talk any more French, Bunter, we'll burst you."

"Beast!"

The Greyfriars party followed their baggage to the waiting train. Seats had been reserved in advance, which was rather fortunate, for the delay in the Customs left the party only time to catch the train. Billy Bunter settled down with a grunt, but the other fellows remained in the train corridor, watching the crowd on the platform with interest, wondering, too, whether among the innumerable passengers and loungers there was any spy watching the party. But no one, so far as they could see, gave them any special attention—except the baggy-trousered porters in quest of tips.

The train rolled out of Boulogne at last, and Billy Bunter put his head out of the doorway of his carriage and blinked at the juniors in the corridor.

"I say, you fellows, how long is it to Paris?" he asked.

"Three or four hours."

"What about grub?"

"Nothing about grub."

"Beast!"

And Bunter grunted and sat down again.

THE TWELFTH CHAPTER.

The Hand of the Enemy!

LORD MAULEVERER yawned.

The train clattered on through the North of France. Billy Bunter, as he had nothing to eat, went to sleep. Harry Wharton and Hurree Jamset Ram Singh played chess with the nabob's pocket set. Johnny Bull and Frank Nugent found entertainment in looking from the windows, and Bob Cherry put in a little practice with a "yo-yo."

Lord Mauleverer, like Gallio of old, cared for none of these things. The schoolboy millionaire had spent many vacations abroad, and foreign travel had lost its novelty for him, which was one of the penalties of being a millionaire. His lordship yawned and strolled up and down the corridor, while the train bumped and rattled and clanged on its way.

In one of the compartments that he passed, as he walked up and down the train corridor, there were only two passengers.

Lord Mauleverer might have noticed that circumstance had he been an observant youth, for the train was crowded; yet these two passengers had a carriage to themselves.

No doubt all the seats in the carriage had been reserved, which accounted for it. Still, the circumstance might have struck Mauly had he been observant. But Lord Mauleverer was not particularly observant; also he had an infinite capacity for minding his own business. He did not glance once into any of the carriages he passed in his stroll, and did not even notice whether the doors on the corridor were open or shut. In that particular carriage the door was open.

The two passengers were dark-faced men, and had Mauly noticed them, he would have noticed that they were foreigners. He might even have guessed that they came from the South of Europe by their looks; and even guessed that they were of Greek race. But he remained unaware even of their existence, as he passed them again and again.

Mauleverer was suddenly and unexpectedly made aware of the existence of the two swarthy men.

He was passing their doorway with his hands in his pockets and thinking of anything but danger, when a dusky hand reached out, grasped him, and dragged him headlong into the carriage.

Bump!

Mauleverer went down on the floor with a gasp of surprise, one of the swarthy men holding him there, with a hand over his mouth. The other swiftly closed the door on the corridor.

"Oooough!" gasped Mauleverer.

He stared up at the dark face above him.

The swarthy hand over his mouth kept him silent. He attempted to struggle, but a knee on his chest pinned him to the floor. The second man turned swiftly on him, grasped his wrists, and held them together, knotting a cord round them. Then the dusky hand was taken from his mouth, but a gag was

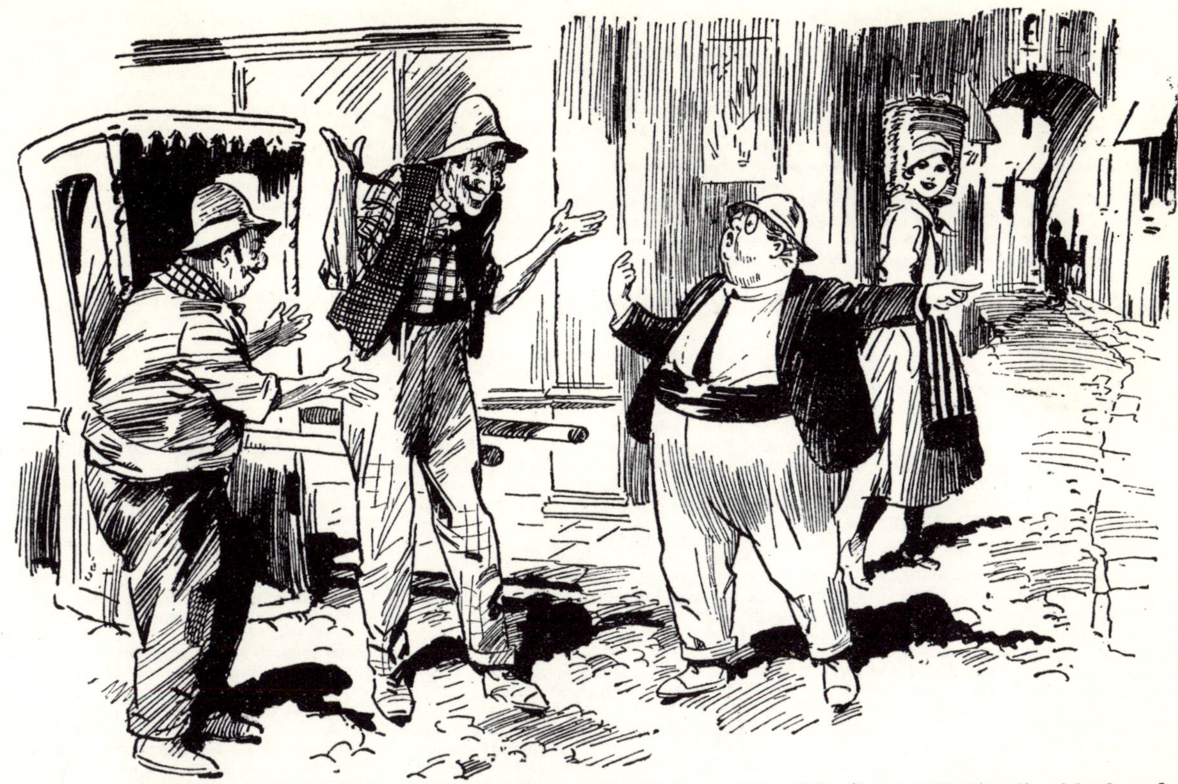

The two smiling Italians hailed Bunter. "Signore ! You wanter chair, yes ?" "Yes," gasped Bunter, "and buck up ! Find my friends in the place yonder—an old gent and six fellows, one of them a nigger—quick !"

thrust in so swiftly that he had no chance to utter a cry.

Not a word was spoken by either of the dark-skinned men. But there was no need of words. Mauleverer knew that they were agents of the Greek of Cairo, and he knew what they were after. The arm of Kalizelos was reaching after the Greyfriars party on their journey to Egypt.

Mauleverer ceased to struggle.

He had no chance, and he accepted the situation with his usual cool philosophy. There was a faint grin on his face.

But for Hurree Jamset Ram Singh's suggestion, the Golden Scarab would have been in his pocket or hanging about his neck, and indubitably it would have fallen into the hands of the enemy. But the Golden Scarab was safe in Harry Wharton's keeping, and Wharton was safe with his friends in the carriage along the booming train. Mauly was quite well aware of what the two rascals were after, and he was aware also that they were going to be disappointed.

Thievish hands went through his pockets as he lay on the floor of the carriage, shut from the sight of all other passengers on the train.

The two foreigners muttered together in a language of which Mauly did not understand a word—except one—the word "scarabaeus." That one word would have told him that they were of Kalizelos' gang, if he had not guessed it before.

Evidently Kalizelos did not care to be seen personally on the track of the party for Egypt. It was not likely that he was on the train; the sight of him would have warned the party of danger at once. The Greek was keeping behind the scenes, and acting by the hands of the rascals in his pay. The two spies were evidently tracking the party, watching for an opportunity, and it had come sooner than they could have anticipated—and they had acted with prompt audacity. Had the Golden Scarab been on Mauleverer it would have been lost for ever. But the thievish hands that sought through his pockets sought in vain.

But the two rascals were not satisfied with turning out his pockets. They proceeded to search him with the utmost care, ruffling his lordship considerably in the process. It was a dishevelled Mauleverer that lay on the rocking floor when they had finished. His money—of which Mauly had a good deal—they put aside; that was not what they wanted. It was the golden scarab they were seeking, and the scarab they evidently expected to find. But they did not find it.

The search finished at last, and they muttered together in their own tongue. Then one of them spoke in English.

"You are Lord Mauleverer?"

Mauly nodded.

"There is no mistake. I knew it. Then where is the scarab? Was it not in your keeping?"

Mauleverer shook his head.

"The truth!" snarled the dark-skinned man, his eyes gleaming with menace. "Is it in your guardian's hands—the old man's?"

Another shake of the head.

"One of your schoolboy friends?"

Mauly made no sign.

"Yes or no!" hissed the threatening voice. "Nod, or shake your head!"

Still Mauleverer made no sign.

"Fool!" muttered the man. "If you do not answer, it is the same as if you answered yes!"

He rose to his feet, and muttered with the other in his strange tongue. Both of them cast black looks at the bound schoolboy lying at their feet, as the train rocked and clanged on into Rouen.

They had gained nothing by their search—except the knowledge that the scarab was not in Mauly's keeping, and the guess that it was in the keeping of one of his friends. And the two rascals had no more time to lose—at any moment Mauleverer's friends might come looking for him; it was certain that they would look for him at once if they missed him from the corridor.

For a minute or more they muttered together, in low, savage tones, and then left the carriage, shutting the door on the corridor after them.

The train was slowing to a stop.

Mauly had no doubt that they had intended to quit the train at Amiens, with the scarab in their possession. Now they had to quit without it and they had no more than time. In a few minutes, passengers would be swarming in and out of the doors, and interruption was certain.

Mauleverer scrambled to his feet. Now that he was no longer held, he was able to get the gag from his mouth with his bound hands, and then to work his hands free from the cord. The train clattered to a stop, and he looked from the window on the side towards the platform, and had a moment's glimpse of his two assailants vanishing in the crowd there. They were gone in a moment, and he saw no more of them. He stepped out into the corridor, and walked back to the carriage where Harry Wharton & Co. still sat, making his way through hurrying passengers.

"Hallo, hallo, hallo!" Bob Cherry, still busy with his yo-yo, stared at Mauleverer as he looked in. "What's up? Been rolling along and collecting the dust on the train?"

Mauleverer grinned.

"Begad, I want a brush down," he remarked. "I've had a frightfully excitin' time, you men—frightfully! You've got that jolly old beetle safe, Wharton, old bean?"

"Yes, rather!"

"Inky's saved its bacon," said Mauleverer. "They'd have had it, if I'd kept it about me."

"What the thump——"

The train was rocking on as Mauly drawled out his tale.

"Oh, my hat!" exclaimed Bob. "After this, we're not letting you out of our sight, Mauly."

"That's what nunky will say when I tell him," groaned Mauleverer. "But it's really all right, as I've not got the jolly old beetle. Keep your eye on Wharton—he's got it! I'll stroll along the train——"

"You jolly well won't!"

Bob grasped Lord Mauleverer, and plumped him down into a seat.

"Sit there!"

"But, really, old bean——"

"If you move before we get to Paris, I'll catch you in the eye with my yo-yo!"

"Oh gad!"

And Mauleverer sat and yawned till the train ran into the Gare du Nord.

THE THIRTEENTH CHAPTER.
An Alarm in the Night!

NUNKY took the schoolboy party in hand again when they got out of Paris.

Billy Bunter blinked round him through his big spectacles, and his fat face lighted up at the sight of the word, in large letters, "Restaurant."

As if by instinct, Bunter's feet turned in that direction. But all the party, as a matter of fact, were ready for refreshments, and the fat Owl was given his head. When they sat down, Sir Reginald was told of what had happened on the train, and his face became very grave. As Mauly expected, he announced that he would not allow his nephew out of his sight again.

The old gentleman was evidently considerably perturbed by the knowledge that the party was followed and watched. But the juniors were not alarmed. Even Billy Bunter was not alarmed, being too busy in dealing with the foodstuffs to give thought to lesser matters. The fat Owl was still going strong, when Sir Reginald rose and announced that it was time to go.

Bunter gave a snort.

"I'm hungry!" he said warmly.

"Poor old Bunter!" said Bob. "He's only eaten enough for three fellows, so far! You can get a meal on the next train, old chap!"

"Come!" said Sir Reginald, without heeding Bunter. "The car is waiting now to take us across to the Lyons station."

"I'm not finished yet," said Bunter.

"Get a move on, fathead!" said Harry Wharton.

Bunter snorted.

"Look here, I don't see getting into another beastly train to-day," he said. "What's the matter with stopping in Paris a day or two?"

"We're going to Egypt, old fat man! If we stop everywhere between Boulogne and Naples, we shan't get to Cairo before the end of the vac."

"Well, I believe in taking it easy!" said Bunter. "And the fact is, I'm jolly well not going to bump along day and night in these beastly French trains. Besides, I'm hungry. I'm not coming yet."

"Get up, idiot!"

"Shan't!"

Sir Reginald was already going.

Billy Bunter blinked after the tall, stiff figure of the old baronet.

"Look here, Mauly——" he barked.

"Yaas?"

"Tell the old fossil to wait a bit!"

"The what?" ejaculated Lord Mauleverer.

"The old fossil—that old ass Brooke—here, I say, leggo!" yelled Bunter, as Lord Mauleverer, departing from his usual calm, took him by the collar and banged his head on the table. "Yoop! Stoppit! Oh, my hat! Yarooh!"

"Ha, ha, ha!"

"Ow! Beast! Leggo!" howled Bunter. "I didn't mean old fossil—I—I meant to say—whooooop!"

"Ha, ha, ha!"

"Come on, you men!" said Lord Mauleverer. "If Bunter isn't finished yet, he can hang on. This way."

The Famous Five followed Lord Mauleverer, and Billy Bunter—deciding that he had, after all, finished—followed on promptly. The foodstuffs were attractive, but the fat Owl certainly did not want to be left on his lonely own in the Gare du Nord.

The party packed in a big car, and it rolled away with them, the juniors keeping their eyes alert, wondering whether any of the confederates of the man from Egypt had watched for them in Paris. Whether there was a spy among the crowds round the Gare du Nord, however, they were unable to discover.

They arrived at the southern station, and took their places in the Lyons-Mediterranean train—Billy Bunter grunting and grousing, and not finding comfort until he learned that there was a restaurant car on the train. After which Bunter disappeared from sight for some time—though the other fellows could guess where he was, and how he was occupied.

If Billy Bunter left off feeding before bed-time, the intervals of repose were short. He had quite a happy feeling of fullness when he rolled into his sleeping-berth.

There he sank at once into the embrace of Morpheus, and his deep snore mingled with the rumble of the train as it rolled on through the starry summer night.

Harry Wharton, who had the other berth, did not find it so easy to woo slumber. In the Remove dormitory at Greyfriars, Billy Bunter's tremendous snore was devastating, but in the close quarters of a sleeping-car it was simply terrific. Between the rumble of the train and the Gargantuan snore so close at hand, it was some time before Wharton fell asleep, and then his slumber was uneasy and haunted by dreams.

The golden scarab, hung on the silk ribbon round his neck, figured in his dreams, with the dark, olive face of the man from Egypt.

Sir Reginald had warned the juniors to lock the doors on the corridor when they turned in, and he was keeping Mauleverer under his own eye. It was possible—indeed, probable—that some confederate of Kalizelos was on the train.

Harry Wharton, as the bearer of the precious scarab, was the one that needed most to keep on his guard, and he had carefully secured the door and placed a bag against it.

It was past midnight when Wharton awoke suddenly from an uneasy slumber. The lights of some station through which the express had boomed, were disappearing behind.

He had been dreaming of the golden scarab and of Kalizelos, and the glittering, black eyes of the Greek were in his mind's eye as he stared in the darkness.

There was a movement close to him.

A thrill ran through the junior.

The train was rumbling noisily, and he did not notice for the moment that the resonant snore of Billy Bunter no longer mingled with the rumble. Locks could be picked even on trains, and Wharton's heart thumped as he heard a movement in the darkness close by him and a hand groped over him.

For a few seconds he lay quite still, his heart leaping, staring hard into the dark in which a dim shadow stirred.

The hand groped over his berth, and a dim figure moved before his eyes. Suddenly, swiftly, Wharton moved, lifting himself on one elbow and striking out with the other hand. His clenched fist landed on the dark figure, and there was a startled gasp and the sound of a heavy fall on the floor.

In an instant Wharton had reached out and flashed on the light, alert and prepared for a struggle. On the floor of the carriage a fat figure in pyjamas lay sprawling and gasping, and Wharton's eyes almost started from his head as he stared at it.

It was not a dark-skinned foreigner in quest of the golden scarab. It was William George Bunter, of the Greyfriars Remove.

Both Bunter's fat hands were pressed to his extensive equator, and he was mumbling and gasping and gurgling wildly.

"Bunter!" gasped Wharton blankly.

"Ooooogh! My tummy! Ooooogh!"

"What the thump——"

"Woooooough!"

"You howling idiot——"

"Yoooough! Oh, my tummy! Grooooooogh!" moaned Bunter.

"You silly chump!" roared Wharton. "What were you doing out of bed?"

"Ooooooooooooogh!"

"What were you up to, you dangerous maniac?"

"Gooooough!"

Bunter sat up. He pressed his fat hands to the place where his many meals were packed away and moaned.

"Oooough! Beast! I woke up—oogh! I was hungry—grooogh! I remembered I had a packet of chocolates—grooogh! I laid them on your berth. Wooogh! I was looking for them—wooogh! I couldn't find the switch to turn on the light—ooooogh! Wharrer you hit me in the tummy for—groooogh!"

"Ha, ha, ha!" yelled Wharton.

"Ow! Beast! I'm winded—woooch! I'm dying—grooogh! Oh, my tummy! Yooooooogh!"

"Ha, ha, ha!"

"Gug-gug! Oh dear! Ooooough!"

"You silly owl, I thought it was one of those rotters after the scarab! What was I to think, you frabjous ass?"

"Ow! Fathead! Wow! Oooogh!"

Harry Wharton chuckled, turned out the light, and settled down to sleep again. But it was quite a long time before the hapless Owl left off moaning and mumbling and crawled into his berth again. Then once more Bunter's hefty snore awoke the echoes of the South of France, and he was still going strong when the rest of the party turned out to breakfast.

THE FOURTEENTH CHAPTER.

Southward-Ho!

BLUER skies by day and brighter stars by night greeted the Greyfriars party as they rolled on their journey southward.

The steamer for Alexandria was to be taken at Naples, at the other end of the Italian peninsula, and every mile of the long journey had interest for the schoolboys. Under a blazing sun they crossed the frontier from France into Italy, and rolled on through a land of dreamy beauty—with which Bunter, however, was not quite satisfied.

Azure skies, soaring mountains, fertile valleys, smiling faces, and musical voices did not appeal much to the Owl of the Remove. Billy Bunter declared that the grub was not so good since France was left behind, and that the smells were much more distinct. There is no doubt that the more a traveller in Europe progresses southward, the more his nose is assailed, however much his eyes may be delighted.

There was a halt for a day in Rome, where Nunky took the juniors for a ramble to see the Colosseum and the Forum and St. Peter's and a few more sights, followed by a drive on the Pincio, where there was tea under shady trees; this being the part of the day's entertainment that was thoroughly enjoyed by Billy Bunter.

Roman ruins did not interest Bunter much, but he proceeded to make a ruin of an immense pile of sweet, sticky cakes, and found great enjoyment in the process. The hand of Time had not fallen so heavily on Rome as the fat hand of Billy Bunter fell on that stack of cakes; and though he moved with a little difficulty when the party went back to the car, he was happy and shiny and sticky, and, upon the whole, satisfied with his day in the ancient capital of the world.

Indeed, when the party boarded the train for Naples the next day, Billy Bunter blinked back at the Eternal City through his big spectacles with real regret.

"Might have put in another day in Rome," he said. "I don't see rushing away like this from a place like Rome!"

The other fellows looked at Bunter. They were rather surprised to find the fat Owl taking an interest in such things. Certainly a city like Rome might have appealed to any fellow's imagination, but they had not expected Bunter to bother about it. But even Bunter, apparently, had been impressed by the city of the Cæsars.

"Topping place," agreed Bob. "I'd like to put in a few weeks there, rooting around. Still, we've got to get on our way. So you liked Rome, Bunty?"

"Yes, rather!"

"The jolly old Colosseum, what?" asked Bob.

"Eh? What rot!" said Bunter.

"The Forum——" said Nugent.

"Beastly lot of silly stones," grunted Bunter.

"St. Peter's——" said Wharton.

"Rubbish!" grunted Bunter.

"The Tiber——" said Johnny Bull. "When a fellow thinks of all that's happened on the banks of the Tiber——"

"Oh, was that dirty-looking river the Tiber?" said Bunter indifferently. "I don't think much of it."

"Well, what the dooce was it you liked in Rome, then, old fat man?" asked Lord Mauleverer, puzzled.

Bunter, evidently, had not been interested in the wonderful sights that had interested the other fellows.

"That was a jolly good feed we had in those gardens on the Pincian Hill!" said Bunter.

"Eh?"

"Those cakes were jolly good——"

"Cakes?" repeated Mauly.

"Yes; they make jolly good cakes in Rome."

"Oh gad!"

"Ha, ha, ha!" yelled the Famous Five. They were apprised at last of what had really interested Billy Bunter in the City of the Seven Hills.

Bunter blinked at them.

"They were simply topping cakes," he said. "I ate only eleven of them; I wasn't really hungry. But——"

"Ha, ha, ha!"

"Blessed if I see anything to cackle at! I can tell you that they were simply ripping cakes! I wish I had a few now! Rather fatheaded, if you ask me, to rush off like this—from a place like Rome! You don't go to Rome every day; and those cakes——"

"Ha, ha, ha!"

"Of course, it's a beastly noisy place, and seems to be chiefly a lot of silly old stones," said Bunter. "But they can make cakes. I can tell you fellows I've never tasted better cakes! Look here, you fellows, let's stop at Rome again on our way home. I like Rome!"

And Billy Bunter gave another regretful blink back at the Eternal City, his fat mind dwelling on the one glory of Rome that appealed to him.

The last lap of the railway journey was now before the Greyfriars party. Nothing had been seen of the enemy, and though they had not forgotten Kalizelos, he was relegated to the backs of their minds.

Nunky hoped that they had seen the last of the man from Egypt, but Harry Wharton & Co. did not doubt that Kalizelos would turn up again sooner or later. But it seemed probable that, knowing their destination, the Greek was biding his time, scheming to deal with them when they landed in Africa.

That prospect did not worry the cheery chums of the Remove. They had no doubt of being able to keep their end up if the enemy hunted for more trouble.

Meanwhile, they were enjoying themselves, delighted with the sights of Italy if not with the scents.

There was to be another day's halt at Naples, with a visit to Mount Vesuvius and the lost city of Pompeii, after which they were to take the steamer for Alexandria. Bella Napoli burst on them like a vision of beauty when they arrived in that famous city, with its glorious bay, and the island of Capri in the distance, and Vesuvius smoking against the blue sky. Even Lord Mauleverer sat up and took notice as they drove up the hill to their hotel.

"Toppin'!" said Mauly.

"The topfulness is terrific," declared Hurree Jamset Ram Singh.

"What do you think, Bunter?" asked Bob Cherry, with a chuckle. "How do you like Naples?"

"Eh? I don't know yet," answered Bunter, blinking at him. "Do you fellows know what the grub's like?"

"Ha, ha, ha!"

"A fellow told me once, who had been here, that they cook macaroni a treat in Naples," said Bunter. "I can't tell till I've tried it, of course. I say, you fellows, I'm jolly hungry! What on earth are you stopping the car for, Mauly? We're not at the hotel."

"Lookin' at the sunset over Capri, old bean!"

"You silly ass!" hooted Bunter. "Looking at a fatheaded sunset over a silly island when a fellow's hungry! Are you off your rocker?"

The car rolled on again. Sunsets over the Bay of Naples did not interest

Bunter; but fortunately he found that he had not been misinformed about the macaroni. The Greyfriars fellows slept soundly that night, and turned out early in the morning to see the sunrise on the bay—Billy Bunter snoring on, as indifferent to sunrises as to sunsets.

Bunter snored on till the car came round to take the party to Pompeii; and then he would have gone on snoring, had not Bob Cherry assisted him out of bed, and squeezed a wet sponge down his fat neck, which effectually awakened Bunter.

With the rest of the party waiting, Bunter had hardly time for a couple of breakfasts before he started; but he was comforted by the information that there was an hotel at Pompeii where a fellow could get a snack, while less intelligent fellows were rooting over silly old ruins. But the fat junior eyed the column of smoke rising from the summit of Vesuvius rather uneasily as the car ran on to the buried city.

"I say, you fellows, does Vesuvius ever erupt now?" he asked.

"Every now and then," answered Bob Cherry. "Might happen any minute, in fact. The people round about here build their houses of the stuff that's chucked out of the volcano, and they get lots of building materials cheap."

"Rather a catch if we happened to be here in an eruption," said Johnny Bull. "Something to tell the fellows about at Greyfriars next term."

"You silly chump!" said Bunter. "Look here, I don't like the look of that volcano. I think we'd better go back. We can just stop at the hotel for a snack, and then get back to Naples—never mind the ruins—see?"

The juniors chuckled, but apparently they did not "see." The car stopped at the hotel, close by the buried city, in a blaze of brilliant sunshine, and Bunter rolled into the shade with a grunt of relief. He was seated at a table enjoying a third breakfast, with a fourth in happy prospect when a guide was secured, and the other fellows were ready to start for the ruins. Bunter did not stir.

"You're coming, you ass?" asked Harry Wharton.

Bunter shook his head.

"What is there to see?" he asked.

"City buried two thousand years ago by an eruption of Vesuvius."

"Well, you fellows tell me about it when you come back," said Bunter.

And he devoted himself to the foodstuffs, while the other fellows, perhaps not greatly saddened by the loss of his society, walked off to the buried city.

THE FIFTEENTH CHAPTER.

Danger!

"SON io, signore!"

Billy Bunter blinked round with annoyance.

Bunter was taking a rest.

He needed it.

He had kept several waiters very busy at the hotel, and when he had finished he had left them staring, and he heard the head-waiter murmur, "Dio mio!" as he rolled away. Bunter's performances in the gastronomic line had surprised them. Bunter was feeling that he had done well—perhaps a little too well—and he wanted a rest. He sauntered, slowly, to a shady grove near the building, looking for a comfortable spot for a nap till the party came back from the ruins. He found a shady spot where he leaned his back against a tree, shaded and screened by high, thick bushes.

There he closed his eyes behind his spectacles, and would probably have dropped at once into a happy slumber, but for the flies. There were plenty of flies, and they all seemed to like Bunter. But in spite of the buzzing flies the fat junior would have napped at last, but just as he was dropping off, a voice close at hand came to his fat ears from the thick grove. It really was irritating, for Bunter had selected a very secluded spot so as not to be disturbed. Some beastly Italian, of course, was bound to come jawing just when a fellow wanted to go to sleep. Bunter's eyes, which had closed behind his spectacles, opened again with an angry blink.

"Son io, signore!" murmured the soft Italian voice.

"Speak English!" came another voice; and Billy Bunter gave a jump as he heard it.

He knew that low, musical voice—the voice of Konstantinos Kalizelos, the Greek. He gave a convulsive start, and then sat very still. The Greek and the Italian were not two yards from him on the other side of the tree, and evidently unaware that he was there. A shiver ran through Billy Bunter. He was not thinking of sleep now. He sat transfixed.

"Si, signore—yes, sir," came the other voice. "I forget zat you have no Italian, signore."

"What have you to tell me, Giuseppe?"

"They are here, signore—il vecchio—the old gentleman—has taken i ragazzi—the boys—to the ruins, except one—the fat one—who has remained in the hotel to eat. Dio mio! How he eat!"

"The fat one matters little. He is not likely to be trusted with what I seek. He is a fool—an ass—an imbecile!"

Billy Bunter's eyes gleamed behind his spectacles.

"The others, signore, are now in the ruins. I learn that they will come back to the hotel for lunch."

"Are there many people in the ruins?"

"The usual tourists—English, American. But in this hot weather, not a large crowd."

"You have your men at hand?"

"Si, signore."

"Listen to me, Giuseppe. It will be risky, but you will be well paid—you and your friends. Find what I seek, and you shall receive five hundred pounds—that is nearly fifty thousand lire in your own money."

"Oh, signore!" gasped Giuseppe.

The Greek gave a curt laugh.

"It will not be easy," he said, "with the tourists about, and the custodians of the place. But you can do it. Listen! One of the boys—I cannot say which—carries a jewel—an ornament—in the form of a golden beetle. That is what I want. It is a thing of little value in itself—perhaps three or four thousand lire—that is all. Give it into my hands, and the sum I have named is yours. There are lonely places in the ruins. The boys may be seized, one by one perhaps, and searched, bound or stunned, as you find convenient. Or with a dozen men to help you, you may surround the whole party, and seize on them and search them."

"Leave it in my hands, signore. The days of the brigands are over in Naples, but fifty thousand lire is not picked up every day."

"Bring the golden beetle to me in Naples, and it is done," said Kalizelos.

"Si, signore."

There was a rustle in the grove. Billy Bunter, sitting frozen with terror, heard the Greek and the Italian depart in different directions.

"Oh crikey!" breathed Bunter.

The fat junior did not stir.

He was too terrified to stir, even after the rustling and the footsteps in the silent grove died away.

Long minutes passed before the fat junior ventured to rise to his feet.

Kalizelos, evidently, had gone back to Naples to wait there for the bravo to bring the Golden Scarab. Giuseppe had been set to watch the Greyfriars party, and the Greek had met him in the grove near the ruins to hear his report, and to give him his instructions. Bunter realised that he had nothing to fear from the Greek, whose appearance on the scene would have given the alarm at once. Kalizelos was working from behind the scenes.

But the thought of Giuseppe and a gang of Neapolitan lazzaroni at his heels made Bunter shiver. The fat Owl was powerfully tempted to steer clear of what was to happen in the ruined city where, at any moment now, enemies might be gathering round the unsuspecting sightseers.

But though Billy Bunter was chiefly concerned for the safety of his own fat skin, he was not quite capable of leaving the other fellows in the lurch to that extent.

He rolled out of the grove, blinking round him through his big spectacles, the perspiration thick on his podgy brow. It was hot—very hot—and Bunter was loaded over the Plimsoll line; but he started at a run for the ruined city. There was time yet to warn the Greyfriars party of their danger; but there was no time to lose. And Bunter had to run. A voice hailed him as he plugged breathlessly on.

"Signore, you wanter chair—yes? Tre lire, signore!"

"Oh, good!" gasped Bunter.

Two smiling Italians with a sedan-chair, looking for customers, spotted the fat Owl! Bunter plumped into the sedan. Never had a lift been so welcome to the Owl of the Remove.

"Buck up!" he gasped. "Find my friends in the place yonder—an old gent, and six fellows, one of them a nigger—quick! Look here, here's a hundred lire! Buck up!"

Bunter crammed a hundred-lire bill into the surprised Italian's hand.

"Oh, signore! Tante grazie"

The sedan chair was rushed off.

The chairmen did not often pick up a hundred lire so easily. They went at a rapid trot, realising that the fat signore was in a hurry to find his friends. Other sedans, with tourists in them, were on the road; but Bunter passed them swiftly.

In a few minutes he was passing through the ancient gateway into the city of the dead.

Round him were the roofless houses of the ancient inhabitants of Pompeii, uncovered by the excavations that had been going on for more than a century. The feet of his bearers clattered on the cobbled ways where Romans once had trod. But Billy Bunter had no eyes for the dismantled dwellings of the ancient Pompeians. He blinked round eagerly for the Greyfriars party.

Tourists, with red-covered guide books, were sprinkled among the ruins. Every time Bunter's eyes fell on a dark

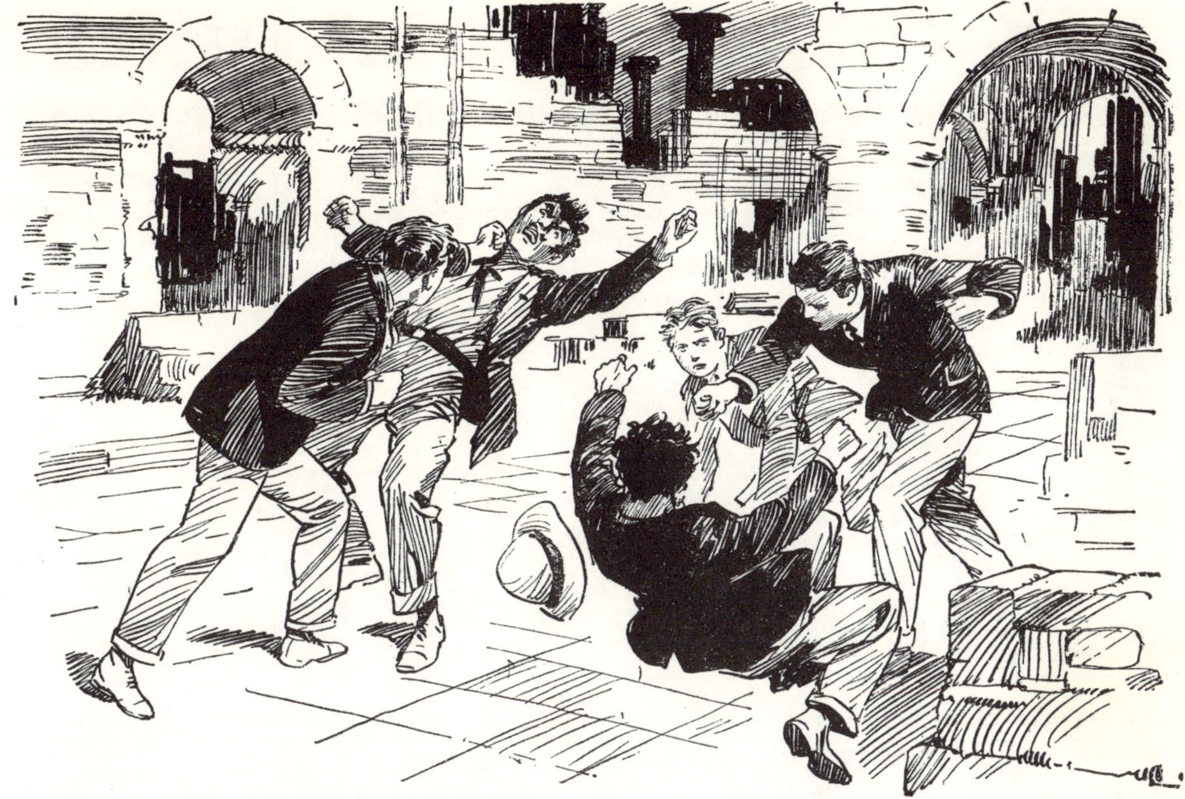

" Back up, Johnny ! " yelled Bob. The two Neapolitans leapt up from Wharton, as Bob Cherry and Johnny Bull rushed at them. But they did not gain their feet—crashing fists sent them spinning over, yelling. " Quick, you fellows—get out of this ! " panted Wharton, scrambling up breathlessly.

Italian face, he wondered whether it was the face of Giuseppe or one of his gang.

"Hallo, hallo, hallo !"

It was Bob Cherry's voice.

Bunter rolled out of the sedan.

"I say, you fellows ! Oh dear !" he gasped. "Oh crikey ! Oh lor' ! I say, you fellows, get out of this ! You're in danger—— Grooogh——"

"My esteemed, idiotic Bunter——"

"What do you mean, Bunter ?" asked Sir Reginald Brooke sharply. "Nunky" was giving his young charges some valuable information with regard to the manners and customs of the old-time inhabitants of Pompeii, when the fat Owl barged in. "What——"

"Danger !" gurgled Bunter.

"Nonsense !"

"I heard them—Kalizelos——"

"Kalizelos here !" exclaimed the old baronet, with a start. "Have you seen him ?"

"I heard him !" gasped Bunter. "He's got a gang of rotters to get after you here—they may be here any minute—I came to warn you——"

The fat Owl panted for breath.

"Oh gad !" said Lord Mauleverer.

The juniors gathered round in amazement, as Bunter panted out his tale.

Sir Reginald frowned grimly.

"We had better leave the ruins at once, my boys," he said. "I can scarcely think that there is danger here, but I cannot take chances with you. Are you all here ? Where is Wharton ?"

"He went into that giddy atrium, back along the street——"

"Call him at once," said Sir Reginald. "You and Bull go, Cherry—the rest remain with me."

"Right-ho !"

And Bob Cherry and Johnny Bull ran quickly along the cobbled "via," the rest of the party waiting for them, while Billy Bunter mopped his perspiring brow, and puffed and blew.

THE SIXTEENTH CHAPTER.

A Narrow Escape !

"SILENZIO !"

The word was hissed in Harry Wharton's ear; but it was hardly needed, for a brown hand was clapped over his mouth as it was spoken.

The captain of the Remove gave a violent start.

He was standing in an ancient "atrium," open to the blue sky above, but shut off from the general view by the remains of the massive old walls.

Only a few minutes before the whole party had been there, gazing at the pictures painted on the old walls, in colours as bright as when they had been laid on two thousand years ago.

Wharton had lingered behind, when the rest went on, looking at the paintings, and never dreaming of danger. He did not even glance round at the sound of footsteps entering the building, only supposing that other tourists were coming in; and he was taken completely by surprise when his arms were grasped from behind and a hand clapped over his mouth.

Strong hands were grasping him. He twisted round, his startled eyes staring at two dark Neapolitan faces. Two men had followed him into the old atrium, and seized him there; but he did not, for the moment, think of Kalizelos. The men were Italians, and he supposed that they were pickpockets from their actions.

He made an attempt to shout to his friends—hardly a dozen yards distant, though hidden from sight by the massive walls between. But his mouth was gripped hard, and he could utter no cry. He struggled; but the sinewy hands forced him to the stone floor, and a knee was planted on his chest. Then dusky hands searched rapidly through his pockets.

"Dove e, dove e ?" muttered Giuseppe, as he searched. "Signorino, dove e ? Where is it—the beetle ?"

Then the junior understood.

He made a terrific effort to throw off the two ruffians. But it was in vain. One of them held him silent and helpless, while the other searched his pockets, one after another.

Whether they knew that he had the scarab, or whether they had taken the opportunity of getting hold of one of the party singly, he could not tell; but it was certain that they would find it on him.

His pockets having been drawn blank, Giuseppe searched further, and there was a grin of triumph on his dusky face as he found the silk ribbon round the schoolboy's neck.

"Buono ! Buonissimo !" he chuckled.

He pulled at the ribbon. In a moment more the golden scarab would have been pulled in sight. Wharton made another effort with all his strength. But it was in vain. And then, like music to his ears, came a shouting voice in the narrow "via" without.

"Hallo, hallo, hallo ! You here, Harry ?"

Bob Cherry came tramping into the atrium, with Johnny Bull at his heels.

"Cospetto !" panted Giuseppe.

(*Continued on page* 28.)

OUR GREAT ADVENTURE STORY.

THE ISLAND TRADERS!

By FRANK RICHARDS

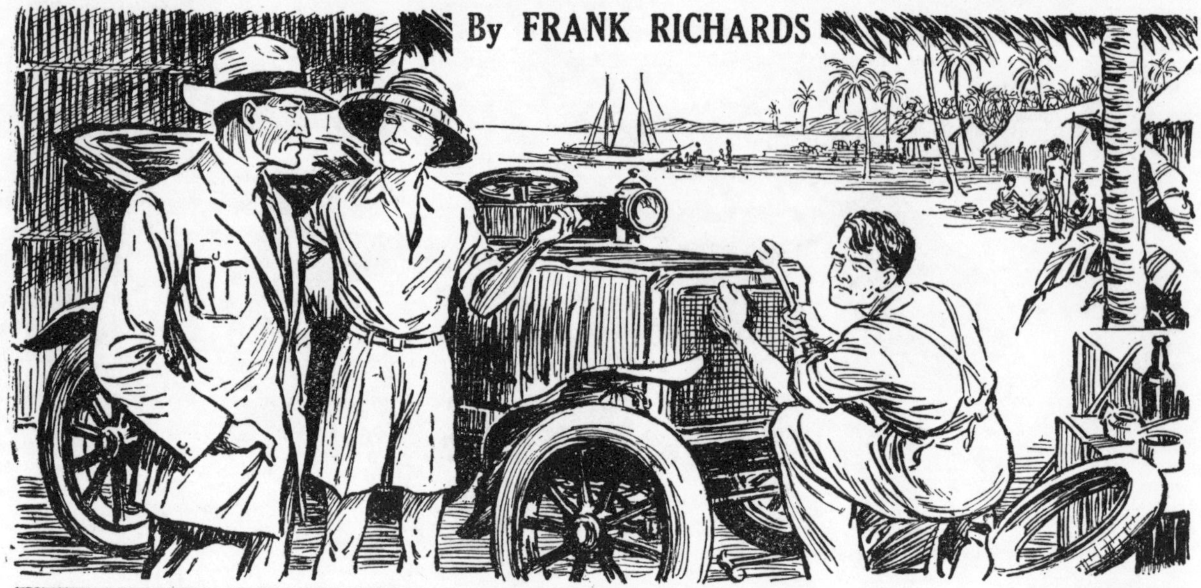

READ THIS FIRST.

BOB HARRIS AND BILLY McCANN, TWO YOUNG BRITISHERS TRADING UNDER THE NAME OF "BOB, BILLY & CO."—THE "CO." BEING AN ANCIENT AND BATTERED FORD CAR—ARE OWNERS OF A STORE ON KALUA ISLAND. KNOWING THAT A VAST TREASURE LIES HIDDEN ON THE SITE, DAVID BONE, A RASCALLY AMERICAN TRADER, OFFERS TO BUY THE STORE, BUT THE ISLAND TRADERS REFUSE TO SELL. AFTER SEVERAL FRUITLESS ATTEMPTS TO DRIVE THE PARTNERS OFF THE ISLAND, BONE BRIBES A BEACH-COMBER TO FIRE THE STORE, AND THEN OFFERS TO BUY THE SITE.

Good News For Bone!

"NOTHING doing," said Bob, with a smile. "We're sticking to that site, Mr. Bone, for old associations' sake. You see, a royal palace stood in that spot once, and we're rather snobs. We like the royal associations."

"No, we're not selling," said Billy, shaking his head—"not in your lifetime, Mr. Bone. We're sticking to that old spot."

David Bone looked at them.

Keen as he was, he could not read those two smiling, good-humoured faces.

"But I'll tell you what," said Bob. "If you're looking for a chance of putting up money on Kalua, what about a pearling proposition?"

"Pearls?" said Bone.

"I fancy you've heard that there's oyster beds on the other side of Kalua. We're going over to the other side," explained Bob. "You see, with the store burned and trade dead we're practically down and out. A man's got to live—and we can't comb the beach. We're trying pearls."

"I'll buy all the pearls you find on Kalua," said David Bone derisively.

"A man might be weeks before he found a single pearl," said Bob. "You don't feel like financing a pearling outfit?"

"I don't!" said Mr. Bone.

"If we could raise a schooner, or even a ketch——" said Billy.

David Bone laughed. He was quite at his ease now. Two down-and-out traders, who were taking up such a desperate resource as pearling on Kalua, need not worry him. He almost ceased to be sorry that he saw them alive.

"I guess if you want to raise a schooner or a ketch, or as much as a whaleboat, you want to look for a sucker," he said. "I'll put money into a pearling proposition when I see the pearls—not before."

"But——"

"So-long!" said David Bone.

And he walked on.

Bob and Billy looked at one another, and both smiled.

That day Mr. Bone spent a good deal of time ashore. He was lounging about the beach when Billy McCann filled up the old car, and the young traders packed her with a camping outfit and food, and helped Pete Purkiss in.

He had talked a good deal with the Kalua planters during the day, and knew all about the way the partners had befriended the beach-comber. He told himself cynically that they couldn't know who had fired their store. David Bone seldom allowed his leathery countenance to express any emotion. But he looked pleased when the old Ford honked away and disappeared.

All Kalua knew that Bob, Billy & Co. were going to try their luck with the pearling on the other side of the island. That was fifteen miles away, and David Bone was pleased to know that the firm would be fifteen miles distant from the site of the burned-out store during his stay on Kalua.

Kalua men shook their heads over the enterprise; pearls had been found on the island, but few and of little value. Still, Bob and Billy looked cheery and hopeful enough when they started.

David Bone, at all events, was pleased. He even wished the partners he had ruined luck in their hunt for pearls. And he smiled after the vanishing Ford—a sardonic smile.

Taking possession of the site of the burned-out store, "jumping" land that belonged to the partners was impossible—while they lived. But if David Bone had a free hand there for one night, unwatched by the partners, he was content to leave the site in their possession.

Now that the store was destroyed it was only necessary to shift a heap of old black embers to uncover the spot that the Santa Cruz boy knew. With Bob, Billy & Co. fifteen miles away across the lagoon, it was as easy for David Bone as if the death spiders had done their work. They could keep the site of the store—when he had taken out of it what the earth hid.

Mr. Bone glanced at the sky, and smiled.

"There'll be a moon to-night," he said—and he dispatched a native into the interior to bring Loo, the Santa Cruz boy, from Tu'uka's village.

Loo joined him at sunset.

Far away across the island the Co. was honking merrily on its way, with the partners and Pete Purkiss on board.

But it did not reach the farther side of Kalua.

Far out of sight the ancient Ford was backed into an opening of the high bush. When the sun sank into the Pacific Purkiss made himself comfortable in the old car and went to sleep.

But not so Bob and Billy. They were tramping under the starlight back round the lagoon.

Golden Sovereigns!

HIGH over Kalua soared the full, round moon.

It was midnight on the Pacific island.

Long ago the last of the bungalow doors had shut. Every white man in the row of buildings was asleep behind his mosquito curtains. The native dance on the beach had long ceased. The brown men were slumbering in their grass houses. On the cutter anchored in the lagoon a riding-light burned; otherwise all was dark and silent.

Any planter on Kalua, had he given the matter a thought, would have supposed that David Bone was fast asleep in his cabin on the Osprey. Never, however, had the American trader been more wide awake.

By the deserted hut, close by the burned ruins of the store, the tall palm-tree cast a long shadow. Two shorter shadows fell by its side. And in the silence of the night there was the muttering of a nasal voice.

"All clear, I guess!" muttered David Bone.

"Me tinkee, sar!" said Loo.

Bone gave a low, dry chuckle.

"You got that feller spade and pick?"

"Yes, sar."

"You know where to look?"

The black face of the Santa Cruz boy wrinkled in a grin.

"Me savvy plenty, sar, Mokatoo bury feller gold piece along palace belong him. He bury him along floor belong room he sleep. Me see um, eye belong me, sar, along me prisoner and slave along Mokatoo. Kalua boy no savvy nothing. Me, Loo, me savvy everything."

Bone nodded.

He had not doubted the Santa Cruz boy's tale when Loo had told him, long weeks ago, on A'ao. At first he had doubted. He had heard too many tales of buried treasure in Pacific Islands to believe easily. But close questioning of the Santa Cruz boy had convinced him.

Mokatoo's slave had buried the golden sovereigns for his master. Again and again he had opened the hidden store to add fresh sovereigns as they came into the old miser's hands.

The old King of Kalua had trusted no man of his own tribe. He had had to trust someone, and he had chosen the slave whose life depended on his nod.

He had paid for his hoarding with his life. Tu'uka had risen up against him and slain him, and there had been wild fighting among the tribesmen, and in the confusion, Loo had stolen a canoe and escaped from the island. He had never dared to return. The Kaluans would have eaten him. But, later, when white men settled on the island, Loo had come, only to find that a Dutchman had built his store on the very spot where the old king's palace had stood in the savage days.

Loo had nursed his secret.

Later, the Dutchman had sold the store to two newcomers, but it was as impossible as ever for Loo to get at the treasure. At last, knowing David Bone's reputation for unscrupulous use of his power, he had taken his story to the American trader.

As soon as David Bone was convinced of the truth of it, he had entered into the "proposition" coolly, ruthlessly. It was for the man from 'Frisco to get rid of the island traders, for Loo to point out the burial-place of the gold. Then they were to take equal shares—if they kept faith! David Bone had given his word. But in his own private thoughts David Bone guessed that Loo might fall overboard from the cutter when he had outlived his usefulness. And perhaps some similar thought worked in the cunning brain of the Santa Cruz boy.

Loo cast a quick, searching glance round—at the beach glimmering in the moonlight; the silent, distant bungalows; the hut where the partners had lived since the burning of the store. He stepped to the hut, opened the door, and peered into the gloom within.

David Bone muttered impatiently.

"It's all clear! Them two suckers are on the other side of Kalua, looking for pearls." He chuckled—a dry chuckle. "I guess they'd get richer looking nearer home, if they knew it! Get to it, you feller boy!"

"Makee all sure, sar," said Loo. "No wantee eye belong any feller see plenty too much gold, sar."

"Get to it!"

Loo, with the pick in his hand, sorted among the ruins of the store. Little clouds of ashes rose from the raking pick. For long minutes the Santa Cruz boy raked and searched and paused and calculated.

David Bone watched him impatiently.

"Me savvy!" said the Santa Cruz boy at last.

He stopped, evidently having located the spot where old Mokatoo's sleeping-room had been in the days when a grass-built palace stood on the site of the island store.

He raked away ashes and dead embers, and the surface of the ground was disclosed.

"Get to it!" muttered David Bone.

"Me gettee plenty quick, sar!"

The muscular Santa Cruz boy plied the pick.

David Bone's sunken, flinty eyes watched him with greedy eagerness.

How many thousands of golden sovereigns had old Mokatoo stored away in the course of forty years' trading? Thousands, certainly; perhaps ten thousand—perhaps twenty thousand. David Bone was a rich man; but as his wealth grew, so grew his hunger for more riches. He was not even thinking of keeping faith with the wretched black man who had led him to a treasure. A handful of the golden sovereigns he would have given him as a reward. But half! He laughed silently at the thought. His eyes burned with greed as he watched the black man dig.

Loo was using the spade now, turning out a heap of earth. He worked hard and rapidly, the sweat streaming down his black limbs.

David Bone glanced round at the star-glimmering lagoon, the sleeping bungalows. Not a sound, save the distant murmur of the surf on the reef, and the dull thudding of the spade in the hands of the Santa Cruz boy. Overhead the soaring moon gave ample light.

This was easy—easier than he had dreamed. This was "pie" to the greedy trader from 'Frisco. He had ruined the island traders for this. He had schemed their death as coolly as he would have crushed a mosquito. Had they been still in his way, he would have stopped at no treachery to rid himself of them. They had saved him a crime by taking themselves out of his way. He cared little whether they lived or died, even with the marks of Billy McCann's lawyer-cane on his back. He cared only for the treasure.

Thud, thud, thud! went the unceasing spade.

A pile of earth was growing beside the excavation.

Clink, clink!

It was not necessary to dig deep. Mokatoo's hoard had been in a shallow grave. Often and often the hoard had been opened to be added to. On that spot, rich with gold, the sleeping-mat of the old king had been laid. Later, it had been covered by the burned ruins of his palace; later, by the store, and then by burned ruins. Now it was open to the moonlight, and the clink of metal on metal told that the hoard was reached.

Many on Kalua had searched for that treasure—in the high bush, in hollows of trees, among crevices of the coral rocks. It was reserved for David Bone to unearth it. Even old Soo-oo, the devil-doctor, believed that it was hidden in the bush. The cunning old King of Kalua had told him so. And it had waited here for David Bone!

Clink, clink!

Loo dropped the spade at last. He threw himself on his knees beside the shallow excavation, his black eyes blazing. David Bone threw himself on his knees also. In the bright moonlight the yellow glimmer of gold dazzled his eyes. The old goatskin sack had rotted away. The sovereigns lay there, as bright as when they had been struck in the Australian Mint.

"By gum!" breathed David Bone

"Plenty much feller gold, sar!" chuckled Loo.

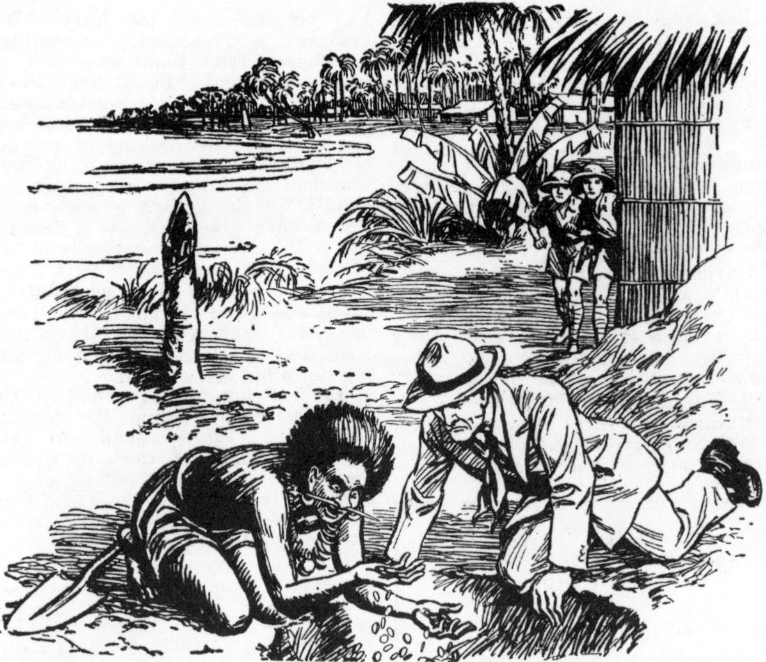

"Plenty much feller gold, sar!" chuckled Loo, running a stream of coins through his black fingers. "Ten thousand at least," said Bone. Neither of them noticed that the two island traders were watching them from the back of the hut.

He ran a stream of the coins through his black fingers.

David Bone drove his skinny fingers through the stack of them. He panted for breath.

"Ten thousand at least! Ten thousand!"

Neither of the treasure-seekers, bending over the excavation, gazing with dilated eyes at the gleaming gold, saw the two black shadows that detached themselves from the back of the hut. Neither of them heard soft footfalls that came noiselessly. But both of them leaped up with startled cries as a voice fell on their ears:

"Thanks!"

Treasure for Two!

"THANKS!" said Bob Harris pleasantly.

"Thanks!" chuckled Billy McCann.

David Bone sprang up, his eyes ablaze. His hand went to his hip, but did not grasp the weapon there. A revolver that gleamed in the moonlight was levelled, and Bob Harris' finger was on the trigger.

"Better not!" said Bob.

The black claw of the Santa Cruz boy was on the knife in his loin-cloth. He did not release it, but he did not draw it, as Billy McCann shoved the muzzle of a gun almost into his black face. He panted, eyeing Billy like a wild beast about to spring.

"Drop that feller knife, you black swab!" said Billy McCann. "I'm not going to tell you twice!"

Loo, with a gurgling mutter, dropped the knife. It clanged on the heap of sovereigns.

"Stand back!"

The Santa Cruz boy stood back.

David Bone was trembling from head to foot with passion. The rage in his sunken eyes was almost demoniac as he glared at the partners of Kalua.

"Quite a pleasant surprise, what?" asked Bob, with a smile. "Don't touch that gun, Bone! I warn you that it won't be healthy!"

"You!" breathed David Bone. "I—I guessed——"

"You guessed we were on the other side of Kalua, hunting pearls?" Bob nodded. "Yes, that's what we wanted you to guess, Mr. Bone. You see, we'd tumbled to it what you were after, but we didn't know exactly where to dig for the treasure, and we didn't want to dig around over three acres or so——"

"Plenty too much hard work for this feller," explained Billy McCann, with a chuckle.

"So we stepped out and let you go ahead," drawled Bob. "And I'm bound to say, Mr. Bone, that we're obliged to you. And if you're still keen on buying this spot, with its royal associations, we'll sell at a reasonable figure—after we've taken out the quids."

"After!" chuckled Billy. "Not before!"

"Double-crossed!" breathed David Bone. "You durned, doggoned——"

He choked with rage.

"If Loo had come to us," said Bob, "we'd have given him a good whack for what he could have told us. But I reckon he wanted the lot."

The Santa Cruz boy gave him a wolfish look.

"You feller Loo," said Bob, with a smile, "you plenty bad feller. You savvy too much along death-spider. But take a double handful of that gold, and beat it!" He glanced at his partner. "You say the same, Billy?"

"Suffering cats!" snorted Billy. Then he grinned. "It's our gold, in our ground. But you hear what feller white master say, you feller Loo, ear belong you? Take it and go!"

The Santa Cruz boy stared at the partners of Kalua almost unbelievingly for a moment. Then he threw himself down and scooped up a double handful of glimmering sovereigns. He stacked them into his loin-cloth, grinning. Then, as if fearing that the feller white masters might change their minds, Loo darted away and vanished into the distant bush.

Bob gave the panting American trader a cheery grin.

"I reckoned that Loo ought to have a whack," he said. "But you, David Bone, all you'll get is the happy knowledge that you've guided us to a treasure that belongs to us. Not a continental red cent over that! Feeling good?"

David Bone gritted his teeth.

"You durned, doggoned Smart Alecs!" he ground out. "You figure you're getting away with this? You reckon——"

"Just a few!" said Billy McCann cheerfully. "And you—— Look out!"

The enraged man from 'Frisco was dragging out his revolver.

Bob's eyes gleamed over his levelled barrel.

"Drop it!" he ordered.

David Bone, with a ringing oath, dropped his gun, and it crashed on the ground. It was only in time to save his life.

Billy McCann, with a grim face, stepped towards the American trader.

"Now I'm going to talk to you, David Bone," he said. "Put up your hands! Bob'll see fair play—a thing you'll get, though you never give it! Put up your paws, you thief!"

In his rage and fury David Bone put up his "paws" willingly enough. He sprang like a tiger at Billy McCann.

The next ten minutes were wild and whirling.

Bob Harris looked on with an approving eye as his partner dealt faithfully with David Bone.

Billy McCann had marks to show when he had finished. But it was a wrecked and almost unrecognisable David Bone that went crashing at last into the excavation, scattering golden sovereigns right and left in his fall.

"Any more?" asked Billy a little breathlessly.

A groan was the only answer.

"Your turn, Bob," said Billy McCann, "though I haven't left a lot for you."

Bob laughed.

He picked David Bone out of the treasure-hole.

"Get going!" he said tersely.

And the American trader, groaning, crawled away to the beach.

Printed and published every Saturday by the Proprietors, The Amalgamated Press, Ltd., The Fleetway House, Farringdon Street, London, E.C.4. Advertisement offices: The Fleetway House, Farringdon Street, London, E.C.4. Registered for transmission by Canadian Magazine Post. Subscription rates: Inland and Abroad, 11s. per annum; 5s. 6d. for six months. Sole Agents for Australia and New Zealand: Messrs. Gordon & Gotch, Ltd., and for South Africa: Central News Agency, Ltd.— Saturday, August 13th, 1932.

It was a nine days' wonder on Kalua.

Seven thousand sovereigns were picked out of the treasure-hole by the partners of Kalua. Seven thousand golden sovereigns, stacked away long ago by old Mokatoo, had fallen into white men's hands at long last. And all Kalua agreed that they could not have fallen into better hands.

At dawn the cutter Osprey lifted the hook and put to sea, carrying away a bruised, sore, and savage David Bone. His business on Kalua was finished—not in the way he had expected. Billy McCann rubbed a swollen nose, and grinned as he watched the cutter glide out of the reef passage into the Pacific.

"We're done with David Bone!" he remarked.

"You've said it!" said Bob.

Fortunate days followed for the island firm. The store was rebuilt, and Pete Purkiss put in charge of it. The beach-comber had had his lesson, and he swore to make good, and a generous share of Mokatoo's treasure helped him to get back his self-respect. The fat and prosperous man in spotless white ducks who sat on the counter of the new store and smoked expensive cigars would hardly have been recognised as the waster who had combed the beach of Kalua.

"Now we're in clover, Billy——" said Bob Harris one day.

"Go it!"

"We'll get a new car."

"Eh?"

"A new car."

"What's the matter with the old bus?" asked Billy unpleasantly.

"You mean what isn't the matter with it?" asked Bob.

"I mean what I say, Mr. Harris."

And Bob chuckled and gave it up. Fortune had changed, but there was no change in Bob, Billy & Co.

THE END.

HIGH JINKS HIKING!

(*Continued from page* 15.)

"Quiet!" hist Jack Jolly, with a glarnse through the winder of the sedan. "I really beleeve he's going to sleep at last. If he does, it'll give us a charnse to escape!"

"My hat, yes!"

The juniors tramped on, with renewed hoap in their breasts. Sure enuff, within the next five minnits, a series of deep, rumbling snores, somewhat resembling a distant earthquake, broke out within the sedan, and the juniors knew that the Head was asleep.

"Now for it!" wispered Merry.

"Half a minnit!" interposed Jack Jolly. "If the sedan stops rocking, the old buffer'll probably notiss it and wake up again. What about hitching it up to those two mokes in the field over there?"

"Oh, grate pip!"

"Ripping wheeze!" declared Frank Fearless enthusiastically. "You fellows carry on slowly while I catch the mokes!"

Grinning all over their dials, Jolly and Merry and Bright carried on with the sedan while Frank opened the gate leading to the field.

Frank Fearless, who had been a skoller at sevveral grate public skools, had an intimate nollidge of donkeys, and soon made friends with the two mokes in the field. He led them out into the road, and, with the aid of sevveral lengths of rope, attached one to the front part of the sedan and one behind.

Evenchually, the job was completed, and Jack Jolly & Co. stepped back to survay their handiwork. The site of the majestick headmaster of St. Sam's sitting fast asleep in a sedan-chair carried by donkeys was awfully comical, and the juniors had to hold their handkerchiefs to their mouths to stop their larfter.

"Better send him back in the direction of St. Sam's!" grinned Frank Fearless. "We can carry on with the toor, then. Gee-up, Ned!"

Fearless gave the leading donkey a slap with his open palm, and, although the moke gave a loud nay, he promptly did what Fearless required—broke into a trot.

Jack Jolly & Co. watched the weerd-looking vehicle out of site. Then, larfing fit to bust, they turned their footprints in the opposite direction.

. . . . .

Meanwhile, two donkeys, carrying another donkey in the shape of Dr. Alfred Birchemall, galloped along the road in the gathering dusk at ever-increasing speed. Farm laberers, walking home to their cottages, scattered in alarm as they thundered past, motorists swerved violently, and chickens flew, shreeking, to their roosts.

Dr. Birchemall slept on for about half an hour. Then a particularly violent bump roused him, and he sat up with a jerk.

"Jolly! Fearless! What the merry dickens are you doing of?" he roared, with his usual faultless grammar, poking his head out of the winder as he spoke.

Then he spotted the donkeys, and a howl of sheer terror arose from him.

"Help! Murder! Perlice!" he hooted. "Some evil spirit has changed my stretcher-bearers into donkeys. Yarooooo!"

For a time his yells remained unanswered. Then suddenly he herd the roar of a powerful car behind him, and reckernised the familiar uniforms of the mobile perlice.

(*Continued on next page.*)

SOUTHWARD BOUND!

(*Continued from page 23.*)

"What—what—— My hat!" yelled Bob. "Back up, Johnny!"

The two Neapolitans leaped up from Wharton, as Bob Cherry and Johnny Bull rushed at them. But they did not gain their feet—crashing fists sent them spinning over, and they sprawled on the mosaic floor, yelling.

Harry Wharton scrambled up breathlessly.

"Quick—get out of this!" he panted.

"But what——" gasped Bob.

"Come on! They're after the scarab——" panted Wharton.

"Oh!"

The three juniors ran out of the building, while Giuseppe and his companion were scrambling up. They heard the footsteps of the two bravos pattering in pursuit on the cobbles as they rushed up the street. But the two rascals pursued them only a few paces.

As the juniors reached the Greyfriars party the bravos dodged away among the ruins and disappeared.

"What has happened?" exclaimed Sir Reginald Brooke. "Wharton—— Have you——"

"They got me—they'd have had the scarab if these chaps hadn't come back for me!" gasped Wharton. "Two of them——"

"Follow me at once!" said the baronet. "Keep together!"

Billy Bunter had clambered back into his sedan. It started, and the rest of the party walked quickly after it. In a few minutes they were outside Pompeii, and walking back to the hotel.

On the well-frequented road, with guides and tourists passing every moment, there was little danger, but "Nunky" was glad when they reached the hotel, and he ordered the car at once to return to Naples.

The excursion was cut short—not to the satisfaction of the juniors. But Nunky's word was law. There was no doubt that Giuseppe and his associates were still hanging about, looking for a chance, and Nunky sagely decided not to give them a chance.

"I say, you fellows!" Billy Bunter was grinning as he packed his podgy person into the car. "I say, I wonder what would have happened to you fellows if I hadn't come on this trip—what?"

"Well, Bunter's saved the scarab," said Harry Wharton. "They'd have had it, if you fellows hadn't come back for me—and it seems that it was Bunter who warned you——"

"The right man in the right place, as usual," said Bunter. "Lot of use you fellows would be without me! You'd have lost that scarab, Mauly, if I hadn't stayed behind to keep watch, while you went rooting about among those fat-headed ruins!"

"You've come in useful for once!" grunted Johnny Bull. "After all, why shouldn't you? You'll never be ornamental!"

"This is the thanks I get for keeping watch and saving you fellows from danger, and all that!" said Bunter. "Well, I'm used to it—and I'll go on looking after you, and protecting you, all the same. You'll be jolly glad I'm with you in Egypt, if we get attacked by dahabiyeh, or a dragoman, or something——"

"Ha, ha, ha!" yelled the juniors, quite overcome by the idea of being attacked by a dahabiyeh, which was a Nile boat; or a dragoman, which was a Cairo guide. Apparently, Billy Bunter supposed them to be fearsome beasts that haunted the banks of the Nile.

"You can cackle!" snorted Bunter.

"Thanks—we will!" chortled Bob Cherry.

And they did!

Whether Giuseppe & Co. were still looking for them the juniors never knew, as the swift car carried them back to Naples. At all events, it was certain that the bravo would never hand the golden scarab over to Kalizelos; the Greek had failed once more.

And the following morning the Greyfriars party boarded the steamer for Alexandria, and churned out into the Tyrrhenian Sea. Under hotter and hotter suns, they steamed on through the blue Mediterranean, looking eagerly forward to Alexandria, and to setting their feet, at last, on the banks of the Nile, in the mysterious and fascinating land of Egypt.

THE END.

(*Whatever you do, chums, don't miss "HARRY WHARTON & CO. IN EGYPT!" the next yarn in this novel holiday series. You'll vote it absolutely GREAT!*)

HIGH JINKS HIKING!

(*Continued from previous page.*)

"Thank hevvan!" he gasped, sinking back on his cushions, with grate releef.

In a matter of minnits the perlice car brought the donkeys to a halt.

Dr. Birchemall stepped out of the sedan, fairly beaming with grattitude.

"Thanks awfully, officers!" he said. "I'm afraid I haven't much change on me, but I feel I must acknollidge your brave deed. If you'll axxept tuppence each——"

"Silence!" roared one of the officers, grately to the Head's serprize. "What is your name?"

"My name?"

The Head of St. Sam's stood nonplussed.

"Yes!" roared the officer, producing a notebook and pencil. "And just you be sharp about it!"

"Alfred Birchemall. But——"

"Then, Alfred Birchemall, you may consider yourself under arrest for exceeding the speed limit! Put the bracelets on him, Jim!"

Dr. Birchemall felt cold steel closing round his wrists. He was handcuffed like a common felon.

"M-m-my hat!" he stuttered, as the officers led him to their car and bundled him ruffly into the corner. "This is what mite be termed the end of a perfect day! Instead of spending the nite in a posh hotel, I look like spending it in some fowl dungeon! What a cell!"

Dr. Birchemall's mental fourcast was correct. He passed that nite on a bare board in a perlice cell, while Jack Jolly & Co., many miles away, slept in comfort.

But nobody can say that it was too harsh a punishment for the hiker who miked.

THE END.

(Don't miss the next yarn in this amusing "hiking" series, chums! It's entitled "THE INN OF MYSTERY!" and will send you into fits of laughter when you read it.)

"THE RED FALCON!" Thrill-packed Highwayman Story Starts To-day!

The MAGNET 2D

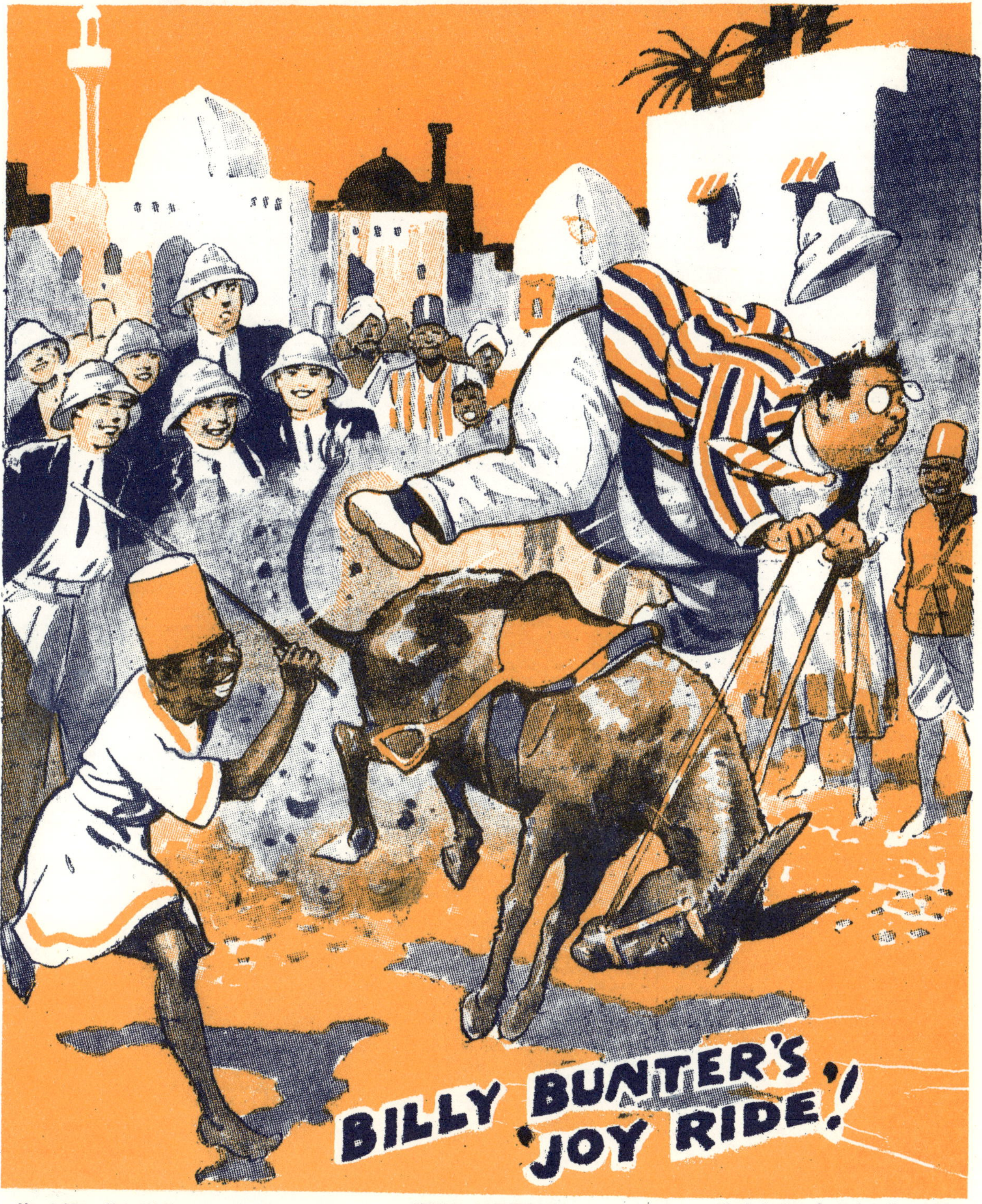

No. 1,279. Vol. XLII. EVERY SATURDAY. Week Ending August 20th, 1932.

ITEMS OF INTEREST FROM ALL QUARTERS !

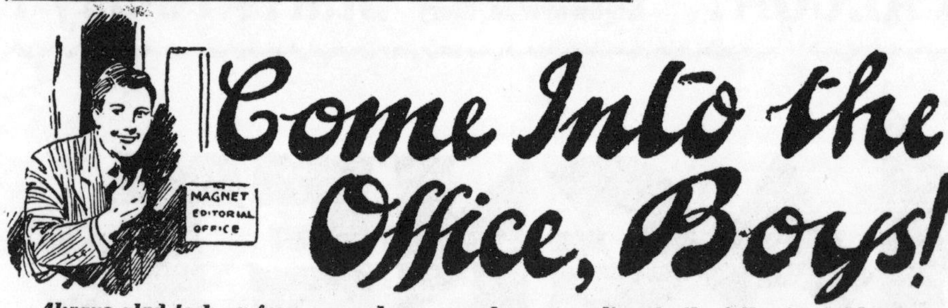

Always glad to hear from you, chums, so drop me a line to the following address: The Editor, The " Magnet " Library, The Amalgamated Press, Ltd., The Fleetway House, Farringdon Street, London, E.C.4.

IN this issue appears the first magnificent instalment of Arthur Steffens' new serial: "The Red Falcon," and I am quite anxious to know what you think about it. I believe it is going to be one of the most popular serials I have ever published—for what boy is there who doesn't revel in a stirring yarn of the " good old days " ? As this story progresses it will keep you guessing at the mystery which surrounds Hal Lovett; and his adventures, and those of his pal, Jerry McLean, will hold your interest until the very end. Tell your chums about this rattling fine serial —and see that you don't miss a single instalment of it yourself ! Take my tip, and tell your newsagent to reserve you a copy of the MAGNET regularly !

Do you know which are

THE LARGEST PASSENGER-CARRYING AEROPLANES IN THE WORLD ?

Jack Harford, of Dumfries, asks me to tell him. The " Heracles " and the " Hannibal " types hold this distinction. Both are owned by Imperial Airways, and the following particulars concerning them may be of interest to many readers. Both have a span of 130 feet, a length of 89½ feet, and a height of 27 feet 3 inches. Both, also, carry a crew of three, but the " Heracles " type carry 38 passengers as against the " Hannibal " type's 24. Here are the technical details of both types:

" Hannibal ": Four Bristol " Jupiter XIF " engines, 9-cylinder air-cooled radial, each 490 h.p. Maximum speed 127 m.p.h. Cruising speed 100 m.p.h. Normally employed between Cairo and Karachi. Built by Handley Page. There are four machines of this type; Hannibal (G-AAGX); Hanno (G-AAUD); Hadrian (G-AAUE); and Horsa (G-AAUC).

" Heracles ": Four Bristol " Jupiter XFBM " engines, 9-cylinder air-cooled radial, with medium ratio supercharger and airscrew reduction gear, each 550 h.p. Maximum and cruising speeds the same as " Hannibal " type. Normally employed between London and Paris. There are also four machines of this type, as follows: Heracles (G-AAXC); Horatius (G.AAXD); Hengist (G-AAXE); and Helena (G-AAXF). These, too, were built by Handley Page.

NOW comes a query concerning

MOTOR-CYCLE RACING.

Bernard Barclay, of Nottingham, wants to know if a foreigner has ever won the British Tourist Trophy Race ? The answer is " No." Although foreigners have tried their best to do so, none have ever been successful. On the other hand, Great Britain has won every foreign road race of importance this year ! The Belgian Grand Prix, which was the last of the big Continental Grand Prix races, and was run recently, resulted in Great Britain winning each of the four classes. The Senior Class was won by Stanley Woods, of Dublin, who also won the last Senior Tourist Trophy Race.

This country is certainly

PILING UP THE SPEED RECORDS !

On land, water, and air we hold the records ! Here they are, up to date. Air: Flight-Lieut. Stainforth's 408.8 m.p.h.; Land: Sir Malcolm Campbell's 246.09 m.p.h.; and Water: Kaye Don's recent 119.81 m.p.h. In addition to that, four railway records were broken by British trains last month. The natives of the land of Fisher T. Fish will have to " pull up their socks " if they want to beat that bundle !

One of our lucky readers this week is Harry Dean, of 7, Tanybryn Street, Aberdare. I have just had the pleasure of sending a top-notch Sheffield steel pen-knife to him in return for the following rib-tickling joke:

Diner: " This milk is very weak, waiter! Can you account for it ? "

Waiter: " Maybe the cow got caught in the rain, sir ! "

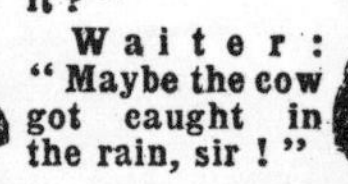

Pile in with your attempts, chums ! You may be one of the lucky ones in a week or two !

HAVE you ever been puzzled as to

HOW " ROTTEN ROW " GOT ITS NAME ?

George Martin, of Poplar, asks me if I can tell him. Well, years ago, the king used to use this drive, and it became known as the " Route du Roi," or the " way of the king." As the years passed the words became corrupted to " Rotten Row," by which name it is called to-day. Many of the London streets have curious names whose origins go far back in history. Birdcage Walk, for instance, was called that because Charles II used to keep an aviary there. Pall Mall received its name because it was there that the game of Paille-Maille was first played in London. The hunting packs of Old London were kept in Houndsditch, and Hoxton was once called Hogsdon, because it was a famous pig market.

There are many

CURIOUS STREET NAMES

in London. Fancy a place called " Of Alley." Its name was recently changed to York Place. It was originally called after George Villiers, Duke of Buckingham, whose estate was sold on condition that his name and title must be remembered. Consequently the streets were named: George Street, Villiers Street, Duke Street, Of Alley, and Buckingham Street. " Adelphi " is a Greek word for " brothers," and Adelphi, in London, was so called because it was built by two brothers, Robert and John Adam. There are, therefore " Robert," " John," and " Adam " streets in the Adelphi. Perhaps the most curious street in London is in Hoxton, and is called " The Land of Promise." The " promise " doesn't seem to amount for much, because at the end of the street there is—a workhouse !

HARRY FOREST, of Wivenhoe, tells me he is making a collection of those interesting paragraphs which I have passed on to you on various occasions, and he wants some more of them. So here are a few more

THINGS YOU'D HARDLY BELIEVE !

The Crystal Palace is Longer in Summer than in Winter ! It is built of glass and iron, both of which expand in heat. On a hot summer's day, the expansion amounts to as much as ten inches !

A Man Once Swam Four Thousand Miles ! He started from the source of the Mississippi River, and swam all the way to its mouth, even swimming the numerous rapids. Needless to say, he came out of the water for periods of rest, and it took him five months to complete the job. As yet, he is the only swimmer to have accomplished this task !

" Portuguese men-o'-war " are NOT Portuguese—Nor are they men-o'-war ! The term is one given by sailors to the Nautilus, which is a genus of cuttle-fish !

Human Beings With Tongues Like Snakes ! Although very rare, human beings have been known to have forked tongues like snakes ! One German woman, whose tongue forked out into two at the end was unable to speak a word !

I have just room left to print this Greyfriars limerick, for which H. Harris, of 33, Shere Road, Ilford, Essex, gets a real leather pocket wallet:

Poor Bunter ! He generally kicks
When Quelchy hands out to him " six."
But this lucky day
He just grinned away—
He'd stuffed his check breeches with bricks !

LOOK out for next week's issue, chums. In the long complete tale—

" THE LURE OF THE GOLDEN SCARAB ! "
By Frank Richards,

you will learn more about the amazing adventures which overtake Harry Wharton & Co. during their holiday in Egypt. There's plenty of fun in the yarn, too, and it is certainly one of the best which this most popular author has ever given us. This splendid holiday series gets better and better every week. Now's the time to introduce your chums to the MAGNET.

In addition to a long instalment of our new serial, there will also be another cheery yarn of Doctor Birchemall, entitled: " The Bogus Hero ! " and the usual shorter features.

Cheerio until next week, chums !

YOUR EDITOR.

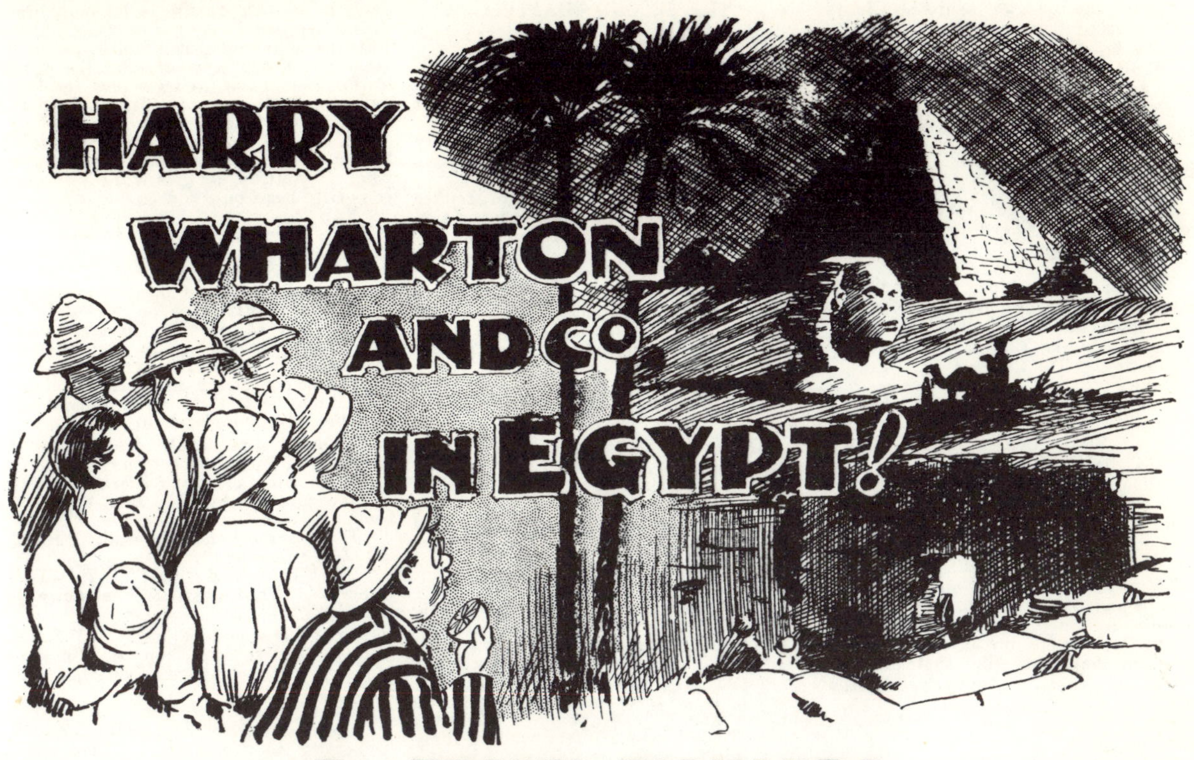

HARRY WHARTON AND CO IN EGYPT!

BY FRANK RICHARDS.

THE FIRST CHAPTER.

Bound for Egypt!

BILLY BUNTER removed Lord Mauleverer's best Panama hat from his bullet head, mopped his perspiring, podgy brow with one of Harry Wharton's handkerchiefs, and gasped.

It was hot!

Harry Wharton & Co. had rather expected to find it warm in the Mediterranean Sea in summer. They found it, perhaps, a little too warm for comfort; except Hurree Jamset Ram Singh, who basked and revelled in the sun-blaze that reminded him of his native land. But they looked very cheery and bright. Billy Bunter, on the other hand, seemed to regard the heat as a special unkind trick purposely played on him by Nature, and he was annoyed.

"Oooooogh!" said Bunter.

Bob Cherry glanced round at him, with a cheery grin.

"Hallo, hallo, hallo, old fat bean! Enjoying life?" he inquired. Warm as it was, Bob Cherry ,at least, seemed to have lost none of his usual energy. Instead of sitting in a deckchair like the other fellows, on the deck of the steamer, Bob was actively engaged with a "yo-yo," putting in a little practice, rather to the peril of his near neighbours. Bob had a skilled hand with a cricket bat; but he had not yet acquired skill with a "yo-yo," and he seemed rather to use it as a weapon of offence.

"Oooogh! No!" grunted Bunter. "It's hot! Beastly hot! I wish I was in Margate!"

"I wish you were, old bean," said Bob cordially.

"Hear, hear!" assented Johnny Bull.

"The wishfulness is terrific!" concurred Hurree Jamset Ram Singh.

"This trip to Egypt," remarked Frank Nugent thoughtfully, "needs only one thing to make it perfect. If only Bunter was at Margate——"

"Ha, ha, ha!"

Grunt from Billy Bunter.

There was no doubt that it was cooler at Margate, and Bunter wished that he was there. But he did not seem pleased, somehow, to find his wish so heartily echoed by the other fellows.

"I say, Mauly!"

"Yaas?" murmured Lord Mauleverer. Stretched in a long cane chair, with his second best Panama tilted over his eyes, his lordship was dozing away the sunny hours.

Ancient and mysterious Egypt holds many attractions for Harry Wharton & Co.—not the least of them being an exciting hunt for a buried treasure worth a king's ransom!

"This idea of a trip to Egypt was simply fatheaded, Mauly."

"Yaas."

"You're a silly ass, Mauly."

"Yaas."

"And a burbling idiot!" hooted Bunter.

"Yaas."

"We could have had a ripping time at Margate——"

"Yaas."

"I'm simply frying!"

"Yaas."

"Beast!"

Billy Bunter fanned himself with Mauly's best Panama, grunted, and blinked round him morosely through his big spectacles. Hot as it was, the other fellows found their surroundings pleasant enough. The Greyfriars party had travelled by train to Naples, and taken the steamer for Alexandria there. Now they were half-way on their journey to the Egyptian port, and the mountains of Crete loomed against the blue sky, on the port quarter—the last land they were to see until the shores of Egypt came in sight.

Later in the season when the rush for the Nile began, the steamers would be crowded, but in the hot weather there was no crowd. Round the churning steamer, rolled the Mediterranean, wide and blue, stretching, apparently, to infinity, inland sea as it was. Only the Cretan hill-tops broke the line where the sea met the sky. At a little distance from the schoolboys Sir Reginald Brooke, Mauly's uncle, was pacing the deck slowly, in conversation with an American tourist. Other passengers were leaning on the rail, or sitting in the deckchairs, reading newspapers, or consulting red-covered guide books. Stewards came and went with cooling drinks. There was hardly a breath of air; and the throb of the engines sounded with loud distinctness, and there was rather an oily scent from the engine-room. Billy Bunter's blink landed on the blue hill-tops against the blue sky.

"I say, you fellows! Is that Egypt?" he asked.

Harry Wharton laughed.

"Not quite!" he answered. "That's Crete!"

"Are we far from Egypt?"

"Only about three hundred miles."

"Oh lor'!" groaned Bunter.

The island of Crete faded away on the port quarter. Out of sight of land, the Naples steamer churned on towards the distant shores of Africa.

"I say, you fellows——"

"Don't say it's hot!" said Bob Cherry. "We've had that one!"

"It's beastly hot——"

"Wait till you get to Egypt! You're only frying here! You'll bake there!"

"The bakefulness will be terrific!" chuckled Hurree Jamset Ram Singh. "The esteemed Bunter will melt away into ridiculous tallow!"

"Beast!"

"Buck up, old fat man," said Bob encouragingly. "Like to take a turn with my 'yo-yo'?"

"Yah!"

"I'll show you how to handle it," said Bob. "You see, you make the spool run down the string like that—and it comes back like that—and you run it down again like that——"

Bang!

"Yaroooooooh!"

"Did that hit your nose, Bunter?"

"Ow! Wow! Beast!" roared Bunter.

"Ha, ha, ha!"

Billy Bunter left off fanning himself, and clasped both fat hands to his fat little nose, and roared. The "yo-yo" had established contact there, perhaps by accident, and perhaps not!

"You shouldn't put your nose in the way when I'm showing you how to handle a 'yo-yo'," said Bob Cherry chidingly. "Let's try again! You run it down the string like that——"

"Keep off, you beast!" yelled Bunter, dodging the whizzing spool.

"And like that——"

"Yoooop!"

"And like that——"

"Wow!"

Billy Bunter jumped out of his chair. The "yo-yo" caught him on a fat ear as he jumped. There was another roar from Bunter.

"Will you keep off, you beast?" he yelled.

"But I'm showing you how to handle a 'yo-yo,' old chap! You see, it goes like this——"

Bang!

"Yarooooh!"

"And like this——"

"Ha, ha, ha!"

Billy Bunter hopped and jumped like a fat kangaroo. Harry Wharton & Co. chortled, and Lord Mauleverer sat up and grinned. Bob, with undiminished energy, continued to instruct the fat Owl of the Remove in the use of a "yo-yo"—his idea of the use of it, apparently, being to deliver a series of sharp taps all over Bunter.

"Leave off, you beast!" roared Bunter, dodging round the chairs. "Keep that beastly thing away, you rotter! Whooop!"

"Ha, ha, ha!"

The fat Owl clutched up a cushion from his chair. He whirled it aloft with both hands, and took aim at Bob, and hurled it with all the force of two fat arms.

Bob Cherry grinned and dodged, and the missile flew over his head and shot along the deck.

But every bullet, it is said, has its billet. The same rule applied to the cushion. It missed Bob Cherry by a foot, whizzed on, and caught a plump Egptian gentleman who was coming along the deck, landing fairly in his dark-skinned face. There was a howl of astonishment from the plump Egyptian gentleman; a red tarboosh flew in one direction, a sun-umbrella in another, and the plump Egyptian gentleman sat down on the deck, with a bump that almost shook the steamer.

THE SECOND CHAPTER.

Bumps for Bunter!

HARRY WHARTON & CO. leaped to their feet.

The Egyptian gentleman sat and blinked.

"You fat chump!" roared Harry Wharton.

"Oh, my hat!" gasped Nugent.

The Famous Five rushed to render first-aid. Bob Cherry picked up the sun-umbrella. Nugent captured the tarboosh. Wharton and Johnny Bull grasped the dark gentleman by either arm and helped him to his feet. He was a plump gentleman, and a good weight, and Hurree Singh and Lord Mauleverer lent a hand each to get him back to the perpendicular.

He stood gasping.

"Awfully sorry, sir!" gasped Wharton.

"Quite an accident!" said Johnny Bull.

"The sorrowfulness is terrific, esteemed sahib."

"Here's your hat, sir!" Nugent held up the tarboosh.

"Here's your umbrella, sir!"

"Hope you're not hurt, sir!"

The dark gentleman gasped spasmodically. He seemed to be winded. He passed a dark hand over his dark features. Fortunately they were not damaged; the cushion was a soft one, though it had hit rather hard. The juniors were full of apologies. A Greyfriars "rag" was all very well in their own select circle; but it was not the thing to floor an unoffending stranger. Billy Bunter, on the other hand, turned up his fat little nose and curled his podgy lip. Billy Bunter considered this an absurd fuss to make about a "nigger." In Billy Bunter's lofty estimation all coloured gentlemen were "niggers," and Bunter had a lofty and superior contempt for them—though he was not himself, as a matter of fact, a remarkably creditable specimen of the white race.

"I say, you fellows——" grunted Bunter.

"You clumsy ass!" hooted Bob Cherry. "Haven't you manners enough to say you're sorry?"

"Oh, rats!" said Bunter. "Lot of fuss to make about a darkey!"

"Shut up, you fat villain!"

"Oh, really, Cherry——"

"All right now, sir?" asked Harry Wharton. "We're awfully sorry, sir. I hope you'll excuse that clumsy owl; he didn't mean it to get you."

The Egyptian gentleman recovered his composure. It was plain that he was annoyed and offended; but he made the juniors a polite bow and moved away to a vacant chair without speaking a word.

He sat down rather heavily in the chair, replaced the tarboosh on his head, and took no further notice of the Greyfriars party. Harry Wharton & Co. resumed their seats, considerably perturbed by the unfortunate accident. Whether the dark gentleman understood English or not, they could not tell, as he had not spoken, but they hoped that he understood, at least, that they had been apologising for the accident. Obviously he was annoyed, which was not surprising in the circumstances.

"What about kicking Bunter?" asked Johnny Bull. "We haven't kicked him since we broke up at Greyfriars, and Bunter can't do without a certain amount of kicking."

"Beast! I say, you fellows, what the dickens does it matter about the darkey?" said Bunter peevishly. "I don't believe in wasting a lot of politeness on niggers."

Harry Wharton cast a quick, anxious glance at the Egyptian. But the dark brown face gave no sign that he had understood Bunter's words, or, indeed, heard them at all.

"You fat, frowsy frump!" said Harry. "The man may understand you. If you say another word I'll bang your silly head on the deck."

"Yah!"

The Egyptian was dressed in European clothes, with the exception of the red tarboosh. He looked like a wealthy man of good position; though to Bunter's lofty eyes he was only a nigger, and of no more account than one of the darkies in the engine-room. He sat with an expressionless face, as if unconscious of the English schoolboys near him, and they could only hope that he did not understand Bunter.

A dark, slim Arab dressed in a galabyeh of fine white cotton came along the deck with a tray of sherbet. Billy Bunter blinked at him and waved a beckoning fat hand.

"Just what I want!" he said. "Here, steward, this way!"

"You benighted owl!" said Bob Cherry. "That chap isn't a steward. Shut up!"

"Rot!" snapped Bunter. "I'm not asking you to pay for it, Cherry! Mauly's standing the exes on this trip, ain't you, Mauly?"

"Yaas."

"Here, steward!" hooted Bunter, still beckoning to the Arab. "This way! Bring it here."

The man did not heed him. He stopped before the plump Egyptian gentleman and bent low as he presented the tray to him. Billy Bunter blinked at that proceeding with great indignation. There were native stewards on the steamer, and the Arab might have been mistaken for one of them; but all the fellows except Bunter could see that this particular Arab was the Egyptian gentleman's servant. He was attending to his master's wants, and probably did not even realise that the fat Owl was speaking to him at all.

"Cheek!" snorted Bunter. "This is what comes of giving them Home Rule, and all that rot! It makes them cheeky! Fancy that cheeky blighter having the nerve to serve a nigger before a white man!"

"Mightn't recognise you as a white man," suggested Johnny Bull. "You haven't washed since we broke up at Greyfriars!"

"The whitefulness of the esteemed Bunter is not terrific. But the grubbiness and the greasiness are preposterous!" remarked Hurree Jamset Ram Singh.

"Oh, really, Inky! Of course, you'd sympathise with other niggers," said Bunter. "Birds of a feather, you know! I've jolly good mind to kick that cheeky blacky!"

The Arab with the tray gave quite a start, and his black eyes turned on Bunter for a second. It looked as if he understood English, whether his master did or not.

The Greyfriars fellows coloured with vexation.

Billy Bunter's manners were never modelled on those of Lord Chesterfield; but when he was among foreigners Bunter really was the limit.

The Egyptian spoke to the servant in a language totally incomprehensible to the schoolboys. They caught the word "Ali," which they guessed to be the Arab's name; but the rest was impenetrable.

Ali, if his name was Ali, salaamed to his master, and carried away the tray and disappeared. He shot another glance at the juniors with his sharp black eyes as he went.

Billy Bunter snorted.

"Cheeky lot of niggers!" he grunted. "I say, you fellows, which of you is going to fetch me a lemon-squash?"

"The whichfulness is terrific."

"Are you going, Bob?"

"I don't think!"

"What about you, Nugent?"

"Fathead!"

"Selfishness all round!" said Bunter bitterly. "I've turned down a lot of invitations for the hols to come out to Egypt with you fellows to protect you, and this is my reward! Blessed if it isn't enough to make a fellow chuck up being generous and kind-hearted."

"Oh crumbs!"

"I shouldn't wonder if you fellows make me selfish, like yourselves, in the long run," said Bunter morosely. "Here I am, hot and thirsty, and not one of you will fetch me a lemon-squash!"

"You can't fetch it yourself?" asked Bob.

"Oh, really, Cherry!" Apparently that resource had not occurred to Billy Bunter's fat mind. "Where's a beastly steward? They buzz round like flies when they're not wanted. Think that nigger would fetch me a lemon-squash if I asked him?" Bunter jerked a fat and not very clean thumb at the Egyptian gentleman.

"What?" gasped Wharton.

"I can't speak his idiotic lingo, of course, but I dare say I could make him understand," said Bunter. "I'll give him a franc—one of you fellows lend me a franc——"

"If that chap could understand what you are saying, you fat porker, I'd jam your silly head on the deck," said Harry Wharton. "Lucky for you he can't."

"Oh, really, Wharton!"

"Shut up!" hooted Bob Cherry.

"I suppose we mustn't drop him into the sea," said Johnny Bull thoughtfully.

"You'll be jolly glad to have me with you if that Greek blighter Kalizelos turns up again," sneered Bunter. "I shouldn't wonder if he's on this steamer, or some of his gang, after the scarab. He jolly nearly got it at Naples, and I saved you——"

"If you thought Kalizelos was on this steamer, you fat funk, you'd be hiding under your bunk!" growled Johnny Bull.

"Yah! I've looked over the passengers, and Kalizelos isn't among them," said Bunter. "But any of these darkies might be in his gang, and you jolly well know he's after Mauly's scarab—that idiotic golden beetle that Mauly's pater dug up somewhere in Egypt, that belonged to some nigger named Washtub, or something——"

"A-Menah, you fat chump!"

"If Mauly had any sense he would give me the scarab to mind, instead of you, Wharton. It would be safe then. If there's any darkey on this steamer after it, I'm the man to handle him, as you jolly well know. You can cackle. But if you fellows get into danger, who's going to pull you through?" demanded Bunter. "That very darkey sitting there looking like a black gargoyle might be after it, for anything you know."

The Egyptian gentleman rose to his feet. He turned to the schoolboys, made a polite bow, and, to their surprise—and horror—spoke in excellent English.

"Young gentlemen," he said quietly, "as you appear to be discussing affairs of a private nature in my hearing I feel compelled to warn you that I speak your language."

With that the plump Egyptian gentleman sat down again and resumed gazing at the sea, his dark face as expressionless as before.

Harry Wharton & Co. looked at one another.

Obviously every word that had been uttered in his hearing had been understood by the Egyptian. He had given no sign until the talk turned on matters which were evidently not for a stranger's ears, when he had felt compelled to "put them wise"—which was certainly a decent and honourable proceeding on his part. Never had the chums of Greyfriars felt so utterly disconcerted and discomfited, and even Billy Bunter was a little abashed.

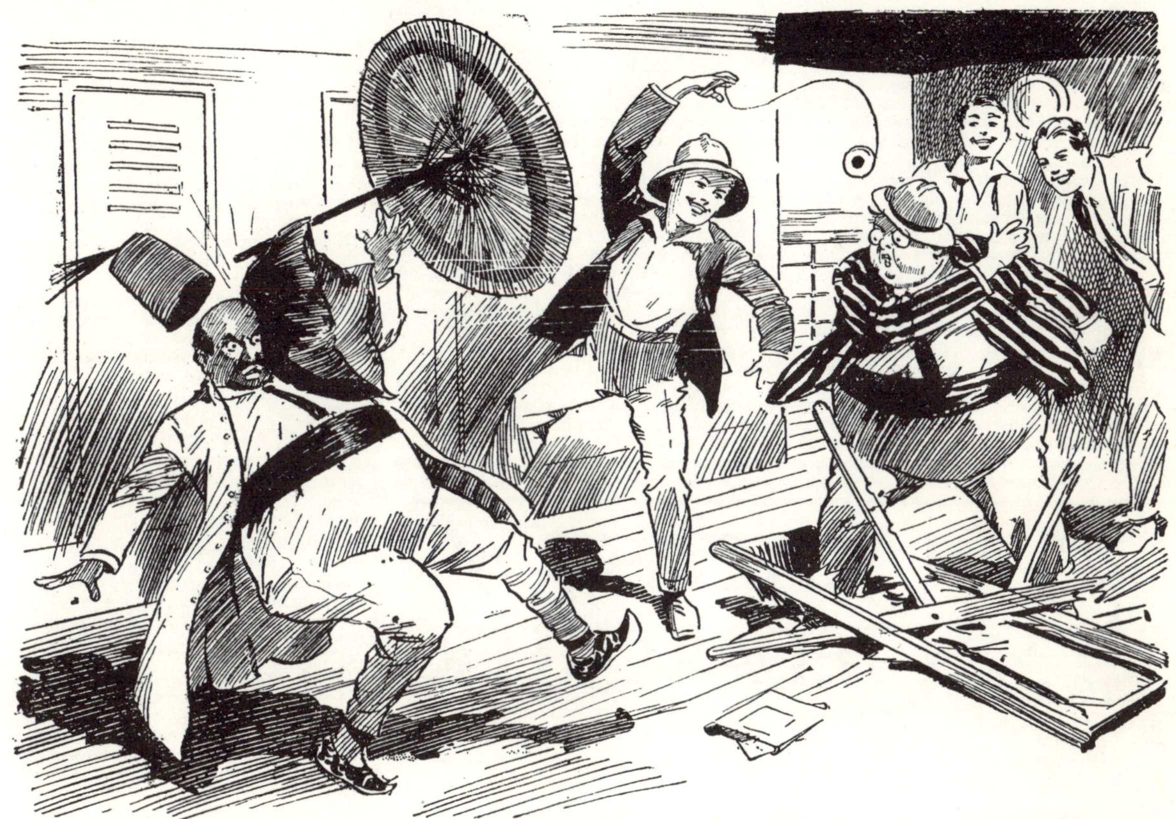

As Billy Bunter hurled the cushion, Bob Cherry dodged, and the flying missile landed fairly in the dark-skinned face of the plump Egyptian. There was a howl of astonishment from the fat gentleman as he lost his balance and staggered backwards!

"Gentlemen, chaps, and fellows," said Bob Cherry, breaking a painful silence, "that fat idiot, that frowsy frump, that unwashed, benighted tick has been asking for it—begging for it—praying for it! Now let him have it!"

"Yes, rather!"

"Hear, hear!"

The Famous Five jumped up. Billy Bunter jumped up, too, in alarm.

"I say, you fellows! Keep off, you beasts! How was I to know that the beastly nigger understood? And what does it matter about a blinking nigger, anyhow? I say—— Yaroooh! Whoop!"

Bump!

In the grasp of many hands Billy Bunter smote the deck. His roar woke every echo of the steamer and caused passengers to stare round in astonishment.

Bump!

"Yooooop!"

"Give him another!"

"I say, you fellows—— Whooooop!" Bump!

"Yow-ow-ow-ow!"

"Now kick him off the deck!" exclaimed Bob Cherry. "First kick to me! See if I can land him down the stairs with one go! Stand steady, Bunter!"

Billy Bunter did not stand steady. He did not stand at all. He fled for his fat life and vanished from the deck, roaring. And for a second a smile flickered over the face of the plump Egyptian gentleman.

THE THIRD CHAPTER.

A Sudden Blow!

"HOT!" murmured Frank Nugent.

It was evening, and the sun was sinking in a blaze of fire in the west. Eastward the blue had faded out, and a steely grey was spreading up from the rim of the sea. It had been a hot day, but with sunset the heat seemed to increase, instead of the usual coolness coming.

Billy Bunter sat in a deckchair and moaned. Bunter had done well at dinner, as usual—remarkably well—and he seemed to have found some difficulty in crawling on deck afterwards. Once there, he collapsed in his chair and moaned. Even Hurree Jamset Ram Singh admitted that it was hot. To the other fellows it seemed like a furnace with the lid off. Not a breath of wind came across the glassy sea; and the stillness, broken only by the throb of the engines and the faint wash of the water against the ship's sides, seemed somehow ominous. Many of the passengers were below, and Sir Reginald Brooke, Mauly's uncle and guardian, who was in charge of the Greyfriars party, had retired to the smoke-room. The plump Egyptian gentleman came along and glanced at the Greyfriars fellows, paused a moment, and then addressed Wharton.

"You will excuse me," he said with his elaborate politeness. "No doubt you are new to these waters, my young friend. There is a change in the weather coming, and you boys would be better below."

"Thank you," said Harry; and the Egyptian bowed and passed on.

The warning was evidently kindly meant, but the Greyfriars fellows had no desire to go below. It was hot on deck, but it was hotter in the cabins. They had noticed, however, that most of the passengers had gone down.

"I suppose this is the jolly old calm before the storm, from what that sportsman says," remarked Bob Cherry. "My hat! I'd be glad to feel the wind, if it blew nineteen to the dozen!"

"Yes, rather!" gasped Nugent.

Storm or no storm, it seemed to the juniors, baking in the heat, that any sort of a wind would have been welcome. And, although the Egyptian had warned the juniors to go below, he was not going down himself. He stood by the rail looking into the leaden east, his tarboosh a red spot against the steely sky. His servant, Ali, came softly on deck, but remained at a little distance from his master, his black eyes every now and then seeking the juniors, though he dropped them at once if the schoolboys happened to glance at him.

"Hallo, hallo, hallo!" ejaculated Bob suddenly, as the steamer gave a sudden shake. "What——"

There was a far-off murmur of the coming wind. A swell had risen on the glassy sea, and the steamer, which had been gliding on a perfectly even keel, rolled and pitched. Billy Bunter gave a convulsive jump.

"Oooh!" he gasped.

"It's coming!" said Johnny Bull. The leaden sky in the east was turning black. "Like to go down, Bunter?"

"Shan't!" grunted Bunter.

"There's going to be a blow, fathead——"

"I'm not afraid of a blow," grunted the fat Owl. "You fellows had better go down if you're funky."

"You fat chump!"

The swell had risen on the sea with startling suddenness. No passengers were to be seen on the deck now, except the Greyfriars juniors and the Egyptian gentleman and Ali. The wind came abruptly and hit the steamer and swept over the deck with a delightfully cold breath.

"I say, you fellows!" gasped Bunter. "I say, what's the matter with this beastly ship? What's it pitching about for? I say, I—I—I've got a queer feeling inside——"

"That's what comes of packing away six dinners one after another, old bean," said Bob. "When you're at sea you should only scoff three or four."

"Grooogh!"

Billy Bunter's complexion had hitherto been like that of a freshly boiled beetroot. Now it changed to a mixture of white and yellow and green. The sudden rolling of the steamer seemed to disturb the immense quantity of foodstuffs that Bunter had parked inside his extensive equator. Not for the first time, William George Bunter had fed not wisely but too well.

"I—I say, you fellows, is—is that the captain on the bridge?" gasped Bunter. "Go and tell him to keep the ship still."

"Oh, my hat!"

"Tell him not to let it wobble about like this!" gurgled Bunter. "Tell him—— Oh dear! Look here, you go to him and say—— Gur-gur-gug-gug!"

"Oh crumbs! Poor old Bunter's got it!" said Bob. "Well, I must say he asked for it."

"Gug-gug-gug-gug!"

"Buck up, old chap!"

"Ooooooch! Woooooch! Groooooch! Wug-gug-g-chug-ug!"

Awful sounds came from Bunter. With a steady ship on a calm sea Bunter could have carried his extensive cargo without disaster. But as soon as the steamer began to pitch, the fat junior's fate was sealed. His fat face was now quite green, and he moaned and groaned and gurgled and gasped in a manner that might have moved a heart of stone. Only that afternoon the chums of the Remove had bumped Bunter for his sins, but now they compassionated him sincerely.

"I—I say, you fellows, help me down to my berth!" groaned Bunter. "Call the steward—call the captain—— Oh crikey! I—I'm going to be s-s-sick! Oooooooch! I—I think I'm dud-dud-dying! You beasts, will you help me—gug—down to my—yug-yug—cabin? Wooooch!"

"Lend a hand, you men," said Bob resignedly.

He grasped the fat Owl of the Remove, and Harry Wharton lent a hand, and Bunter was heaved out of his chair.

The steamer gave a wild pitch on the tossing swell, the deck lurched, and Bunter plunged over, spluttering.

There was a gasping howl from Harry Wharton as Bunter's bullet head butted him in the waistcoat, and he sat down with a sudden shock.

"Ow!" gurgled the captain of the

Remove. "Ow! Ooogh!" He spluttered for breath, winded by the shock.

"Ow! Beasts! Hold me!" shrieked Bunter.

Wharton could only sit and gasp for breath. But Johnny Bull grasped the fat Owl on one side, Bob on the other. Bunter flung one fat arm round Bob's neck, the other round Johnny's, and hung between them, a dead weight. The juniors were strong and sturdy, but they almost crumpled up. William George Bunter was not a lightweight.

"Help!" gasped Bob.

Hurree Jamset Ram Singh and Frank Nugent rushed to help. Four pairs of hands grasped Bunter, and supported him. Harry Wharton, for the moment, was hors de combat; but four members of the Co. heaved Bunter along to the companion.

"Ow! Grooooogh! Don't pinch me, you silly idiots; don't pull my hair out, you dummies; don't bang me in the ribs, you blithering cuckoos—— Ooogh!"

"Go it!" gasped Bob.

"Heave ahead, my hearties!" stuttered Johnny Bull.

"The heavefulness is terrific!"

"I say, you fellows—— Grooogh! Beasts I say—— Whoooop!"

With a long pull, a strong pull, and a pull all together, the juniors got the fat Owl to the head of the stairs. The steamer gave a heavy roll, and Bunter gave another, and, clinging frantically to his helpers, he plunged down the steps. Bump, bump, bump, bump!

Wild yells rose from Billy Bunter and from the four hapless fellows who rolled down with him. They landed together in a sprawling, yelling heap at the bottom.

"Yoooop!"

Billy Bunter sat up, on Bob Cherry's face, and roared.

"Ow! Beasts! You did that on purpose! Yarooooooh!"

"Urrrgh! Gerroff! Draggimoff! Urrgh!" gurgled Bob.

"My esteemed idiotic Bunter——" gasped Hurree Jamset Ram Singh.

"Ow! Wow! Beast! Help!"

A steward rushed to help, and Bunter was dragged up. Spluttering wildly, he was navigated along to his state-room, and plumped into his berth. There he collapsed, moaning and groaning, in the throes of sea-sickness, and wishing that he had not had the fifteenth helping at dinner.

"Oooogh! Ow! Gimme a basin! I say, you fellows, don't leave me! Stay here with me, you beasts! Grooogh! Ooooch! I say, I'm dying! I say—— Wooogh!"

"Oh, go and eat coke!" growled Johnny Bull.

"Ow! Beast! I say, I won't be left alone!" howled Billy Bunter. "I say—— Gug-gug-gug-gug-gug!"

Lord Mauleverer looked in.

"You men all here?" he asked. "Nunky says we're to keep below; he fancies it's dangerous on deck in this squall. Where's Wharton?"

"He hasn't come down," said Bob.

"Steward says they're goin' to close the hatches; there'll be seas breakin' over the deck now the jolly old Mediterranean's getting up on its hind-legs!"

"I'll go and tell him," said Bob, and, leaving his comrades to the pleasure—or otherwise—of listening to Billy Bunter's moaning and groaning, Bob Cherry clambered back to the deck.

THE FOURTH CHAPTER.

A Struggle in the Storm!

HARRY WHARTON held on to a stanchion, the deck rocking under his feet, the wind howling in his face. Ten minutes ago the Mediterranean had looked like a pond, glowing in the sunset. Now it was a heaving, wildly tossing maelstrom, and the sunset had been blotted out.

Darkness had spread over the sky like a cloak, and from the darkness came tearing wind and lashing rain.

The roar of the squall drowned the throbbing of the ship's engines, and the steamer rocked and rolled, with fierce seas leaping up on either side, looking every moment as if they would overwhelm the slanting deck.

It was one of the sudden squalls of the Mediterranean, brief but fierce; and there was undoubtedly danger on deck for any fellow who did not keep a cool head and a strong hold.

But, after the suffocating heat, the Greyfriars junior was enjoying the hiss of the rain and the lash of the wind, and the thundering seas had no terrors for him. He could see hardly a couple of yards from where he stood holding on, but from the darkness came the gleaming of white, frothing billows, and from moment to moment a zigzag flash of lightning tore through the blackness of the sky.

Something red whizzed past Wharton's face on the wind and disappeared into the sea; it was the tarboosh blown from the head of the Egyptian, whom Wharton could faintly discern in the gloom.

The Egyptian was holding on, too, and, looking round as his fez blew away, he glimpsed the schoolboy, and smiled at him with a flash of white teeth. Then he moved to get shelter from the fierce wind, and disappeared from Wharton's sight.

The steamer rocked and rolled and plunged in a way that might have been terrifying to a landsman; but Wharton was well aware that the ship was in no danger, and that this was all in the day's work to captain and crew.

Rocking and rolling, the steamer churned on her way, while the rain lashed and the wind buffeted, her red and green lights gleaming through the murk ahead. Something unseen brushed past Wharton in the darkness, and he felt a hand grasp at him.

Supposing that it was another passenger losing his footing on the reeling deck, he released one hand, and grasped at the shadowy figure to help. At the same moment there came a flash of lightning, and, only a few inches from his face, he recognised the dark features and black eyes of Ali, the Arab servant of the Egyptian.

What happened next seemed like a nightmare to Harry Wharton. The Arab recognised him at the same moment, grasped him with both brown hands, and dragged him down to the slanting deck. So utterly unexpected was the attack, that Wharton was taken totally by surprise, and he lost his hold and went down helplessly.

In the grasp of the slim and wiry Arab he rolled on the deck, and for one fearful moment he believed that he was shooting overboard in Ali's grasp; but both of them brought up suddenly against the rail, with a bump and crash.

Amazed as he was, Wharton recovered his presence of mind swiftly. He gave grasp for grasp, and struggled with the Arab.

What the meaning of the attack could be he could not imagine. The man was a stranger to him. He had seen him about the steamer several times, waiting on his master, since the ship had left Naples, but that was all.

Possibly the man had been offended by Bunter's bad manners in the afternoon, but that, of course, could not account for his present actions. It seemed in those terrible moments to the captain of the Greyfriars Remove that he was struggling in the hands of a lunatic. And, worse than that, he was struggling in vain, for, sturdy as he was, the Arab was twice as powerful. It was a grown man against a boy, and the boy had no chance in the struggle.

Wharton was crushed down to the deck, jammed against the rail, seeing nothing of his enemy but the glimmer of the white galabyeh in which he was dressed, and the gleam of his dark eyes. A sinewy knee pinned him to the angle of the deck and rail, and the gasping cries that he uttered were drowned in the roar of the wind.

He was at the Arab's mercy, for the moment, at least; and as the knee pinned him down, thievish fingers groped over him, as if in search of something. And then, in a flash, the junior understood.

It was Wharton who had charge of the sacred scarab of A-Menah—the golden beetle that, according to ancient Egyptian tradition, was a guide to the treasure of Osiris. Again and again Kalizelos, the Greek dealer of Cairo, had sought to obtain possession of Lord Mauleverer's scarab; and this, as Wharton realised now, was one more attempt. Ali, the Arab servant of the plump Egyptian, was in the pay of the Greek, and he had probably been watching for a chance ever since the steamer had left Naples. Now his chance had come, and his thievish fingers were seeking the scarab as he held the schoolboy pinned down under his knee in the darkness and rain and wind on the pitching ship.

Fiercely, desperately, almost madly, the junior struggled. Mauleverer had entrusted the scarab to his keeping. None of the juniors quite believed, as the Cairo Greek evidently did, that it was a guide to the treasure of A-Menah, the ancient Egyptian soldier who had fought under the banners of Rameses the Second three thousand years ago. But whether it was a clue to treasure or merely a curio worth a few pounds, Wharton would not fail in his trust so long as he could struggle.

So fierce was his resistance, that the Arab was forced to leave off groping for the golden beetle, which the junior wore on a silken cord about his neck, and grasp him again with both hands.

For a full minute the desperate struggle went on, and then the junior, exhausted, was crushed down again. There was no help. The struggle was unseen in the darkness, unheard in the roar of the storm.

Breathless, panting, exhausted, Wharton felt the thievish brown hand groping again, and felt the fingers close on the silken cord, felt the golden scarab drawn from him. He could not see, but he knew that the Arab was feeling it, fingering it in the gloom, to make sure that it was the prize he sought; he knew by the man's movement that he had slipped it into a pocket under his loose galabyeh. Through the howl of the wind a voice came to Wharton's ears.

"Hallo, hallo, hallo! Where are you, old bean?"

It was Bob Cherry's shout.

Bob was on deck, but Wharton could not see him. Before he could cry out in answer, a hand was on his throat, and he was choked into silence. A shudder of horror ran through him as he felt himself dragged up, pressed close to the rail, and realised the Arab's murderous intention. It was of little use for Ali to seize the scarab on a ship at sea from which there was no escape, if the schoolboy survived to accuse him and reclaim the plunder. Now that the golden beetle was taken from him, the wretch's intention was clear—it was to toss the boy into the raging sea, and by that murderous act to cover up his tracks.

Once more the schoolboy made an effort, a fierce and furious effort, exerting every ounce of his strength.

It was his life he was fighting for now.

And as he fought he heard again, half-drowned by the wind, the shout of his chum somewhere in the dark of the deck. Bob might have been only a few yards from him, never dreaming that he was struggling in murderous hands. As a matter of fact, Bob was across the deck, holding on to the saloon skylight as he called to Wharton.

Ali the Arab heard him and redoubled his efforts to pitch Wharton over the rail. Wharton dragged an arm loose, and crashed his fist into the dark Arab face, and there was a grunt of pain from Ali. The junior panted out a cry, but it was drowned in the wind. The steamer gave a heavy roll, and the rail against which Wharton was pinned dipped to the sea, down, down below the frothing tops of the billows, till it seemed that the sea must rush over the ship and flood it fore and aft.

A wave broke over the rail, washing the deck, and the water, for the moment, was up to the necks of Ali and the schoolboy in his grasp. It tore them both away from the rail and flung them on the deck, wrenching them apart, and Ali's brown hand clutched the railed back of a deck-seat, and he held on, his glittering eyes seeking the junior.

From the blackness came a glare of lightning, and it showed Harry Wharton, with outflung arms, washing away helplessly on the wave. The flash died out and blackness followed; and in the darkness the Arab grinned. The schoolboy was gone—gone to death—and the Arab crept and crawled away, nothing doubting that the depths of the sea had swallowed his victim, and that the secret of his crime was for ever buried in the deep waters.

THE FIFTH CHAPTER.

Saved from the Sea!

A HAND in the darkness fastened on Harry Wharton, but he was scarcely conscious of it. The desperate struggle with the Arab had exhausted him, and his hands, as he flung them out, swept only the roaring water that tumbled over the slanting deck. A moment or two more, and the helpless schoolboy would have been washed over the dipping rail, hurled to death in the sea; but in those fearful moments an unseen hand held him back from destruction.

Spent and dizzy, blinded and deafened by the roaring water, the Greyfriars junior hardly knew that he was held, hardly knew that he was still on the ship, and not plunging into the maddened sea. But the grasp on his collar was firm, and as the ship's side heaved up from the sea, he found that he was sprawling half across the rail, his legs over the side in space, but with some-

thing that he could not see holding him back from death.

He was dragged back, and found himself on the deck again. His hands caught the edge of the rail, and held. A shadowy figure was close to him, he had a glimpse of eyes from a dark face. For a second he supposed that it was the Arab who had seized him again, but he realised that it could not be the murderer who was saving him from death, and it was not Bob Cherry. One of the seamen, perhaps——

"Hold on, my young gentleman!" came a voice in the wind, and he knew it was the plump Egyptian who had saved him. He remembered that the Egyptian had been on deck, he remembered the red tarboosh that had blown past him. Ali had sent him to death, and Ali's master had saved his life. The man, evidently, had seen nothing of the struggle, had known nothing of his servant's attack on the schoolboy. The rush of the water had hurled Wharton against him in the darkness, and he had caught him and saved him. The dark brown face was close to him, and Wharton could see it now, and see that there was a smile on it.

"You are safe, young gentleman!" said the Egyptian, his voice hardly audible in the wind. "But you should be below—this is no place for a boy. Did I not warn you?"

Wharton could not speak; he could only gasp. The Egyptian supposed that the wind, or the wash of the wave that had broken over the steamer, had torn him from his hold; he knew nothing more.

The junior, as he held on, still in the plump gentleman's grasp, stared round with dizzy eyes for his enemy. Where was the Arab?

A flash of lightning rived the sky, and for a second, the ship's deck leaped into ghastly illumination. Wharton had a glimpse of a seaman, and of Bob Cherry clinging to the skylight; but he did not see the Arab. Ali was gone—whether overboard, or below, or crouching in some shelter, Wharton could not tell. He was not to be seen. But he had little doubt that the villain, believing him gone to his death, had crept away, the scarab in his possession, safe, as he supposed. Wharton gritted his teeth. He was not sinking in the depths of the storm-tossed Mediterranean as Ali believed, and there was to be a reckoning soon.

Wharton found his voice at last.

"Thank you, sir," he panted. "You've saved my life—I thought I was gone. It's all right now."

"You are safe—you can hold?"

"Yes, yes."

"But you will be safer below, young gentleman."

"Yes, yes; I shall get below at once."

The Egyptian released him, and Wharton lost sight of him the next moment. He knew where Bob was now, and, clambering from one hold to another, he reached Bob Cherry, where he was holding on to the skylight.

"Hallo, hallo, hallo!" He heard Bob's voice as he bumped into him in the gloom. "That you, Wharton?"

"Yes—let's get below."

"Bit exciting up here, what?" chuckled Bob. "I came up for you—nunky's orders to keep below, but I couldn't spot you. Didn't you hear me calling?"

Wharton did not answer; he hardly heard. It was difficult to move about the pitching deck, but the juniors made their way to the companion, groping and grasping in the darkness. The door was closed, but they got it open, and a wash of water followed them down the stairs before they got it shut again. Almost every minute a frothing sea broke over the steamer. The electric light was burning below, and the change from the darkness above made the juniors blink. Bob stared at Wharton in the light.

"You're as white as chalk, old man," he said.

"Am I?" Wharton was not surprised to hear it. "Where are the other fellows—I've got something to tell you——"

"I left them with Bunter—he's sick."

"Come on."

Wharton's eyes were alert for the Arab, but he saw nothing of Ali. A deep groan greeted him as he reached Bunter's state-room. Three of the Co. were gathered in the doorway, and Lord Mauleverer was in the room, beside Bunter's bunk. Billy Bunter looked like chalk, and a succession of hair-raising groans came from him, interrupted every now and then by spluttering and gurgling and guggling. The motion of the steamer had relieved Bunter of most of his dinner; but what remained seemed to be still troubling him.

"You men look wet," said Nugent, as Wharton and Bob Cherry arrived.

"The wetfulness is terrific!" remarked Hurree Jamset Ram Singh.

"It's a bit damp on deck," said Bob cheerfully. "Raining like billy-ho, and the sea seems to have a fancy for coming aboard in chunks. I rather think I'll go and change, and you'd better do the same, Wharton."

"Something else to do first," said Harry quietly. "Have you fellows seen anything of Ali—that Arab blighter—you remember him——"

"The jolly old Egyptian gent's factotum?" asked Johnny Bull. "Yes, he came down about ten minutes ago, looking drowned."

"Where is he?"

"He went into a state-room farther up—his governor's quarters, I suppose. What on earth do you want with him?"

"He's got the scarab!"

"Wha-a-t?"

The juniors stared at Wharton in amazement.

In a low voice, and a few words, Harry Wharton told them what had happened on deck.

"Great pip!" breathed Bob Cherry. "Then while I was looking for you—— Great pip!"

"I heard you calling, while that villain was trying to put me overboard," said Harry. "There's no doubt that he believes he succeeded—as he would have, if his master had not been on deck, and caught me as I was going over. I don't know the man's name; but I'm jolly grateful to him. He saved my life. Kalizelos must have hired that Arab scoundrel to get hold of the scarab, of course. He couldn't have known anything about it otherwise, and couldn't have wanted it, if you come to that. But he's got it. The villain must have been watching for a chance!"

"Good gad!" said Lord Mauleverer. "And I dare say Kalizelos is waiting for him at Alexandria to hand it over to——"

"He won't hand it over to Kalizelos," said Wharton grimly. "He's going to hand it over to us. It's no good waiting to speak to the captain. Ali might hide it where it couldn't be found, or even chuck it out of a porthole to save

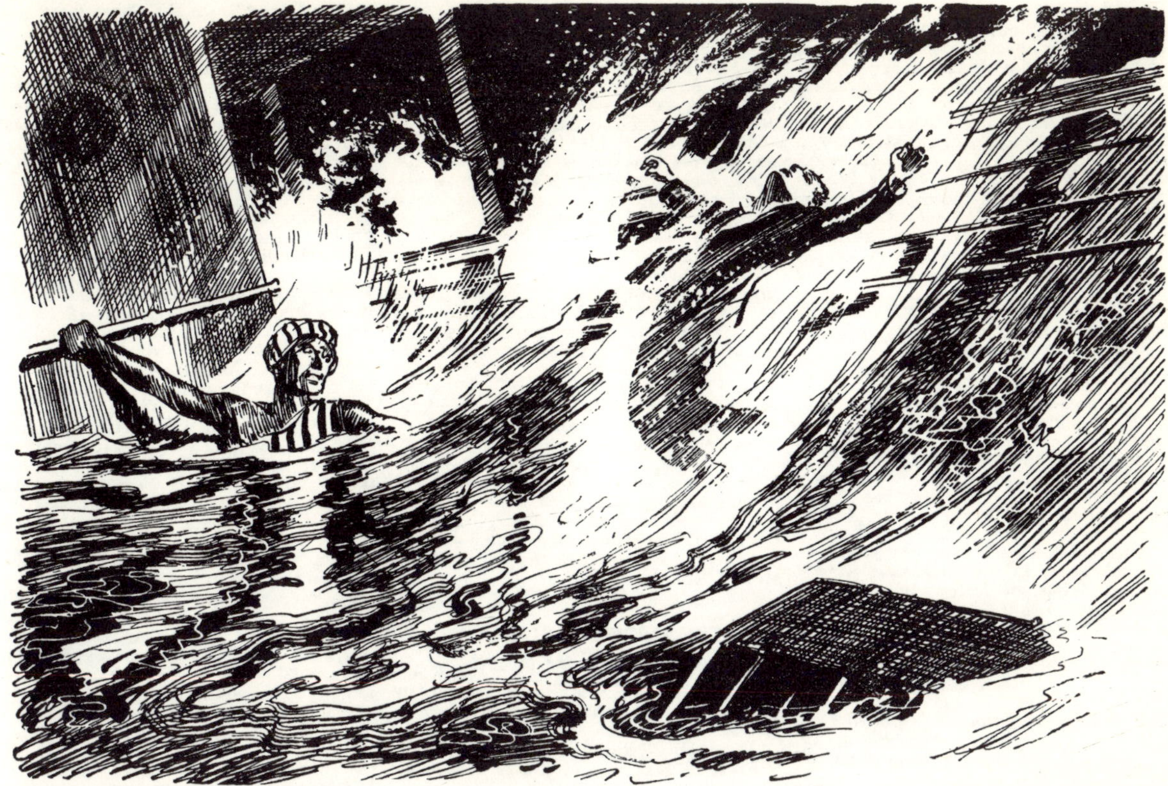

A wave suddenly broke over the rail, wrenching Harry Wharton and Ali apart. Then from the blackness came a glare of lightning, and it showed Harry Wharton, with outflung arms, washing away helplessly on the wave !

his skin. We've got to collar him before he finds out that I never went overboard, as he fancies."

"Right as rain," agreed Nugent. "He must believe that you went over the side, or he wouldn't have come below."

"I should have gone, but for the Egyptian chap; and the villain never saw him save me. Come on! There's no time to lose!"

"I say, you fellows!" groaned Billy Bunter.

But the juniors gave the fat Owl no heed. He was left to groan and gasp and splutter on his own.

Harry Wharton stopped an Italian steward in the cabin passage. Ali had gone into one of the state-rooms, but the juniors were not sure which. It was easy enough to get information from the steward. The wealthy Egyptian gentleman was a considerable person on the steamer, as the juniors had noticed, though they had not heard his name. They heard it now from the steward.

"Si, si, signore! The Egyptian gentleman—Signore Hilmi Maroudi. He has the best cabin; but I think he is on deck."

"It is his servant we are looking for—an Arab named Ali," said Harry.

"His room is next to his master's," said the steward. "I will show you, if the signore will follow me."

Probably the steward was puzzled to know what the English schoolboys wanted with the Arab servant of Mr. Hilmi Maroudi. But a tip of five francs satisfied him, and he pointed out the door and went his way. Harry Wharton & Co. waited till he was gone.

"Now!" said Harry.

And he threw back the door of Ali's cabin.

THE SIXTH CHAPTER.

"Hand Over!"

ALI, the Arab, was sitting on the edge of a bunk, swaying to the pitching of the steamer, a grin on his brown face.

In his dusky hand lay a golden beetle, that glimmered and shone in the electric light.

The Arab was grinning with satisfaction, but his eyes were curious as he scanned the golden scarab. It was such a curio as he had seen many times in Cairo and Alexandria, only uncommon from the fact that it was made of gold, and appeared to be of solid gold. It's value, as metal, could hardly have been more than twenty pounds; as a curio and antique, it might have been worth ten times as much. But there was nothing about it to reveal why Kalizelos, the Greek dealer of Cairo, placed a higher value on it. Yet that he did, Ali knew, for the Greek had paid him three hundred pounds at Naples for his rascally services, and promised him five hundred more at Alexandria when he handed the scarab over.

Ali had a good place as servant of the rich Egyptian, Hilmi Maroudi. His pay was good, and probably he robbed his master of three times as much as his pay. But the Greek dealer's bribe dazzled him, and the life of a Faringhee was not much, in Ali's estimation, set in the balance against such a sum as eight hundred pounds of Faringhee money.

Ever since the steamer had churned out of the Bay of Naples, Ali had been watching for an opportunity, though the Greyfriars fellows had hardly noticed his existence, and certainly never dreamed of suspecting that his eyes were upon them. In the sudden squall on the Mediterranean he had found the opportunity for which he had watched, though no doubt he would have found another before Alexandria was reached had there been no squall. Now he was grinning over his success, gloating over the little golden object that lay in the palm of his dusky hand, and thinking of the shop he would open in the Sok of Cairo with the proceeds of his villainy. And with those happy thoughts in his Oriental mind, he had none to waste on the schoolboy, whose body, as he believed, was washing in the wild waters of the Mediterranean, miles behind the pitching steamer.

It was quite a happy dream for Ali, but unfortunately for him there was to be a rude awakening. As he grinned and gloated over the scarab of A-Menah his door was suddenly thrown open, and a crowd of Greyfriars juniors appeared in the doorway.

Ali's brown hand closed instantly over the scarab, and he started to his feet, his black eyes snapping. Then, with a gasping howl of terror, he staggered back against the bunk, his eyes almost bulging from their sockets as they fell on the schoolboy whom he had believed to be dead and drowned, standing before him, dripping with water, but very much alive. With bulging, unbelieving eyes the Arab stared at Harry Wharton, scarcely able to believe that his sight did not deceive him.

"You scoundrel!" said Harry; and he sprang at the Arab, and dragged him with a crash to the floor. "Collar him!"

"What-ho!"

The startled Arab went down helplessly, and the juniors piled on him. But the next second he was struggling like a wild cat. His eyes blazed, his brown face was distorted with rage, and he fought and tore and bit like a wild animal, but all the time his right hand remained clenched on the scarab.

But the odds were too heavy, savage and lithe and muscular as he was, Johnny Bull's knee was clamped on his chest, pinning him down; a brown arm was grasped on one side by Nugent, on the other side by Hurree Singh. And Bob Cherry fastened both hands in the thick hair, and Lord Mauleverer grasped the brown legs that thrashed out under the galabyeh. Harry Wharton, spotting at once the clenched right hand, had no doubt what was in it, and he grasped the Arab's right wrist with both hands, and twisted it mercilessly till Ali, screaming with pain, opened his fingers.

The next moment Wharton had torn the scarab from him.

"Got it?" gasped Bob.

"Here it is!"

"Oh, good luck!"

"The goodfulness of the luck is terrific," chuckled Hurree Jamset Ram Singh. "The scarab is recovered, my esteemed and idiotic Mauly."

"Blow the thing!" growled Lord Mauleverer. "Wharton, old bean, you can chuck it out of a porthole if you like."

"Fathead!" said Harry, laughing.

"Look here, I'd no idea that it was going to bring you fellows into danger, you know," said Lord Mauleverer. "You've had a fearfully narrow escape, old bean, and it's all through that beastly scarab. I've a jolly good mind to chuck it overboard, and have done with it."

"You jolly well won't!" grinned Bob Cherry. "Ain't we going to dig up the jolly old treasure—if any—when we get to Egypt?"

"Well, I'm not lettin' you fellows take the risk of carryin' it any more," said Mauly. "Hand it over, old bean!"

"You'll lose it, you ass," said Nugent. "You lose everything."

"Well, if I lose it, I shan't worry, if I lose that giddy Greek, Kalizelos, at the same time," answered Mauleverer.

Lord Mauleverer took the scarab, and tucked it into his waistcoat pocket. The eyes of the panting Arab followed it as it disappeared. The juniors looked at one another. Lord Mauleverer had too many possessions to be very careful with them, and he slipped the golden scarab into his waistcoat pocket as carelessly as if it had been a sixpence. But it was Mauly's property, and it was for Mauly to decide—and that was that! His lordship had made up his mind that his friends should not be endangered by the scarab. And as for the danger to himself, his noble intellect did not seem to consider that at all.

"Now what about this scoundrel?" asked Bob, with a glare at the Arab, who was writhing like a snake in the many hands that held him.

"I suppose he ought to be handed over to the captain, and charged with the robbery," said Harry doubtfully. "But——"

"But what, fathead?" asked Johnny Bull. "We're jolly well not letting the villain get off!"

"We've got the scarab back, and we've rather taken the law into our own hands in getting it," said the captain of the Remove, with a smile. "But I'm thinking of the Egyptian chap—Hilmi Maroudi, the steward said his name was. This rotter is his servant, and he saved my life! He can't have the faintest idea what a villain this man is, of course. He seems a thoroughly decent man himself. I think we'd better tell him how the matter stands, and let him decide what's to be done with this rotter!"

"Well, he can't get off the ship, anyhow," said Johnny. "He can be found when he's wanted."

"That's so! Let him rip!"

The Arab was released, and left sprawling on the floor, as the juniors crowded out of the room.

Ali sprang to his feet, panting for breath, his black eyes blazing, and his white teeth gleaming in a savage snarl. He looked, for the moment, as if he would spring at the schoolboys; but no doubt he realised the futility of such a proceeding.

He watched them go, muttering to himself in Arabic; and it was perhaps just as well that the juniors did not understand that tongue, for there was no doubt that the words were far from suitable for youthful ears.

Leaving the defeated rascal to curse in the fluent Arabic, the Greyfriars fellows departed, and Wharton and Bob Cherry went to change their wet clothes.

The steamer thumped on through the tossing sea, to an accompaniment of groans and gurgles from Billy Bunter; and the groaning and the gurgling went on, like the unending melody in Wagnerian music, till the squall blew itself out.

THE SEVENTH CHAPTER.

Bunter Asks for More!

HILMI MAROUDI sat silent in the deckchair, his dark, grave face almost expressionless, only his dark eyes searching Wharton's face as the junior talked to him.

It was late in the evening, and the Mediterranean shone like a sheet of silver in the light of a soaring moon. The storm had vanished, leaving hardly a trace; only a swell on the sea followed the steamer swiftly churning onward. A sky of blue velvet, dotted with fleecy white clouds, that looked like fine lace in the moonlight, stretched over the shining sea.

It was difficult for the Greyfriars fellows to realise that, only a few hours since, the Naples steamer had been pitching in the midst of a pandemonium of wild waters. Now the vessel glided on an even keel, and even Billy Bunter was not troubled by inward qualms.

Under the gleaming moon the chums of the Remove strolled on deck, where they sighted the Egyptian gentleman; and Wharton had dropped into a vacant chair by his side, while his comrades continued their promenade.

Mr. Maroudi had to be told what had happened, and the sooner the better, and the captain of the Greyfriars Remove took this opportunity.

The Egyptian gave him a smile of polite welcome as he sat down in the vacant chair; and though the smile disappeared, his dark, impassive face expressed little or nothing, as he listened to what the junior had to tell him. His eyes were keenly on Wharton's face all the time, but he did not speak till the Greyfriars junior had finished.

"This is a very strange tale, my young friend," said the Egyptian at last. "Why do you tell me, instead of asking the captain of the steamer to place my servant Ali under arrest?"

"Only because the man is your servant, sir," said Harry. "You saved my life, Mr. Maroudi."

"That is true, I think," smiled the Egyptian. "But I little fancied that it was my servant's hand that had placed you in danger. I saw nothing of all this—and others, I think, saw nothing."

"Nothing," agreed Harry.

"And if Ali should deny your tale, how will you prove it?"

Wharton crimsoned.

"It never occurred to me that you might not believe me," he said quietly. "I suppose it would be my word against his; but my friends, at least, can prove that the scarab was taken from him, after he had robbed me of it."

"Do not be offended, little friend," said Maroudi, smiling. "I do not doubt a single word you have told me. But it would be difficult for you to prove this against Ali in an Egyptian court. If you are content to leave the matter in my hands, I will see that the rascal does not escape punishment; and it will save me much disagreeable unpleasantness—for Ali is my servant, and his shame reflects on me, his master."

"I thought of that," said Harry, "and we are more than willing to leave it to you, sir. I have asked Sir Reginald Brooke, and he says the same. I had to tell you, especially to warn you that the man is a murderous villain. So far as we are concerned, it is at an end, if you wish."

"On my head be it!" said Hilmi Maroudi gravely. "Ali, the son of Abdullah, is an unworthy follower of the Prophet; and in my house in Cairo he shall receive many strokes of the kourbash, and then be cast forth. And you need fear him no more, for my eye will be upon him."

The Egyptian was silent for a few moments. Wharton made a movement to go; but Maroudi signed to him to remain, and he sat down again. His friends passed and repassed, chatting as they sauntered up and down the deck in the bright moonlight. There was a thoughtful shade on the brow of the plump Egyptian gentleman.

"You have spoken of a scarab, little friend, which you call the scarab of A-Menah," he said at length.

"Yes," said Harry. "Perhaps you had heard of it?"

Hilmi Maroudi smiled.

"Many have heard of it," he said. "It is said that it tells a secret—the secret of the Eye of Osiris, the great diamond that is mentioned in writings of the time of Rameses the Second, a king of the nineteenth dynasty of the kings of Egypt.

"I have many old papyri in my house at Cairo, and I have often read, in the picture-writing of my forefathers of this great and precious stone, which A-Menah is said to have brought back from Syria, after the great battle of Kadesh, in which Rameses defeated the Hittites.

"I have seen paintings of the scarab of A-Menah, and read what is inscribed thereon, but it tells nothing but the name and title of that soldier of King Rameses. To me it seems impossible that it can give guidance to the lost stone."

"To me also," said Harry, with a smile. "But Kalizelos told Lord Mauleverer that he had learned the secret from some old document—a papyrus of ancient Egypt."

"It is possible," said Maroudi musingly. "I know this man Kalizelos well, and have often bought curios in his shop in Cairo. He is a keen man, and clear-headed—he has made a fortune in business. He is not the man to believe a fable. Yet the story of the scarab must be a fable. But if it should be a true tale——"

Maroudi paused.

"The Eye of Osiris was worth more than a king's ransom," he said slowly. "It is a great fortune if it is found. My little friend, you will do well to keep on your guard when you reach my country. Kalizelos is an unscrupulous man—but, bismillah, you have already learned that! And in the East life is cheap!"

"We shall be careful," said Harry.

"You have been in great peril already," said Maroudi gravely, "and this is on my head, for it was my servant's hand that was raised against your life. In me you have made a friend, for it was the will of Allah that I should save your life, and perhaps I may save it again, my little friend. You will see me again in Cairo."

"You live in Cairo?" asked Harry.

"I have a poor dwelling there," said Maroudi. "But much time I spend up the Nile—sometimes in my dahabiyeh, and sometimes on my sugar and orange plantations. You shall come to my poor house in Cairo, and bring your friends, even the little fat one whose manners are so bad."

He smiled.

"There are many Egyptians who do not love the English—but I am not one of them. The days of the great Rameses are gone for ever; and to those of us who are intelligent, it is known that the dervishes of the Sudan would have over-run Egypt, even to the mouths of the Nile, had not the English stood in the way, even as the Hyksos over-ran us—the shepherd kings in the time of the fourteenth dynasty. Of whom," added Maroudi, with a smile, "you have never heard, my little friend."

Wharton smiled, too.

The long, almost endless history of ancient Egypt was fascinating to his imagination; but he had to admit that he knew very little about it.

"The history of your country is so much longer than ours," he said. "You count almost as many dynasties as we count kings. Thirty dynasties, isn't it, up to the time of Alexander the Great—and that was more than two thousand years ago. A fellow would have to swot pretty hard to mug it all up."

Maroudi laughed.

"I say, you fellows!"

Billy Bunter rolled into view. He blinked round him through his big spectacles, which flashed back the light of the moon, and spotted the Greyfriars fellows.

"Hallo, hallo, hallo!" roared Bob Cherry. "Is that you, Bunter? What the thump do you mean by being alive?"

"Oh, really, Cherry——"

"You told us you were dying!" said Bob, accusingly. "Do you call it playing the game to come to life again like this?"

"Look here——"

"I call it letting us down! Raising a fellow's hopes for nothing!" said Bob, with great indignation.

"Beast!" roared Bunter.

"Ha, ha, ha!"

"Lot you care for a fellow lying in his berth—lying at death's door——"

"Dash it all, Bunter, if you were at death's door, you ought to have chucked lying," said Johnny Bull.

"Ha, ha, ha!"

"I was frightfully hungry. You never thought of bringing me anything to eat. I just managed to stagger along and get some supper. Did you fellows give me a single thought?" asked Bunter bitterly.

"We guessed that you'd snaffled some supper," chuckled Bob. "That was an easy one to guess."

"Ha, ha, ha!"

"I've a jolly good mind to take the first steamer back at Alexandria and leave you fellows on your own," said Bunter, "and I jolly well would, only you're in danger, and I feel bound to look after you. I say, you fellows, I've asked the steward about that nigger, and he says his name is Hilly Moody, or something—he says he's frightfully rich, and has a palace in Cairo. Well, I'll tell you what I think about that nigger. My belief is that he's after the scarab, see?"

"Shut up, you silly owl!" hissed Bob.

Bunter had not observed that he was standing within six feet of the Egyptian.

"Shan't!" answered the fat Owl. "I heard Wharton telling you about the nigger's nigger getting hold of him. Well, my opinion is that the nigger put the other nigger up to it, see, and—yarooooop!"

Harry Wharton rose from his chair, reached out with his foot, and landed it on Billy Bunter's tight trousers. There was a roar from the fat Owl as he scudded along the deck.

"Whooop!"

A LAUGH A DAY KEEPS THE DOCTOR AWAY!

Herewith a sample for which Leslie Creed, of 42, Blenheim Road, Stratford, E.15, has been awarded a USEFUL POCKET KNIFE.

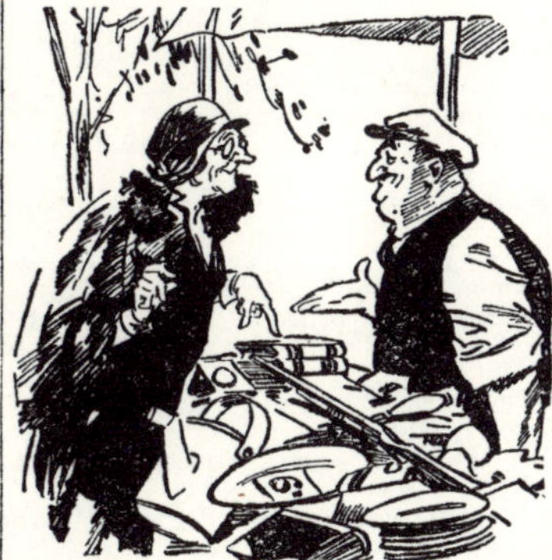

Old Lady (rummaging over second-hand stall): "What's that?"
Stallkeeper: "An air-gun, madam. It shoots slugs."
Old Lady: "Oh, I'll take it, then; my garden's full of slugs!"

You turn in the laugh, and I'll supply the prize!—Ed.

Bunter brought up against the rail and sat down with a bump.

"Goal!" chuckled Bob.

"Ha, ha, ha!"

Hilmi Maroudi rose to his feet. With a grave salaam to the juniors, he went below. Billy Bunter sat and roared.

"Look here—ow! Look here, you rotters—wow——"

"You fat idiot!" hissed Wharton. "Mr. Maroudi heard your silly cackle——"

"I didn't see the beast! Anyhow, what does it matter? He's only a nigger, isn't he? Yaroooh! You kick me again, you beast, and I'll jolly well chuck the lot of you when we get to Alexandria!" roared Bunter.

"Mean that?" asked Bob.

"Yes, you beast!"

"Then here goes! Too good a chance to lose!"

"Yaroooh! Keep off! Yooooop!"

"Ha, ha, ha!"

"I say, you fellows—I say, old beasts—I mean, old chaps—leave off kicking me, you rotters—oh crikey!"

Billy Bunter fled below in indignant wrath. But there was still balm in Gilead, so to speak. He found comfort in another supper!

THE EIGHTH CHAPTER.
Egypt at Last!

"ALEXANDRIA!"

"Here we are!"

"Founded, my dear boys, by Alexander the Great," said Bob Cherry, assuming the manner of Mr. Quelch, the Remove master at Greyfriars, imparting instruction to his pupils, "in the year—blessed if I haven't forgotten the year—but it was a jolly long time ago."

"Three, three, two B.C.," said Nugent.

"That sounds like Alexander's telephone number," said Bob. "My dear boys, in the year 332 B.C. Alexander of Macedon extended his conquests to the ancient kingdom of the Pharaohs, and founded the city of Alexandria, which was named after himself, and—and—and here it is!"

"The herefulness is terrific," agreed Hurree Jamset Ram Singh.

"I say, you fellows——"

"Hallo, hallo, hallo! Bunter, old fat man, that's Alexandria—founded by Alexander the Great in the year——"

"Three, three two B.C.," chuckled Nugent.

"Blow Alexander the Great!" grunted Bunter.

"Well, you ought to have a fellow feeling for jolly old Alexander," said Bob. "He lived in Greece—and you live in grease now that there's nobody to make you wash of a morning——"

"Beast!"

"Alexandria is rather a modern city, for Egypt," continued Bob. "Not much more than two thousand years old. But it's full of antiquities for tourists—most of them made in Germany! Those spiky things sticking up into the sky are minnows—was it minnows, you fellows? I asked that man Maroudi, and he told me, but I don't think it was minnows——"

"Minarets, fathead," said Harry.

"That's it," said Bob. "Minarets! Bunter, old bean, those spiky things sticking up into the sky are minarets."

"Blow 'em!" said Bunter.

"From the minarets," went on Bob, "the jolly old what-do-you-call-him calls the faithful to prayer—what do you call him, Wharton?"

"The muezzin!" said Wharton, laughing.

"That's it—the muezzin! Listen to me, Bunter, and improve your knowledge. You are the most backward boy in the Remove, Bunter," said Bob, in the severe manner of Mr. Quelch. "Your objection to the acquisition of knowledge is almost beyond belief! Remember, Bunter, that in a Mahomedan country, the what-do-you-call-him goes up the thingummy to call the followers of the prophet——"

"For goodness' sake, shut up!" said Bunter peevishly.

"This is for your own good, Bunter! Lend me your ears—or one of them will do, as it's as big as any two I've ever seen——"

"Shut up!" roared Bunter. "I say, you fellows, where's that old ass Brooke? They have to go through the passports before you can get away from the silly niggers. Where's that old dummy——"

"Are you speaking of me, Bunter?"

asked the icy voice of Sir Reginald Brooke behind the fat Owl.

Bunter spun round.

"Oh, I—I didn't see you, sir! I—I wasn't calling you an old ass, sir! I—I was speaking of another old ass——"

"Keep with me, my boys," said Sir Reginald, after a glare at the fat Owl. "There is a very great crowd. One of you take hold of Bunter's arm—that foolish boy will get lost if he is not taken care of——"

"Oh, really, sir——"

"That will do, Bunter!"

"Baggage, sar! Carry a baggage! Speak English, sar! Carry you a baggage!" A brown hand plucked a bag from Bunter, and the fat junior gave a yell.

"Here, stop him! He's got my bag—that black thief in a nightshirt!" yelled Bunter.

"Ha, ha, ha!"

Bob Cherry jerked the bag from the Arab porter. Porters innumerable had already invaded the steamer as soon as she came to her berth in the Inner Harbour of Alexandria. There was a babel of voices, speaking in innumerable languages. Round the steamer rocked boats of all sorts and sizes, bearing more porters, and the numberless hangers-on, touts, and officious meddlers of an eastern port—with eager, greedy eyes, extended hands and screaming voices. Billy Bunter dropped his bag, and before he could pick it up again, five or six energetic natives pounced on it, and one, luckier than the rest, grabbed it and presented it to the fat junior, with a grin that displayed a splendid set of teeth, flashing white from a brown face.

"Backsheesh, sar!"

"Go and eat coke!" said Bunter, grabbing the bag.

"Come on, Bunter!" Bob Cherry dragged the fat Owl on.

The Arab followed, gesticulating.

"Backsheesh!" he howled.

It was the juniors' first acquaintance with a word they were to hear many times in Egypt. Billy Bunter did not know that "backsheesh" meant a tip or gratuity; he fancied that the man was insulting him. He snorted, and turned his back, and rolled on; and the Arab's brown face appeared first over one shoulder and then over the other, and he fairly howled into Bunter's ears:

"Backsheesh!"

"Go away!" yelled Bunter. "Shut up! Look here, if you use such language to me, I'll call a policeman."

"Ha, ha, ha!"

"Blessed if I see anything to cackle at," howled Bunter. "I'm not going to have a nigger insulting me."

"Ha, ha, ha! You fat ass," roared Bob. "Backsheesh means a tip—it's the principal word in all Oriental languages, and the one they use most. Give him a tip and get shot of him."

"Backsheesh, sar!" wailed the Arab. "Backsheesh!"

"I'm not going to waste money on niggers," said Bunter. "Look here, you black beast, you sheer off, see?"

"Backsheesh!"

"Go and eat coke!"

"Backsheesh!"

"Kick him, Bob!"

"Backsheesh!" The Arab porter's voice rose to an indignant shriek. He picked up a bag, and if he was not tipped, it was time for the skies to fall, in the opinion of an Arab porter of Alexandria. He clutched at Bunter's fat arm, shoved his brown face into Bunter's, till his long, aquiline nose almost collided with Bunter's little fat one, and screamed: "Backsheesh!"

"Beast!" roared Bunter. "Gerraway!"

"Give him a piastre, and let him rip," said Bob.

"You give him one, blow you!"

Bob Cherry groped for Egyptian money in his pocket, and found a piastre, and dropped it into the brown hand. A piastre is worth twopence-halfpenny, and Bob considered twopence-halfpenny enough for a troublesome person who had done nothing but butt in where he was not wanted. But the Arab did not seem to think it enough.

"Ten piastre!" he exclaimed. "Ten! Yes! Ten! Backsheesh!"

"Oh, hook it, you sweep!" said Bob indignantly. "Get out!"

"Backsheesh! Ten piastre! Yes!"

The man clung to Bunter's fat arm. Bunter wriggled. Several more porters gathered round, adding their voices. A tall man, in a red tarboosh, with a gold tassel, blue loose trousers, gold-braided jacket, and crimson sash, interposed. He tapped the Arab porter on the shoulder, spoke to him in Arabic, and the man slunk away. Then the tall man, who, in his many colours looked rather like a tropical butterfly, bowed and grinned to the schoolboys, and addressed them in English.

"You want a dragoman, gentlemen lords! Yes! Hassan is your dragoman! All English gentlemen lords like Hassan! He know everything. He show you Pyramids, tombs, ruins, museums, mummies, all things he show! Yes! Hassan is your dragoman!"

The juniors were aware that a dragoman was a guide, and that the most difficult thing to accomplish in Egypt is not to have a guide.

Hassan bowed and smiled and showed all his teeth.

"Hassan is your dragoman!" he said, with conviction.

"I say, you fellows, let's get out of this!" wailed Bunter. "I'm being squashed!"

"Come this way, my boys!" called out Sir Reginald Brooke.

"You want a dragoman, gentlemen lords——"

"No, thanks!" grinned Bob. "Much obliged, but try next door!"

And the juniors followed Sir Reginald, and Hassan followed the juniors. He had relieved them of the importunate porter, and evidently he intended that his further services were not to be dispensed with. From that moment onward, no member of the Greyfriars party could glance round without meeting the amiable grin of Hassan and the flash of his white teeth. He haunted them like a highly coloured ghost, and it was evidently a settled thing in his mind that they were going to have a dragoman, and that Hassan was going to be the dragoman.

THE NINTH CHAPTER.

The Dragoman!

"BABEL must have been a bit like this!" remarked Harry Wharton.

"Yes, rather!"

"Anteek, sar—genooine noo antique!" A tray was shoved almost under the chins of the Greyfriars fellows, displaying "antiques" of Egypt that had obviously been manufactured in Europe at a recent date. "You buy, sar—genooine scarab of Tutankhamen, sar!"

"You want a guide, sar——"

"You want a carriage, sar—best first-class arabeyeh, sar—drive you some—anywhere, sar——"

"You buy a hairbrush, sar——"

"Genooine anteek——"

Harry Wharton & Co. might, had they liked, have expended all the cash they had brought from England, and accumulated a vast collection of worthless articles, before they had been five minutes off the steamer. At the first glance, Alexandria seemed to be chiefly populated by importunate persons in shabby nightgowns, with something to sell. They all talked at once, and pushed their wares almost on the noses of the travellers, and so far from taking "no" for an answer, a hundred "noes" one after another had not the slightest effect on them.

A merchant with a tray full of strings of amber beads—which might have been made of anything but amber—planted himself fairly in the path of the smiling juniors, and refused to be waved off. As they tried to pass him, he backed like a horse, still keeping in front of them, talking in a mixture of Arabic, French, and English, with an incessant stream of words of which few were comprehensible.

A red tarboosh with a gold tassel danced above the crowd, and the tall figure of Hassan, the dragoman, pushed through, and he hurled a volley of Arabic at the amber merchant. What he said, the juniors did not know, Arabic being a sealed book to them, but it had the effect of withering the amber merchant, and he backed away and sought fresh victims.

Hassan grinned at the juniors.

"No such trouble for my gentlemen lords," he said. "I, Hassan, manage all things! These peoples are troublesome peoples! All that you want you ask Hassan! Hassan is your dragoman."

After which, Hassan walked beside the Greyfriars fellows, and "shooed" off the innumerable merchants. Hassan, apparently, was a well-known and respected dragoman, for the porters and itinerant merchants treated him with great respect, and fell back at the wave of his brown hand.

"Hallo, hallo, hallo!" exclaimed Bob Cherry suddenly, as a face he knew appeared in the crowd—an olive-skinned face with jetty black eyes, that glittered searchingly at the juniors. "There he is!"

"He—who?" exclaimed Nugent.

"Kalizelos!" answered Bob.

"The Greek?"

The juniors looked round quickly. Their eyes fixed on the handsome, olive face of the Greek of Cairo.

But the next moment Kalizelos disappeared in the crowd.

"That was the rascal!" said Harry, setting his lips. "I suppose he's hanging about to see Ali come off the steamer."

"With the jolly old scarab?" grinned Bob. "Well, he won't get it from Ali. Still got it safe, Mauly?"

"Eh? Yaas! I believe so!" answered Lord Mauleverer.

"I say, you fellows, there's that nigger!" said Billy Bunter. "Look at his car! Whacking car for a blinking nigger, isn't it?"

Hilmi Maroudi was stepping into a magnificent car at a little distance. The juniors had said good-bye to their Egyptian friend on the steamer, and promised to see him again in Cairo. Maroudi glanced round as he sat down in the car, sighted the juniors, and waved a plump hand to them, with a friendly smile, and the Greyfriars fellows politely raised their hats. The car rolled away with the Egyptian, and Hassan stared after it, and then at the juniors with a new respect in his manner.

"My gentlemen lords are friends of the great Maroudi?" he asked.

"Oh, you know Mr. Maroudi, do you?" said Bob.

"Hassan know everybody and everything in Egypt," answered the dragoman modestly. "Hassan know all things!

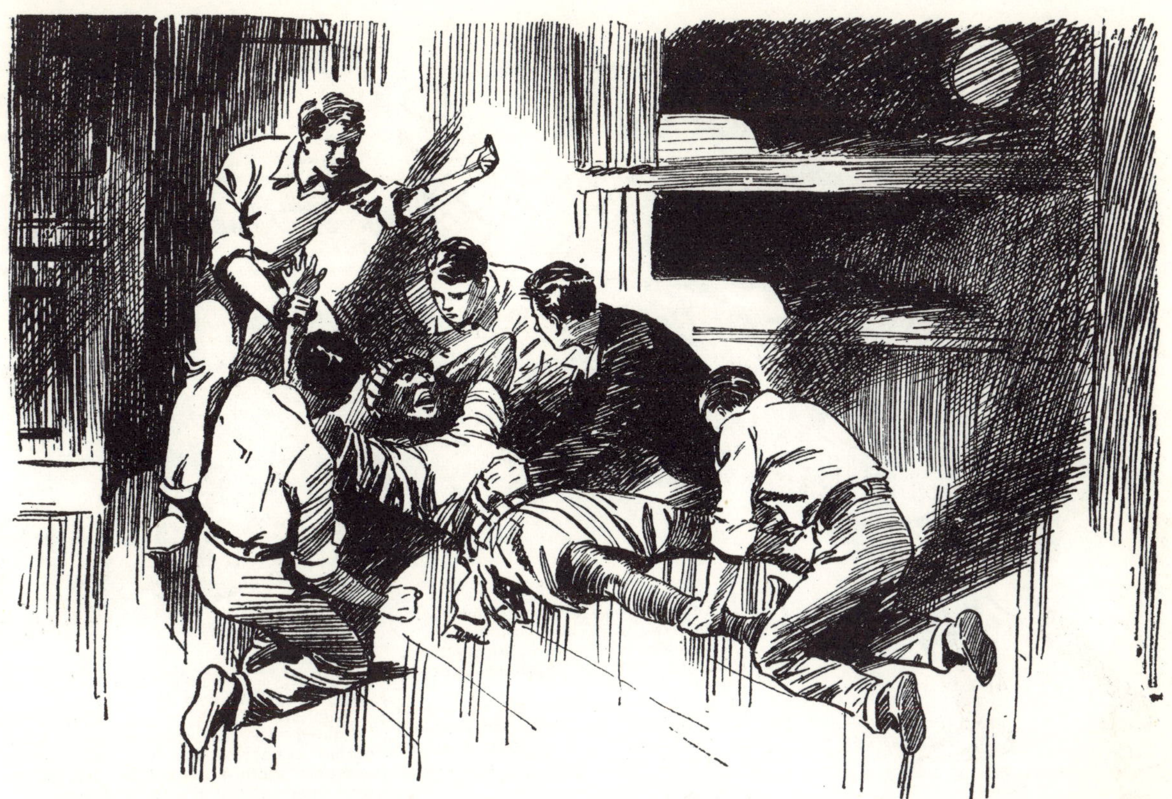

Savage and lithe and muscular as he was, Ali was pinned down by the Greyfriars juniors. Grasping the Arab's right wrist, Wharton twisted it mercilessly, till Ali, screaming with pain, opened his fingers. The next moment Wharton had torn the scarab from him. "Got it?" gasped Bob Cherry. "Good!"

Maroudi, he is a great man—very rich—so rich——" Hassan spread out both brown hands, to indicate how enormously rich Maroudi was. "He have palace in Cairo, in Luxor, plantations on the Nile, in the Fayyum—everything! If my gentlemen lords are friends of the rich Maroudi, they are fortunate ones."

"Here is the car from the hotel," said Sir Reginald Brooke. "Are you all here? Who is this man?" The old baronet stared at Hassan through his eyeglass

Hassan salaamed.

"Hassan, the son of Suleiman, is your dragoman, gentleman lord!" he answered. "He tell you everything."

"Have you engaged this man, Herbert?"

"I don't remember engagin' him, nunky," answered Lord Maleverer. "Did I engage him, you men?"

"I think he's engaged himself!" chuckled Bob Cherry.

"Please go away," said Sir Reginald. "We do not require a guide." He waved the multi-coloured dragoman aside.

"Gentleman lord, I show you everything in Alexandria, in Cairo, in Luxor, in all Egypt. I read you the picture-writing in the tombs. I hook you up the Pyramids! All the English say Hassan he one splendid rascally guide, sar. All these young gentlemen lords say they want Hassan. I take you to first-class hotel——"

"Please go away!"

"I take you to see Pompey Pillar and see huge catacombs chock-full of dead persons——"

"Go away!"

Sir Reginald waved the dragoman off, and Hassan salaamed and retreated a few paces. The juniors packed into a big car that came from the Hotel Magnifique for them, and Hassan jumped forward and closed the door. He stood salaaming, as if worked by a spring, as the car started, the gold tassel on his tarboosh dancing in the air. The juniors could not help grinning, and Hassan grinned, too, showing all his teeth. He vanished from sight as the car rolled off. But a few minutes later Harry Wharton, glancing back, saw a gold tassel fluttering over the crowd in the street. He laughed.

"He's after us!" he said.

"These Egyptian guides are extremely pertinacious!" said Sir Reginald.

"They're stickers!" grinned Bob.

"He won't let us off, especially now that he knows we know Mr. Maroudi," said Harry, laughing. "Maroudi seems to be a great gun here."

"A very eminent man," said Sir Reginald. "He has an estate in the Fayyum, adjoining my own property. I have had some very interesting talks with him on the steamer. It is his desire to show us some courteous attention while we are in his country. A very agreeable gentleman."

Mr. Maroudi seemed to have made a very good impression on the rather stiff and formal old baronet.

"I say, you fellows, I believe that nigger was after the scarab——"

"Shut up, you fat idiot!"

"Well, you mark my words," snorted Bunter.

"I'll mark your nose if you don't dry up!" said Bob.

"Yah!"

The car drew up in the courtyard of the hotel. When the juniors alighted, one of the first things they saw was a gold tassel fluttering over the heads of the crowd in the court. Hassan grinned at them with a flash of white teeth.

"Tracked down!" grinned Bob Cherry.

"I follow my gentlemen lords," said Hassan, grinning. "To-morrow you see Alexandria. I show you everything. You shall rejoice to see catacombs chock-full of dead persons!"

"Must be a jolly sight," said Bob.

"Go away!" said Sir Reginald severely.

"Hassan is your dragoman, sar. All these troublesome people are liars, and desire only backsheesh. But Hassan is truth-speaking. Hassan is the only dragoman speaking the truth——"

"Go away!"

Sir Reginald marched his flock into the Hotel Magnifique. Hassan was left in the courtyard. Later, when the juniors came out on the balcony in the cool of the evening to watch the endless, ever-moving, ever-changing crowd, a red tarboosh and a gold tassel danced under the railing as Hassan salaamed like clockwork.

"Hallo, hallo, hallo! Here he is again!" chuckled Bob.

"Ha, ha, ha!"

The juniors could not help laughing. Hassan grinned up at them.

"Gentlemen lords come to see Alexandria by night?" he asked. "Hassan show you everything."

Sir Reginald leaned over the railing and waved his cigar at the dragoman.

"Go away!" he said.

"Sar, Hassan is your dragoman."

"Go away!"

"To-morrow, at sunrise, Hassan will be here, sar, to show you everything."

"Go away!"

"Hassan awaits your commands, my gentleman."

Hassan was still there when the Greyfriars fellows went to bed. They might have fancied that he camped for the night before the hotel in the open air; for when they looked out in the morning, the gold tassel on his tarboosh was

(Continued on page 16.)

THE INN OF MYST

By DICKY NUGENT

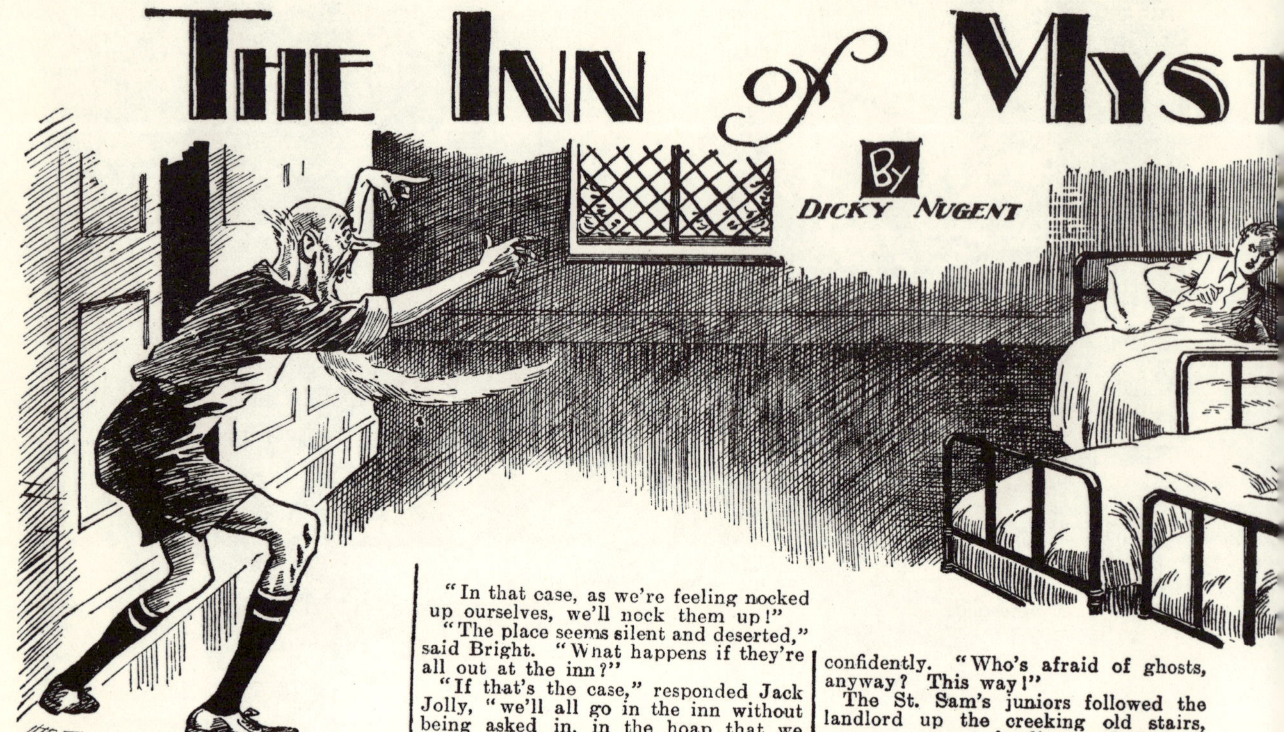

I.

"Hay-ho, here we go!
Sing Ho for the life of a hiker!"

JACK JOLLY & CO. of the Fourth at St. Sam's, sang that little ditty out of sheer joy of spirits as they tramped along the moonlit highway. They were on a hiking toor round some of the bewty spots of England, and, since getting rid of Dr. Birchemall the day before, they had been having a rattling good time. At present they were looking for an inn where they could spend the nite.

"Who wouldn't be a hiker?" sighed Frank Fearless contentedly. "I reckon it's a grand life myself!"

"Same here, old chap!" corussed Merry and Bright, while Jolly nodded in full approval.

Everybody would not have agreed with the St. Sam's juniors just at that moment, however. There was something rather sinnister and weerd about the moonlit lane down which they were tramping. The trees russled misteriously, owls blinked down with green, shining eyes from the branches, bats flew about with many an earie squeal, rats scuttled across the road, and, now and again, the juniors thought they herd distant peels of feendish larfter.

Under such sercumstances, most hikers would have felt their neeze nock together and their hair stand upright on their heads. But Jack Jolly & Co. knew not the meaning of fear, and their weerd, uncanny surroundings only made them all the merrier.

"Here's an inn!" cride Jack Jolly suddenly, pointing to a dark building standing back from the road. "We'll see if they can take us in the inn!"

"Suppose they're all asleep in the inn?" asked Frank Fearless.

Jack Jolly larfed.

"In that case, as we're feeling nocked up ourselves, we'll nock them up!"

"The place seems silent and deserted," said Bright. "What happens if they're all out at the inn?"

"If that's the case," responded Jack Jolly, "we'll all go in the inn without being asked in, in the hoap that we shan't be found out. Here goes, anyway!"

With that, Jack Jolly gave the old oak door a series of sharp wraps.

Bang! Crash! Wallop! Boom!

For a minnit, silence was the only answer. Then there was a rattling of chains and a crashing of bolts being drawn, and the door swung slowly open.

An evil-looking old man, wearing a black skull-cap, peered out from the inn. The flickering light of the candle he carried showed that he had a hawk-like nose, eagle eyes, crow's feet, a swallow-tail coat, and pigeon toes. He looked a very misterious old bird.

"What do you want at the Hawnted Inn?" he snarled, making horrible grimaces at the hikers of St. Sam's.

The juniors nudged each other meaningly.

"So it's hawnted, is it?" larfed Jack Jolly. "Well, never mind; I like a few ghosts to liven up the nite myself. What's your name, landlord?"

"Coyning Luker!" snarled the evil-looking jentleman. "What bizziness brings you to this ghost-ridden spot, where spooks and spirits make the nite hiddeous with their spectral sport?"

"Well, Mr. Luker, we've nocked you up becawse we want a nite's lodging!" grinned Jack Jolly. "Can you put us up?"

To the serprize of the St. Sam's juniors, the misterious Coyning Luker immejately broke into a howl of feendish larfter.

"Har, har, har!"

"Grate pip! Has he nocked his funny-bone against the door?" asked Frank Fearless wonderingly.

"Har, har, har! The Hawnted Inn has guests!" roared the landlord, rubbing his bony hands together. "Welcome, jentlemen! You want to stay here, and so you shall—in the Hawnted Room, from which no guest has ever emerged alive! Har, har, har!"

"I'm dashed if I quite like this chap's sense of humer!" remarked Merry, as they all went into the inn. "Do you think it's altogether safe to stay here?"

"Safe as houses!" replied Jack Jolly confidently. "Who's afraid of ghosts, anyway? This way!"

The St. Sam's juniors followed the landlord up the creeking old stairs, across a narrow landing, and through sevveral gloomy passidges, till at last they reached the Hawnted Room.

"Har, har, har! Here you will sleep for the nite!" chuckled Coyning Luker, leering at his guests. "I trussed you will enjoy your rest! Har, har, har!"

With that, he left them and walked away, larfing hiddeously as he went.

"Well, chaps, I'm tired," said Jack Jolly. "I sujjest we turn in now."

"Good wheeze!"

They turned into their respective beds and were soon in the Land of Nodd.

It must have been some time after midnite when they were awakened by a misterious muffled scratching sound.

"What's that?" wispered Jack Jolly, sitting up in bed.

"D-d-do you think it's the g-g-ghost?" asked Merry, somewhat nervussly.

Despite their bravery, Jack Jolly & Co. felt the blud freeze in their veins at the thought.

All of a sudden, Bright pointed a trembling fourfinger at the wall.

"Look!" he cride horsely

They looked. As they did so, a panel in the wall slid back slowly, and, by the earie light of the moon, a tall, bearded figger stepped into the Hawnted Room—a figger which was somehow familiar to them all.

"The Head!" cride Frank Fearless. "It's the ghost of Dr. Birchemall! We're bewitched!"

II.

"PRISONER at the bar! You are charged with exceeding the speed limit in a sedan-chair supported by two donkeys! Have you anything to say in your defence?"

Thus, the magistrate in the perlice court, the morning after Jack Jolly & Co. had watched their sleeping headmaster galloping away in his sedan.

Dr. Birchemall klutched the spikes of the dock in which he stood and licked his dry lips.

"Your honner, all I can say is this here!" he cride, with his usual faultless grammar. "In the first place——"

ERY!

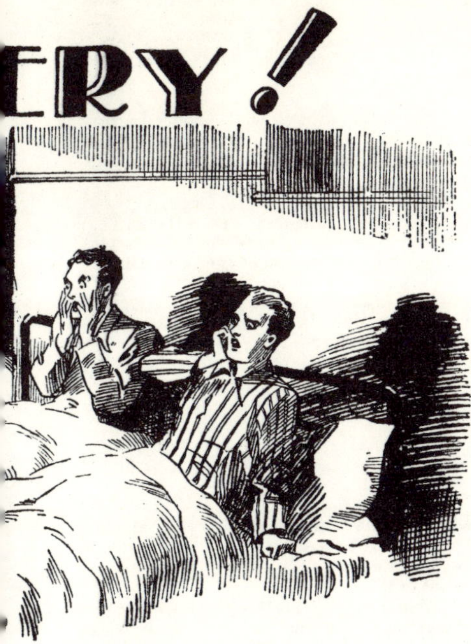

"Fined half-a-crown!" snapped the magistrate. "Next case!"

"But I haven't got half-a-crown!" gasped the Head of St. Sam's. "Owing to thoughtlessly leaving my wad of ten-pound notes at home, your honner——"

"Make it ten years' hard laber, then!" snorted the magistrate. "Remove the prisoner!"

"M-m-my giddy aunt!" stuttered Dr. Birchemall, as burly perlicemen seezed him and dragged him below. "Ten years' hard! I can't possibly do it just now. I've got a lot of bizziness appointments next week, and besides I——"

"Got the manacles ready, Jim?" asked one of the perlicemen, as they reached the cells.

The Head let out a yelp as his eyes lighted on the manacles and handcuffs that were waiting for him.

"Help! Lemme go!" he cride. "Reskew, St. Sam's!"

It was a cry of despair on the part of Dr. Birchemall. But, strangely enuff, it was answered. A refined-looking jentleman, who was grinning all over his dial, pushed his way through the perlicemen—and the Head of St. Sam's uttered a shout of joy.

"Lickham!"

"Yes, sir, it's me!" said Mr. Lickham, in his best English. "I happened to be passing through this town on my way to the coast when I notissed them taking you out of the Black Maria. I came into the Court to lissen to the case—and it seems I came just in time. Shall I lend you half-a-crown?"

"Thanks, awfully!" eggsclaimed the Head, full of gratitude.

A silver coin changed hands, then Dr. Birchemall passed it on to the perlice-sergeant who was in charge.

"Here's your munny, officer!" he cride. "I trussed that you will now let me go in peace!"

"Certainly, sir!" said the sergeant, saluting. "Good-day, sir!"

And so it came about that Dr. Birchemall walked out with the master of the Fourth a free man once again.

Mr. Lickham then buzzed off rather hurriedly, and the Head, muttering to himself, turned his footprints in the direction he fansied Jack Jolly & Co. had taken in their hiking toor.

It was a long and tiring jerney for Dr. Birchemall after that, with never a sign of the St. Sam's hikers to cheer him up.

Nite came on, and the Head began to feel awfully fed-up—which was just as well, in a way, for he had had nothing to eat since his froogal breakfast at the perlice station.

Evenchually, Dr. Birchemall reached an inn standing back from the road. Feeling desprit for food and shelter, he nocked on the front door.

There was no reply, and after waiting for a few minnits, the Head, with the aid of a jemmy he always carried for emergencies, opened the door and walked in. In pitch darkness he groped his way up the stairs till, without knowing it, he reached a secret recess behind the Hawnted Room.

Finding he couldn't get out, Dr. Birchemall began to kick and nock violently on the wall. Then suddenly he found a panel opening before him. Walking through the apercher, he found himself in a moonlit bed-room occupied by the very fellows he was seeking—Jack Jolly & Co. of St. Sam's!

"My giddy aunt!"

It was an eggsclamation of serprize and plezzure from the Head, as he reckernised Jack Jolly & Co.

The St. Sam's hikers' yells died away as they herd it.

"Grate pip!" eggsclaimed Bright. "It's the Head himself! How ever did you get here, sir?"

Dr. Birchemall scowled at the reckerlection of his trials and trubbles.

"Only by a series of very paneful eggsperiences, Bright!" he answered sternly. "You juniors treated me shamefully; I can only describe your behaviour as an infernal-machine in an ox—that is to say, a bomb in a bull! When we get back to St. Sam's I'll birch you all black and blew, bust me if I—— Hallo, hallo! What's happening?"

"Yarooo! The floor's moving!" yelled Merry.

Merry had not eggsaggerated. Not only was the floor moving—the entire room was descending through the house as though it was nothing but a grate lift—which, in point of fact, it was!

Right down into the bowels of the earth went the hikers of St. Sam's. As they drew near the bottom they herd peels of feendish larfter wringing out.

"The landlord!" gasped Jack Jolly. "That villan Coyning Luker is waiting at the bottom with some fowl serprize for us!"

And so it proved. When the lift stopped the St. Sam's juniors found themselves staring with horror at an underground coiner's den, in which Coyning Luker was standing with an ortomatic in one hand, a shot-gun in the other, and a crool, glittering dagger in the other!

III.

"HAR, har, har!"

It was a peel of mocking larfter from the landlord of the Hawnted Inn.

"So this is the secret of this devilish place!" remarked Jack Jolly grimly. "A coiner's den, eh? No wonder the villan likes to frighten visitors, when the inn is only a cloak for Coyning Luker's criminal activities!"

"Walk into my parler, jentlemen!" leered Coyning Luker, flurrishing his deadly weppons of war. "It's not often I get a chance of practissing marksmanship on so many guests! Har, har, har!"

"Back up, you fellows," said Frank Fearless fearlessly. "Let's show this skoundrell we can die like men! Coyning Luker, do your worst! Fire!"

"Yaroooo!" yelled Dr. Birchemall, who was hanging behind and misunderstood Frank's meaning. "If it's a fire, call the fire brigade at once and get some water!"

"Who's that?" asked Luker, at the sound of Dr. Birchemall's voice. "I thought there were only four of you."

At that moment the Head of St. Sam's advanced to the four, making the fifth. And then Jack Jolly & Co. saw an amazing thing happen.

Coyning Luker and the Head eyed each other for a moment. Then they uttered a simultaneous cry of reckernition.

"Luker!"

"Birchemall!"

"Bust me!" eggsclaimed the Head, beginning to grin all over his dial. "It's my old college pal, Coyning Luker! Do you remember our happy days at Borstal when we were boys together, old chap?"

Coyning Luker dropped the weppons he was carrying and began to smile quite a plezzant smile.

"Well, I'm jiggered!" he cride. "This is a serprize, and no mistake! Are these boys friends of yours, then, Birchy?"

"Friends and pupils, Coyning!" answered the Head, eyeing them with something like pride. "But what's all this bizziness about shooting them?"

Coyning Luker grinned.

"Well, Birchy, this is a coiner's den where I mint counterfeet coin of the relm—bogus pennies and imitation ha'pennies, you know. Natcherally, like all coiners, I make a sideline of luring people to their deth. But in this case, as they're friends of yours, I shall, of corse, let them off. Please axxept my sincere apologies, jentlemen!"

"Right-ho!" said Jack Jolly, after a pawse. "We still think you're a hartless villan, but we'll say no more about it for the present!"

"Good! And now, jentlemen, you must come upstairs and have supper with me," said Coyning Luker briskly. "Follow me!"

Dr. Birchemall rubbed his hands.

"Now, that's what I call a really brilliant sujjestion!" he said. "A whacking grate feed, followed by a long sleep, is just what I am most in need of! Lead on, Macduff!"

It took a lot to put Dr. Birchemall off his grub. The amount he mannidged to eat when they got upstairs serprized even Jack Jolly & Co.

Supper being over, Coyning Luker showed the Head to his room, then led Jack Jolly & Co. to their apartment—which was not the Hawnted Room on this occasion! But the hikers of St. Sam's had had about enuff of the Hawnted Inn by this time, and as soon as they herd the snores of Coyning Luker and Dr. Birchemall echoing through the house they tiptoed downstairs and shook the dust of the inn from their feet.

In the interests of other hikers who mite call there, Jack Jolly & Co. thought it advisable to inform the perlice of their eggsperiences at the first town they entered; and they had the satisfaction of seeing a perlice-car set off, carrying officers armed to the teeth!

Thanks to Jack Jolly & Co., there was likely to be an early end to the evil happendins at the Inn of Mystery!

THE END.

(The next story in this novel "hiking" series. "THE BOGUS HERO!" is funnier than ever. Watch out for it, chums, in next week's MAGNET.)

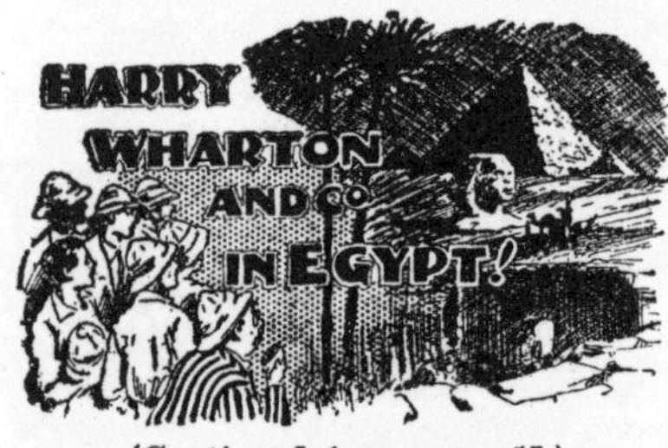

(*Continued from page* 13.)

gleaming in the sun. He was waiting for them with a grinning, brown face, and it was evident that there was no escape for them. Hassan had constituted himself their dragoman.

THE TENTH CHAPTER.
A Cocktail for Mauly!

ALEXANDRIA shimmered in a blaze of sun. Harry Wharton & Co. looked from the hotel balcony, in the brilliant morning, at the ever-varying crowds and the strange buildings, and their faces were merry and bright. They were in Egypt at last, though Alexandria was not the real Egypt. They were on the threshold of the land of the Pharaohs—the dim, mysterious, immemorial land of the Nile. Only a couple of days were to be spent in the ancient city of the conquering Alexander; then they were going on to Cairo, to the Sphinx and the Pyramids, the Nile and the desert, Luxor and the tombs, perhaps even a glimpse of the Sudan. It was a glorious prospect, and they were going to enjoy every minute of it, in spite of the heat and the flies and the dragomans.

Even Billy Bunter forgot to grouse that brilliant morning, possibly because he had found the provender good at the Hotel Magnifique and had parked away enormous quantities of the same. He was ready to go forth and see Alexandria, and his spectacles gleamed cheerily under the brim of Lord Mauleverer's best Panama hat.

Mauly had sat down in a long cane chair on the balcony, with one elegant leg crossed over the other, and his hands clasped behind his noble head. His lordship was apparently content to see Alexandria sitting down and without moving.

"Buck up, Mauly, old man!" said Bunter. "Don't slack, old chap! Can't possibly leave you behind."

"It's rather restful here," murmured Lord Mauleverer.

"Don't you want to see the sights?"

"I'm seein' lots of them through the railin'."

"There's a lot of things to see, fathead. The Sphinx. Is the Sphinx at Alexandria, you fellows?"

"That's at Cairo, fathead!" said Nugent.

"Well, there's the great Pyramid of Chops," said Bunter.

"The whatter?"

"The Pyramid of Chops. Chops was a king, or something."

"Oh, Cheops!" said Harry. "The Pyramid of Cheops is on the other side of Cairo."

"I dare say it is. But I'm talking about Chops."

"Ha, ha, ha!"

"Blessed if I see anything to cackle at. I'm not going to miss seeing the Pyramid of Chops, I can tell you. I say, Mauly, get a move on! Ain't you interested in Chops?"

Lord Mauleverer grinned.

"You've simply got to come, Mauly," said Bunter. "We shouldn't think of going out and leaving Mauly behind, should we, you fellows?"

"No fear!"

"You see, old chap, we want you to pay for admission to all the places," explained Bunter.

"Oh gad!" ejaculated Lord Mauleverer. He had rather wondered why Billy Bunter was so keen on his company. Now he knew!

Sir Reginald Brooke came along the balcony. What looked like a tropical butterfly fluttered behind him. It was Hassan, the son of Suleiman, salaaming as he came, as if he had a steel spring in his back. How a man could keep on folding himself up like a pocket-knife was rather a mystery to the juniors. But no doubt Hassan had had a lot of practice.

The old baronet had met some acquaintances at the Hotel Magnifique, also he had been in Egypt many times, and was past the age for active and strenuous sight-seeing in a hot climate. Perhaps that was why he had yielded to the blandishments of the son of Suleiman. Evidently Hassan had succeeded in hooking on. Sir Reginald was going to take a rest, in the company of his elderly friends, while the juniors saw the sights.

"I have engaged this guide, my boys," said the baronet. "The hotel manager recommends him, and you will be safe under his guidance."

"All hotel managers in Alexandria and in Cairo please to give personal recommend," said Hassan, salaaming. "They know Hassan, the only one Arab in Egypt who speaks the truth."

"I have given this man his instructions," said Sir Reginald, "and you will be careful not to wander away from him, and he will bring you back to the hotel for lunch."

"Hassan is your dragoman, gentlemen, lords," said the guide, his flexible back going again like clockwork. "You trust Hassan! All other guides are liars and thieves!"

"I say, you fellows," said Billy Bunter, as the old baronet left them with the dragoman, "mind you keep together, and don't get out of my sight. That blighter Kalizelos is in Alexandria, you know, and goodness knows what may happen to you if you get wandering away from me."

"Ha, ha, ha!"

"Blessed if I see anything to cackle at! Got the scarab safe, Mauly?" asked Bunter.

Lord Mauleverer's hand went to his waistcoat pocket.

"Yaas," he answered.

"Are you going to tell all Egypt about it, Bunter?" asked Johnny Bull sarcastically. There were at least a dozen people within hearing of Bunter's voice.

"Oh, really, Bull——"

"Hadn't you better leave it with your uncle, Mauly, for safety?" asked Harry Wharton.

Mauly shook his head.

"Somebody might get after it, and worry nunky," he said. "It's all right."

"Well, let's have a cocktail, and start," said Bunter. "Where's that waiter? Here, waiter!"

Lord Mauleverer sat up.

"Let's have a which?" he ejaculated.

"A cocktail," said Bunter breezily. "Lots of the people here are drinking cocktails. It's all right here, Mauly—no masters or prefects about—he, he, he! And old Brooke has cleared off! I'll stand the cocktails all round. You lend me some money——"

"Ha, ha, ha!"

"Here, waiter!" called out Bunter. "Cocktails!"

"Yessar!"

"You frabjous owl!" roared Bob Cherry. "If the waiter brings you a cocktail, I'll pour it down the back of your neck."

"Now, look here, Bob Cherry," said the fat Owl, blinking severely at Bob through his big spectacles, "I want it understood, once and for all, that I don't want any of your Remove passage tricks here. Remember, you're travelling now in decent company, and try to do me credit."

"Oh crikey!"

"If you namby-pamby fatheads prefer lemonade, have lemonade, and be blowed," said Bunter. "I'm having a cocktail! Here, waiter—six lemonades, and one cocktail. And mix it strong."

"Yessar!"

"We can shake a loose leg here, you know," said the fatuous Owl. "What's the good of being on a holiday in a foreign country if we can't shake a loose leg? What?"

"You howling ass!" exclaimed Harry Wharton. "If you mopped up a cocktail we should have to roll you along, or wheel you on a barrow."

"Yah!"

"The esteemed cocktail is not the proper caper, my idiotic Bunter," said Hurree Jamset Ram Singh.

"Rats!"

Billy Bunter evidently meant business. He had ordered a cocktail, and he was going to drink a cocktail; if only to show the other fellows that he could do what he liked—which was a rather important consideration with the Owl of the Remove. The opinion of the other fellows was that Billy Bunter couldn't do as he liked—not, at all events, to the extent of absorbing cocktails.

The waiter came back with a well-laden tray. Six lemonades were placed on the table, and one cocktail. Billy Bunter, with a defiant blink at the Co., reached out a fat hand to his glass. Bunter, certainly, had no knowledge of the probable effects of a cocktail taken internally. Taken externally, it was not agreeable; but, undoubtedly, ever so much better than taken internally. And the chums of the Remove were quite determined that if Bunter took that cocktail at all he was going to take it externally.

"Here's how!" said Bunter recklessly, as he lifted the glass. Bunter had no doubt that he looked quite a man of the world.

Bob Cherry grabbed his fat wrist.

"Ow! Leggo, you beast!" howled Bunter.

"Sure you want this cocktail?" asked Bob.

"Yes; blow you!"

"It will be jolly bad for you if it goes down the inside of your neck!"

"Leggo!"

"So it's going down outside——"

"Ha, ha, ha!"

Billy Bunter struggled as Bob twisted his fat paw, with the glass in it, round to the back of his neck. The contents of the glass shot out in a stream, and landed just under Lord Mauleverer's chin, and streamed down him. Lord Mauleverer bounded to his feet. For once, he forgot the calm repose that stamps the caste of Vere de Vere. He roared.

"Oh, my hat!" gasped Bob.

"You clumsy ass, Bunter!" exclaimed Wharton.

"Leggo! I say, you fellows—whoooop!" roared Bunter, as he sat down on the balcony, with a bump that almost shook the Hotel Magnifique.

"Oh gad!" gasped Lord Mauleverer. "I'm soaked! I'm drenched! I shall have to go and change! Kick Bunter while I'm gone."

"Certainly, old chap!"

"Yaroooh!"

Lord Mauleverer disappeared into the hotel, dripping with Bunter's cocktail. The fat junior squirmed away from several lunging feet. After about a quarter of an hour his lordship emerged again, and the Greyfriars fellows followed Hassan, the son of Suleiman, down the steps from the balcony, and started to see Alexandria.

THE ELEVENTH CHAPTER.

The Pickpocket!

"THE Kom-el-Chogafa——"

"Oh, my hat! The which?"

"The Kom-el-Chogafa!" said Hassan beaming. "Magnificent catacombs chock-full of dead persons—yes!"

"Oh! The jolly old catacombs!" said Bob Cherry.

"Hassan tell you everything. Here you pay for admission—it is only five piastres for every gentleman lord. Nothing! To see catacombs chock-full of dead persons is worth many piastres. Yes! Hassan tell you the truth."

The juniors had seen the busy Place Mohammed Ali; and the shops in the Rue Cherif Pasha; and had stared up Pompey's Pillar, once supposed to be the burial-place of the great Pompey. Hassan, indeed, had assured them that Pompey was there; a statement the juniors took the liberty of doubting, as they did many other statements of the only truth-speaking Arab in Egypt. They had had Pompey in history-class with Mr. Quelch at Greyfriars, so they knew all about the hapless Roman general whose head was cut off when he landed in Egypt long ago. So they only smiled when Hassan told them that he was a great sheikh of ancient times, and the very King of Egypt who had oppressed the Children of Israel. After which, they arrived at the catacombs, and followed their guide down the modern steps which led to the ancient entrance, glad to get out of the glare of the sun.

"I say, you fellows, I think they might put in a lift here!" grunted Billy Bunter, as the explorers descended a long winding staircase. "Look here, I'm going to sit down and rest. Wait for me."

"Oh, buck up, fatty!" said Bob.

"Shan't!"

Billy Bunter sat down, half-way down the winding staircase. His fat little legs were fatigued.

The rest of the party followed Hassan down.

"I say, you fellows, wait here for me!" yelled Bunter. "I won't keep you half an hour!"

"That's all right, old fat bean—you won't keep us half a minute!" said Bob Cherry, over his shoulder.

"Beast!"

The Greyfriars party and the dragoman disappeared below.

Bunter sat and grunted, and fanned himself with Lord Mauleverer's Panama.

He sat in the middle of the winding staircase, fanning himself, oblivious of the fact that he was in the way of anyone else who happened to be coming down to the catacombs.

There was a sound of running feet on the stair above him, as if someone was coming down in a hurry.

Bump!

"Oh crumbs!" gasped Bunter, as the man running down from above, landed on him, and sprawled over him.

The fat junior roared. He was rather hurt. But the man, who had lost his footing and tumbled down the steps, was more hurt than Bunter. He sat up, several steps below the fat Owl, and glared up at him with black eyes from a brown face, and poured out a stream of infuriated Arabic.

Bunter rubbed the back of his head, and glared at the native through his big spectacles.

"You clumsy nigger!" he roared.

The Arab scrambled up, clutched up the tarboosh that had fallen from his head, and clamped it down on his thick dark hair, glaring savagely at Billy Bunter.

"Fat fool!" he panted, breaking into English. "Why you sit on a stair?"

"Clumsy ass!" retorted Bunter. "Can't you look where you're going?"

OUR 10,000-GIFT PLAN
RESULT.

Our recent huge coupon-collecting scheme, in which many thousands of Fine Gift Books were offered, proved a tremendous success, and as a result readers all over the country are now enjoying the topping books they have won.

We congratulate them on the many magnificent totals of points scored—prizes were awarded for totals ranging from 32,700, sent by H. Legetter, of Luton, down to 3,000—and we only regret that it is not possible to give all their names in the paper. All prizes for Home readers were, however, sent off promptly, and also personal letters from the Editor to all unsuccessful entrants.

The remaining 500 of the Prize Books offered are, of course, being reserved for Overseas readers—for whom there is a later closing date—and these will be awarded and sent as soon as possible after that date.

The dark-brown face stared up at him evilly.

The Arab was a short, thick-set muscular man, with the scar of an old knife-cut across one brown cheek. As Bunter blinked at him it dawned on his fat brain that he had seen the man before—hanging about the balcony of the hotel that morning.

Brown faces, red tarbooshes, and dingy galabyehs girdled round the waist, were too numerous to be noticed, but he had noticed the livid knife-scar that ran across the brown cheek from nose to ear. The scarred man had approached the Greyfriars party several times with picture postcards for sale. His tray of picture postcards, however, was not with him now.

"Faringhee fool!" said the Arab, between his teeth, and he made a motion to come up the steps again, apparently to deal with the fat junior.

But if that was his intention, he changed it. With a black look at Bunter, he turned away and ran down the lower stair.

Billy Bunter was glad to see him go. The look on the scarred face had been rather alarming.

"Beast!" grunted Bunter.

The running footsteps died away below.

Why the man was in haste was a mystery to Bunter. There was nothing but the catacombs at the bottom of the stair, in which natives were not interested like foreigners who came to see the sights. Anyhow, the place was open all day to visitors.

Billy Bunter grunted, rubbed his head again, set Lord Mauleverer's Panama on it, and resumed his way down—at a much slower pace than the scarred Arab's.

Tourists and guides were moving about the chambers cut in the rock, and Bunter blinked round for the Greyfriars party. It was the voice of Hassan that guided him to them at last.

"Here is bier in shape of lion," came the sing-song voice of Hassan, "the three gods which stick around are Horus, Thoth, and Anubis—great famous gods of ancient times! Here is priest of Isis, who made the sacrifice, carved in rock, which is very wonderful. Here in sarcophagus is dead person of——"

The Greyfriars fellows were standing round Hassan, as he expounded.

At a little distance from them a thick-set figure in tarboosh and galabyeh stood half hidden in a niche in the rock wall, the black eyes fixed on the Greyfriars party.

As they moved on the thick-set figure moved after them, at a distance, still watching, and behind him rolled Billy Bunter—with a grin on his fat face now.

It was the scarred Arab who had fallen over him on the stair who was following the juniors and keeping them under observation, and, as he did not look back, he did not observe Bunter coming on behind.

Billy Bunter's fat brain was not quick on the uptake; but he could guess that the scarred man had followed the party on their excursion that morning, and he could guess the reason

Kalizelos, the Greek, had not ventured to let himself be seen; but it was easy enough for him to set a spy on the party, and Bunter had no doubt that the scarred man was the spy. That was why he had been running down the winding stair—having momentarily lost sight of the party when they went down into the catacombs.

Bunter grinned a fat grin.

Bunter wondered whether he was looking for a chance to pick Mauleverer's pocket of the scarab. If he did, Billy Bunter was prepared to butt in, and to demonstrate once more to the Famous Five how helpless they were without him.

Hassan, with an incessant stream of talk, led the way down a lower staircase, into a lower story of the catacombs. After them went the scarred man, keeping well behind, and after the scarred man went Bunter, grinning. The juniors, keenly interested in the strange relics of ancient times, had no suspicion that they were being shadowed.

"Here it is more dark!" chanted Hassan, at the corner of a passage cut in the solid rock. "But my gentlemen lords will be able to see wonderful sarcophagus, from which mummy removed, now in museum. Beyond there is gallery chock-full of dead persons!" added Hassan, by way of consolation, in case his charges were disappointed at finding one of the sarcophagi empty.

The Greyfriars fellows went into the corridor, which was dusky and dim, getting only a glimmer from the light-shafts of the larger apartments. They gathered before the sarcophagus, which lay in a deep niche in the rock wall.

The huge stone coffin was empty, and the lid, which was also of solid rock, stood back on its edge.

The juniors peered into the dim interior, in which a mummified Egyptian had lain for, perhaps, two thousand years, his name and age being painted, in red paint, on the rock tomb—still visible, and readable, if the juniors could have understood it.

The mummy, as Hassan told them, had been removed to the museum. Although the lid stood up on edge and the sarcophagus was kept open, a musty smell lingered in it, and one glance was enough for the juniors.

Hassan was telling them that it was the tomb of some early Alexandrian citizen, whose name was Psah, when there was a bustle in the dusky corridor, and the scarred Arab pushed rudely through the group of schoolboys. He shoved against Bob Cherry, who promptly pushed him back, and he staggered on Lord Mauleverer, pressing that youth to the wall, and falling against him.

"Here, you bad-mannered person, what you do?" exclaimed Hassan, loudly and indignantly. "You push one gentleman lord, son of five hundred pigs?"

"Oh gad! Gerroff!" gasped Lord Mauleverer.

Harry Wharton caught the man by his galabyeh, and pulled him away from Mauleverer.

The scarred man tore himself loose, and hurried on, without speaking a word, and disappeared into the gallery at the end of the rock passage. He was gone almost in a moment.

"I say, you fellows!" Billy Bunter rolled up behind the juniors. "I say, stop that man! He's got it!"

"Hallo, hallo, hallo! You turned up again?" exclaimed Bob Cherry.

"I tell you he's got it!" exclaimed Bunter, in great excitement. "He's been following you, and I've been watching him. I jolly well knew what he was after. He's picked your pocket, Mauly!"

"Oh gad!" ejaculated Mauleverer.

"I'll bet you he's got the scarab!" said Bunter. "That silly ass Mauly had it in his waistcoat pocket; and I tell you that darkey has been following and watching you——"

"Is that why he bumped into us?" exclaimed Wharton. "Look if the scarab's safe, Mauly—quick!"

"Yaas, old bean!"

Lord Mauleverer slid his slim fingers into his waistcoat pocket. They came out empty.

"Gone?" exclaimed Nugent.

"Oh gad! Yaas!"

"I say, you fellows, I told you so!" grinned Bunter. "Look here, you can stop him before he can get out of the catacombs. I say——"

"My gentleman lord he has been robbed!" exclaimed Hassan, in dismay.

"I say, you fellows——"

"Get after that Arab scoundrel!" exclaimed Wharton hastily.

"Hold on!" exclaimed Lord Mauleverer. "It's all right!"

"Have you got the scarab?"

"No; but——"

"Fathead! Then we haven't a moment to lose——"

"It's all right!" gasped his lordship. "You see——"

"I say, you fellows, that nigger was watching us at the hotel, and he knew Mauly had the scarab in his waistcoat pocket all right," said Bunter. "He's been after us all the time, and I spotted him——"

"Yaas, I fancy he knew where the scarab was," assented Lord Mauleverer cheerfully. "I felt him poke me in the ribs when he shoved me at the wall, and I've no doubt he was fishing for the jolly old scarab in my waistcoat pocket. But, you see, I changed my waistcoat before we left the hotel——"

"What?"

"You remember Bunter's cocktail was spilled over me," chuckled his lordship. "Well, I had to change my waistcoat, you know—and the scarab's in the other waistcoat."

"You left it in the other pocket?" yelled Bob Cherry. "Left it in your room at the hotel?"

"Yaas! Forgot all about it, you know."

"You silly ass!"

"Well, a fellow can't remember everythin'," said his lordship. "I forgot all about the dashed scarab when I changed my waistcoat. Lucky I did, as it turns out! That sportsman would have had it!"

"Well, my hat!" exclaimed Bob Cherry.

Lord Mauleverer chuckled.

"What a sell for the jolly old pickpocket!" he said. "Trackin' us all over Alexandria—to shove his paw into an empty pocket, what?"

"Ha, ha, ha!"

The pickpocket had vanished—probably the most disappointed rascal in Alexandria. Evidently he had been following the juniors and watching for a chance to pick Lord Mauleverer's pocket of the scarab—and his chance had come when the party were in the dim underground corridor. But for the fact that Mauly had changed his waistcoat before leaving the hotel—and forgotten to transfer the scarab—there was no doubt that the rascal would have secured it. Bunter's cocktail, and his lordship's forgetfulness, had saved the scarab once more from the hands of Kalizelos.

THE TWELFTH CHAPTER.

In a Living Tomb!

LORD MAULEVERER sat on the edge of the empty stone sarcophagus and leaned back against the rock wall of the niche. Hassan, the son of Suleiman, was saying his piece, so to speak, reciting the history of Psah and his tomb, and translating—or, more probably, pretending to translate—the strange inscription painted in red on the rock. Mauly's eyes closed under the brim of his hat, and he nodded drowsily while Hassan's sing-song voice ran on, seemingly like the little brook in the poem, which went on for ever. But the Famous Five soon had enough of the stuffy corridor and the history of Psah, and they made a move onward.

"Wake up, Mauly, old bean!" chuckled Bob Cherry.

"Eh?" Lord Mauleverer opened his eyes. "I wasn't asleep; I heard all you fellows were saying. Anythin' more to see?"

"Lots and lots!"

"The lotfulness is terrific, my esteemed Mauly."

"Innumerable dead persons, my gentleman lord," said Hassan. "We next proceed to great gallery newly excavated, chock-full of dead persons."

"Right-ho!" yawned Lord Mauleverer. "I'm comin'."

The juniors followed the dragoman and turned out of the corridor into the wide, open gallery lined with rock shelves, on which the tombs were laid with the mummies in ancient days. Lord Mauleverer made a movement to rise and follow, and then sat down again.

His lordship was tired. He had put in an unusual amount of exercise that morning, and he was getting a welcome rest. And his interest was not deep in the "innumerable dead persons" which Hassan considered so attractive.

Harry Wharton stopped at the corner of the corridor and looked back.

"Come on, Mauly!" he called.

"Yaas," yawned Mauly.

And the Greyfriars fellows followed the dragoman along the gallery, Hassan's sing-song voice going on like the little brook.

Lord Mauleverer remained sitting on the sarcophagus in the dim passage enjoying a rest. But at the sound of footsteps he made an effort and rose, supposing that one of his comrades was coming back for him.

"All right, old bean, I'm comin'!" yawned Mauly, as he slipped from the stone rim of the sarcophagus. "I——Oh!"

It was not one of the juniors coming along the corridor from the gallery, as he had supposed.

It was a man dressed in European clothes, with a tarboosh, whose dark face was almost hidden from sight by a large beard and a pair of blue-tinted sun-glasses.

Mauleverer glanced at him, and would have passed him; but the man stopped directly in his way, his black eyes gleaming through the tinted glasses.

What happened next took Mauleverer completely by surprise.

The man in the tinted glasses glanced swiftly over his shoulder to make sure that there was no one in the corridor behind him, and the next instant grasped at the schoolboy earl.

Before Mauleverer could resist, or even think of resisting the sudden attack, he was swept off his feet in the grasp of two powerful hands and whirled into the deep niche in the rock wall where the sarcophagus lay.

Bump!

"Oh!" gasped Mauleverer in utter amazement, as he was bumped down into the empty sarcophagus.

He landed on his back, and his assailant plunged in after him, pinning him down.

A hand grasped his throat, choking back the cry he would have uttered.

Mauleverer stared upward in sheer stupefaction at the face bending over him.

"Silence, my lord!" said a soft, musical voice.

Mauleverer started violently.

He did not know the face disguised by the beard and the big, coloured glasses, but he knew the voice.

It was the voice of Kalizelos, the Greek, of Cairo.

It was hardly needed for the Greek to bid him be silent; the grip on his throat silenced him. Mauleverer's heart throbbed. He had lingered behind his comrades only for a few minutes, but those few minutes had been enough for his watchful enemy. Now he was out of sight of his friends, even if they looked back along the passage, for the sarcophagus was deep in the niche cut in the rock wall, and could only be seen close at hand.

The Greek grinned down at him.

"I have found you again, my lord!" he said. "Did I not tell you at Mauleverer Towers that you would meet me again in Africa?"

Mauleverer could only stare up at him.

"The scarab!" whispered the Greek. "Give it to me and save your life, my lord! Hamza failed to pick it from your pocket. But you have it about

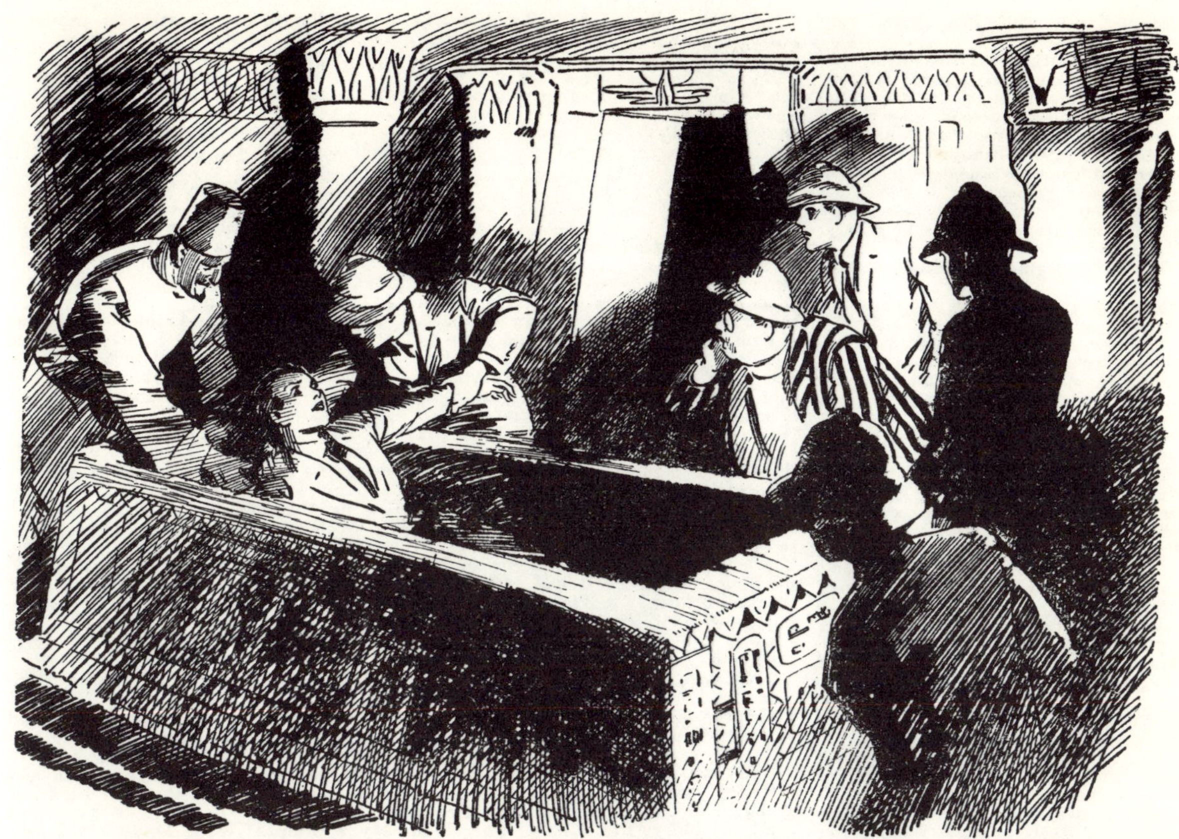

In the combined grasp of Harry Wharton & Co. the heavy stone lid of the sarcophagus swung up and back, and the juniors stared into the dim interior. "Mauly!" panted Wharton, assisting the schoolboy earl to rise.

you, I am sure of that! In which pocket, my lord?"

He relaxed the grip on Mauleverer's throat.

"Speak—in a whisper!" he hissed.

"You scoundrel!" panted Mauleverer.

"Where is the scarab?"

"You won't get it! I've not got it on me, as it happens!" gasped Mauleverer. "Your thieving pickpocket would have got it if I had!"

The Greek's eyes blazed.

His grip tightened on the schoolboy earl's throat again, silencing him. There was a sound of footsteps.

But they passed in the rock gallery at the end of the passage. The Greek listened intently.

At any moment tourists and guides might come along the corridor to look at the tomb of Psah. But for the moment the corridor was deserted, and Mauleverer was at his enemy's mercy. He was sturdy, but his strength was as nothing in the muscular grip of the Greek.

Kalizelos bent lower over the junior sprawling on his back in the hollow tomb.

"Waste no time, my lord!" he hissed in Mauleverer's ear. "There may be interruption any moment. I cannot afford the time to search you. Give me the scarab! Quick—quick—or I will close the tomb on you, and return to take it from your dead body!"

Again he relaxed his grip on Mauleverer's throat for the schoolboy to speak. But as Mauleverer attempted to shout he tightened it again, his eyes blazing.

"Fool! Die, then!" he breathed. "Die in the tomb of Psah, and I will take the scarab from your body when death keeps you silent!"

He sprang up and leaped from the tomb. A crashing blow felled the junior as he scrambled up, and he sprawled in the sarcophagus. The next moment the Greek's sinewy hands had dragged over the stone lid, and it fell into its place with a thud.

Instantly the dim light was blotted from Mauleverer's eyes. He stretched his hands upwards, and they touched the cold stone above him.

A shudder ran through him from head to foot.

He shouted, filling his narrow prison with booming sound; but he knew only too well that no sound could penetrate beyond the thick, heavy stone.

"Oh gad!" gasped Mauleverer.

He braced himself against the floor of the sarcophagus and pushed upward with his whole strength. It seemed to him for a moment that the stone above him stirred a little; but if so, it was only a little. His strength—or twice his strength—would not have lifted it.

Panting with his effort, his head spinning, Mauleverer sank back again. No sound reached him. Whether the murderous Greek was gone he could not tell. There might have been tourists gathered round the tomb of Psah, and a dragoman expounding the history of the mummy to them, and he would have heard no sound. Silence as of the grave lay heavy upon him—silence and overpowering darkness. And, with a shudder, he realised that the air in that narrow space would not last long.

Again he made a terrible effort to lift the stone lid; again he failed and sank back exhausted.

He was lost!

How long he might live, in that living tomb, till the air failed, and he was suffocated, he could not tell. But not long—not long! If the stone lid of the sarcophagus was not lifted, he was doomed—and it would not be lifted till the Greek came to search him for the scarab—not till all was sure!

He was lost—in the blackness of the tomb where a mummy once had lain! Where, long centuries ago, Psah, the Egyptian of Alexandria, had been laid in death, he was laid in life—till life flickered out like a candle! And his friends, wandering among the rock-galleries, deep in the dusky catacombs, never dreamed that the sands of his life were running swiftly out!

THE THIRTEENTH CHAPTER.

Startling!

"I SAY, you fellows!"

"In every which tomb, when recently of late times excavated, were found three mummies——"

Hassan was going strong in the rock-gallery.

"I say, you fellows——" hooted Bunter.

"Shut up, Bunter!"

"What about lunch?"

"Three bootiful specimens of mummies were found in every one of all these wonderful tombs, my gentlemen lords!" said Hassan. "And, further on, there are still more enormous numbers of dead persons——"

"I'm hungry!"

"My esteemed, idiotic Bunter——"

"Old Brooke told us to get back to the hotel for lunch," said Bunter. "He's rather an old ass, and I can't say I like his manners. Still, he's in charge of us, and we're bound to respect him, see?"

"At meal-times, anyhow!" grinned Bob. "Perhaps it's time we got a move on, you men! It's a good step back to the hotel."

"Oh, my gentlemen lords, do not be in pressed hurry!" exclaimed Hassan. "There is much more to see—huge numbers of dead persons. To return to hotel we take arabeyah, which, in English, is called 'cabby.' Yes, there is plentiful time to take leisurely look at wonders of catacombs."

"It's a jolly interesting place, and we shan't be here again," said Harry. "If you're hungry, Bunter——"

"I jolly well am!" said Bunter, with emphasis.

"Then you can go and eat coke!"

"Why, you cheeky beast——"

"Where's Mauly?" asked Nugent, glancing round. "Have we left him behind? I suppose he won't lose the scarab, as we left it at the hotel; but he will lose himself."

"Sitting down somewhere for a rest, I suppose," said Johnny Bull. "We'll pick him up as we go back."

"I say, you fellows, let's go back now! I'm hungry. Never mind Mauly—if he's lost himself, he can follow us—anybody will tell him the way out. Look here, if you jolly well don't come, I'll jolly well go without you!" declared Bunter. "I'm not going to die of hunger in these beastly catacombs to please you, see?"

Harry Wharton looked back along the rock-gallery. A good many people were in sight, tourists and guides and touts, but he could not see Lord Mauleverer among them.

"The old duffer must be still sitting where we left him, in that corridor between the galleries," he said. "I thought he was coming after us. Gone to sleep, as likely as not. We'd better go back and fetch him—Nunky told us not to get separated."

"I say, you fellows——"

"Shut up, Bunter!"

The Famous Five retraced their steps along the rock-gallery to the corner of the corridor where the tomb of Psah lay in the excavated niche. Dim as the corridor was, they could see through it, to the lighted rock-chamber at the other end, and there was no one to be seen.

"Not there," said Bob, "unless he's sitting on the jolly old tomb in the wall. Hallo, hallo, hallo! Mauly!"

Bob's powerful voice boomed along the corridor. But there came no answer, save a thousand echoes from the rock walls.

"I say you fellows——"

"Shut up, Bunter!"

"I dare say Mauly's got hungry, and gone back for lunch——"

"Fathead!"

Harry Wharton ran back along the rock-corridor, as far as the tomb of Psah.

As he came to the deep niche cut in the wall, he saw that a man was leaning on the tomb, of which the stone lid was now closed. He was dressed in European clothes, save for the tarboosh, and his face could hardly be seen, under a large beard and a pair of large, blue-tinted glasses. As he leaned on the stone top of the sarcophagus, he was lighting a cigarette, and he did not even glance at Wharton as he came up.

There was nothing to be seen of Lord Mauleverer. Wharton noticed that the stone lid of the sarcophagus was closed; but certainly it did not occur to him for a moment that it had closed over the junior he was looking for. He supposed, without thinking about it, that some custodian of the place had closed the tomb.

"Not here," said Harry, as his friends came up. "He must have followed us, I suppose, and we shall find him somewhere in the gallery."

"I say, you fellows——"

"Dry up, Bunter!"

"Look here, you beasts, we're not going to root all over these putrid catacombs, looking for Mauly, when I'm hungry!" hooted Bunter. "He will find his way back all right!"

"Shut up!"

"Shan't!" roared Bunter. "I tell you I want my lunch! Look here, ask that nigger if he's seen him—it's not five minutes since we left him here, and he can't be far away."

The bearded, spectacled man leaning on the sarcophagus was taking no notice of the schoolboys—openly, at least. But from under the cover of the big, blue-tinted glasses, he watched them as he smoked the cigarette.

Harry Wharton turned to him.

"Excuse me, sir," he said politely. "We are looking for a friend. Perhaps you have seen him?"

The spectacled man shook his head, to indicate that he did not understand English. Hassan came along the corridor after the juniors, his gorgeous raiment making a bright splash of colour in the gloomy place.

"Let Hassan ask him," said Bob. "Hassan, old bean, ask this chap if he's seen Mauleverer."

The dragoman addressed the spectacled man in Arabic. In what seemed to the juniors a surly way, the man shook his head, still without speaking, and, turning his back, proceeded to light a second cigarette from the stump of the first.

"This person has not seen the gentleman lord," said Hassan. "Without doubt he has walked along to gallery, and my lordly gentleman will find him gazing at mummified dead persons——"

"Well, we'd better find him at once," said Harry. "I suppose there can't be any danger in a place like this, except from pickpockets; but we can't be too careful. That pickpocket may not be the only man that that rotter Kalizelos set to watch us."

"I say, you fellows——"

"Shut up, Bunter!" roared Bob Cherry.

"I tell you I jolly well won't go round rooting after that silly idiot Mauly!" yelled Bunter. "I'm going back to lunch, see? Mauly can go and eat coke! I warned you that you'd get lost if you got out of my sight—you can't say I didn't! Well, Mauly's got lost, and he can stay lost, and be blowed to him! Now let's get back to lunch!"

"Kick him!" growled Johnny Bull.

"Beast!"

The juniors started up the corridor again. They were not alarmed for Lord Mauleverer; but they had made up their minds to look for him and find him at once. They little dreamed, as they started, that they were turning their backs on the hapless junior, and they did not see the mocking glitter in the eyes under the blue-tinted glasses of the man leaning on the tomb.

"Look here, I'm not coming!" roared Bunter.

"Come on, you silly owl!" snapped Bob, over his shoulder.

"Shan't!" roared Bunter. "I'm jolly well going, and you can root about after that silly idiot Mauly as long as you jolly well like! I'm jolly well going back to lunch!"

"Come with us, you fat idiot!" exclaimed Harry Wharton. "You will lose yourself in two ticks, and we shall have to hunt for you as well as Mauly."

"Yah!"

"Oh, yank him along by his ears!" exclaimed Nugent. "We can't leave the fat dummy on his own."

Bob Cherry strode back towards Bunter. It was more likely than not that the fat Owl, left on his own, would have lost himself in the catacombs, and the chums of the Remove certainly did not want two lost fellows to hunt for, up and down the passages and galleries and rock-chambers. Bob Cherry grabbed at the fat Owl's collar.

"Come on, you silly chump!" he grunted.

Bunter squirmed.

"Leggo!" he yelled. "Beast! I'm not coming!"

"This way, idiot!"

"You cheeky rotter——"

"Get a move on, fathead!"

Billy Bunter made a terrific effort to

wrench himself loose. Bob's grasp did not yield; but Bunter's collar did. It flew off in Bob's hand, and he staggered against the rock wall. Billy Bunter spun away like a fat humming-top, crashed into the spectacled man leaning on the tomb, and clutched at him wildly for support.

The man, taken utterly by surprise by that sudden and unexpected crash, staggered and stumbled over, Billy Bunter sprawling on the floor with him, clutching frantically. One of his fat hands caught the stranger's beard—which came off in his grasp. Bunter, hardly noticing in the excitement of the moment what had happened, rolled spluttering with the false beard clutched in his fat fingers.

Bob Cherry jumped forward to help the stranger up, and the other fellows ran back to the spot. The next moment there was a yell of astonishment from the Famous Five—almost of stupefaction, as their eyes fixed on the face of the man breathlessly scrambling up. The blue-tinted glasses lay smashed on the rock-floor; the false beard was in Bunter's clutch—and now that the beard and the glasses were gone, a clear-cut olive-skinned face was revealed—a face they knew.

"Kalizelos!" yelled Bob.

"Oh, my hat! Kalizelos!" panted Wharton.

"I say, you fellows—yarooh! I say—— Whoop!" spluttered Bunter. "I say, I've banged my head—yaroop!"

The Greek was on his feet, agile as a cat, his black eyes burning, his olive face convulsed with rage.

For a second he glared at the Greyfriars fellows; then as they made a movement towards him, he turned and ran.

Almost in a twinkling of an eye he vanished out of the rock corridor, leaving the juniors staring blankly, and Billy Bunter sitting up, spluttering, and blinking at the beard clutched in his fat hand.

THE FOURTEENTH CHAPTER.

Saved from the Tomb!

HASSAN, the dragoman, stood staring after the vanished Greek, more astonished than the Greyfriars fellows. He knew the dealer of Cairo; though he had not recognised him in his disguise. Hassan's eyes almost bulged from his brown face in his astonishment.

"That is Kalizelos, the rich dealer of Cairo!" he ejaculated. "Why does he wear a beard that does not belong? Why does he run? My gentlemen lords, this is one astonishment—a knock into a cock-hat, as you say in your magnificent language. Yes."

"I say, you fellows——"

"It was Kalizelos," said Harry Wharton. "He has been spying on us, of course—got up like that so that we should not know him."

"Well he's gone," said Bob. "We'd better look for Mauly! The sooner we find him the better, with that Greek scoundrel knocking about."

"Come on," said Johnny Bull. "Mauly can't be far away; but we'd better find him at once."

"Hold on!" said Harry Wharton.

He stood quite still, his eyes fixed on the tomb on which the disguised Greek had been leaning.

An almost scared look was on his face, and the colour wavered in his cheeks.

But for the discovery that the man at the tomb was Kalizelos, the juniors would have left the spot unsuspecting. But now a strange and terrible suspicion was in Wharton's mind. Mauleverer had been left at this spot, sitting on the sarcophagus, and they had found the Greek there! And the sarcophagus, which had been standing open when they left it, was closed. Wharton had attached no importance to that circumstance—till now! But now——

"What——" began Bob, startled by the look on the face of the captain of the Remove.

Wharton caught his breath.

"Mauly!" he breathed. "If that villain found him here——"

"Mauly's not here——"

"Hassan!" Wharton pointed to the tomb of Psah. "Is that tomb ever closed—or——"

"No, sar, I have not seen this tomb closed before this time," said the dragoman. "Wonderful mummy being removed to museum, tomb is left open for honourable inspection by inquisitive tourists."

"But what——" began Nugent.

"If Kalizelos closed it——" muttered Wharton.

"But why——"

"Mauleverer——"

"Good heavens!" gasped Nugent, as he read Wharton's thought. "Harry—it's impossible—even that villain——"

"Get it open!"

"Yes, rather!"

"Thank goodness that Bunter played the fool, and we found Kalizelos out," panted Wharton. "But for that we should have gone—— Lend a hand. Get the thing open! Hassan, help us!"

"Yes, sar! Lid of sarcophagus being very heavy indeed, but Hassan is strong as King Rameses," said the dragoman, and he added his muscular grasp, and helped the juniors to lift the heavy stone lid of the sarcophagus.

The same thought was in the minds of all the juniors now—though it seemed almost too terrible to believe. The great mass of stone swung up, and back, in their combined grasp, and they stared into the interior.

"Mauly!" panted Wharton.

A white face glimmered from the shadow within the stone tomb.

"Mauly!"

Many hands seized the schoolboy earl and lifted him out of the sarcophagus. He was conscious, but his face was white as chalk. He leaned heavily on Harry Wharton's shoulder, as the juniors set him on his feet, and his breath came in gasps.

"Mauly, old man——" breathed Wharton.

"Oh crumbs!" gasped Billy Bunter, his eyes almost popping through his big spectacles. "It—it—it's Mauly! What the thump did you get into that beastly hole for, Mauly?"

Lord Mauleverer stared at him, and a faint smile came over his colourless face.

"Oh gad!" he murmured. "I—I'm glad to see you fellows! I—I thought I was a goner! Oh gad!"

"But what did you get into the tomb for?" asked Bunter. "You must have been a silly ass, Mauly."

"I was chucked in, fathead!" said Mauleverer.

"Kalizelos——" said Bob.

"Yaas! You've seen him?"

"He was here—disguised; but that idiot Bunter butted into him, and——"

"Oh, really, Wharton——"

"How long have I been in there?" asked Mauleverer, in a low voice. "I—I thought the air wouldn't last; but it must have lasted all the hours I've been shut up in that horrible place——"

"Hours!" repeated Bob Cherry. "My dear old chap, it's not a quarter of an hour since we left you here."

"Good gad! Sure of that?" ejaculated Mauleverer. "My hat! It's the longest quarter of an hour I've ever known then!" He glanced at his wrist-watch. "Great Scott! You're right! But it seemed——" His voice shook, and he broke off.

"And—and we never guessed—never imagined——" muttered Nugent. "If we hadn't found Kalizelos here, we should never have guessed——"

"If I hadn't found him here, you mean," interrupted Billy Bunter. "I don't want to rub it in, but I'd like to know what would have happened if I hadn't been with you? I ask you."

"Oh, dry up, Bunter!"

"And now," continued Bunter, "as I've saved Mauly's life the least you can do, I think, is to come back to lunch at once. I've told you I'm hungry."

"Let's get out of this," said Bob. "Come on, Mauly!"

"My gentlemen lords, there are still large numbers of dead persons——" said Hassan.

Lord Mauleverer grinned.

"There'd have been one more dead person, if you fellows hadn't hooked me out of that jolly old tomb," he said. "I'm rather fed-up on tombs and things. If you fellows don't mind, I'd rather chuck these jolly old catacombs."

"Come on!" said Harry Wharton.

Mauleverer leaned on Wharton's arm as they made their way back to the staircase out of the catacombs. His face was still pale; but he was recovering now. The juniors were glad to find themselves above the earth and in the brilliant sunshine again. Hassan followed them with rather a sorrowful expression on his face. They had not seen half the sights of the Alexandria catacombs; and Hassan was quite pained by their loss of interest in the innumerable dead persons. But after what had happened, the juniors had had more than enough of the catacombs.

"My gentlemen lords return to hotel?" asked Hassan.

"Yes—get us an arabeyeh," said Harry.

"Yes, sar! But if my gentlemen lords walk, there is an enormous Arab cemetery for my gentlemen to see——" said Hassan persuasively. "It is on the way to hotel—one great tremendous cemetery—all visitors come to see this enormous cemetery——"

"Call an arabeyeh!"

Hassan sadly obeyed. Wharton helped Mauleverer into the arabeyeh and got in with him. Two more arabeyehs were called for the rest of the party, and they started on their homeward way, Hassan trotting after the carriages, his gold tassel dancing in the sun. As the carriages rolled along the Rue de la Colonne Pompee, Hassan called out to his gentlemen lords, and pointed with his stick.

"Here is great cemetery, my fine gentlemen—you look out of an arabeyeh and see tremendous cemetery——"

But the chums of Greyfriars had lost their interest in sight-seeing, for the present, and they did not even glance at the celebrated Arab cemetery. The arabeyehs rolled on through the busy streets of Alexandria, the juniors thinking, not of the sights of the city of Alexander, but of what had happened in the catacombs—excepting, of course, Bunter. Bunter was thinking of his lunch. To his immense relief, they arrived at the Hotel Magnifique in good time for lunch—and, so far as Billy Bunter was concerned, at least—all was calm and bright!

THE FIFTEENTH CHAPTER.

Off to Cairo!

"GO away!"

"But, my fine gentlemen——"

"Go away!"

"Noble and magnificent lord——"

"Go away!"

Harry Wharton & Co. looked from the train window and grinned.

There was a tone of mingled sorrow and affectionate persuasion in the voice of Hassan, the son of Suleiman, as he stood by the train in the station of Alexandria. But Sir Reginald Brooke was inflexible. The Greyfriars party were leaving Alexandria for Cairo; and Hassan had been dismissed, with a liberal backsheesh for his services—such as they were. But Hassan, though he was dismissed, seemed to consider that he was still attached to the party. Perhaps the liberality of the backsheesh strengthened his attachment. The dismissed dragoman was rather like the gentleman in the old story, who was dead but would not lie down. Dismissed or not dismissed, Hassan had made up his mind that the Greyfriars party could not possibly dispense with his valuable services.

Sir Reginald entered his carriage. A Coptic porter closed the door. Hassan looked in at the window, while from the adjoining carriage the Famous Five watched him, with amused faces.

"Fine and splendid gentleman!" urged Hassan almost tearfully. "Hassan is your dragoman."

"Go away!"

"At Cairo you will want Hassan—at Luxor—everywhere! Hassan knows all things."

"Go away!"

"Yaas, get off, old bean," said Lord Mauleverer, who was in the carriage with his uncle. "Good-bye! Here, shove this in your pocket and clear."

Hassan's black eyes almost popped out of his brown face as the schoolboy earl dropped a banknote into his brown hand. Lord Mauleverer sat down, supposing that he was done with the dragoman. But giving an Egyptian dragoman a banknote was not the way to have done with him. If Hassan had been attached to the party before, he was doubly and trebly attached now. Visions of unlimited backsheesh danced before the eyes of Hassan, the son of Suleiman. He salaamed, and salaamed, till the juniors, watching him, wondered that his backbone did not go.

"Noble gentleman, Hassan is your dragoman! He will serve you for ever! At Cairo, at Luxor, everywhere——"

"Go away!" said Sir Reginald.

He snapped the window shut.

"That jolly old dragoman is a sticker!" grinned Bob Cherry.

"The stickfulness is terrific!" chuckled the Nabob of Bhanipur.

"Hallo, hallo, hallo, we're off!"

Hassan's crimson tarboosh, with its gold tassel, disappeared in the crowd. The train rumbled out of Alexandria on its journey southward to Cairo. Billy Bunter, in a corner of the carriage with the Famous Five, grunted.

"Beastly hot!" he remarked.

"It's not chilly!" agreed Bob.

"And it's dusty——" grunted Bunter. "Blessed if I ever saw so much dust anywhere."

"That's the jolly old desert," said Bob.

"And the flies—look at the flies——" said Bunter. "There's a beastly fly keeps settling on my nose."

"I expect he takes it for a strawberry."

"Beast!"

There was no doubt that it was hot; and there was a great deal of dust from the desert. And there were plenty of flies—all sorts of flies—and the flies seemed to like Billy Bunter very much. Perhaps his fat perspiring face attracted them—though, generally speaking, it would not have been called attractive. Or perhaps the traces of his last meal had a fascination for them. Since breakfast, Bunter had disposed of a large supply of Turkish Delight, and he was sticky. The flies seemed to like Turkish Delight as much as Bunter did.

It seemed to William George Bunter that one, at least, of the ancient plagues of Egypt was still on—the plague of flies. He dabbed, and smacked, and smacked, and dabbed, but quite a large party of the flies of Alexandria seemed to have made up their minds to accompany him to Cairo. Like the dragoman, they were stickers.

"Did you fellows bring a mosquito net?" asked Bunter. "I think you might have brought a mosquito net for me—you jolly well knew that I should want a nap in the train! Selfishness all round! Do you fellows ever think of anybody but yourselves?" added Bunter sarcastically.

"My esteemed idiotic Bunter——"

"Well, shut up, anyhow," said Bunter. "The train makes enough noise, without you fellows jawing when a fellow wants to go to sleep. Wake me up when we get to Cairo."

Billy Bunter settled back in his corner and closed his eyes behind his big spectacles.

"Don't you want to look at Egypt, fathead?" asked Bob Cherry.

"Blow Egypt!"

Harry Wharton & Co. looked from the window with tireless interest while Bunter settled down to snore. Alexandria was only the gateway of Egypt; but the real Egypt was unrolling before their eyes as the train ran on to the south. Alexandria and the great Lake Mareotis disappeared behind. Wide fields of barley and rice began to appear, and groups of date-palms—and they stared at the sight of a camel and a donkey yoked together to a plough. The new and the old jostled one another on all sides. On the road that ran beside the railway a man in a tarboosh and a djubbah was driving an Austin Seven. A brown-faced Copt navigated a bicycle, winding among camel-riders and donkey-boys. Brown children, catching sight of the foreign faces in the train, held out brown hands and shrieked "Backsheesh!"

"Urrrrrrgh!"

It was a sudden snort from Billy Bunter.

The juniors looked round at him. He was awake again, and coughing and spluttering wildly. It was Bunter's elegant custom, when he shut his eyes, to open his mouth. One of the flies had started investigating the spacious interior.

"Oooogh! Oooop! Grooogh!" spluttered Bunter. He got rid of the fly, who was probably sorry he had entered by the time he left. "Ow! I say, you fellows, if you're not going to sleep, I think you might fan the flies off a fellow while he has a nap! I really think that!"

"Anybody feel inclined to sit by Bunter and fan the flies off him?" asked Bob Cherry. "Don't all speak at once."

"Ha, ha, ha!"

"Blessed if I see anything to cackle at! After all I've done for you——"

Bob Cherry chuckled, and picked up a little feather brush from the floor of the carriage. It had been left there by the man whose duty it was to flick the dust from the seats.

"All serene, old fat man—I'll fan you!" he said. "Go to sleep—you're nicer when you're asleep."

"Well, keep those beastly flies off me!" grunted Bunter; and he closed his eyes again behind his spectacles.

The flies were not long in settling. The smears of Turkish Delight on Bunter's fat countenance seemed to have an irresistible attraction for them. A dozen flies, large and small, buzzed over the fat face of the Owl of the Remove as he began to snore, and Bob lifted the feather brush. As it had been used for dusting the carriage it was well charged with the fine, almost impalpable dust that blew from the desert. That, however could not be helped. Perhaps Bob did not notice it, or perhaps he did. Anyhow, he fanned Bunter with the feather brush.

The flies fled. There was a gurgling roar from Billy Bunter, and he woke up again quite suddenly.

"Ooogh! Grogh! Oooch! Wooch! Ow! I'm chook-chook-choking! Yurrgh! Wharrer you doing, you beast, smothering a fellow with — oooogh! — dust? Yurrrrgh!"

"Fanning you, old fat bean——"

"Yurrrrrgh! Keep off!" shrieked Bunter. "Keep that thing away! Ooooooch! My nose is full of—wooogh—dust! My mouth's full of—gerrrgh—beastly dust! I say—grooogh!"

"Ha, ha, ha!"

"There's another fly," said Bob cheerily, "just settling on your nose. There—got him!"

"Yurrrrggggh!" spluttered Bunter, as the dust-brush whopped on his fat little nose. "Atchoo — chooop — choooop! Atchew—woop! Gug-gug-gug!"

"Ha, ha, ha!"

"Ow! Beast! Stoppit!" yelled Bunter. "Keep that thing away, I tell you! Ow! Groogh! Atchooo—whoop!"

"Don't you want me to fan the flies off?" asked Bob.

"Ow! Beast! No!" roared Bunter. "Leave them alone! Mind your own business! Oh crikey! Atchoo—chooop! Billy Bunter sneezed frantically. Ow! Grooh! Leave a fellow alone, you beast! Ooooooch!"

"If that's the way you thank a chap for fanning the flies off——"

"Ow! Beast! Yurrggh!"

"Ha, ha, ha!"

"Some fellows never seem to know what they want," remarked Bob Cherry. "First he wants to be fanned, and then he doesn't want to be fanned! There's no pleasing some people. I shan't fan you any more, Bunter!"

"Beast!"

The plague of flies continued to give

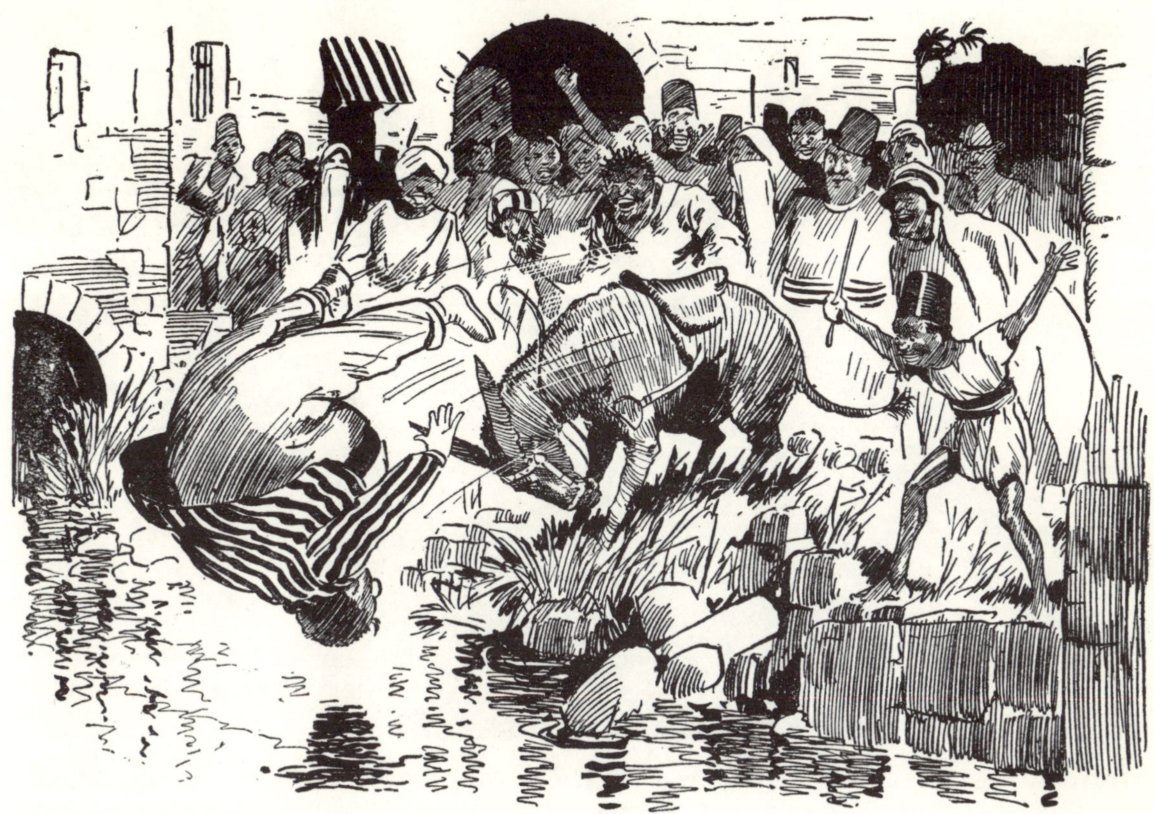

The more tightly Billy Bunter clung to William Shakespeare's neck, the faster the donkey careered. At the sight of the gleaming water, however, the animal stopped—suddenly lowering its head. The next moment Bunter was shooting through the air like a bullet !

Billy Bunter their best attention as the train hummed on southward. But Billy Bunter did not ask to be fanned any more. He had had enough fanning.

THE SIXTEENTH CHAPTER.
Bunter on a Donkey !

"CAIRO !"

"Wake up, Bunter !"

The train clanged into Cairo. From the windows Harry Wharton & Co. had their first view of the Pyramids of Ghizeh, towering over the desert in the distance, blue-grey against the burning sky of Egypt. The train clanged on into the station and stopped, and Harry Wharton shook Bunter by a fat shoulder.

"Lemme alone, you beast !" mumbled Bunter. "'Tain't rising-bell !"

"Fathead ! It's Cairo !"

Billy Bunter rubbed his eyes, set his spectacles straight on his fat little nose, and grunted. The carriage door flew open, a swarm of porters appearing, clamouring for baggage.

The juniors descended, brown hands fairly clutching at bags, sticks, everything they could clutch at. They joined Sir Reginald and Mauleverer, surrounded by jostling, gesticulating, babbling porters, black and brown. Over the crowd appeared a crimson tarboosh with a dancing gold tassel, and a familiar voice was heard. A volley of Arabic, which sounded remarkably like fuming to English ears, drove back the porters, aided by sharp raps from the stick carried by Hassan, the son of Suleiman, and the grinning dragoman salaamed to the Greyfriars party, looking more than ever as if he had a spring in his backbone.

"Here, sar ! Hassan is your dragoman. You leave all things to Hassan. He keep away these very troublesome peoples."

"Oh, my hat ! We haven't lost Hassan, after all !" chuckled Bob Cherry.

"Hassan is your dragoman, sar."

"Go away !" rapped Sir Reginald. "Come, my boys. The hotel porter will see to the baggage."

"Hassan take care of everything !" protested the dragoman.

"Go away !" roared Sir Reginald.

"Ha, ha, ha !"

"But, sar, very fine gentleman, Hassan is your dragoman !"

"Go away !" hooted the baronet. "Go away !"

Evidently the dragoman had travelled on the train from Alexandria, determined not to be shaken off by his gentlemen lords. The juniors chuckled, rather entertained by the pertinacity of the son of Suleiman. But Sir Reginald glared at him and stalked off, shepherding his flock out of the station. But the juniors, glancing back, saw the gold tassel in pursuit. The dragoman was following on.

Whether they liked it or not, Hassan gave them his services, driving off importunate porters with volleys of Arabic or waves of his stick, shoving back the crowds of black and brown boys with things to sell—things of every imaginable kind — roses, newspapers, amber combs and beads, strings of sweetmeats, writing-paper and postcards, even live pigeons, tooth-brushes, and hairpins. Hassan drove them back ruthlessly, escorting the party out of the swarming station like a very brown and very decorative guardian angel.

"Donkey, sar ? Very fine donkey !" A black donkey-boy shouted and gestured imploringly, leading a donkey up to the party so suddenly that there was nearly a collision. "You ride a donkey, sar ! His name William Shakespeare, sar. A very fine old donkey, sar !"

Arabic volleyed from Hassan, and the donkey-boy volleyed back and receded. But Billy Bunter turned his spectacles on the sturdy donkey, and signed to the black boy.

"You fellows can get in the taxi," said Bunter. "I'll ride. Haven't ridden since the last time I backed a hunter at Bunter Court, you know."

"Oh, my hat !"

"Fine old donkey, sar !" said the donkey-boy eagerly. "Me Mustapha, sar. Best donkey-boy in Cairo, sar. William Shakespeare best donkey, sar. You ride um, sar. Handsome gentleman ride a donkey !"

"You troublesome peoples, you go 'way !" exclaimed Hassan, waving his stick. "My noble gentlemen no want donkey."

"This handsome gentleman, this great lord, he say he ride a donkey !" yelled Mustapha angrily ; and he volleyed in Arabic, with a sound like nuts in a nut-cracker.

Billy Bunter nodded. He rather fancied riding while the other fellows packed in a taxicab. But if he had been undecided, Mustapha's description of him as a handsome gentleman and a great lord would have settled the point. A donkey-boy who saw at a glance that Billy Bunter was a handsome gentleman and a great lord was a donkey-boy to be encouraged.

"That's all right," said Bunter. "I'm riding the donkey. You go and eat

(*Continued on page* 28.)

OPENING CHAPTERS OF A THRILLING OLD-TIME ROMANCE!

The Red Falcon!

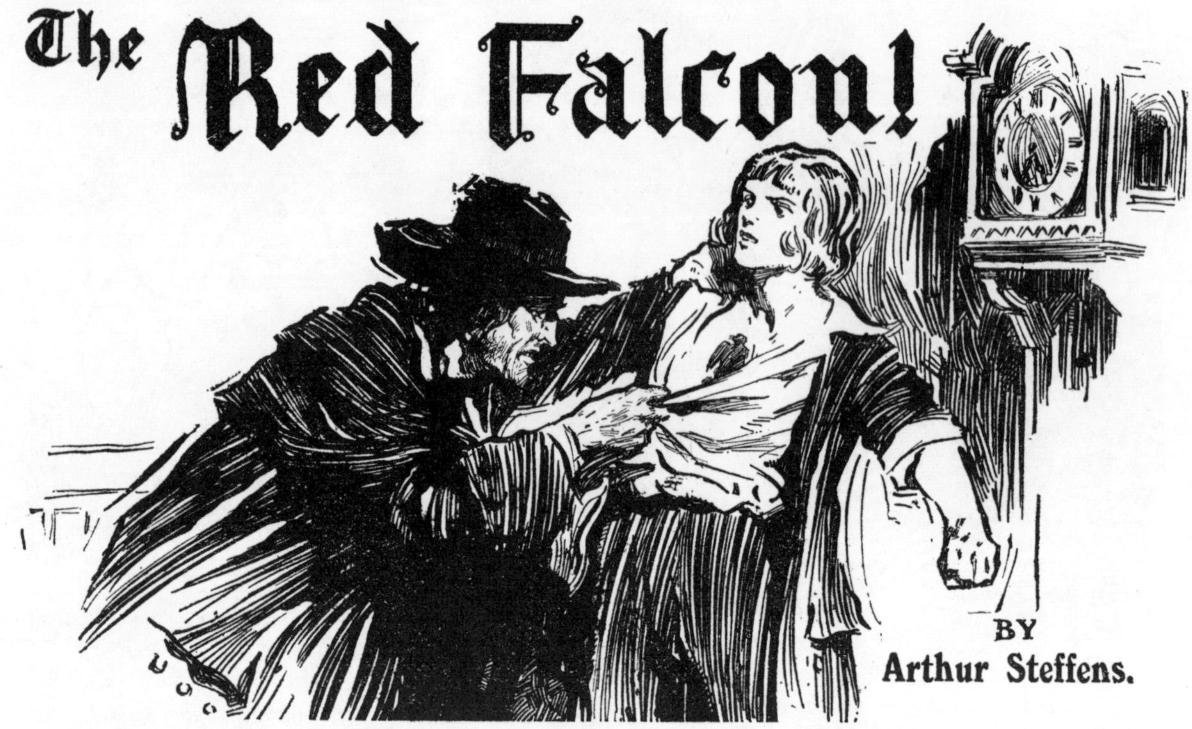

BY

Arthur Steffens.

Introducing HAL LOVETT and JERRY McLEAN, Knights of the Road.

CHAPTER I.

The Mysterious Stranger!

A YOUNG and strongly built boy pumped water from a well, and when his bucket was full he carried it into the scullery and set it on a stool. Ragged though his clothes were, they were cared for and free from stains. The frayed ends of his knickerbockers had been neatly sewn up.

The youngster's legs were bare, and his arms naked to above the elbow. Divesting himself of his coat and drawing off his shirt, he plunged his head into the water and splashed his naked body and then rubbed it until it glowed. He dried his hair, his face, and his body, rubbing until his skin was red, and then, straightening his hair with a broken comb. he eyed himself in a square of cracked looking-glass.

Tumbling reddish curls, a straight nose, two bright intelligent blue eyes, and shapely lips, which, parted, showed two rows of even teeth—this is what he saw.

And below, upon his glowing skin, a tattooed mark, a red falcon which stood with one foot raised, marvellously depicted.

For some time the youngster studied the bird as he had so often done before, then he slipped into shirt and tattered coat, emptied out the dirty water, and brought back the bucket—just as the street door bell rang.

Hal Lovett, for such was the youngster's name, hastened out into the shop.

There, blocking out the sunshine which filtered into Wych Street, he saw a broad-shouldered, big-limbed man.

"Samuel Lovett in?" demanded the intruder.

"No," answered the boy.

The man strode farther into the shop. His keen, brown eyes swept the counter littered with a piled disarray of second-hand clothes, roamed the shelves packed with articles of all kinds, hats and boots and shoes, canes and swords and odds and ends of discoloured finery—everything second-hand; studied the cheap and faded furniture.

His three-cornered hat was pushed back on his head, his scarlet waistcoat showed a brilliant patch of colour against the sombre hue of his coat. Riding-breeches, brown-topped boots with spurs, and a newly-starched cravat completed his attire.

Hal looked at the celebrated Bow Street Runner in awe.

"Anything I can do for you, Mr. Cosgrave?" he asked.

"No, my lad," answered the Runner, as he pulled out one drawer after another behind the counter and studied carefully the contents. "I wanted a word with him; that's all, just a word."

Mr. Cosgrave's keen eyes still wandered. He peeped into the scullery, walked up three stairs into the parlour and looked around, then came down again, fumbling his staff with the royal crown on top as he completed his survey. Then back to the door he went, and pulled it open to a brazen clang.

His eyes held Hal's.

"Just you tell your father that Martin Cosgrave called, will you, me lad?" he said. "Martin Cosgrave the Runner."

"That all, sir?" asked the boy.

"No! Add this. A little bird has whispered. Warn him to be careful, or one of these fine days I'll be nabbin' him for thieving and receivin'. And you know what that'd mean, boy."

"No," answered Hal.

"Transportation," said the Bow Street Runner. "Transportation; or else a ride to Tyburn Tree." Then Mr. Cosgrave's hard face relaxed into a smile. "You're a bright boy, Hal," he added. "I've allus liked you. And bust me if I know how you came to be like you are with sech a father as Sam Lovett."

With that, he pulled the door to with a slam and went off with slow and measured strides beneath the overhanging gables of the houses in Wych Street, followed by a hundred furtive eyes.

Martin Cosgrave had visited Samuel Lovett's shop in Wych Street before, and Hal had never been afraid of him. But he was uneasy now. He delivered the warning, and cleverly ducked the smashing blow his father hurled at him for giving it. But he could not get it out of his mind.

Hal was a clever boy. He noticed things. His father did very little trade in his rag shop, but there were times when he had plenty of gold to squander in drink.

Hal almost knew that his father was a receiver and a thief.

The boy scarcely slept a wink the night after the Runner had called. Cosgrave's visit worried him.

The very next day Hal experienced another shock.

His father was upstairs in the parlour, recovering from a drinking bout. His mother had gone out, and the boy was glad, because her constant nagging fretted him more than his father's blows.

Hal had been told to look after the shop.

He was sitting on the counter swinging his bare legs when a shadow darkened the glass panes of the shop door, and a hand lifted the latch.

The man who entered the shop was a beggar. There was nothing remarkable in that. Such men had often called before.

But the thing that did strike Hal as strange was the way in which the beggar peered at him out of eyes that seemed all a-fire.

Slowly the man came towards him with his head bent as if to see the better.

Hal stopped breathing. He was not afraid, only there was something uncanny about the man.

"So," said the stranger, "you are Sam Lovett's boy?"

"Yes," said Hal.

For a minute they looked at each other. And as the boy studied the beggar he noticed many things; for instance, that the features of the man's dirty face were not those of a gutter rascal, that the begrimed hand which held the weather-stained rag of a cloak close about him was smooth, and the nails carefully trimmed. The boy's eyes travelled to the man's feet. His shoes were filthy. They had not been cleaned for a long time, Hal judged, but they were expensive shoes and soundly soled and heeled.

"Ah!" said the stranger, breaking the silence. "Take me to your father, boy."

Hal slipped off the counter and dodged away.

"What name?" he asked.

"The name doesn't matter," answered the stranger, as he pulled the brim of his battered felt hat down farther to shield his eyes. "Tell him Mr. Who."

Hal held his breath. His eyes had caught the flash of a diamond as the man raised his right hand. Mr. Who's voice was smooth and cultured, too, in spite of his attempts to coarsen its tone.

The boy turned to deliver the message—and saw his father standing at the head of the three steps leading to the parlour.

Gaunt and ugly, his hair tumbled, his clothes stained and unbrushed, Samuel Lovett towered over Hal as he took a pinch of snuff.

"If you're not livelier delivering a message next time, I'll whip you till you bleed, you young villain," said Lovett, glaring through bloodshot eyes at his son. "Look after the shop. Come in, Mr. Who."

The murmur of voices from the parlour where the door stood ajar worried Hal as he remained in the shop whilst the shadows deepened.

A droning murmur of lowered voices talking about whom and what?

After a while, the boy crept up the three stairs and drew as near to the open door as he dare.

Hal was growing up. Only a few days back the thought of fleeing from home had entered his mind for the first time. He thought of it again now. After all, why should he stay with a father whom he hated and who hated him, and a mother who was forever scolding him and depriving him of food—a favourite form of punishment, and always undeserved?

The words that came to him made him shiver and his heart beat fast.

"And so—that's the boy." It was the stranger speaking.

"That's the boy."

"I shall want to make sure of it. You say he bears the mark?"

"He does. You shall see it before you go."

"I would like to see it now."

Hal scuttled like a startled rabbit, noiselessly and on tiptoe, back into the shop, and he was bunched lazily on the counter top when his father came to fetch him.

Samuel Lovett's clutching hand hurt as he dragged Hal into the dingy parlour.

The boy almost fell as his father hurled him towards Mr. Who.

"Look and see!" growled Lovett, glaring savagely at his son.

Mr. Who seized Hal by the collar of his coat and drew him with surprising ease—such was his strength—into the dim light that streamed through dirty window-panes.

There, as he held the lad tightly with his left hand, he tore Hal's shirt back with the right, and the boy saw again the flash of the diamond ring.

A beggar with a diamond ring!

As the man bent Hal backward his eyes greedily devoured every detail of the tattooed falcon, which showed up vividly on the boy's bare chest.

"So!" he muttered, and Hal knew that an active brain was busy behind the mask of that grimey face. "So! H'm! It was nice of you to ask me to come and see your boy, Lovett, but I'm afraid he will not do—no, assuredly, he will not do."

Some boys would have been frightened, but not so Hal Lovett, he had never been afraid. He kept on wondering what had brought Mr. Who to his father's shop, and why he should figure in the pretended beggar's calculations at all.

Once again their eyes met and held their gaze. Then the stranger released Hal, and Samuel Lovett, grasping him savagely by the collar, spun him through the door and cuffed him into the shop.

"You stay there and watch the door," Hal's father growled. "And let me know the moment anyone calls."

He strode back into the parlour again, closing the door behind him.

Hal did not stay in the darkening shop. Instead, he crept back to the parlour door. After all, he felt safer with the door closed.

The boy had never listened before. There was something mean about eavesdropping; but the visit of the mysterious stranger intrigued him, and he set his ear to the keyhole.

Hadn't he the right to listen, since he knew they were discussing him?

Mr. Who was talking in a low voice, but his tone was so rich Hal could hear almost every word.

"It is the boy, right enough, Lovett; which is as well for you, for if you'd lied I'd have sent you to the hulks. Since it is he, can you contrive anything?"

The listening boy held his breath.

"No doubt. If you could tell me your movements, why——"

"I shall attend Drury Lane Theatre to-night. Kemble is appearing in 'Hamlet.'" Mr. Who's voice was cultured now.

"And shall you be carrying anything on your person worth the priggin'?" It was Samuel Lovett speaking.

"Assuredly. Even a diamond——"

Hal lost the last word as Mr. Who lowered his voice, but it sounded like "star."

"I'll see the boy is there. I'll be there myself. But——"

"You want your pay before you've earned it—eh?" Hal heard the stranger's voice shrill. "Well, I don't mind. But this time see that you properly earn it!"

The listening boy heard the dull chink of money, and, peeping in at the keyhole, saw Samuel Lovett snatch a bag purse up from the table and pour out of it into his palm a rain of golden guineas.

In his excitement Hal had held his breath. He let it go now with a sobbing gasp, and both men wheeled and faced the door.

"What was that?"

Hal tore like the wind along the passage, turned into a darkened room, snatched a rushlight from a greasy candlestick, and raced with this up the steep stairs, up and up to his garret above.

The Boy Becomes a Man!

It was a poverty-stricken garret Plaster had fallen from the ceiling, exposing the laths, and through the holes water dripped. A damp, musty den, lit only by a small recessed window.

Hal sat on the end of a shaky bed with a book upon his knees. The rushlight burned upon a broken chair, and he bent double in order to read the close print.

The boy had borrowed the mouldy volume from a pile in the shop, for he had taught himself to read. The ting-a-ling of the street door bell sounded clearly, but he did not move or run to the window to watch Mr. Who going home. His reading absorbed him. For the same reason he did not hear his father's heavy tread upon the creaking stairs.

The door whined open on rusty hinges, and Samuel Lovett came in. He held a stout whip in his hand, and smiled evilly as he felt its wicked interlaced thong.

Hate smouldered in his eyes as he studied the boy. Why should Hal read and write when he and Mrs. Lovett could not even scratch their names?

For a moment Samuel Lovett was silent. Then his rough voice boomed through the tiny room.

"Didn't I tell you to mind the shop?"

With a start Hal set the book down, then, when he saw the whip and read his father's intention in the gleam of cruel eyes, he backed away.

"I couldn't stay in the shop," said Hal. "I did not like that man. I had to come up here and read."

"Had to—eh? And you didn't like that man?"

Samuel Lovett cracked the whip.

"I didn't like him. You were plotting something about me. He didn't come to find me employment." Hal crouched back against the wall, watching nervously the stealthy approach of the powerfully-built man. "You shan't use that whip on me!"

"Shan't I?" said Samuel Lovett. "We'll see, then!"

The whiplash leapt from the driving hand; but, with a lightning-like leap, Hal sprang aside, and the swishing thong struck against the wall.

The next moment the boy had dodged the cumbersome bully, and was close to the window.

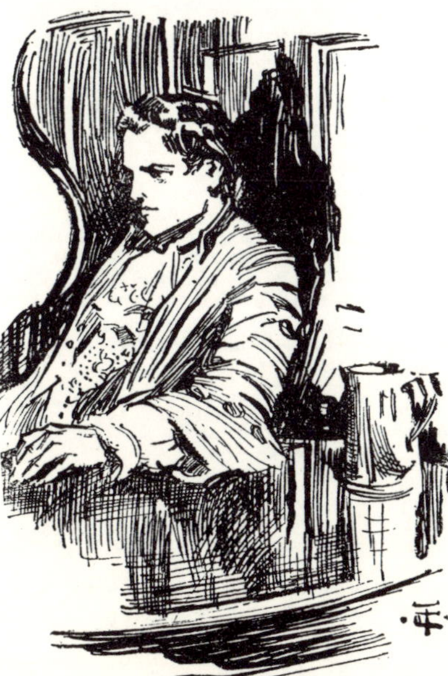

JERRY McLEAN Hal's bosom pal.

But Samuel Lovett was agile—quick. He cleared the truckle bed and barred the way to the door. Then leaping in, he swung the biting thong about Hal's middle.

Hal did not cry out—did not wince. Long years of endurance had hardened him to Samuel Lovett's cruelty. He scarcely felt the cutting bite of the lash.

Something had happened to Hal to-day. He had risen from his poverty-stricken bed a boy. But now he felt that he had suddenly become a man.

Back he sprang, his eyes flaming with hate, for love and respect for this man had died in him long ago.

"Don't strike me again!" he cried fiercely. "You'll be sorry if you do——"

Lovett laughed. Not strike—eh? Why, he loved to whip this boy of his! It would be sweet to keep on lashing until he made him cry. And so the thong flashed out again, biting deep into the boy's shoulder.

This time Hal felt pain. Springing aside, he stooped, and, picking up the broken chair, hurled it at the man's head.

His aim was true and the chair hard. Lovett dropped as if he had been pole-axed and lay half stunned upon the dirty boards.

The boy snatched the whip out of his hand, and, standing within distance, lashed the bully as fast as he could ply the thong.

"You are not my father," he told the writhing, squirming villain. "I couldn't have such a father as you. I'm not like you! I don't think like you! I don't look like you! I hate you! You're a thief, a receiver, a drunken loafer! I'm—not—going—to—stay—here—any—more! I'm—going—away!"

Every word was punctuated by a blow, and, as the thong bit deep in the man's soft flesh, Samuel Lovett rolled over on his hands and knees and unsteadily regained his feet.

"You beggar's brat!" he screamed. "I'll make you pay for this!"

With arms raised to protect his face Lovett plunged in, but Hal sprang to the door and beat him off with the lashing whip.

Tripping over a knot in the boards, Lovett tumbled heavily, and lay, panting, leering up at the boy out of bloodshot eyes. The blow from the chair had weakened him.

"I'm leaving the house. I shall not come back any more," said Hal, as he hurled the whip into a darkened corner of the garret. "I'm going away!"

"You'll come back to-night, d'ye hear?" mumbled the dazed man.

"I'm your father. You'll be at Drury Lane Theatre to-night when the play-goers turn out. I want you there!"

Setting his arms akimbo, Hal stared down with a smile at the man he had whipped.

"Because of what you plotted with Mr. Who?" he asked jeeringly.

"You listened, you thieving pup!" said the bully, as he rose unsteadily. "Why, yes, because of that. It means money——"

"Perhaps," mocked the boy, "I'll be there!" And then, as Lovett made a sudden spring, he crashed the door to so that the man fell against it, and pelted down the steep, winding stairs and through the shop, out into the narrow, cobbled street.

Day had gone. A moon hung up above the overhanging eaves of the gabled houses.

Hal hurried on past dimly illuminated windows, whistling.

He was no longer a boy, he reckoned, for he had beaten Samuel Lovett; he was a man, and he was free!

The Diamond Star!

HAL wandered about the streets adjoining Clare Market, until it began to rain. Then, his naked feet growing numbed, he wandered under the piazza of Covent Garden for shelter. It was there that he met Jerry McLean.

McLean was leaning against one of the columns, hands in pockets, staring out at the drizzle.

His fine clothes were shabby, only his cravat being clean. His weatherworn hat was set sidewise on his curly head, and his hands were thrust deep into his pockets.

McLean's young and handsome face was marked and lined from the effects of dissipation, but his hard expression relaxed and softened as he recognised the ragged, bare-footed boy.

"Whither away, Hal?" he asked. "How's your bully father?"

Hal told his tale breathlessly.

"Funds are low, lad," said McLean, as soon as the boy had finished, "but we must have a cup of coffee and talk over this."

In the shelter of a cosy pew in a common coffee-house frequented by Covent Garden porters McLean asked a hundred questions, and pondered over the boy's tale.

"Strap me, but it's deuced odd," he said, his blue eyes sparkling. "You talk of a beggar with a diamond ring, a bag of gold and an appointment at Drury Lane Theatre to-night. H'm! Let's look at that falcon, lad!"

Hal bared his body, and McLean stared long at the tattooed sign.

"Queer!" he muttered. "Now, lad, there are two courses to pursue. The first and safest is to get right away from these parts. You could come and share rooms with me—only, like you, I'm homeless and penniless. I haven't any rooms. My last coppers have gone to pay for the coffee."

"I'm sorry," said Hal impulsively.

"Never be sorry, boy. It gets you nowhere. A year ago I was rich. But I ran through a fortune, and now I'm—poor. But I had a good time, and I'm not sorry."

McLean sprawled back in his pew, handsome, smartly dressed in stained and dirty clothes that were slightly out of fashion, the wreck of a dandy who once had been.

"Since we have no home, and money can be made among the dandies when the theatre turns out, boy," he went on, "we come to course number two. That is we can go to the theatre as your father urged and see what game he means to play. There, boy, we can have another look at the mysterious Mr. Who."

The coffee had warmed Hal. His bright eyes danced as he leaned upon the table between them.

"That's what I want," he said breathlessly. "I want to know who this Mr. Who is."

McLean drummed his fingers on the table.

"A beggar with a diamond ring, who gives your father a bag of gold, and attends a theatre wearing a diamond—star, didn't you say, my boy? Why, yes, I think I'd like to know him, too!"

It was nearly midnight when Hal and Jerry McLean left the cheap coffee-house and hurried to near-by Drury Lane. Rain was dripping down and the cobbled roads were full of puddles.

No stranger association than that between McLean, the broken man about town, and Hall, the bare-legged, ragged boy could ever be imagined.

Their friendship had begun three weeks ago when a gusty wind had blown McLean's hat from his head. Hal had run in chase of it, had saved it from going into an open gutter, and had brought it back to its owner. McLean, having nothing to do, had stayed to gossip with the boy, liking his intelligence, his good looks, and his happy, bright eyes. They had met many times since.

Now, as they came in sight of the theatre, hackney carriages and coaches moved onward to the portico. Chairmen bore their heavy Sedans—a fast dying fashion—with braced shoulders and straining arms, shouting "by your leave!" as they went by.

Loafers hung about watching the well-dressed audience with envious eyes.

As McLean and Hal pushed their way to the front, the boy could see men and women of fashion crowding the theatre foyer. Diamonds flashed. Rich silks and fine laces and radiant beauty made a glowing picture, mellowed by the soft light of countless tapers.

"We're here, boy," laughed McLean. "But we must be wary. There's danger in the trap this Mr. Who and your rascally father have set for you. Have you thought of that?"

"I don't care!"

Hal's keen eyes searched the crowd, and, in the background, he saw the burly figure of Martin Cosgrave, the Bow Street Runner, propped against the theatre wall. Then his eyes, wandering on, picked up the figure of Samuel Lovett as his father came lurching along, fuddled with liquor, and his feet unsteady.

"My father's coming," whispered the boy.

"Ay," answered McLean, with a nod; "but if he's wise, he'll keep his hands off you."

Lovett came closer and caught sight of Hal. But the boy had no eyes for him now, for he had caught sight of a tall and elegant man, who pushed his way courteously among the theatre throng until he passed the yawning doors.

There he stood, dressed in the height of fashion, diamonds flashing on his fingers, his powdered head thrown haughtily back, a gold-mounted cane in his right hand, a small sword dangling by his side, the mysterious Mr. Who!

Hal stared at him in wonder.

Upon the man's left breast blazed a diamond star, the Star of the Garter, and across his silk waistcoat swept the Garter ribbon.

Very handsome indeed looked Mr. Who, very graceful, his shapely legs, clad in silk stockings, ending with elegant buckled shoes.

McLean bent forward seeing Hal so absorbed.

"What's the matter, boy?" he asked.

Hal turned his curly head and lifted up his startled eyes.

"It's him—it's Mr. Who——"

A heavy hand suddenly dropped on Hal's shoulder and urged him forward. Samuel Lovett had found his boy!

Printed and published every Saturday by the Proprietors, The Amalgamated Press, Ltd., The Fleetway House, Farringdon Street, London, E.C.4. Advertisement offices: The Fleetway House, Farringdon Street, London, E.C.4. Registered for transmission by Canadian Magazine Post. Subscription rates: Inland and Abroad, 11s. per annum; 5s. 6d. for six months. Sole Agents for Australia and New Zealand: Messrs. Gordon & Gotch, Ltd., and for South Africa: Central News Agency, Ltd.—Saturday, August 20th, 1932.

"So, I've got 'ee at last, have I?" he stormed. "I'll teach 'ee, you gallows brat!"

Hal was urged forward in the direction of Mr. Who, who stepped down to meet a splendid carriage, at whose open door stood a flunkey bowing low.

Hal broke away from Lovett, but was instantly seized again.

A moment later Hal found himself struggling among the well-dressed men and women of the theatre. He looked up into the devilishly handsome face of Mr. Who, whose eyes smouldered evilly as he looked down.

It seemed to Hal that a sign flashed between the swell and Samuel Lovett. Then Hal found himself hurled right against the elegant Mr. Who, who had played the role of beggar in the afternoon, and rich lord at night.

Mr. Who staggered, recovered himself and seized Hal in an iron grip.

In one brief second the diamond star had been torn from his silk coat by the dirty, greedy, grasping hand of Samuel Lovett and thrust into the gaping pocket of the boy's ragged jacket.

Just as swiftly as he had ripped the diamond star from tearing silk, Samuel Lovett backed away

Hal tried to free himself, but Mr. Who's hands were like iron.

"Call the watch!" cried Mr. Who. "This boy has robbed me!"

"The watch! Police!" yelled the crowd. "Fetch the Runners!"

"By gad, no!" bawled McLean, who had seen everything, and now came bursting through the excited crowd.

He found himself close to Sam Lovett, and smashed a heavy punch into the rascal's evil face as it bobbed near him, dropping him heavily to the ground.

Hal, with a desperate effort, broke away from Mr. Who.

"I've done nothing!" he cried.

With a lightning spring, the dandy closed with him and gripped him again, twisting his coat collar so tightly round his throat as to almost choke him.

"You robbed me of my diamond star!" hissed Mr. Who.

"It's not true—it's not true——"

Hal fought desperately, but the crowd closed in.

Then, with heaving shoulders, half a dozen Runners from up the street shouldered the crowd aside and seized Hal and held him fast.

"What's the trouble, my lord?" asked Martin Cosgrave, as he confronted Mr. Who.

"This gutter boy robbed me of my diamond star. You will find it in his pocket," answered Mr. Who, wiping his lips with a dainty lace handkerchief.

Martin Cosgrave's big, fat hand went into Hal's pocket, and came out again holding fast the diamond star.

"And I called to warn your father," said the Runner, with a twisted grin. "I allus liked you, boy. But I might have known you were brought up wrong, and would end on the gallows. This will mean the hulks or transportation, as sure as I'm a Runner!"

"But I didn't steal the star! It was——"

"He came right up to me and snatched it from my coat!" said Mr. Who. "I have never known such daring! Take him away!"

"No, by thunder, no!"

McLean came again, fighting his way to Hal's side. With a hefty punch, he knocked a Runner down, then tore Cosgrave's hand from Hal's coat.

An instant later, as the Runners closed in, with head down, shoulders heaving, and fists flying, he was fighting like a madman to try to rescue Hal.

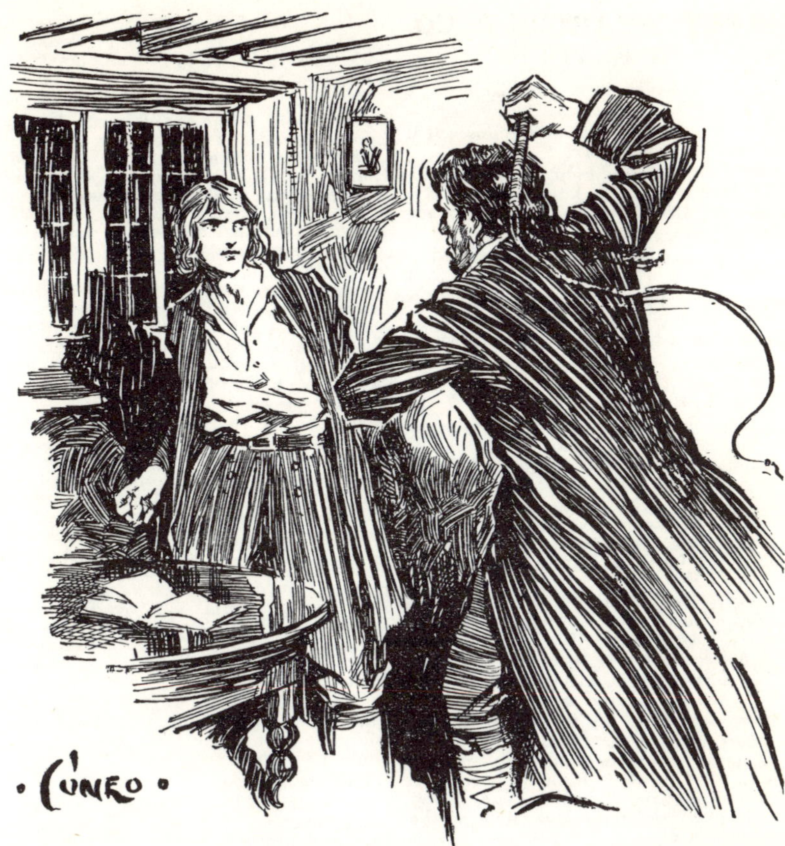

Hal Lovett crouched back against the window, watching nervously the stealthy approach of the powerfully built man. "You shan't use that whip on me!" he cried. "Shan't I?" said the bully. "We'll see, then!"

Hal did his best to help, but was dragged aside. Handcuffs snapped upon his wrists, and he was half-stunned by a savage blow.

Then McLean, still fighting hand and foot, with a handcuff dangling from his left wrist, legs spread wide, and head butting, made his last game stand.

Six Runners bore him down, using him brutally because of his desperate resistance, and a few minutes later he was hurried to Bow Street Police Station and charged.

Hal, dazed, and with handcuffs on his wrists, looked wonderingly at McLean, whose handsome face was cut and bruised and bleeding.

"Courage, boy!" said McLean, licking dry lips.

And then the stranger, known to Hal as "Mr. Who," looking remarkably distinguished in a sinister way, drawled out his story.

"The boy had brushed into him and stolen his diamond star. He hoped and trusted the young villain would be hanged!"

"It's a plot!" shouted Hal, scarcely able to speak in his excitement. "That man is Mr. Who! He came to my father's shop to-day disguised as a beggar. They planned to do this to me!"

"The boy is dangerous!" drawled the splendidly dressed gentleman. "I am the Earl of Huntford. See to it that your prisoners are properly ironed, for, should they escape, some of you would pay dearly for it!"

"Yes, my lord," said Cosgrave, the Runner, nodding his head and casting a surprised glance at Hal Lovett.

McLean tried to speak, but he was seized and borne away. His voice rang in defiant protest, and Hal heard him call out, but the gruff voices of the Runners drowned his words.

Two burly men hurried Hal to a prison cell, into which they hurled him.

The boy dropped on one knee, regained his balance, and rose.

As he turned, the heavy door swung to with a clang, and Hal found himself in utter darkness. He heard iron bolts shot home and a key turn, then the sound of retreating footsteps.

The cell measured about twelve feet by six, and Hal found a coarse mat thrown against an angle of the walls. On this mat he threw himself, lying as comfortably as his handcuffed wrists would allow.

As he lay there, he pondered upon the amazing double identity of the Earl of Huntford and the mysterious Mr. Who, and wondered what had brought an earl to Samuel Lovett's rag shop that day, and why the earl should have plotted with his father to lay this trap for him. For that the earl and Mr. Who were one and the same person Hal had not the slightest doubt.

He had found no solution of the puzzle when, towards the morning, he ceased his restless turning and tossing, and mercifully fell fast asleep.

(Here's an intriguing start to one of the most thrilling highwayman stories ever written. Mind you read next week's sensational chapters. Meanwhile, introduce Hal Lovett and Jerry McLean to your pals—they'd just love to read of their exciting adventures.)

HARRY WHARTON & CO. IN EGYPT!

(*Continued from page* 23.)

coke, Hassan! I say, you fellows, I'll follow you in that taxi."

With the eager help of Mustapha, Billy Bunter mounted the donkey. Sir Reginald Brooke glanced round to see that all the party was there.

"Where is Bunter?" he exclaimed.

"Oh gad! There he is, nunky," said Lord Mauleverer, "on that donkey!"

Sir Reginald's eyeglass fixed on Bunter in astonishment. He frowned.

"Bunter!" he rapped out. "Get off that donkey, you absurd boy! Get into the cab! Bunter——"

"Here, hold him!" roared Bunter, in alarm.

Bunter had settled down quite comfortably into the red saddle while Mustapha held the donkey. But William Shakespeare, the donkey, did not seem so comfortable. Probably he had never borne a weight like Bunter's before. He was a strong and sturdy donkey, and looked quite fresh and frisky. But Bunter's weight was more than a joke, and William Shakespeare did not seem to like it.

He turned his head round inquiringly at Buuter and stared at him, and then jumped and threw up his heels.

There was a roar from Bunter as he began to play cup-and-ball in the saddle. Up went Bunter and down again, up again and down again, and he dropped the reins and clung to the donkey's neck.

"I say, you fellows!" yelled Bunter. "Help!"

"Ha, ha, ha!"

"Yarooh! Stoppim! Lemme gerroff! Help!" roared Bunter. "Catch hold of his legs! Catch hold of his tail! Yaroooop!"

Mustapha crashed his stick on the donkey to reduce him to order. But William Shakespeare seemed only to get more excited. He flung out his heels wildly, and Mustapha dodged away. Another crash of the stick started William Shakespeare off at a gallop.

"I say, you fellows!" howled Bunter, clinging frantically to the donkey's neck. "I say! Help! Yaroooop!"

"Ha, ha, ha!"

Howls of laughter followed Billy Bunter, as he disappeared on the donkey into the crowds of Cairo. Sir Reginald snorted—and the juniors chortled. Bunter vanished, clinging to the neck of his mettlesome charger, and they started for the hotel, hoping that the Owl of the Remove would arrive there in one piece.

It seemed like some fearful nightmare to Billy Bunter. There are many strange sights in the streets of Cairo—but the streets of Cairo had never seen a stranger sight than that of William Shakespeare, the donkey, careering along with the fat Owl clinging frantically to his hairy neck.

That desperate clutch on his neck seemed to add the last straw to William Shakespeare's excitement. He dashed among motor-cars, taxi-cabs, camels, water-carriers, sherbet-sellers, donkeys and donkey-boys, with Bunter clinging to his neck like a limpet to a rock. Mustapha was lost in the crowd. But behind the runaway donkey gleamed a red tarboosh, and a gold tassel danced—Hassan, the dragoman was in pursuit. But Hassan could not overtake the donkey. William Shakespeare was on his mettle, and he gave an exhibition of speed seldom equalled by a Cairo donkey.

"Ow! Wow! Ow! Help! Rescue! Yoooop!" gurgled Bunter. "I say, you fellows—— Oh crikey! Stoppim! Shoot him! I say, help! Yaroooh!"

William Shakespeare careered onward.

The streets of Cairo passed Bunter like a kaleidoscope. He whisked past motor-cars and trams, camels and bicycles! The faster the donkey careered the more tightly Bunter clung to his neck, and the more tightly he clung to the donkey's neck, the faster William Shakespeare careered.

There was a gleam of water in front of Bunter. It was the Nile! And William Shakespeare, at long last, halted. Had not the Nile been there the donkey might really have carried Bunter onward, past the Sphinx and the Pyramids, into the Libyan Desert. Fortunately the Nile was there! William Shakespeare stopped—suddenly, lowering his head.

Bunter shot off over his head like a bullet.

Splash!

"Ooooooooch!"

William Shakespeare trotted away, no doubt relieved to be rid of his extraordinary burden. Billy Bunter sat in mud and shallow water and roared.

A brown hand dragged him out.

"My fine gentleman, you trust Hassan. Hassan is your dragoman!"

"Grooogh! Ooooch! Wooogh!"

. . . . . .

"Where's Bunter?"

"Lost!"

"No such luck!"

"Hallo, hallo, hallo! Look!"

Harry Wharton & Co. had lunched and come out on the balcony of Shepheard's Hotel, in Cairo. Bunter had not turned up yet. But as they looked down from the balcony at the motley crowd below, they sighted him—turning up at last. He was muddy, he was dusty, he looked tired, and he looked cross. It was evident that his donkey-ride had not agreed with him. Hassan, with a grinning brown face, was bringing him in, and he helped Bunter up the steps to the balcony, where innumerable eyes were fixed on him, and innumerable faces were wreathed in smiles.

"Hallo, hallo, hallo! Enjoyed your ride?" roared Bob Cherry

"Beast!"

"Had a good time?" chuckled Lord Mauleverer.

"Yah!"

Bunter rolled into the hotel. Hassan salaamed to the Greyfriars fellows. He salaamed to Sir Reginald.

"Hassan is your dragoman, my gentlemen lords!" he said. "When you want Hassan, he always here!"

Sir Reginald opened his lips to say "Go away!" but he closed them again. Hassan had established his claim. So long as Harry Wharton & Co. remained in Egypt, Hassan was going to be their dragoman. And that was that!

THE END.

(*The next yarn in this grand holiday series is better than ever chums. Make a note of the title: "THE LURE OF THE GOLDEN SCARAB!" It's full of fun and amazing adventures.*)

THRILLING HOLIDAY ADVENTURES OF HARRY WHARTON & CO. IN EGYPT!

The MAGNET 2^D

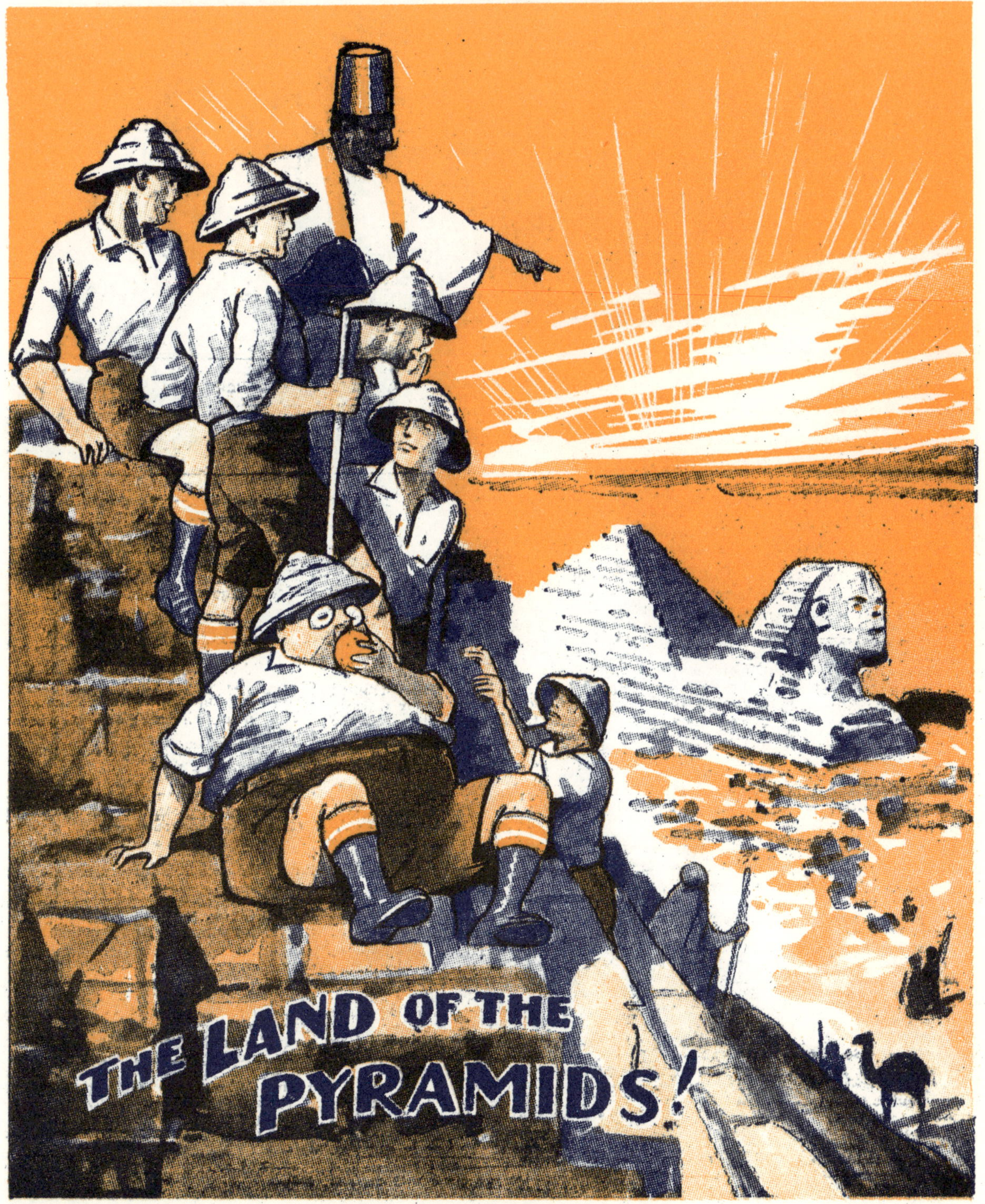

No. 1.280. Vol. XLII. EVERY SATURDAY. Week Ending August 27th, 1932.

JUST STARTING—A STIRRING STORY OF THE "GOOD OLD DAYS."

The Red Falcon!

Introducing HAL LOVETT and JERRY McLEAN, two Knights of the Road.

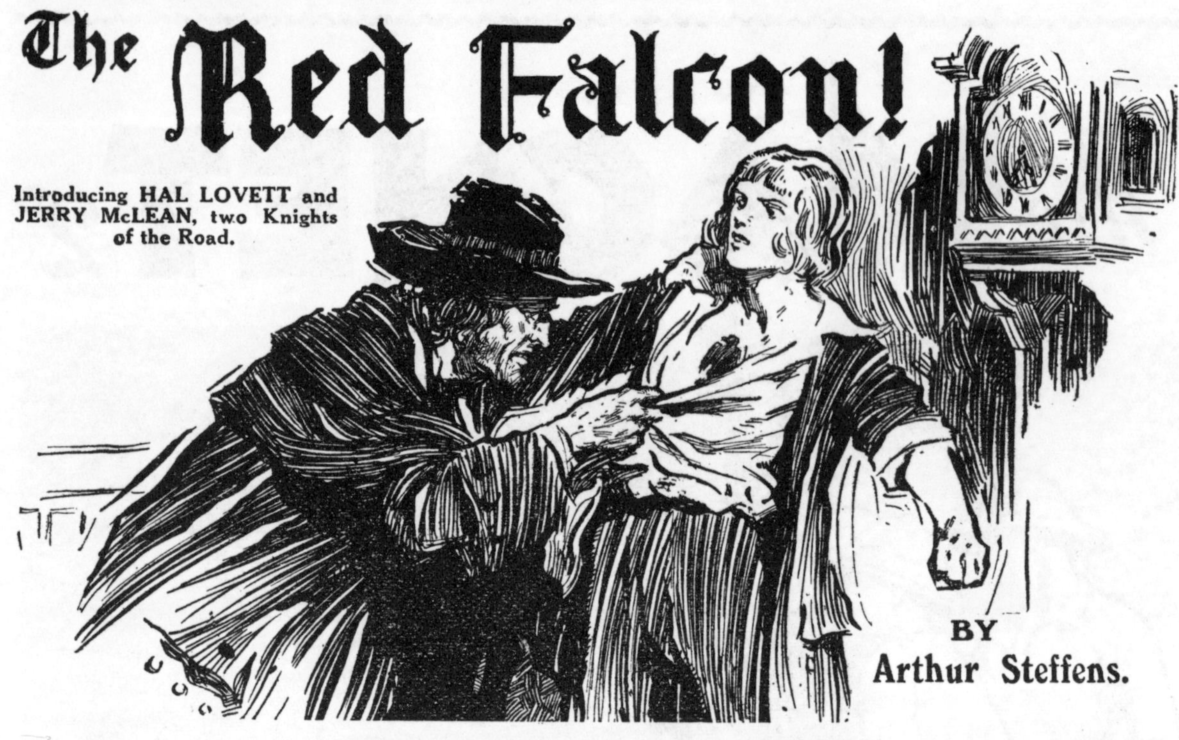

BY Arthur Steffens.

HAVING OVERHEARD HIS RASCALLY FATHER AND MR. WHO, A MYSTERIOUS STRANGER, PLOTTING AGAINST HIM, HAL LOVETT RUNS AWAY FROM HOME. HE IS BEFRIENDED BY JERRY McLEAN, A ONE-TIME DANDY, TO WHOM HE UNFOLDS HIS STRANGE STORY. HAL AND JERRY ARE OUTSIDE THE DRURY LANE THEATRE THAT SAME NIGHT JUST AS THE PLAYGOERS ARE LEAVING, WHEN THEY ARE BOTH ARRESTED FOR CONSPIRING TO ROB THE EARL OF HUNTFORD—WHO IS NONE OTHER THAN MR. WHO—OF A DIAMOND STAR!

Up for Trial!

IT seemed to Hal Lovett that years had passed since the night of his arrest outside Drury Lane Theatre. It seemed ages since he had appeared before the Bow Street magistrate with McLean and they had been committed for trial at the quarter sessions.

Their confinement in Newgate Prison had steeped McLean in gloom, and nearly broken the boy's proud spirit. Hal loathed contact with the coarse and ribald prisoners. He hated the never-ending quarrelling and fighting, the hard drinking, and the thousand and one degrading brutalities that marked the gathering together of the prisoners in the common-rooms of the gaol.

If Jerry had not appealed to some rich friends, who bribed the governor to give them special privileges, Hal felt that he might have died.

But they were permitted to share a room to themselves in the governor's quarters, and they avoided contact with the rest of the wretched prisoners as much as possible.

Hal often discussed with McLean the events which had led up to their misfortune, and it never occurred to McLean to question the boy's story, though he was doubtful as to whether they would be able to prove their innocence.

"You'll never get judge or jury to believe that the Earl of Huntford came to Samuel Lovett's rag-shop in Wych Street and gave him a bag of gold to play that trick of the diamond star on you, boy," said Jerry, as they sat in their cell the night before the Old Bailey trial.

"But it's true!" said Hal passionately. "You remember I told you about it that night in the coffee-shop in Covent Garden."

"Of course you did," rejoined Jerry McLean, shifting the position of his double irons so as to ease his cramped limbs, "and then, though we knew the trap was set, we foolishly went to the theatre and walked right into it."

"The Earl of Huntford was the beggar who called himself Mr. Who!" said Hal excitedly. "I recognised him at the theatre in spite of his fine clothes."

Jerry McLean nodded his tousled head.

"Ay," he said grimly, "they framed you, boy. Gad! I saw your rascally father snatch the diamond star from the earl's breast and plant it on you before the Runners seized you. That's why I tried to rescue you. But they refused to listen to our story at the police court, lad, and I don't suppose they'll give us a hearing at the Old Bailey to-morrow. We can only hope for the best and prepare ourselves for the worst."

"But why did my father do it?" asked Hal. "And why did the Earl of Huntford come to his rag-shop disguised as a beggar and pay him one hundred golden guineas to lay such a trap for me?"

McLean pulled Hal's shirt wide open so that his flesh was bared, and there, vividly tattooed in red on the white flesh, was a falcon jessed and belled and hooded—as real as life. Jerry's handsome face set as he studied the tattoo mark.

"Who knows but what this red falcon had a great deal to do with it?" he growled. "How came you by the mark, boy?"

"I don't quite know. I believe my father pricked it into the skin when I was very young, Jerry."

McLean stared at the boy in surprise. "You remember that, eh? Boy, that's devilish odd. Do you know why Samuel Lovett did it?"

"He said so that he should know me again should I ever get lost," answered Hal.

"It's a dashed queer thing for a father to do," mused Jerry McLean. "But worrying about it won't help us now. I can't see the earl's connection with it. But we know that your father is a thief and a fence, boy. There's something odd here, and if ever I get free I'm going to probe it."

"What sentence shall we get if they convict us to-morrow?" asked Hal Lovett, looking wistfully at McLean.

The man shrugged his broad shoulders.

"Transportation! If we escape the other thing, I guess!"

Hal shuddered, for he knew the alternative was—hanging. Drawing the shirt over his naked flesh, he leaned back against the stone wall with a shiver of dread, and looked around him in horror. Though money had been paid for it, the cell was damp and dark and horrid.

From the common-room, where men were drinking hard, rang echoing oaths and voices raised in ribald laughter.

A drunken man was screaming out a song. Hal could hear women shrieking in high-pitched voices. There came an echo of blows, the sound of ringing curses, and the gruff voice of a turnkey raised in threatening anger.

A cell door banged, a lock clicked, and rusty bolts were shot home. Somewhere close by, a man was moaning as if in agony, and on every hand rang the clank of chains.

The air was foul, stifling.

Hal closed his eyes and felt sick and faint.

It was then that Jerry McLean's gentle hand sought his and pressed it.

(*Continued on page 26.*)

AN AMAZING STORY OF PERIL AND ADVENTURE IN EGYPT—

THE LURE OF THE GOLDEN SCARAB!

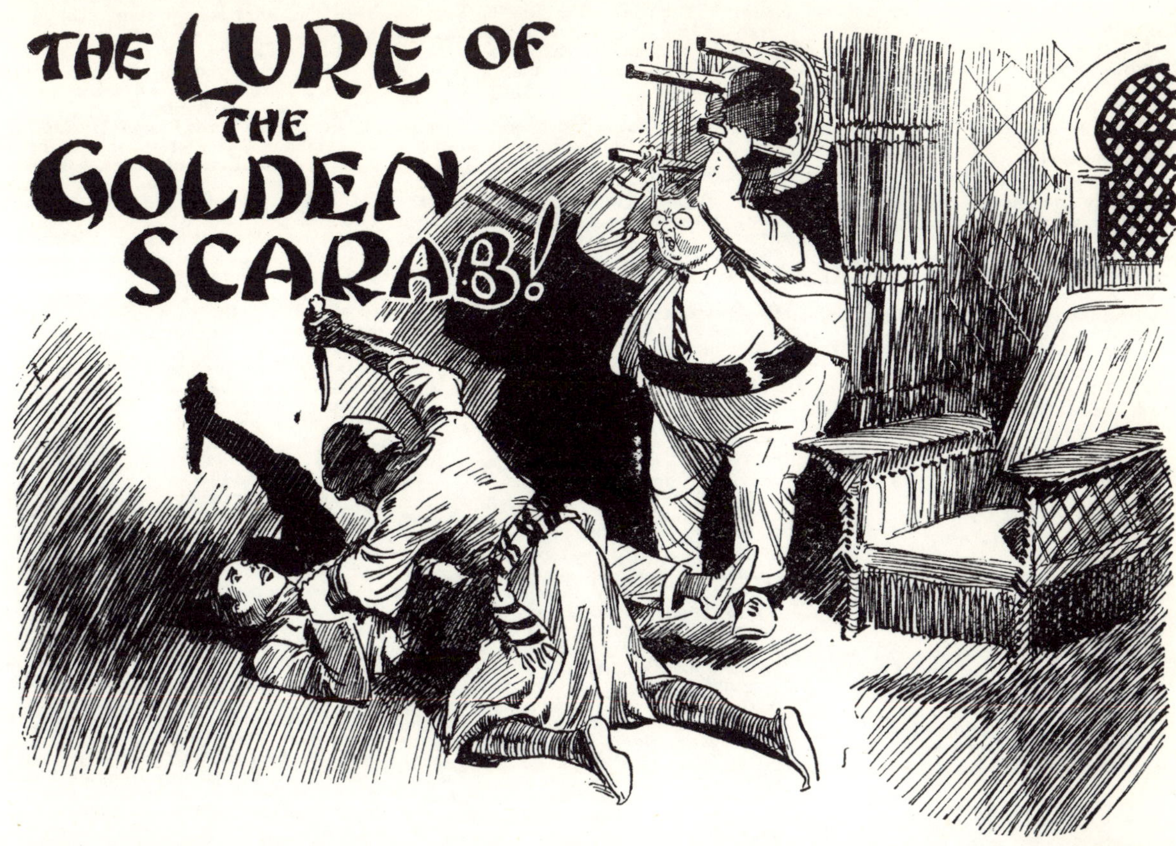

Featuring Harry Wharton & Co., the chums of Greyfriars. **By FRANK RICHARDS.**

THE FIRST CHAPTER.

Beastly for Bunter!

"BEAST!" murmured Billy Bunter.

Bunter was annoyed.

Billy Bunter was standing before an open wardrobe in Lord Mauleverer's room in the Cairo hotel.

He was just about to make a selection from the numerous—or rather, innumerable—garments belonging to the schoolboy earl of Greyfriars.

Naturally at such a moment Billy Bunter did not want to be interrupted. So the sound of a footstep at the door was quite annoying.

Mauly was the best-tempered fellow in the Greyfriars Remove. He was a long-suffering youth. Otherwise, certainly Billy Bunter would not have been a member of the Greyfriars party that had gone out to Egypt for the holidays. Still, even Mauly's good temper and patience had a limit. It was quite possible that if he found Bunter rooting over his things, he might kick him—quite likely that he might kick him hard.

Bunter did not want to be kicked. Kicking had often come his way, though not so often as he deserved. Still, he did not like it. Custom had not made it grateful or comforting.

So Billy Bunter turned from the wardrobe, and fixed his eyes and his big spectacles on the door with an apprehensive and annoyed blink.

He had really chosen his moment well. Harry Wharton & Co. were on the hotel balcony, discussing the excursion for the day, which was to be to the Pyramids and the Sphinx, with Hassan, the guide. Lord Mauleverer had been taking part in the discussion to the extent of nodding his head at every suggestion. Bunter had taken it for granted that Mauly would not stir till the latest possible moment, and even then probably not till Bob Cherry tilted him out of his chair. The fat Owl of the Remove had supposed that he had ample time for making his selection among the belongings of the schoolboy earl. And he had barely started when that footstep was heard at the door of Mauly's room, which meant—he concluded—that Mauly was coming in. And only the day before, when Bunter had annexed Mauly's best

If all that be said about it be true, the quaint golden scarab in Lord Mauleverer's possession is the key to a fabulous treasure!

trousers, Mauly had solemnly promised him a kicking next time. This was next time—and the kicking was due.

"Beast!" breathed Bunter.

The doorhandle turned.

Billy Bunter backed behind a handsome screen of Cairo mushrabeyeh work that stood by the window.

He was out of sight when the door opened.

Behind the mushrabeyeh screen he grinned.

Whatever Mauly had come up for, he was not likely to look round behind the screen; and Billy Bunter sagely decided to wait till he was gone. Then that selection from his extensive wardrobe could be made without danger.

The door closed.

There was a soft footstep crossing the room.

Billy Bunter started.

He blinked through the openings of the mushrabeyeh, which was a kind of lattice, and his little round eyes widened behind his big round spectacles.

It was not Lord Mauleverer who had entered Mauly's room. His lordship was still taking his ease in the cane chair on the balcony, as Bunter had supposed. It was a native who had entered—a thick-set man with a dark Arab face, in a turban, with a white cotton galabyeh girdled at the waist. He stopped in the middle of the spacious room, looking round him with keen black hawkish eyes.

Bunter blinked through the mushrabeyeh, startled. The man looked like one of the native hotel servants to Bunter's eyes, at least. But what did he want in Lord Mauleverer's room? He had not come there to perform any duty, that was plain. He stood silent, with a strange stealthiness in his look and manner, scanning the room with searching eyes. And it dawned on the fat junior that he was not an hotel servant, but an hotel thief!

Bunter suppressed his breathing.

Evidently the dark-faced Arab supposed the room to be empty, but for himself. Like Bunter, he had selected his moment carefully, when the Greyfriars party were busy in their discussion with Hassan, the dragoman, on the balcony. Billy Bunter did not like that hard, dark face, with its cruel lines and hawkish eyes. He had no doubt that the man had a knife about him somewhere. He only hoped that the Arab, if he was looking for loot, would not look behind the mushrabeyeh screen for it.

Only for a few moments the hawk-faced Arab stood there; then he moved swiftly towards the wardrobe Bunter had so recently left. Standing there, he examined the garments within, running his dark thievish fingers through all the pockets.

He was likely enough to find plunder; for Mauly was careless with his money. There might be Egyptian piastres or pounds, or English banknotes, in the pockets. Bunter, blinking through the latticed screen, saw him draw something from a pocket—it was a handful of piastres—and then, to Bunter's great surprise, put the money back again. It was not loot in the form of money that he was seeking.

He turned from the wardrobe and gave his attention to a suitcase. The suitcase was locked, and Bunter heard a faint click. Then it came open. Evidently the hawk-faced Arab was an expert thief. He had picked the lock of the suitcase.

Kneeling by it, he proceeded to search through the contents, lifting out silver-backed brushes and other things, but—as Bunter noted with increasing surprise—replacing everything that he moved as he had found it.

"Mafish!"

Bunter heard him mutter the Arabic word.

He locked the suitcase again and stood with a wrinkle of thought in his dark brow. Then he turned to the bed, on which a jacket had been carelessly thrown, and ran his fingers through the pockets.

Bunter, silent, watched.

But he guessed now what the man was after. It was not money or jewellery.

"The scarab!" flashed through Billy Bunter's fat mind.

He hardly dared to breathe.

It was the scarab—the sacred scarabæus of A-Menah—that the man was seeking—the scarab that had belonged to Mauly's father, and that the schoolboy earl had brought with him to Egypt. The strange scarab of gold that had a secret—known only to Kalizelos, the Greek dealer of Cairo! The Golden Beetle, which, according to legend, was an infallible guide to the great diamond known as the Eye of Osiris—told of in many an ancient Egyptian papyrus, but never seen since the reign of Rameses the Second, three thousand years ago!

Peril by sea and land had haunted the Greyfriars party through the desperate attempts of Kalizelos to obtain possession of the mysterious scarab. And Bunter realised now that this was one more attempt to seize on the scarab of A-Menah—that the hawk-faced Arab was one more emissary of the Greek of Cairo.

His fat heart thumped.

But there was no need for Bunter to intervene, even had he ventured to think of it. For he knew that the Golden Scarab was in Lord Mauleverer's pocket, and that the searcher could only draw blank.

The hawk-faced Arab seemed to realise it. He ceased his search at last and crossed to the window and looked down.

Billy Bunter cast a longing blink towards the door. But he dared not move—he dared make no sound. The Arab was only a couple of yards from him as he looked down from the window. It overlooked the long, wide balcony, and Bunter knew that the man was watching the Greyfriars party below. They were all there—the Famous Five of the Remove, with Mauly, and Mauly's uncle, Sir Reginald Brooke, and the dragoman. A voice floated up from below. Bunter recognised the voice of Bob Cherry.

"Time we got a move on! Where's that fat frump Bunter?"

The hawk-faced Arab turned from the window and crossed to the door again. Billy Bunter, watching through the interstices of the mushrabeyeh, hoped from the bottom of his fat heart that the man was going. The Greyfriars juniors would be coming up to their rooms to get ready for the excursion; the thief could not remain without discovery.

But he did not go.

He stood back against the wall, behind the door, so that in opening it would conceal him.

Billy Bunter saw a dark hand slip under the loose cotton galabyeh, and his eyes bulged behind his spectacles as he caught a glimmer of steel.

But the Arab's hand came empty from the galabyeh again. He had only been making sure that the dagger was there, in readiness, if he wanted it.

Then he waited; silent, like a cat about to spring; his black eyes glittering as there were footsteps and voices in the corridor without. He was waiting for the schoolboy earl to enter—unsuspecting. Billy Bunter's eyes, almost bulging through his spectacles with terror, were fixed on him through the lattice of the mushrabeyeh, the fat Owl's heart thumping so hard that he feared that the Arab would hear it. Five minutes—ten minutes—that seemed like hours to the terrified Owl—and then the door-handle was turned from without.

THE SECOND CHAPTER.
Caught Napping!

"JOLLY!" said Bob Cherry.

Probably there were few sights in the wide world that Robert Cherry of the Greyfriars Remove would not have described as "jolly!"—his nature being merry and bright. But really it was rather jolly, looking from the hotel balcony at the varied, ever-shifting crowd—with Cairo all round, and tall graceful minarets piercing the deep, intensely blue sky, and the Nile and the desert in the distance.

Cairo was noisy, and Cairo was hot; but the Greyfriars fellows were having—and going to have—the time of their lives. Egypt was new and strange to their eyes—strange and delightful—and even the pertinacious sellers of unwanted and worthless antiquities, the persistent guides who were not to be denied, and the endless Bedouin beggars, did not worry them—they were all part of the novel Eastern scene. They were told that there was hardly anybody in Cairo; the crowd did not come till the winter. But it seemed to them that there were plenty of people about—in fact, the narrow streets swarmed, and almost every known language was incessantly heard—and the cries of water-sellers, sherbet-sellers, sweetmeat-sellers, were continual.

"The jollifulness," said Hurree Jamset Ram Singh, "is terrific!" Hurree Singh's dusky face wore a perpetual smile, in the bright sunshine, which was like that of his native land.

"Glad you came, Mauly?" asked Harry Wharton.

"Eh? Yaas," yawned Lord Mauleverer.

"Keen to climb the pyramids?" grinned Nugent.

Lord Mauleverer, stretched in the long cane chair, did not look as if he was keen on exertion in any shape or form."

"Oh! Yaas!"

"We'll hoist you up, old bean," said Johnny Bull. "But we shall want a steam crane for Bunter."

"Gentlemen lords," said Hassan, the dragoman. "The start should be of early punctuality, otherwise there is enormous heat of a sun. Large car of luxurious appointment is waiting with readiness."

"Ready, Mauly?" asked Wharton.

"Yaas. But——" His lordship yawned portentously. "I'll tell you what, you men. I've got rather an idea! It's jolly here, sitting in this jolly chair, you know, and watchin' things! You can see quite a lot of Cairo from this jolly old balcony. Look here, what about you fellows bumpin' along to the Pyramids and the Sphinx and things, and tellin' me all about it when you come back? What?"

"Ha, ha, ha!"

"Good idea, what?" asked his lazy lordship.

"Feeling that you'd like a rest?" asked Bob Cherry.

"Yaas."

"You think it a ripping idea, to travel out to Egypt and see the sights from a chair on a balcony?"

"Yaas."

The juniors chuckled; but Hassan, the dragoman, looked quite shocked. Hassan, the son of Suleiman, had appointed himself dragoman, or guide, to the Greyfriars party with so much determination that he had got away with it. Hassan, no doubt, was thinking chiefly of "backsheesh"; but he was deeply in earnest in displaying the wonderful sights of Egypt to his clients. He was accustomed to eager tourists who wanted to see everything, and a little over; and Mauleverer was a new experience to him. He spread out both brown hands in gesticulating remonstrance.

"Oh! My lordly gentleman!" exclaimed Hassan. "You must see Pyramids of Ghizeh—you must see a sphinx! All the world comes to Egypt to climb pyramids and see a sphinx! Hassan will show you all things—Hassan knows everything! You shall be struck with admiring wonderfulness when you see glorious pyramids."

"I'll take your word for it, old bean," answered Mauleverer. "You men get off—tell the waiter to bring me a cool drink, and I'll have a jolly time waitin' for you, see?"

"Poor old Mauly feels as if he can't get out of that chair," said Bob Cherry sympathetically. "This is where he finds it useful to have a pal with him who's full of beans. I'll help you up, old chap."

Bob helped Mauly up—by the simple process of tilting the back of the chair and shooting his lordship out on the balcony in a heap.

Lord Mauleverer sprawled and roared.

"Whooooop!"

"Ha, ha, ha!"

"Now, if Mauly can't walk up to his room, we'll help him," said Bob. "I'll take one ear and you take the other, Franky."

Lord Mauleverer jumped up.

"Keep off, you silly ass! I'll go and get ready! I—I'm rather keen to see the jolly old pyramids, really."

"Come on, then," said Harry Wharton, laughing.

And the juniors went into the hotel to get ready for the trip. Sir Reginald Brooke had left the hotel, to make a call upon Mr. Hilmi Maroudi, the Egyptian gentleman whose acquaintance the Greyfriars party had made on the steamer to Alexandria. The schoolboys were left in the care of the drago man for the trip to the Pyramids.

In earlier days, visitors to the Pyramids had to go on donkey-back or camel-back, or on Shanks' pony; but in more modern days, it was an easy trip. There was an electric tramway to Mena House, which stood close by the Pyramids; and there was a good road for arabeyehs and cars. Harry Wharton & Co. would have been satisfied, like most tourists, with the tramway; but Lord Mauleverer was running the show, and Mauly was a millionaire; and did things always in style.

Hassan, the dragoman, rejoiced greatly in the possession of this munificent client. Backsheesh fairly rained on Hassan. If a car was wanted, Hassan engaged it—camels or donkeys or Faringhees were sent into the world specially to be robbed by faithful followers of the Prophet. If Hassan had passed a whole day without cheating a foreigner, he would have mourned over a day wasted.

Harry Wharton & Co. were quite well aware that Hassan was a rogue; but they did not expect a Cairo guide to be anything else; and he was good-natured, good-tempered, obliging, attentive, and eternally smiling. Since he had found out that Lord Mauleverer was very rich, and that the juniors were friends of Mr. Maroudi, the wealthy Egyptian, Hassan had worn a smile that would not come off. Like all dragomans, he lived and moved and had his being in "backsheesh"; and backsheesh being plentiful, Hassan was as happy as a sandboy.

that one surprised stare. The hawk-eyed man was on him with the spring of a tiger.

Mauleverer went heavily to the floor on his back, the Arab over him. A brown hand gripped his throat and choked him into silence.

He stared up blankly at the dark, menacing face glaring down at him.

In the corridor he could hear the voices of his friends as they went to their rooms. But the closed door was between; they could not see him, and he could make no sound to draw their attention.

The dark face bent closer.

"Silence! Give me the scarab!" breathed the Arab. "Quick, unbeliever! Give me the scarab—the scarab of A-Menah—the golden beetle!"

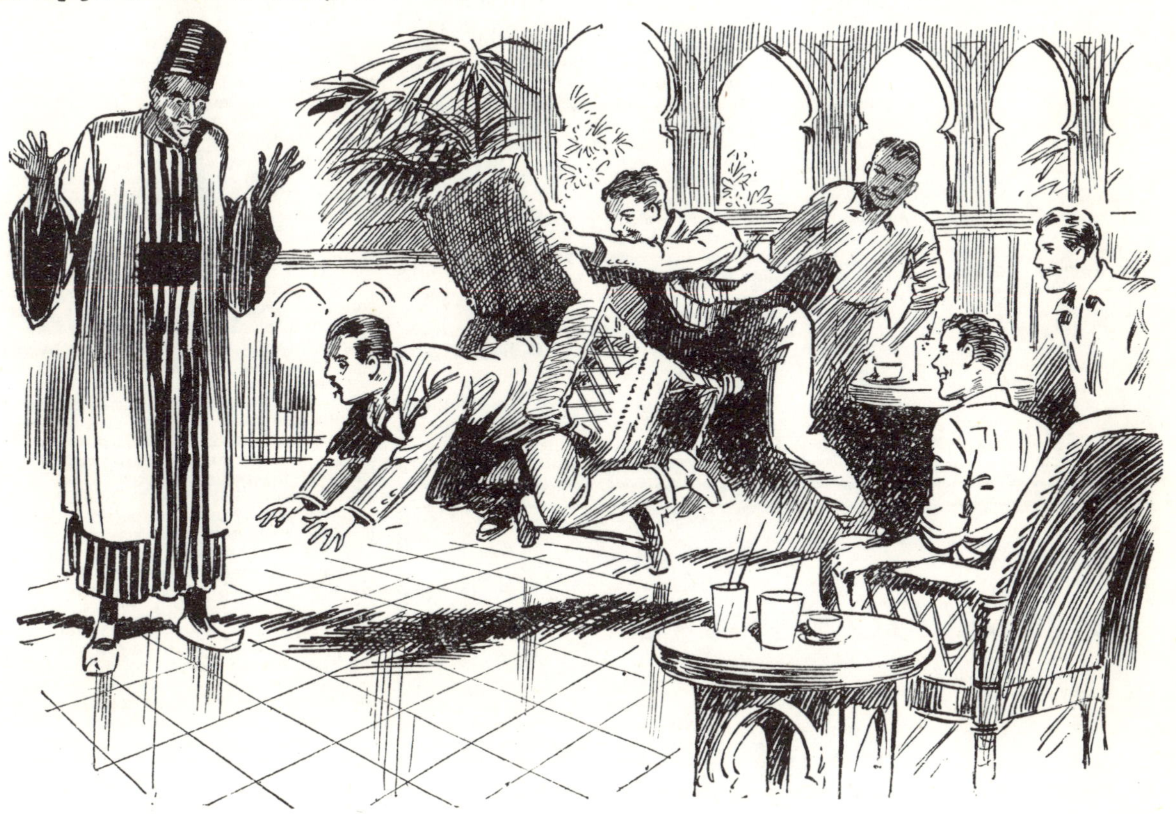

"Come on, Mauly," said Bob Cherry, cheerily, "Hassan wants us to see the Pyramids. I'll help you to get out of that chair." Tilting the back of the chair, Bob shot his lordship out on the balcony in a heap. "Whooop!" Lord Mauleverer sprawled and roared.

anything else; and everything that Hassan touched meant a profit for Hassan—like Cassius of old, he had an itching palm. No tourist ever stepped in Egypt without being "done" by his dragoman; but Lord Mauleverer was proving a gold-mine to the son of Suleiman. Every day Hassan returned thanks to the Prophet for having delivered this wealthy Faringhee into his hands.

And Hassan was a very useful man. He was a prominent guide; he had good recommendations; he knew Egypt from the Delta to the Cataracts of the Nile; and while he cheated his clients to the uttermost possible extent, he thoughtfully intervened to prevent others from cheating them—except in cases when the others handed over "backsheesh" to Hassan. When he shared the loot, of course, Hassan let them go ahead. Hassan may have had a conscience, among his own people, but it was an article of his faith that

Leaving the faithful Hassan waiting at the steps of the balcony, the juniors went up to their rooms.

"Give you ten minutes, Mauly!" said Bob Cherry, as Mauleverer stopped at the door of his room. "If you go to sleep instead of getting ready, rely on me to come and wake you up."

Lord Mauleverer grinned.

"Yaas, old bean," he said. "I'll be ready!" As a matter of taste, his lazy lordship would rather have looked at Egypt from a chair on the balcony; but he had made up his noble mind to the trip to the Pyramids. He did not want any more help from the energetic Bob.

He turned the handle of his door and went in, closing the door after him. Then he jumped.

The closing of the door revealed the figure that was standing behind it. For a second Lord Mauleverer stared blankly at the hawk-faced Arab.

But he had no time for more than

Lord Mauleverer could not speak. In the muscular grip of the thick-set, brawny Arab he could not struggle. He was helpless, at the mercy of the hawk-faced wretch. But though he read the threat of death in the gleaming eyes above him, his courage did not falter. He knew that he was in the hands of an emissary of Kalizelos, the Greek—the man who was now hunted by the Egyptian police, and who had disappeared from his shop in Cairo. Hunted as he was, with prison awaiting him if he was caught, Kalizelos had evidently not given up his quest of the Golden Scarab.

A look of contempt flashed over Mauleverer's face. Not to save his life—not to save a hundred lives—would he have yielded to the threat of the hawk-eyed ruffian.

He made a fierce effort to tear himself loose, but the grasp on him was

like that of a steel vice. He was powerless.
"The scarab!" hissed the man in the turban. "The scarab!"
With his left hand gripping Mauleverer's throat, his knee planted on the schoolboy's chest, the Arab groped under his galabyeh. From the folds of the cotton garment a bright blade flashed out.
"The scarab—or I will take it from your dead body, dog of an unbeliever!" hissed the Arab.
And the dagger flashed before Mauleverer's eyes.

——

THE THIRD CHAPTER.

Bravo, Bunter!

BILLY BUNTER shuddered.
Through the interstices of the mushrabeyeh screen that concealed him the Owl of the Remove blinked in horror at the scene.
Terror seemed to chain him.
To reveal his presence while that hawk-faced, desperate-eyed wretch was in the room seemed impossible to Bunter.
But as the Arab flashed the dagger from his galabyeh and flung up his brown hand, with the flashing weapon in it, Billy Bunter moved.
That was too much even for Bunter. In Mauly's place Bunter certainly would have handed over the scarab, or anything else, with the dagger flashing before his eyes. But Mauleverer's face had set hard, and it was clear that he was not going to yield. Shuddering with terror, the Owl of the Remove pulled himself together somehow. The Arab's back was to him as he crouched over the prostrate Mauleverer, and Billy Bunter stepped out from behind the screen—with terrified stealthiness.
An Oriental stool, with short, carved legs, was near at hand. The fat junior caught it up, and, taking his courage in both hands, as it were, jumped at the Arab.
The wretch heard some sound behind him, and turned his head—and as his head turned the heavy stool crashed on it.
It landed with a heavy thud.
The Arab gave a gasping howl and pitched over, the dagger flying from his hand.
"Oooooh!" gasped Bunter.
"Oh gad!" gurgled Mauleverer. The instant he was released the schoolboy earl bounded to his feet; though he was as much astonished as the Arab by Bunter's unlooked-for intervention.
The hawk-faced ruffian had sprawled helplessly over, his head spinning from the crash. But he was on his feet with the swiftness of a tiger.
His eyes flashed round for the dagger, and Bunter, in sheer terror, dropped the stool and jumped away. Lord Mauleverer jumped, too. But it was towards the Arab. And as he jumped he shouted:
"Help! Help!"
His shout rang far beyond the room. And the desperado, realising instantly that the game was up, bounded for the door. Already there were footsteps in the corridor.
The brown hand tore the door open, and the man rushed out before Lord Mauleverer could reach him.
"Oh gad!" gasped Mauly.
"Ow! Help! I say, you fellows, help!" yelled Billy Bunter. "Oh crumbs! Oh crikey! Help! Yarooooh!"
"Hallo, hallo, hallo!" Bob Cherry stared in at the open door. "What the jolly old thump——"
"Is he gone?" gasped Mauleverer.
"He—who? I saw an Arab running for the stairs. He's gone——"
"Ow! Help! Help!" yelled Bunter.
"Shut up, old bean!" said Lord Mauleverer placidly. "It's all right now; he's gone. Safe as houses, old fat man!"
"Oh dear! Oh crikey!" gasped Bunter. "I wish I hadn't come to Egypt! Oh lor'!"
"But what——" gasped Bob.
Lord Mauleverer picked up the dagger. Bob stared at it blankly. By that time the rest of the Co. were on the scene, as well as several hotel attendants.
"What's happened?" exclaimed Harry Wharton, staring at the dagger in the hand of the schoolboy earl.
"A jolly old darky after the scarab," drawled Lord Mauleverer. "Hidin' in my room, waitin' for me—and he snaffled me as I hopped in! If Bunter hadn't been here—— By the way, what on earth were you doin' in my room, Bunter?"
"Oh dear! Oh crikey!"
There was a babble of excitement from the hotel attendants. They gathered that a thief had attacked Mauleverer in his room with the intention of robbing him, and hurried away to search for the man and report to the manager. There was little likelihood, however, of the hawk-faced Arab being found. He had had some time to get clear, and there was no doubt that he had already vanished into the teeming crowds of Cairo.
"No need to make a fuss, you men!" yawned Lord Mauleverer. "I'm gettin' rather used to Kalizelos' stunts by this time. Let them think it was just a common or garden hotel thief. They'll never get him, anyhow. He's done the jolly old vanishin' trick before this!"
"The scoundrel!" said Harry. "Mauly, old man, we were thinking that the danger was over, now that Kalizelos is being searched for by the police and has run from Cairo. But—— After this, old man, you're not going to be left alone. And you're not carrying that scarab about any more, either. We'll ask the hotel manager to lock it up in his safe before we start for the Pyramids!"
"One of us will share your room after this, and keep an eye on you," said Bob Cherry.
"Leave that to me, you fellows!" Billy Bunter had recovered now. The danger being over, Bunter's courage had returned with a jump. "I'll look after my pal Mauly. I'll sleep in this room to-night, Mauly."
"You jolly well won't!" said his lordship emphatically. "I get enough of your jolly old snore in the Remove dorm at Greyfriars. Can't stand it on vac. Much obliged. But I really couldn't!"
"Oh, really, Mauly——"
"But what were you doin' here, anyhow?" asked Lord Mauleverer. "I'm jolly glad you were on the spot, old fat bean, but——"
"That's me all over," explained Bunter. "The right man in the right place, you know! I never came to this room to borrow your clobber, Mauly, and I never hid behind the screen because that beastly Arab butted in!"
"Oh gad!"
"The fact is that I was keeping guard over you," explained Bunter. "As I've told you often enough, I only came out to Egypt with you to protect you from danger. I never had the least idea of bagging a holiday on the cheap."
"Ha, ha, ha!"

"Blessed if I see anything to cackle at! I'd like to know where you would be if I hadn't been here!" exclaimed Bunter warmly. "I've shaved Mauly's wife—I mean, saved his life! You fellows would have been scared stiff. Not me! Pluck's my long suit, as you know!"

"Oh, my hat!"

"And after this, Mauly," added Bunter severely, "I hope you won't make a fuss if a fellow borrows a pair of trousers and a waistcoat or so, and a few socks and neckties and things. There's such a thing as gratitude. Not that I came here after your clobber, you know. I wasn't just going to sort over your things when that beast sneaked in —and I never got out of sight because I was afraid of him. And if you fellows can't do anything but cackle——"

"Ha, ha, ha!"

"Well, Bunter did butt in, and I fancy that jolly old Arab has carried away a bump on his jolly old coconut!" chuckled Lord Mauleverer. "And you can jolly well borrow anythin' you like, Bunter! Leave me a shirt or two, won't you, old man, and a change of socks?"

"Ha, ha, ha!"

"Well, I'll borrow a few things, old chap, as you're so pressing," said Billy Bunter amiably. "I'll do the same for you when you come to stay with me at Bunter Court, you know."

"Oh gad!"

"I mean it, Mauly. When you stay at Bunter Court I shall place the whole of my extensive wardrobe at your service—all my suits of clothes——"

"Both of them?" asked Bob Cherry.

"Ha, ha, ha!"

"Beast!"

When the Greyfriars party joined Hassan, for the excusion to the Pyramids, anyone looking at Billy Bunter might have supposed that he was dressed in his best. But that would have been a slight error. He was dressed in Lord Mauleverer's best.

THE FOURTH CHAPTER.

The Pyramids!

CAIRO hummed and buzzed round the cheerful Greyfriars party as they drove away in the big car.

Lord Mauleverer sat contented and placid, apparently having forgotten the episode in his room, and the grasp of the hawk-faced Arab; at all events, having dismissed it from his noble mind. The other fellows could not dismiss it quite so easily, and they had resolved not to let his lordship out of their sight during the day.

Billy Bunter, it was certain, was not thinking about his lordship's peril, or the hunted Greek's desperate attempts to get hold of the scarab of A-Menah. Bunter was in possession of a huge chunk of Turkish Delight—which he slowly but steadily devoured as the car rolled on through the streets of Cairo—and Bunter's thoughts, naturally, were concentrated on his provender.

He was not likely to think of anything else till the Turkish Delight was finished; and, in the meantime, he was happy and sticky, and forgot even to grumble at the heat and the flies. And really there was plenty of heat, and lots and lots of flies. Likewise, there were a good many smells in Cairo, as in all Eastern cities, and not all of them were like unto attar-of-roses.

Hassan sat beside the Coptic chauffeur, grinning round at the Greyfriars fellows every few minutes, with a brown finger pointing out some object of interest, and his active tongue going almost continually.

Outside Cairo at last, and over the bridge on the Nile, the car ran on by a good modern road towards the Libyan Desert. It was strange enough to the juniors to know that a great and populous city like Cairo was so close to the desert—the real desert, where there was endless sand, and nothing grew save in the rare oases—the Libyan Desert, which extended right away westward, and was, in fact, the beginning of the great Sahara Desert, stretching across Africa.

The Pyramids were built on the edge of the desert, which was so clearly marked that one could almost stand with a foot in the desert, and the other foot in cultivated Egypt. For the land of Egypt, after all, was only the banks of the Nile, and, but for the Nile, would never have existed.

The hour was still early, and the juniors watched men and women at work in the fields—work which would cease as the heat of noon drew near. Men in blue cotton, women in black, labouring with the industry of the Egyptian fellaheen! They passed camels on the road, and donkeys, and shaggy black buffaloes, and innumerable beggars who held out grubby hands and squeaked "Backsheesh!" at the sight of white faces and pith helmets in the car. "Backsheesh," or "backshish," was the Arabic word with which they had grown most familiar.

Billy Bunter, having finished at last his cargo of Turkish Delight, bestowed a blink on the Pyramids rising over the desert in the distance.

"What are those pointed things sticking up there?" he asked.

"Oh, my hat! They're the jolly old Pyramids, fathead!" answered Bob Cherry. "The jolly old Pyramids of Ghizeh, which are the jolly oldest and tip-toppest of all the jolly old pyramids in jolly old Egypt."

"Oh!" Bunter gave those ancient works a rather disparaging blink. "Can't say I think much of them. What did they build them for?"

"To stick their tombs inside."

"Fatheaded idea, what?" said Bunter. "Which one is Chops?"

"If you mean Cheops——"

"I don't mean Cheops," answered Bunter calmly. "I said Chops, and I mean Chops. You fellows don't know much about it. Chops was a king or something, though they call him Coffee or something in their own silly language."

Hassan waved a brown finger.

"On edge of desert, gentlemen lords, are six groups of pyramids," he said, "wonderful works of ancient times—wonderful to excessive and exceeding extent. Oldest monumental works known to mankind, at which gazed with awe ancient persons of Greek and Roman origin, such as Herodotus and Julius Cæsar. The Great Pyramid, or Pyramid of Cheops——"

"You mean Chops?" asked Bunter.

"Honourable lord, Cheops——"

"Chops!"

"Estimable foreign gentleman, Cheops——"

"Chops!"

"Shut up, Bunter!"

"Shan't! I suppose I know more about it than a blinking native!" said Bunter. "The old codger's name was Chops, called Coffee or something——"

"Cheops, honourable admired sar!" said Hassan. "The great king Cheops is called Khufa by native Egyptian——"

"You mean Coffee!"

"Shut up, Bunter!" roared Bob.

"Yah!"

"Great King Cheops, called Khufa in native tongue, built huge Pyramid," said Hassan. "Once covered with total entireness by polished stone, since taken for building mosques in Cairo under Arab rule. Age of Great Pyramid hugely tremendous."

"Supposed to have been put up about 2,680 B.C.," remarked Nugent, who had been reading it up. "Nearly 5,000 years ago. A king of the fourth dynasty. It was about 2,000 years old when Herodotus visited it in 450 B.C., and wrote a description of it. And here it still is—much the same as when Cheops left it——"

"You mean Chops——"

"Shut up, Bunter!"

"What's that show?" asked Bunter, pointing to a large, rambling building at the tram terminus, which the car was now approaching. "Did Chops put that up, Hassan?"

Hassan blinked.

"That is Mena House Hotel, honourable sar, and is quite modern," he answered.

"Oh, good!" said Bunter, evidently more impressed by the hotel than the Pyramids. "A chap can get something to eat there."

"We'll leave Bunter to eat at Mena House, while we go up the jolly old Pyramid," said Bob.

"You jolly well won't!" said Bunter. "I shan't keep you more than an hour while I have a snack."

"I can see us sitting around for an hour while you're making another famine in Egypt!" grinned Bob.

"There are very few peoples, lordly sars," said Hassan. "In the season there are huge numbers of peoples, and Pyramids are crowded, but in hot weathers there are few peoples. Perhaps my noble lords have Pyramid of Cheops all to their admirable selves this hot day. Yes! But in lonely solitude of pyramid top with so few peoples, there is opportunity for solemn meditation. Many lordly gentlemen prefer solitude when viewing Pyramids, to meditate on past greatness and such things which are of interest to Faringhees, and for which there is no extra charge."

"Oh, my hat!" gasped Bob. "If there's no extra charge, you men, we may as well put in some solemn meditation on past greatness and such things."

"Ha, ha, ha!"

"Looks a decent sort of place," said Bunter, as the juniors alighted from the big car. "I like this, you fellows."

"Oh, you like the jolly old Pyramids, after all?"

"Eh? Who's talking about pyramids? I mean the hotel! Looks as if you can get some decent grub here."

"You podgy cormorant, we've come here to explore pyramids, not to scoff tuck. It will be too hot presently."

"You'd like a rest, wouldn't you, Mauly?" asked Bunter.

"Eh? Yaas."

"Look here——" roared Bob.

"I think you fellows ought to be considerate to Mauly, as he's our host," said Bunter. "Here you are, Mauly! Sit down, old chap! I'll see that they bring you something to eat."

"Give the fat villain ten minutes," said Harry Wharton. "I think I could do with a sherbet, now I come to think of it."

The juniors drank sherbet, while Billy Bunter packed away cakes. He was still packing away cakes when the ten minutes had elapsed, and Harry Wharton & Co. got a move on. Lord Mauleverer glanced at the sloping hillside that led up to the Pyramids, sighed, and gave his comrades an appealing glance.

"I've got rather an idea, you men," he remarked.

"Cough it up!" grinned Bob.

"You get a splendid view of the Pyramids from here. Let's sit here and look at 'em."

"I've got a better idea than that, old bean. My idea is to pour this sherbet down the back of your neck if you don't get up on your hind legs in two ticks——"

"Ow! Keep off, you silly ass!" roared Mauleverer, and he was on his feet in a twinkling.

"Come on!" said Harry Wharton, laughing. "Finished, Bunter?"

"No!"

"How long are you going to be?"

"About half an hour."

"Right-ho! We'll pick you up coming back."

"Beast!"

"This way, lords and noble gentlemen," said Hassan; and the juniors started, Hassan having taken the tickets while they were taking the sherbet.

Billy Bunter blinked after them wrathfully.

"I say, you fellows——" he yelled.

"Good-bye, Bunter!"

"I'm coming!" hooted Bunter.

"My dear man, don't trouble——"

"Yah!"

With a cake in either fat hand to eat on the way, Billy Bunter jumped up and followed the party. How any fellow gifted with all his seven senses could prefer pyramids to cakes was a mystery to William George Bunter. Still, he was not going to be left out. He was going to climb the Great Pyramid, if only to tell the fellows at Greyfriars next term that he had done it. He was not yet aware what climbing a pyramid was like. Had he been aware of it he might have stuck to Mena House and the cakes and sherbet.

"I say, you fellows," gasped Bunter, as he laboured up the sandy hill after the juniors—"I say, I'm thirsty! These cakes make a chap thirsty! Did you fellows think of bringing a flask, or anything?"

"The thinkfulness was not terrific, my esteemed Bunter."

"Selfishness all round!" said Bunter bitterly. "It never occurred to you that I might be thirsty, I suppose? Hassan—— Where's that dashed nigger?"

"Lordly gentleman——"

"Oh, here you are! Can't a fellow get something to drink in this beastly place?" demanded Bunter.

"Yes, sar! You trust Hassan. I will call a khamali——"

"You silly ass! What do you think I want a camel for?"

"Mashallah!" ejaculated Hassan. "Khamali, honourable sar, not being one camel, but carrier of water."

There was a "khamali" on the path up the hill—a dusky gentleman with a large earthen jar of water on his back, and a string of brass cups which he tinkled as he walked to draw custom. Hassan beckoned to him, and the water-carrier came up, tinkling more than ever as he salaamed to the Faringhees.

The juniors watched him with interest—he was one of the sights of Egypt, in fact—as he leaned forward to let the water run from the spout of the huge jar, over his shoulder, into a brass cup. Hassan having assured them that the khamali carried filtered water in his jar, which it was safe for even lordly and noble gentlemen like Hassan's clients to drink, the juniors took the brass cups and drank, and were refreshed. They had seen water-sellers of all sorts swarming in Cairo, and in such a climate it was a paying trade. Egypt is a thirsty land.

"Good!" said Bunter. "Now we'll sit down and rest. You'd like a rest, wouldn't you, Mauly?"

"Yaas."

Billy Bunter sat down on a large stone and Mauly followed his example. There was no doubt that Mauly was always ready for a rest.

"March!" said Bob Cherry.

"Shut up, Cherry!" said Bunter, mopping his perspiring brow with one of Lord Mauleverer's best cambric handkerchiefs. "Mauly's taking a rest. I'm bursting with energy myself——"

"You mean with grub!"

"No, I don't!" roared Bunter. "I'm full of energy; I could walk you fellows off your legs, and chance it. But Mauly's going to have a rest. I can be considerate to a chap, if you fellows can't."

The khamali was moving on down the hill, when Bob Cherry tapped him on the shoulder. The khamali's language was an unknown mystery to Bob, but the language of signs was easily understood. Bob held up a dozen piastres in one hand, with the other he tapped the spout of the water-jar and pointed to the back of Billy Bunter's fat neck.

The khamali stared for a moment; then, as he understood, he grinned, with a flash of white teeth. Having secured the piastres first and tucked them away in some recess of his dusty djubbah, he approached Bunter from behind and tilted the jar forward. Bunter, having no eyes in the back of his head, remained unaware of what was happening till a stream of water shot from the spout and landed on the back of his neck.

"Yarooooh!"

Billy Bunter bounded to his feet as if worked by a spring.

"Ooooooch! Woooooch! What—— I'm all wet! Yaroooooh!"

"Ha, ha, ha!"

The khamali, grinning, went on down the hill. Billy Bunter dabbed at the back of his neck and roared.

"Coming on now, old fat man?" asked Bob.

"Ha, ha, ha!"

"Beast!" roared Bunter.

"You coming, Mauly? Or shall I call the khamali back for you?"

"I'm coming!" said Lord Mauleverer hastily.

"Look here, you beasts, I'm all wet!" shrieked Bunter.

"Oh, you'll dry in the sun, old fat man! Come on!"

"I'm going back to the hotel to get dry!" roared Bunter.

"Good egg! Stay there, won't you?"

"Lordly gentlemen, if there is excessive delay there will be exceeding and considerable large heat of sun on a pyramid," said Hassan.

The Greyfriars fellows followed Hassan—and Billy Bunter followed on, snorting with indignation. He was dry by the time the party reached the Pyramid of Cheops, but he was still indignantly snorting.

THE FIFTH CHAPTER.

Bunter Climbs the Pyramid!

"OH crikey!"

That was Billy Bunter's first remark as he gazed, at close quarters, at the Pyramid of Cheops, up which the Greyfriars fellows were to climb.

Seen from a distance the pyramid did not look a difficult proposition; seen from close at hand it looked rather dismaying.

Once upon a time polished stone had covered the pyramid's outer surfaces, but long centuries had passed since that covering had been carried off for building mosques in Cairo. Rugged, irregular masses of the yellowish limestone, ascending in steps that were never less than three feet—and occasionally four or five—faced the juniors, and even Bob Cherry admitted that it was "some" climb, while Hurree Jamset Ram Singh justly remarked that the climbfulness would be terrific.

But it is not customary for a tourist to climb the Pyramids unaided. Three guides help the climber—one holding either hand, and the third shoving behind. Even so, most tourists have had enough by the time they reach the summit.

The perpendicular height of the Pyramid of Cheops is only 450 feet—little more than twice the height of the Monument in London. But the long slope of the sides makes the distance much greater, and the irregularity of the huge steps makes the ascent difficult to the most active climber.

Billy Bunter blinked at it in utter dismay.

"I say, you fellows, how the thump is a fellow to get up there?" ejaculated the Owl of the Remove. "Chops must have been a silly ass to put up that stack of rubbish over his silly old tomb. I say, you fellows will have to carry me up somehow."

"Oh, my hat!"

"Ha, ha, ha!" yelled the juniors.

Getting up the steep pyramid themselves was likely to tax the climbing powers of the Famous Five. Carrying Billy Bunter up was a suggestion that made them yell.

"Blessed if I see anything to cackle at!" said Bunter peevishly. "I'm jolly

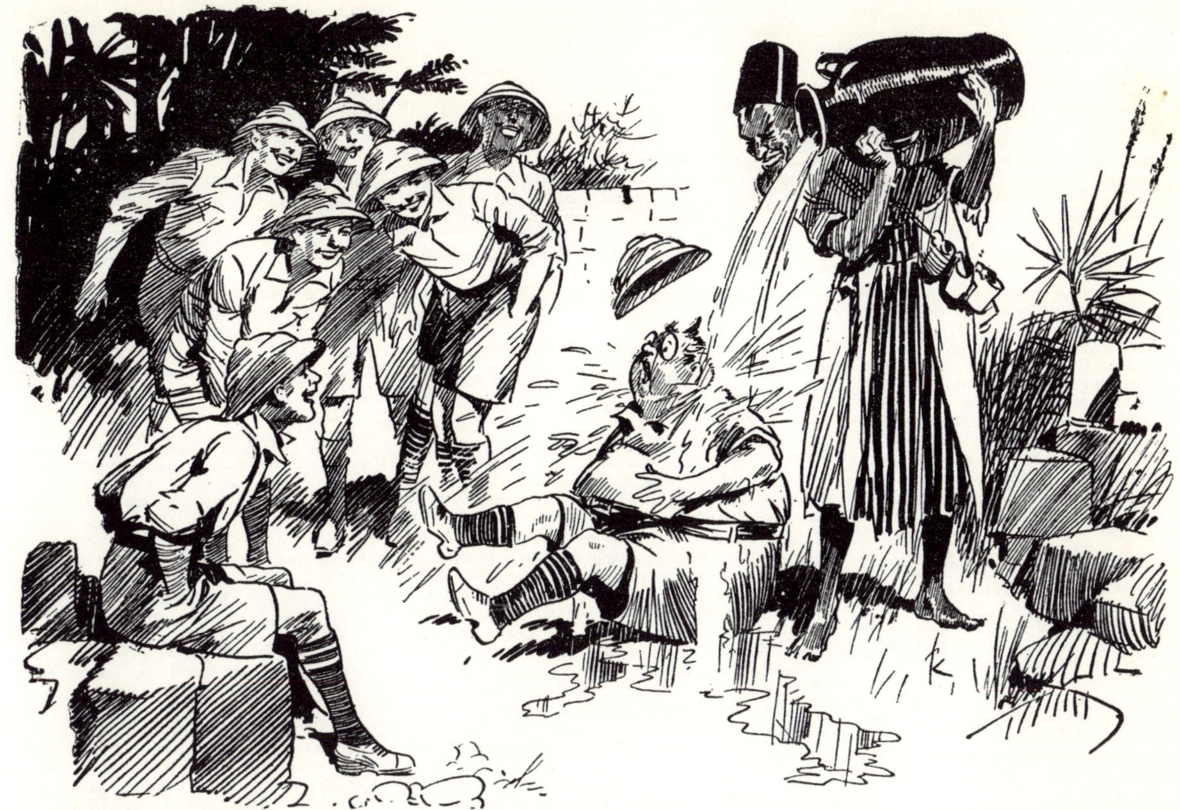

The khamali approached Bunter from behind, and tilted the jar forward. Bunter, having no eyes in the back of his head, remained unaware of what was happening, till a stream of water landed on the back of his neck. "Yarooooh!" he yelled. "I'm all wet—oooooch!"

well going up! I'm not going to have you fellows saying at Greyfriars next term that you left me at the bottom. I'm going up! I fancy you could manage to carry me up if you all stick together and exert yourselves. Don't be slackers, you know."

"Ha, ha, ha!"

"Better sit down and rest, old fat bean, while we go up!" chuckled Bob Cherry. "You'll never carry all those cakes to the top!"

"I'm going up!" snorted Bunter.

"By gad, you know, it looks a bit thick—what?" yawned Lord Mauleverer. "Ought to be a lift, or somethin'—what? I rather think I'll sit down and watch you fellows at it!"

"Think again!" grinned Bob.

"Gentlemen lords, ample muscular assistance to climb is ready and at hand," said Hassan. "You trust to Hassan! Hassan, he manage your business. It is easy as billy-oh, as you say in your noble language!"

Bedouin Arabs, eager for backsheesh, had gathered, accustomed to the peculiar task of hoisting tourists up the Pyramids. Hassan gave them their directions.

A brawny Bedouin grasped the right hand of Lord Mauleverer—another brawny Arab his left—and pulled. A third swarthy gentleman butted him in the back. Up went his lordship, gasping.

"Oh, good gad!" spluttered Mauleverer.

"You see, it is as easy as to wink," said Hassan cheerfully. "By means of to pull and to push, ascent is ridiculously simple and facilitated. Lordly noblemen, the Arabs are ready!"

"Pick out the stoutest lads for Bunter!" chuckled Bob.

"Here are three hugely muscular persons as strong as Rameses the Second!" said Hassan.

"Go it, Bunter!"

"Oh lor'!" gasped Bunter.

It was the only way up, and Bunter "went" it. Hassan had sagely picked out his strongest men to hoist Bunter. But strong men as they were, they found Billy Bunter a big order.

His hands were grasped by the two who had to pull. Behind him shoved the third man. Up went Bunter.

"Yarooooooh! Hold me!" roared Bunter.

The three Arabs were strong. But the man behind had an almost agonised expression on his face as he shoved and hoisted. The hapless three had hoisted fat tourists in their time with success. But they had never had to deal with a member of the Bunter tribe before. William George Bunter was a new experience to them. Judging by their looks, they were not enjoying the new experience.

Lord Mauleverer was going up almost like a bird in advance. But the Famous Five stood and watched Bunter. They wondered whether the three Bedouins would stand the strain.

"Don't let me drop!" yelled Bunter, as the straining trio swayed. "I say, you fellows, help!"

"Those stout lads are going to earn their piastres!" said Bob.

"The earnfulness will be terrific!" chuckled Hurree Jamset Ram Singh.

"I say, you fellows," yelled Bunter, "I'm going to fall!"

"For goodness' sake don't!" yelled Bob. "If you drop on Egypt, you'll knock it right through to Australia!"

"Ha, ha, ha!"

"Beast!" howled Bunter.

"With considerable exertion, lordly fat gentleman will reach top of pyramid!" said Hassan encouragingly.

"I say, you fellows——"

"Mashallah!" groaned the Arab behind Bunter.

He shoved and shoved. The two upper Arabs dragged and dragged. Up went the fat Owl, spluttering.

"Look out!" yelled Bob.

"Oh, my hat!"

The Famous Five rushed to help. But it was too late. The Bedouins cracked under the strain, and Bunter came down again. He came with a bump fairly on the Arab behind him. That unfortunate follower of the Prophet was spread-eagled, and as he collapsed Bunter plumped on him. The wretched Arab broke Bunter's fall. Judging by his horrible gasps and gurgles, Bunter had broken him. The two men above, striving to hold on to Bunter, came down after him. They sprawled over Bunter as he sprawled on the third Arab, and fearful howls and yells rose from the heap.

"I say, you fellows—yaroooh—help!"

"Bismillah!"

"Yurrrrrrgggh!"

"Wahyat-en-nabi!"

"Wallah! Wallahi!"

"Yarooooop!"

"Ha, ha, ha!"

Hassan and a dozen Bedouins rushed to sort out the heap. Harry Wharton & Co. lent their aid.

Billy Bunter was dragged up, spluttering wildly. Two of the Arabs scrambled up, talking explosively in Arabic. But the third man, on whom Bunter had fallen, lay and groaned. His groans were faint and feeble. There was no breath left in him. Four or five of his dusky friends raised him at last, and he leaned heavily on them, gurgling for breath.

"Oh crumbs!" spluttered Bunter. "Beasts! Where's my specs? I say, you fellows—ow, wow! I'm killed! I mean, nearly killed! Ow! Ooooogh!"

"Ha, ha, ha!"

"You've nearly killed that jolly old Arab, anyhow!" said Bob Cherry. "Look at him!"

"Blow him! Bother him! Why didn't he hold me? Ow, wow! Gimme my specs, you beasts! Ow!"

"Hassan, old brown bean, you'd better get a dozen men to hoist Bunter up!" said Bob. "Three can't do it! Better have a dozen fore and a dozen aft——"

"Ha, ha, ha!"

There was a volley of Arabic from the Bedouins, which sounded to the juniors like the cracking of nuts. They all talked at once, and they all talked emphatically, and they gesticulated wildly. Hassan made soothing gestures.

"What's the row about, Hassan?" asked Harry Wharton at last.

"Noble lordly gentlemen, they demand double payment for helping the lordly fat Faringhee up pyramid—also that six men shall conduct the fat lord instead of three," said Hassan.

"That's fair!" said Harry. "Get on with it!"

Six strong men were picked out for the hefty task. Once more Billy Bunter's fat hands were grasped, and his fat elbows also, and two strong men shoved in the rear. Six stout Arabs were equal even to Billy Bunter's weight. Up he went.

Gasps and gurgles and howls floated down from him. The six Arabs seemed to be bumping him a little as they hoisted and dragged and pulled. But really that could not be helped.

After him went the Famous Five, each assisted by two or three Bedouins. Hassan followed on behind, looking like a gorgeous tropical butterfly on the pyramid in his red tarboosh, gold-braided jacket, bright blue trousers, and crimson sash.

"I say, you fellows," howled Bunter, "are we near the top yet?"

"Not half-way up yet, old bean!" called back Bob Cherry.

"Oh crikey!"

"Stick it out, old fat man!"

"Beast!" howled Bunter. "Tell these silly idiots not to keep on pinching me. Ow!"

"My dear old rhinoceros, if they let you fall now, you'll break Egypt into small pieces!" chuckled Bob. "Shall I tell them to hold on to your ears? Lots of room for the lot of them!"

"Yah!"

The Famous Five were soon ahead of Bunter. Lord Mauleverer was already at the summit of the pyramid, and they joined him there. The six Arabs were still struggling up with Bunter. Every step of the innumerable steps required a big effort, and there was no doubt that the six Bedouins were earning double pay. They were earning it hard by the sweat of their brows. When they staggered at last on the summit of the pyramid, and landed Bunter in a gasping heap, they looked as if they had had the time of their lives. Billy Bunter sat and gasped, and the six Bedouins stood round him, held out their brown hands, and said with one voice:

"Backsheesh!"

"Ooooough!" was Bunter's reply.

"Backsheesh!" chorused the gasping half-dozen.

"Yah! Go away! Beasts! Oooogh!"

"Backsheesh!"

"Hassan, old bean, give them some piastres!" yawned Lord Mauleverer. "If ever a jolly old Arab earned backsheesh, I fancy they have!"

"I say, you fellows—oooogh! Blow these rotten pyramids! I wish I'd gone to Margate instead of coming to Egypt. Ooooogh! Those black beasts were pinching me all the way up! Ooooh! Making out that I'm heavy, you know—Ooooogh! Oh crikey!"

"Jump up, old fat man," said Bob. "There's a splendid view from here!"

"Blow the view!" groaned Bunter.

And he sat and gasped and gurgled, regardless of the view from the summit of Cheops' Pyramid.

THE SIXTH CHAPTER.

The Man on the Pyramid!

"HERE is extensive and remarkable view, lordly gentlemen!" said Hassan, waving a brown hand. "All Faringhee tourist gaze with delight on this large and highly interesting view, suggesting thoughts of solemn Nature, such as death and eternity and like matters, all of which included in charge of ten piastres for ascending pyramid."

Harry Wharton & Co. looked with keen interest at the vast prospect from the summit of the Great Pyramid.

Westward stretched the desert, endless sand and barren cliffs. Southward the Pyramids of Sakkara stood against the blue of the sky. North and east were the cultivated lands of the Nile, the Mokattam Mountains, and Cairo in the distance.

Tombs, and tombs, and more tombs, met their eyes. And they gazed at the Sphinx in its hollow—standing in the quarry from which the stone for the Great Pyramid had been taken, where it had been shaped by the orders of Khephron, the successor of Cheops, five thousand years ago. Hassan's babble passed unheeded by their ears as they gazed.

It was strange enough to gaze upon the scene, on which had gazed Herodotus, the Father of History, five centuries before the Christian era began. Strange enough to gaze where Julius Cæsar and Mark Antony had gazed; to look on what had met the dark eyes of Cleopatra.

All human things had changed—the Pharaohs were gone, and the Ptolemics, the Caliphs and the Mamelukes—but the Nile still rolled its fertilising flood, the Pyramids still stood against the intense blue, the Sphinx still looked out over the silence and mystery of the desert!

The place was one for meditation, with a melancholy tinge, so far as the inanimate surroundings went. But the animate surroundings were far from being of a serious nature. Dusky natives of the country, blind and deaf to all considerations but backsheesh, gabbled like geese.

On the plain below, the juniors, looking towards the solemn Sphinx, spotted a couple of German tourists mounted on donkeys—both of them immensely fat, and the hapless donkeys almost tottering under them.

Both of them had red-covered guide-books in their hands, and large spectacles on their podgy red noses that flashed back the rays of the sun. The donkey-boys running behind, whacking with their sticks, howled and yelled, and their howls and yells could be heard by the group on the summit of the pyramid.

From nearer at hand came a nasal voice—that of an American tourist who had climbed after the juniors.

"I surely guess this cost something to erect!" the American gentleman was saying. "I'd surely like to know how it would work out in dullars! I'll say it cost a whole heap of dullars! Yeah!"

Bob Cherry grinned.

"Gentlemen, chaps, and sportsmen," he said, "I think we'll leave the solemn meditations till we get back to the hotel! What?"

"The solemnity of an esteemed meditation in this ridiculous spot would not be terrific!" agreed the Nabob of Bhanipur.

"I say, you fellows——"

"Hallo, hallo, hallo! Bunter, old fat bean, this is where you meditate on the passing of human greatness——"

"I'm thirsty," said Bunter plaintively—"and I'm getting hungry!"

"Think of jolly old Herodotus coming along on his donkey to look at this, two thousand five hundred years ago!"

"Blow Herodotus! It's beastly hot!" said Bunter.

"Think of jolly old Julius Cæsar trotting out here on a donkey—perhaps one of your remote ancestors——"

"You silly chump!" hooted Bunter.

"Yep!" went on the voice of the American gentleman. "I'll say it cost a heap of dullars! I'd surely like to know what it ran old Cheops into! It surely was an expensive stunt!"

Hassan's voice was running on:

"Visit to interior of pyramid is facilitated by modern staircases, after taking lunch at hotel at fixed price. Gentlemen lords having gazed upon unequalled view, with solemn meditation on brief period of human glory, will descend pyramid and take lunch——"

"I say, you fellows, that darky's talking sense for once," said Billy Bunter. "I'm ready for lunch! I hope a fellow can get a decent lunch at the hotel. I say, how are we going to get down?"

"That's an easy one," said Bob cheerfully. "You just lie down on the edge, and we roll you down like a barrel."

"Beast!"

Harry Wharton & Co. strolled about the summit of the Great Pyramid, the space at the top being about twelve yards square. There were a few other tourists on the top, or coming up, each attended by many backsheesh-hunting Bedouins.

Billy Bunter sat and rested his weary, fat limbs, not deigning to bestow a single blink from his spectacles on the "unequalled view." He had other matters to think of—the serious fact that he was thirsty, and the scarcely less serious circumstance that he was getting hungry.

The Arabs who had helped the schoolboys up loafed on the rugged steps, waiting to help them down again, chattering in Arabic. To them the wonderful monuments of the ancient inhabitants of Egypt were simply a means by which they extracted backsheesh from the foreigner.

Billy Bunter blinked at them morosely. He had had a rather rough journey, with the Arabs lugging him up, and he was not looking forward to the descent, with the Arabs lugging him down. He suspected the beasts of having pinched him on purpose while they were lugging him up. Perhaps they had!

A thick-set Arab appeared on the rugged steps, and Bunter blinked at him as he came in sight. The man had a fold of linen across the lower part of his face, apparently to keep off the dust of the desert; above it his black eyes, hawkish in their keenness, scanned the tourists moving about the summit of the pyramid.

He beckoned to Hassan, the

dragoman, who joined him, leaving his lordly gentlemen to themselves for a time—much to their relief.

The two began to speak in Arabic, in low voices.

They were quite near Bunter, and he could hear them plainly, but could not, of course, understand a word they said.

But he blinked at them curiously.

The thick-set Arab seemed to be urging something on Hassan, and the dragoman was shaking his head and gesticulating.

It dawned on Bunter that the newcomer was not unfamiliar to his eyes.

All Arabs were much alike to Bunter; he would have found it difficult to tell one dark face from another. And this man had his face partly concealed.

But there was something in the hawkish glitter of the black eyes that Bunter seemed to remember. And in the eagerness of his talk with Hassan the man shifted the linen from his face, and then the fat Owl had, for a moment, a full view of him.

He started.

He knew the man now! It was the hawk-faced Arab who had been in Lord Mauleverer's room that morning, and who had attacked Mauly. Bunter was sure of it.

A shiver ran through his fat limbs, hot as it was on the pyramid. He forgot that he was tired, and picked himself up hastily, and rolled away to join the Famous Five and Mauleverer on the other side of the summit.

"I say, you fellows——" breathed Bunter.

"Chuck it, old fat man—we know you're hungry," said Bob. "Put on a new record."

"Oh, really, Cherry——"

"And we know you're thirsty!" grinned Johnny Bull. "Don't tell us over again, old fat bean!"

"Oh, really, Bull——"

"And we know you're tired," added Nugent. "And we know it's hot! And we know there are a lot of flies! Give us a rest."

"A rest from the esteemed jawfulness would be a boonful blessing," agreed the Nabob of Bhanipur.

"Oh, all right!" said Bunter. "If you want Mauly to be robbed and kidnapped and murdered——"

"Eh?"

"What?"

"I say, you fellows, it's him!" breathed Bunter.

"Who's him, you fat image?" demanded Harry Wharton.

"See that nigger talking to Hassan over there—well, that's the darky that collared Mauly this morning in his room——"

"Oh, my hat!"

The juniors looked round quickly.

The talk between Hassan and the Arab with the covered face was going on with undiminished emphasis. They were too deep in their argument, whatever it was, to take any notice of the schoolboys.

"Is that the chap, Mauly?" asked Bob Cherry doubtfully. "Can't see much of his chivvy, with that dust-clout on it. You saw him this morning——"

"Blessed if I know!" confessed his lordship. "Might be the same johnny—he looks sort of familiar. Let's go and ask him."

"I say, you fellows, I'm jolly certain——"

"We'll make sure, anyhow," said Harry Wharton quietly. "If it's the man we'll collar him, and there's a police station opposite Mena House where he can be handed over. You'd know the man if you had a good look at him, Mauly?"

"Yaas."

"Come and have a look, then!"

"Yaas," yawned Mauly.

The juniors hastily crossed the summit of the pyramid, towards the top of the steps where the dragoman stood in talk with the thick-set Arab. But the movement caught the Arab's attention at once. The hawkish eyes flashed at the schoolboys for a second with quick suspicion; and then the man turned to descend the steps, breaking off his talk with Hassan in the middle of a sentence.

"That looks——" muttered Bob.

"Hassan! Stop that man!" shouted Wharton. He broke into a run.

The dragoman stared round.

"My noble gentlemen——"

"Stop that man! Tell the guides to stop him!" exclaimed Wharton.

He had no doubt now, for the thick-set Arab with the hawkish eyes was making his way fast down the rugged

WIN A PENKNIFE

like T. Almond, of 21, Mosley Street, Blackburn, Lancs, who has scored a bull's-eye with the following amusing storyette.

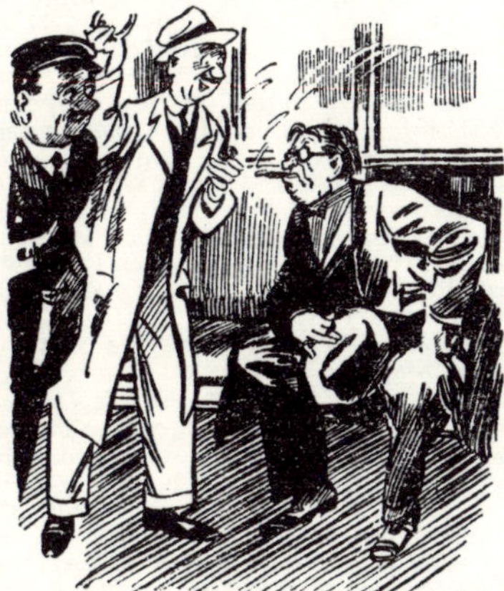

"Say, conductor!" said the American sightseer, travelling on a London bus. "You jest remember I want your St. Paul's Cathedral—and I want it slick! Get me?"

"That's all right," said the harassed conductor. "I ain't forgotten, I'm a-gettin' it wrapped up for you now!"

Now, what about an effort from you, chum?

steps, bounding from one to another at imminent risk of losing his footing and falling.

There was a babble of excitement from the Bedouins as they started to their feet.

Hassan, usually so swift and prompt to obey the orders of his lordly gentlemen, hesitated now; and Wharton, passing him, made a jump down the steps in pursuit of the fleeing Arab. Then the dragoman acted promptly enough—he reached out a quick brown hand, caught Wharton by the shoulder, and pulled him back.

"Let go!" roared Wharton, as he staggered back.

"Oh, my lordly noble gentleman, you will break and injure your admirable limbs by unconsidered hurry on steps of pyramid——" gasped Hassan. "Steps are not safe for running with enormous speed——"

"Let go, you fool!"

Wharton would have wrenched himself away, but Hassan held him fast. Either he was alarmed for the junior's safety, or he had some other motive for holding him back. He held the schoolboy in the grip of a vice.

"My noble gentleman," he gasped, "when you are ready to descend Bedouin guides are to help—Bismillah!" gasped Hassan, as Wharton gave him a fierce shove, and he sat down on the summit of Cheops' Pyramid, with a heavy bump and was forced to release his hold.

Harry Wharton rushed down the steps, his comrades after him. Lord Mauleverer and Billy Bunter watched them from the top, neither of them inclined for such wild exertions in the blazing sunshine. The Famous Five scrambled down half a dozen of the steep, rugged steps, and then came to a halt, panting. The bounding Arab was almost at the bottom, and had disappeared from their sight, and further pursuit was evidently hopeless. Bob Cherry mopped his streaming brow.

"Chuck it," he said. "Nothing doing—it's too jolly hot for a foot-race, old beans, and he's got too good a start. Chuck it."

There was nothing to do, but to "chuck it," and the Famous Five scrambled back, panting and breathless, to the summit of the pyramid.

THE SEVENTH CHAPTER.

Bunter is Fed-up!

HARRY WHARTON fixed his eyes sternly on the face of Hassan, the dragoman. The flight of the hawk-faced Arab was as good as proof to the juniors; they were certain that he was the man who had attacked Lord Mauleverer in his room at the Cairo Hotel. It could hardly be doubted that he had feared recognition, and that that was the reason of his flight. Hassan was staring at his noble gentlemen with a look of astonishment which, if it was assumed, was very well done. But the juniors had their doubts of the faithful Hassan now.

"My noble lordly gentlemen!" exclaimed Hassan. "What is a matter? What is cause of anger? If you run fast in sun of Egypt there is enormous danger of sunstroke! Yes! You trust Hassan——"

"Who was that man?" demanded Wharton.

"The man to which I was speaking?" asked Hassan. "He is donkey-man of Cairo, my gentleman lord, of name Yussef, the son of Hamid. He is one very good donkey-man."

"You know him?" asked Harry.

"Hassan knows all things, and all peoples in Cairo, and in all the Nile as far as the Cataracts, noble sar! Know Yussef very well!"

"What did he want?"

All the juniors were eyeing the "faithful Hassan" very keenly. But the brown face of the dragoman expressed only wondering surprise. From his looks, at all events, Hassan appeared to be amazed by the outbreak of excitement and ignorant of its cause.

"He want my noble gentlemen to hire him donkeys!" explained Hassan. "He offer me backsheesh, much backsheesh, if I hire him donkeys for my noble English lords."

"And you were going to hire them?" asked Harry quickly.

"Oh, no, my noble gentleman! Already I have hired donkeys for a ride to a Sphinx in an afternoon, after my noble lords have rested, and to Yussef I say no, I do not want him donkeys! I say no many times, and Yussef he grow angry and offer more backsheesh, because him want very much to hire him donkeys to my lordly gentlemen. But him donkeys not good donkeys—not good enough for my estimable lords!" Hassan shook his head. "Much better donkeys are hired for my gentlemen."

Wharton scanned the dragoman keenly while he was speaking.

But it seemed likely enough that Hassan was telling the truth.

It was very probable that Yussef, the hawk-faced Arab, would have been glad to get his donkeys hired by the Greyfriars party, for a chance of getting hold of Lord Mauleverer in the desert. It was natural for him to approach their dragoman on the subject—for all such business had to be done through the dragoman, whose palm had to be oiled. There was really no reason to suspect Hassan of knowing anything of the donkey-man's ulterior object.

"Is the man a friend of yours?" asked Johnny Bull.

Hassan made a lofty gesture of denial.

"Oh, sar!" he said, with dignified reproach. "I am Hassan, the son of Suleiman, the most best-known and personal-recommended dragoman in Egypt! Donkey-boys are not friends of such a dragoman as Hassan! No, sar! Bismillah! This man is known to me, like all donkey-boys in Alexandria, in Cairo, and in Luxor! Hassan knows all things and all peoples, sar, from the Delta to the Cataracts! That is Hassan's business, sar! But a donkey-boy is not a friend of Hassan, sar! Oh, no, sar!"

"I say, you fellows. I'm fearfully hungry——"

"Shut up, Bunter!"

"Look here, I've been thirsty a long time, and now I'm getting fearfully hungry as well——"

"Shut up!" roared Johnny Bull.

"Beast!"

"Look here, Hassan," said Harry abruptly. "that man you call Yussef is a thief, and very likely a murderer, and——"

"Oh, sar!" ejaculated Hassan.

"He is the man who attacked Lord Mauleverer in the hotel this morning at Cairo, and the police are looking for him——"

"Wahyat-en-nabi!" gasped Hassan. "Is this possible, my noble lord? I have speak to a man who raise a hand against my noble lord——"

Hassan stared down the rugged slope of the pyramid.

"He has gone," he said. "He run very fast, and why should he run, except that he fear? My noble gentleman is right—he is one villain—for if he is not afraid, why should he run? Now I understand, sar."

Hassan waved both brown hands in his excitement.

"That son of ten thousand pigs!" he exclaimed. "Noble sar, let us descend a pyramid—by Mena House there is police station, and policemans will find that grandfather of five hundred hogs! I, Hassan, will go to policemans, and tell them where to look for Yussef in Cairo, sar! Yes, sar! Now I know why he want to hire him donkeys to my noble lords—why he offer Hassan much backsheesh! Oh, sar, if I have known that he is enemy of my lordly gentlemen, I speak not with him—I strike him with my stick—I bash him, as you say in your noble language!"

"Let's go," said Harry.

Hassan called the Bedouins for the descent of the pyramid. For the moment a suspicion had crossed the minds of the juniors that the faithful Hassan might be in league with the hawk-faced Arab. But the dragoman's explanation was plausible enough, and they dismissed the idea.

The juniors began the descent of the pyramid.

Three of the Bedouins helped each of the party—except Bunter, who gave plenty of work to six.

Getting down the pyramid was almost as hard work as getting up. There was an unending accompaniment of grunts, and gasps, and groans from Billy Bunter. But they reached the foot of the ragged steps at last, and started down the sandy hill towards the Mena House Hotel.

"I say, you fellows"—Billy Bunter turned an indignant and accusing blink on the Famous Five—"I'm fed-up with pyramids! You silly idiots can climb all the beastly pyramids you like, but I'm jolly well not going to climb any more putrid pyramids—see? If you go up any more rotten pyramids, you can jolly well leave me behind!"

"Gentlemen and chaps," said Bob Cherry, "we'd better spend a lot of time climbing pyramids! Seems sort of attractive, doesn't it?"

"Yah!" snorted Bunter.

The heat of the day was coming on as the juniors arrived at Mena House, and they were glad to get into the shade. Harry Wharton went across to the police station opposite the hotel, with Hassan, to be present while the dragoman explained the affair of Yussef, the son of Hamid, to the native inspector. He understood little of what was said; but Hassan's excited volleys of Arabic and earnest gesticulations seemed to leave no doubt of his good faith in the matter. Then the captain of the Greyfriars Remove joined his friends at lunch.

Billy Bunter had recovered his cheerfulness by that time. He packed away one lunch after another with great enjoyment. After which Bunter retired to a shady tree for a siesta; and, the midday rest being a necessity in the Egyptian climate, the other fellows followed his example.

Not till late in the afternoon did Hassan announce that the donkeys were ready for the ride to the Sphinx.

The Famous Five and Lord Mauleverer were ready, too, but Billy Bunter was not ready.

He sat up and blinked at the juniors when they called him.

"If you think I'm going to stir in this fearful heat——" he began.

"The other donkeys are waiting!" said Bob.

"Yah! Call me again in two hours——"

"Oh, all right! We shall be back by then."

"What I mean is, you can wait a couple of hours, and then I'll come," explained Bunter. "If you go now, you go without me! Mind, I mean that! I'm here to look after you and protect you, and all that, but I refuse to stir in this fearful heat! I refuse distinctly! If you go before two hours from now, you go without me, and take your chance! I wash my hands of the matter!"

"Ha, ha, ha!"

"You can cackle!" hooted Bunter. "But I tell you I shall wash my hands——"

"Wash your neck at the same time," suggested Bob; "it can do with it!"

"Ha, ha, ha!"

"Beast!"

"Look here, Bunter, you'd better come!" said Harry. "You want to see the Sphinx——"

"Blow the Sphinx!"

Bunter closed his eyes again behind his big spectacles. The Sphinx did not appeal to him so much as a prolonged nap in the shade.

Harry Wharton & Co. walked over to where the donkeys were waiting with the donkey-boys, leaving Bunter to nap. And the keenest eye could not have detected any sign of grief at the loss of Billy Bunter's fascinating company.

THE EIGHTH CHAPTER.

In the Desert!

WHACK, whack, whack!

The sticks of the donkey-boys whacked and cracked on the backs of the trotting donkeys. Each donkey had its own special donkey-boy, in charge of mount and rider, running beside the animal, objurgating in Arabic and whacking it with a stick.

It was in vain that the juniors told the dusky donkey-boys to "chuck" it. They either did not or did not want to understand. It was their way to whack the donkeys, and they whacked them.

But it was hardly more than a half-mile from Mena House to the Sphinx, so the ride did not take long.

The Famous Five would just as soon have walked the short distance; but Lord Mauleverer undoubtedly preferred to make the trip sitting down, and, still more undoubtedly, Hassan, the dragoman, had to be allowed to hire donkeys and pocket backsheesh for the same from the donkey-owner.

Hassan had declared that the donkeys were the best donkeys that were obtainable in all Egypt, only the very best of all things being suitable for his noble gentlemen. But, as a matter of fact, the Famous Five were provided with rather poor animals, only Lord Mauleverer getting a good one.

But Mauly's mount was a large powerful white donkey, strong and sturdy, and evidently capable of speed. Hassan had specially selected him for his lordship, with his donkey-boy, Mohammed, who was rather a tough-looking Arab, with part of an ear missing, from a knife-slash in some affray. Had Lord Mauleverer "let out" his donkey he would have left the other fellows far behind. But Mohammed kept the white donkey at the same pace as the others, and they arrived at the Sphinx together.

They dismounted near that ancient monument, and the donkey-boys were left in charge of the donkeys while the juniors explored the Sphinx.

Although in the hot weather there were few "peoples," as Hassan said, a dozen or more tourists were round about the Sphinx. The American gentleman who had been on top of the Pyramid of Cheops was there, and the chums of Greyfriars caught his voice:

"I guess it must cost something to keep this clear of sand. I'll say they have to do a lot of sweeping! I sure wonder if a guy could find out what it costs!"

"Wunderbar!" a stout German was saying. "Ach! Wunderbar! Kolossal!"

"Backsheesh!" came several native voices. "Backsheesh!"

"Ma foi, mais ja'i soif!" came a French voice.

There was a snapping of cameras.

"Here, lordly gentlemen." Hassan's sing-song voice started—"here is great and wonderful Sphinx, which is huge lion sitting down, with head of a man, royal head-dress on same head. This place is quarry where stones for Great

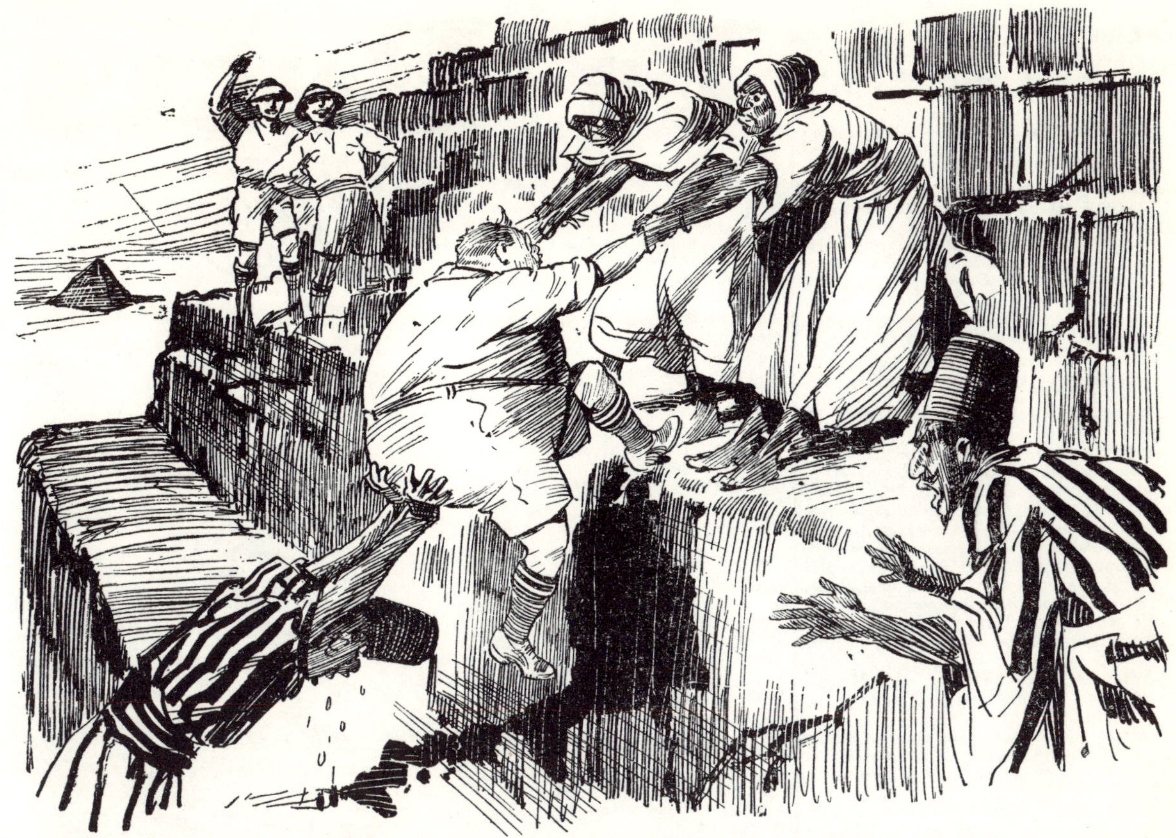

"With considerable exertion, lordly fat gentleman will reach top of pyramids!" said Hassan, encouragingly. One of the Arabs shoved Bunter from behind, while two more dragged from above. "Look out!" yelled Bob Cherry, suddenly, as the Bedouins cracked under the strain. "He's falling!"

Pyramid taken by Cheops. Huge stone remained, and was made into Sphinx on the spot, by order of Khephron, honourable successor of Cheops. Travellers in all ages had admired and wondered. Photographs have been taken in all languages! Yes! Covered many times by sand of desert and hidden from honourable eyes of noble travellers, sar! Now it is keeped clear of desert sand that noble travellers may see! Yes! Hassan tell you all things."

"I suppose a dragoman must be allowed to run on!" murmured Lord Mauleverer. "Next time I come to Egypt I shall go to Cooks, and ask for a dumb dragoman!"

"Mutilations of magnificent Sphinx done by Arabs in time of Caliphs," chanted Hassan. "In year 1380 much damage was done! Yes! Later, Mamelukes used Sphinx as target for firing! All round there are chips from the old block, as you say in your noble language! Many chips have been sticked on again to the old block! Yes! Here, in front of Sphinx, it is customary for noble gentlemen to stand and gaze on majestic monument, and spend some minutes in solemn reflections."

Solemn reflections might very well have been induced by the strange old monument, that with stony eyes had gazed out on the desert for years unnumbered.

But the human surroundings were anything but solemn.

A stout German tourist had clambered on the Sphinx, where his equally stout better half was snapping him with a Kodak.

Dust of the desert had got into the German gentleman's nose, and he was blowing it with a big red handkerchief, and a series of loud reports like pistol-shots. There was no doubt that the German gentleman detracted considerably from the majesty of the Sphinx.

"Height of wonderful Sphinx is sixty feet, feet English," went on Hassan. "Length of same two hundred and forty feet, also English! Gigantic monument of huge size, truly enormous! Nose of Sphinx five feet, English, and mouth of same seven feet."

"Beats Bunter!" murmured Bob Cherry.

"Ha, ha, ha!"

"My noble gentlemen, here you do not smile!" exclaimed Hassan. "Here you meditate with considerable solemnity, all being included in total charge of twenty piastres."

"It was rather a mistake of the Mamelukes to do their shooting practice at the Sphinx," murmured Lord Mauleverer. "They ought to have done it at the dragomans!"

"Now we return to donkeys, and view temples and tombs, also of which some are covered with sand of desert," said Hassan. "My lords shall see everything; for I, Hassan, know all things. Yes, sar! Hassan is your dragoman; you trust Hassan!"

The juniors returned to the donkeys and remounted. Once more the sticks of the donkey-boys whacked and cracked. They looked at pyramids, and rock-tombs and temples; and they were rather curious to see the spot where tombs were covered by the drifting sand of the Libyan Desert, and the donkeys were turned in that direction. Cultivated land was left behind them as they rode into the desert. Even at a short distance the din of tourists and guides was left behind, and the silence of the desert fell upon them.

At a sign from Hassan, the donkey-boys urged on the animals, and the party proceeded at a swift trot.

Each donkey-boy seemed to be doing his best, with the result that Lord Mauleverer, being the best mounted in the party, soon got ahead of the others.

Mohammed whacked and whacked, and had to go all out to keep pace with the swift white donkey.

"Hallo, hallo, hallo! Old Mauly's leaving us behind!" exclaimed Bob Cherry. "We mustn't get separated here. Hassan, tell that fellow Mohammed to slow down."

Hassan shouted in Arabic after the driver of the white donkey.

But Mohammed seemed deaf.

He continued to whack Lord Mauleverer's donkey, and his lordship drew farther and farther ahead of the rest of the party.

"Son of five hundred pigs!" exclaimed Hassan. "He does not hear! By the beard of the Prophet, never again will I hire that donkey-boy!"

"Call him back at once!" exclaimed Wharton sharply.

Hassan put his brown hands to his mouth to make a trumpet, and roared in Arabic.

Still Mohammed did not heed.

Lord Mauleverer glanced back; evidently he heard the shouting. Bob Cherry yelled to him:

"Hold on, Mauly! Wait for us, old bean!"

Bob's powerful voice carried the distance, and Mauly waved his hand in response. The juniors saw him lean towards Mohammed to speak. They urged on their donkeys to overtake him.

(*Continued on page 16.*)

THE BOGUS

By DICKY NUGENT

I.

CRASH!

"What's that?" asked Jack Jolly of the Fourth at St. Sam's, poking his head out of his tent.

"Don't be alarmed, old chap!" called out Frank Fearless, from the depths of his blankit. "It was just the day breaking, I fansy!"

Fearless was right; dawn had just broken over the tent in which the hikers of St. Sam's had spent the previous nite. Now, the woods around them were waking to life. Precipices yawned, weeping willows rubbed their eyes, springs sprang up, and the wind began to whissle. Natcher's day had begun.

"I say, you chaps," cride Merry, who had been seveerly stung by nettles the nite before, "I've got a rash!"

"That's nothing!" said Bright, with a grin. "I've got a rasher! Let's get a fire going, and cook the brekker!"

"Good wheeze!"

Sevveral days of hiking had given Jack Jolly & Co. tremenjous appetites, and they fell to the task of preparing breakfast with a right good will. Before you could say "Jack Robinson," the fire was sizzling, the kettle crackling, and the bacon singing—or, at least, that's what Jack Jolly imajined.

The hikers of St. Sam's waded into breakfast.

"Wonder how the poor old Head's getting on?" said Frank Fearless, between mouthfuls of bacon.

"When we last saw him, he was going up to bed in the Hawnted Inn!" grinned Merry, between mouthfuls of bread-and-butter.

"Hoap the perlice didn't arrest him when they raided the inn!" chuckled Jack Jolly, between throatfuls of coffy.

"One thing's certain—he'll never find us now!" larfed Bright, between mouthfuls of dry biskit. "If you ask my opinion, he's given up the chase as hoapless and gone back to St. Sam's!"

"Good-morning, boys!" broke in a refined, cultured voice at that moment. "Nice weather we're having lately, aren't we? Provided the rain keeps off, it ought to remain dry, I should imajine!"

Jack Jolly & Co. started to their feet in amazement.

"The Head!" they eggsclaimed.

It was Dr. Birchemall himself! The Head was standing before them with a somewhat sinnical smile on his skollerly fizz.

"Uneggspected plezzure for you—what?" he said. "I seem to have come along at just the right time, too; breakfast is just what I need at the moment. Don't cook me too much, boys; just a duzzen rashers of bacon, half a duzzen eggs, a few pounds of sossidges, and anything you happen to have in the way of vegetables!"

Jack Jolly gasped.

"You're not asking much, sir, I must admit, considering what a wacking grate breakfast you usually eat. But, unforchunitly, we can't even mannidge the little you require. We're just eating the last crums ourselves, sir!"

"Oh crums!" eggsclaimed Dr. Birchemall, in dismay. "I suppose that's what I mite have eggspected from you greedy young beggars! Well, since you greedy young rascals have licked the platter clean, so to speak, I'm going to set a trap or two and see if I can't bag a nice fat rabbit!"

"But you can't do that, sir!" eggsclaimed Jack Jolly. "This land all belongs to Lord Broadacres, and anyone caught catching rabbits is liable to fearful penalties for poaching!"

"Ratts!" retorted the Head, fetching out from his poacher's pocket the nets and traps he always carried for emergencies of this kind. "When a man's hungry, all the Lord Broadacres in the country can't stop him bagging a rabbit for his breakfast. Here goes, anyway!"

He stalked off majestically across the clearing and dived into the undergrowth.

An instant later, he emitted a yell of pain and rage.

"Yarooooo! Help! Murder! Perlice!"

"What's the matter, sir?" asked Jack Jolly, in serprize.

"Matter!" yelled the Head furiously. "I'm caught in a man-trap set for poachers—that's what's the matter!"

II.

BEFORE Jack Jolly & Co. had recovered from their first shock of serprize, they herd the sound of tramping feet and deep voices from the woods.

"Poacher ahead!" cride a horse voice. "Caught in a man-trap, I fansy!"

"We'll give the scoundrell 'poacher'!" cride another. "We'll flay him alive before we hand him over to the perlice!"

"Yaroooo!" roared the Head, at the sound of those dreadful threats. "Jolly! Fearless! Help me! Reskew, St. Sam's!"

Jack Jolly & Co. hezzitated, not knowing quite what to do. And even as they hezzitated, two grate hulking gamekeepers burst through the bushes, grinning all over their dials.

"Gotcher!" they cride together.

While one held Dr. Birchemall by his beard, the other released him from the man-trap.

"Name?" snapped one of the gamekeepers, when this little operation had been completed.

"Oh crikey!" gasped the Head. "If you must know, it's Alfred Birchemall."

The gamekeepers larfed harshly.

"Well, Alfred Birchemall, our motter's: 'Search 'em all!' Go through his pockets, Bill!"

Bill went through the head's pockets. Among the varied assortment of buttons, conkers, pieces of toffy, and lengths of string he found quite a complete poacher's outfit.

"My eye!" he remarked, when he had finished. "Lord Broadacres will be pleased about this, and no mistake! His lordship happens to be the local magistrate, Alfred Birchemall, so you'll be sure of getting a good long stretch in chokey, not to mention a jennerous taste of the catterninetales!"

"Oh, grate pip!" gasped the Head. "But I assure you, my good men, I'm not a poacher. As a matter of fact, I had just taken these traps and nets from those boys over there. I was in the middle of lecturing them on the evils of poaching, when by some strange mischance I got caught in this blessed man-trap. That's the truth, isn't it, boys?"

Jack Jolly & Co. were so brethless with indignation at that peculiar version of the "truth" that they couldn't reply at once. Before they had recovered their breth, another jentleman came upon the seen—an aristocratic jentleman, who wore a monocle in his eye.

"Bai Jove! What's all the bally fuss about? Don't you know? Eh—what?" he drawled, in a langwid, cultured voice. "Gunn! Shooter! Tell me what it's all about immejately!"

"Good-morning, your lordship!" cride Gunn and Shooter, grovelling before their lord and master. "If it pleases you, your lordship, we've caught a poacher!"

"Bai Jove! Good biznay—what!

WOULD YOU BELIEVE IT?

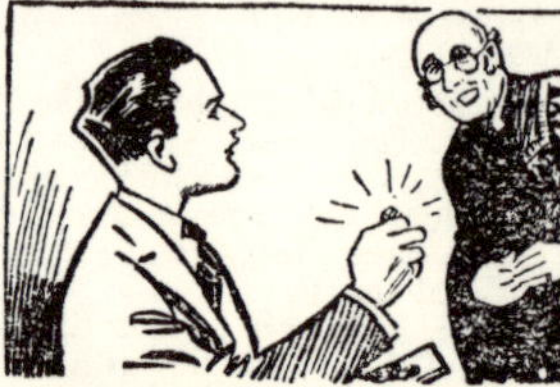

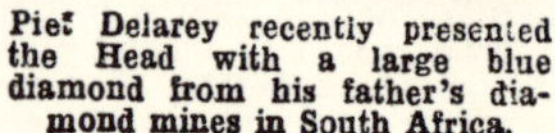

Pie! Delarey recently presented the Head with a large blue diamond from his father's diamond mines in South Africa.

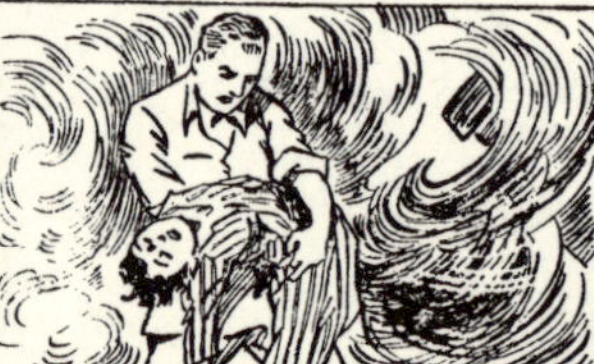

Wingate's first chum was Arthur Courtney, who died from burns sustained in rescuing a fag from a blazing dormitory.

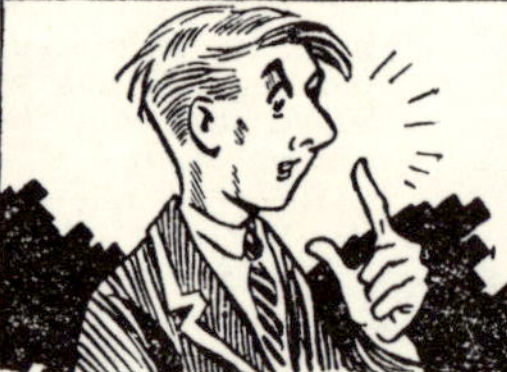

Peter Todd has the distinctio of possessing the largest nose a Greyfriars. His cousin Alonz has a large nose, too.

ERO!

"I'll see if I can't arrange a life sentence for the beggah!" said Lord Broadacres; for that was evvidently the eyedentity of the newcomer. "Take him up to the castle, and fling him into one of my privit dungeons!"

"Certainly, your lordship!"

The two gamekeepers turned on Dr. Birchemall. But the Head was ready for them by this time. What he had herd was quite sufficient to inspire him to fight to the last gasp for his freedom.

Springing into sudden activvity, he turned a summersault, balanced for an instant on the palms of his hands, and lashed out with his feet. One foot caught Gunn full in the fizz, and the other landed with fearful force on Shooter's left ear.

"Woooop!"

"Yarooo!"

Two aggernised yells rang out as Gunn and Shooter collapsed, and though both gamekeepers were game keepers, they weren't game enuff to rise again. They just sat there yelling, while Dr. Birchemall took advantage of their indisposition to land once more on his soles, and take to his heels.

With a cry of "Bai Jove! What a bally nerve, don't you know—what?" Lord Broadacres fixed his monocle more firmly in his eye, and leaped after the fugitive with swift, spasmodic movements somewhat reminissent of the kangaroo.

The St. Sam's hikers came to the conclusion that the chase was a uneek sporting event not to be missed. Larfing fit to bust, they followed on the heels of the Head and his noble persewer.

All six raced through the woods at breakneck speed till they reached a stream spanned by a wooden plank. Then, with a suddenness that none could have fourseen, the little komedy was nearly turned into a tragedy. Dr. Birchemall got across the plank in complete safety; but Lord Broadacres, who was liable to go potty at times, became unbalanced half-way across, and fell into the swirling waters of the streem with a fearful splash.

"Help!" he shreeked, as he disappeared. "I can't swim for nuts, bai Jove! Reskew, somebody!"

The Head pawsed in his flight, and returned to the bank, looking deadly white. Dr. Birchemall was a brave man; but, although the streem was only six feet wide, it was about forty feet deep, and he didn't fancy plunging in. It seemed an occasion when discretion mite prove the better part of valler.

"Reskew him, somebody!" he called out across the streem. "I can't very well do it myself, as I haven't brought a bath-towel with me! What about you, Jolly?"

But there was no need for that rekwest to be made. Jolly, like the rest of the Co. was peeling off his jacket in reddiness to take the plunge.

"Stand back, you fellows!" cride Jack Jolly modestly. "This is a job for one hero, not four!"

Splash!

An instant later he was swimming through the water in the direction of the struggling figger. An instant after that he was reskewing the half-drowned aristocratt for all he was worth. An instant after that he was climbing up the bank with his yewman burden to the plawdits of his chums. An instant after that he was applying artificial perspiration to Lord Broadacres. And an instant after that, Lord Broadacres was sitting up, fixing his streeming monocle into his eye.

"Bai Jove!" he eggsclaimed. "What bally hero reskewed me, I wondah?"

III.

BEFORE Jack Jolly had time to answer that question, someone pushed him ruffly out of the way, and answered it for him.

"Me, your lordship!" said that "someone," who, needless to say, was Dr. Birchemall. "At the risk of my very life, I plunged recklessly into the depths of the boiling waters and brought you in the teeth of the storm safely back to terra firma! Just you see how wet I got in the process!"

Jack Jolly & Co., gaping at the Head, saw that he was farely streeming with water. They realised then what had happened; the old villain had actually walked nee-deep into the streem and slooshed himself with water so as to deceeve the earl when Jack Jolly had reskewed him!

"M-m-my hat!" stuttered Jack Jolly.

But Lord Broadacres was not lissening to Jack Jolly. He was gazing through his monocle at Dr. Birchemall.

"Bai Jove!" he said. "I must say you look more like a Nero than an hero; but, if what you say is correct, I owe you a dett of grattitude, don't you know. Thanks, awfully!"

"Don't mensh!" said the Head smirking.

"But——" gasped Jack Jolly.

Lord Broadacres rose to his feet, and patted the Head on the back.

"I'm awfully sorry now about the other affair, don't you know, my brave fellow!" he remarked. "Forchunitly Fate has given me an opportunity of reckernising your trew worth, and I should like to show you how I appreciate it. Will you honner me by being my guest at the Castle for as long as you care to stay?"

The Head's fizz became one huge grin as he lisenned to those hunneyed words.

"You've sure said it, Lord Broadacres," he cried. "Let's away!"

"Hurrah!" yelled Jack Jolly, when the two had vannished.

"What are you cheering about?" asked Frank Fearless, in surprize.

Jack Jolly grinned.

"Don't you see, fathead?" he cride. "Now that the Head's a guest of a pier of the relm, he'll stick to him like glew. And, that being the case, we can finish our walking toor without the slitest fear of meeting the old buffer again. Hurrah!"

And the Co. returned to break up their camp in high spirits, convinced now that they would see no more of Dr. Alfred Birchemall till they assembulled at St. Sam's for the new term!

THE END

(Boys, you'll find another screamingly funny yarn of Jack Jolly & Co. in next week's MAGNET, *entitled: "BIRCHEMALL'S BENNYFIT!" You'll laugh until your sides fairly burst, when you read it, believe me.—*ED.)

GREYFRIARS FACTS WHILE YOU WAIT.

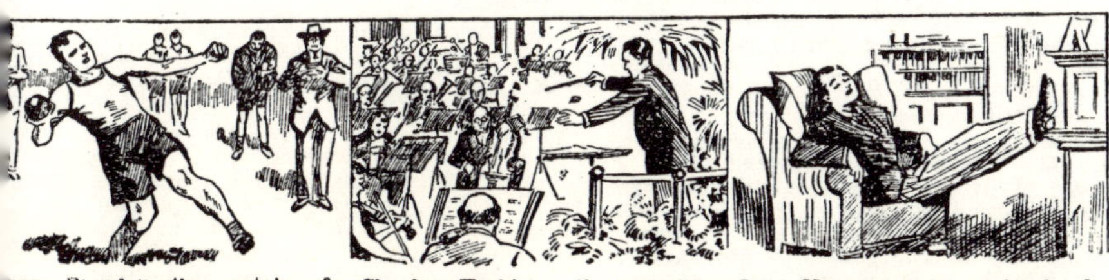

orge Blundell, the captain of Fifth, is a champion at putg the weight. His record is 33 feet 1 inch.

Claude Hoskins, the musical genius of the Shell, recently conducted a new Symphony composed by himself.

Lord Mauleverer has not missed his after-dinner "nap" for terms and terms and terms! He'll be caught "napping" one day!

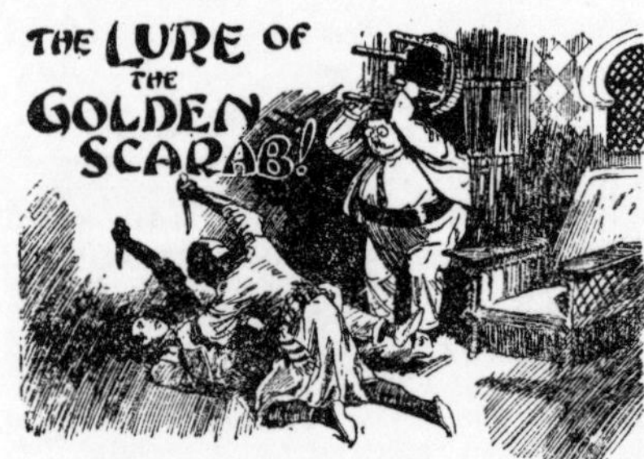

(*Continued from page 13.*)

But if Mauly was telling Mohammed to stop, as no doubt he was, the donkey-driver heeded him no more than he had heeded Hassan. Instead of stopping, Mohammed grasped the donkey's reins, and led him at a gallop round a fold in the sand, which hid donkey and rider and donkey-boy from the eyes of the juniors behind.

"What the thump——" exclaimed Nugent.

"Son of pigs!" exclaimed Hassan. "What does he do? He is the most stupid donkey-boy in all Egypt!"

Wharton compressed his lips.

"Get after him, you fellows!" he said. "We mustn't let Mauly get out of our sight!"

The Famous Five drove on their donkeys as fast as the animals could go. They rounded the ridge of sand where Mauleverer had disappeared, expecting to see him again.

But they did not see him.

Ridge on ridge, fold on fold, of sand met their eyes, stretching away towards a low range of barren, sun-scorched cliffs. Somewhere behind the ridges of sand Lord Mauleverer had disappeared, with the white donkey and his driver.

Hardly a couple of miles from the Pyramids and the Sphinx, where tourists were staring and snapshotting, and bedouins and dragomans babbling and gabbling, the schoolboy earl of Greyfriars had vanished into the desert, and the silent waste of sand had swallowed him from the sight of his friends.

THE NINTH CHAPTER.

Trapped!

"K-K-ALIZELOS!"

Lord Mauleverer fairly gasped.

The action of Mohammed, the donkey-boy, in seizing the donkey's bridle and leading him onward instead of stopping, had taken Mauly by surprise. He rapped out a sharp order to the donkey-boy, but Mohammed did not heed; he ran at full speed beside the galloping white donkey, and they were going so fast now that Mauly had to take care not to be tossed out of the saddle. A fall on the rough sand would have been extremely painful.

Lord Mauleverer, looking back, saw only a high ridge of sand, which hid his friends from his sight, and though he was not alarmed, he was determined to stop till they came up, and he strove to drag in the donkey. From a hollow of the sand, a sort of gully that sank between sand-drifted rocks, a man leaped suddenly and caught at his arm.

In sheer amazement, Lord Mauleverer recognised the jetty-eyed, olive-skinned Kalizelos—the Greek of Cairo, who had travelled to far-off England in quest of the scarab of A-Menah, and who had followed the Greyfriars party back to Egypt, seeking it still.

As Mauleverer stared at him, and stuttered his name, Kalizelos dragged at his arm, and wrenched him from the saddle.

Mohammed, the donkey-boy, did not stop.

The white donkey galloped on, Mohammed running swiftly at his side, and they vanished among the sand dunes almost in a moment.

That Mohammed had led him into a trap was plain enough; but now that he had delivered the goods, as it were, Kalizelos had no further need of him, and donkey-boy and donkey vanished together.

Lord Mauleverer sprawled on the ground, the Greek bending over him, the hoof-beats of the donkey dying away in the distance.

There was a mocking grin on the handsome, olive face of the Greek, and triumph glittered in his jet-black eyes.

"Yussef!" he called sharply.

A thick-set Arab emerged from the gully. Lord Mauleverer, as he struggled with the Greek, recognised him. It was the man who had attacked him in the hotel at Cairo, the man who had been in talk with Hassan, the dragoman, on the summit of the Great Pyramid.

Kalizelos rapped out a sharp order in Arabic. The muscular Yussef grasped Mauleverer, and Kalizelos, lending his aid, the schoolboy was dragged down into the gully.

The hoof-beats of Mohammed's donkey had died out; but from another direction hoof-beats could be heard. Harry Wharton & Co., though still out of sight beyond the sand-ridge, were drawing nearer.

Yussef had drawn a dingy linen clout over Mauleverer's mouth to gag him, and in silence the two rascals lifted the schoolboy and carried him farther down the gully.

They did not go far, however. They stopped where several squared masses of old yellow limestone—evidently part of an ancient building buried in the sand—cropped up. Kalizelos and Yussef crouched among the old blocks of stone, holding Mauleverer down between them.

Clatter, clatter, clatter! sounded the donkeys' hoofs on the hard sand, clattering past the end of the sunken gully at a distance of not more than twenty yards.

Lord Mauleverer listened, his heart beating painfully.

He was powerless to struggle or cry out, but surely his friends would find him, and the Famous Five, with the assistance of the muscular Hassan, would be more than a match for these two scoundrels who had kidnapped him.

But the grin of Yussef's face, the sneer on that of Kalizelos, were not reassuring.

Clatter, clatter, clatter! The sound grew louder—and then fainter, fainter, and fainter!

Mauleverer could have groaned.

His friends had ridden on past the end of the gully. He had been out of their sight when he was seized, and they did not dream that he was dismounted, and held in lawless hands, so close to them. The tracks of Mohammed and his donkey led onward into the desert, winding among the sand-dunes, and the Greyfriars fellows were naturally following. Even if they guessed yet that something had happened to Mauleverer, that the donkey-boy was treacherous, it was the track of the donkey that they would follow in search of him.

They were not likely to overtake it. Lord Mauleverer remembered, with a pang of dismay, that he had been the best-mounted in the party—the white donkey of Mohammed had been worth twice any of the others. Mohammed could lead the pursuers a dance as long as he liked.

Not till the clattering hoof-beats had died away did Kalizelos and Yussef rise and drag Mauleverer to his feet. The rag was removed from his mouth, allowing him to speak; but he did not think of shouting. His friends were beyond hearing now.

"At last, my lord!" grinned the Greek. "You are in my hands at last!"

"Yaas," said Lord Mauleverer. "Looks like it, old bean." Mauleverer was well aware that he was in the deadliest danger, but he was quite cool.

"The scarab, my lord!" Kalizelos held out his hand. "The scarab—and you may rejoin your friends as soon as you please."

Lord Mauleverer smiled.

"You've rather beaten yourself, you rascal!" he remarked.

"What do you mean?" snarled the Greek, his black eyes gittering at the schoolboy earl. "I warn you not to trifle with me!"

"I mean exactly what I say," drawled Lord Mauleverer. "I had the scarab in my pocket this mornin' when that black-jowled pal of yours tackled me in the hotel. I should have brought it out with me if that hadn't happened. But, you see, my friends made me leave it indoors for safety—and I'm jolly glad they did now! They fancied I wasn't safe carryin' it—and it looks as if they were right, what?"

Kalizelos spoke to Yussef in Arabic, and the hawk-faced Arab proceeded to search Lord Mauleverer. Mauly submitted quietly; there was no help for it in the hands of the two rascals. Yussef's thievish brown fingers did their work swiftly and thoroughly; but the result was only to prove that the Golden Scarab was not on the prisoner.

THE TENTH CHAPTER.

No Surrender!

KONSTANTINOS KALIZELOS gritted his teeth.

"You left the scarab in Cairo?" he asked.

"Yaas."

"With your guardian, the old man Brooke?"

"No!"

"The truth!" hissed Kalizelos.

Lord Mauleverer's lip curled.

"My dear man," he said contemptuously, "I shall tell you the truth or nothin'. You surely don't take me for a lyin' rascal like yourself, Mr. Kalizelos?"

"Take care!" muttered the Greek, clenching his hands. "If you have parted with the scarab you have left it with your guardian——"

"Not in the least, old bean! You've been so jolly active after that jolly old scarab, you see," explained Mauleverer. "My uncle's an old man, and I wasn't going to land him in danger from you and your gang. He's advised me several times to let him have charge of the scarab, but I wasn't lettin' him in for anythin' of the sort."

"Then where have you left it? In whose hands?"

"Find out," answered Lord Mauleverer coolly.

"It is usual to hand valuables over to the hotel manager, to be locked in the safe," said Kalizelos. "Is that what you have done?"

That, as a matter of fact, was exactly what Lord Mauleverer had done, though he would hardly have taken the trouble had not Harry Wharton insisted, and walked him off to the manager's room for the purpose.

But he had no intention of telling Kalizelos so.

"I've told you to find out," he answered.

"Will you answer me?"

"No, I won't," said Lord Mauleverer coolly. "The Golden Scarab of A-Menah belongs to me, and belonged to my father before me. Accordin' to your account, it's a clue to a treasure—worth a quarter of a million pounds. I'm not a stingy chap, I hope; but I'm not makin' you presents to that tune, Mr. Kalizelos. You're never goin' to get your hands on that scarab."

"We shall see!" muttered the Greek. "You are in my hands now, Lord Mauleverer! I have failed many times—at Mauleverer Towers in your own country, at Naples, in Alexandria, and in Cairo. Here in the Libyan Desert I have succeeded! Your life for the scarab!"

"Go and eat coke!"

"Your guardian, Sir Reginald Brooke, may make a different answer," sneered the Greek. "He will receive a letter from you, my lord, asking him to hand over the Golden Scarab to my messenger, as a ransom for your life and liberty. What will the old man Brooke do in answer to such a letter?"

"I rather fancy he would hand over the scarab, dear man, if I wrote an' asked him to. But I'm not goin' to write."

"You think not?" sneered Kalizelos.

"I'm quite sure not," yawned Mauleverer.

"We shall see, my lord! To-morrow your answer will be changed, I think."

"I hope I shall be seein' the last of you before to-morrow," said Lord Mauleverer. "You've got me here; but my friends will be searchin' for me, and they'll guess pretty soon what has happened. They'll start every jolly old Arab within a mile of the Pyramids huntin' for me—and every jolly old Arab in the desert, for that matter. You know your own jolly old country, Mr. Kalizelos, and so you know that every Arab in Egypt will jump on his hind legs and hunt for me at the word 'backsheesh.'" Mauleverer grinned. "You've got me here, but you can't get me away!"

"That is true," said Kalizelos. "If I carried you away into the desert, Lord Mauleverer, you would not remain long in my hands. The offer of a reward would set hundreds—nay, thousands—of greedy Arabs searching for you. But it is not my intention to carry you away into the desert. My plans have been laid, as you will see."

The Greek spoke again in Arabic. Yussef stepped to one of the blocks of limestone, and, to Mauleverer's astonishment, grasped it in his brawny hands. The muscular Arab exerted his strength, and the limestone block rolled aside, revealing a narrow, oblong opening in the pile of masonry behind.

It was the entrance to an ancient tomb, half buried in the sand.

Kalizelos pointed to the opening.

"Enter, my lord!" he said mockingly. "If you are curious about the antiquities of this strange land, you may spend your time exploring this tomb, where mummies still remain that have lain hidden from all knowledge for 3,000 years. But perhaps your lordship will not care to explore in the dark—and I regret that I can leave you no light! Do not fancy that you may be found here, my lord; this lost tomb is known only to me and to my friends."

"Oh gad!" murmured Mauleverer.

"All the backsheesh in Egypt will not cause you to be found here," grinned Kalizelos. "And Yussef will remain, with orders to drive his dagger to your heart if there should be a chance of rescue. But that, as you will see for yourself, is not likely."

Lord Mauleverer was silent, gazing at the gloomy portal of the half-buried tomb.

"Perhaps your lordship would prefer to write?" sneered Kalizelos.

"Never!"

"In twenty-four hours, I think, your lordship will give a different answer," said Kalizelos. "I can wait—and we shall see! Now enter!"

Mauleverer clenched his hands hard. He knew now that there was no hope of rescue by his friends. In that lost tomb, unknown even to the guides who plied their trade at the Pyramids, he could never be found. The cunning Greek's plans had been carefully laid, and the schoolboy earl was trapped.

But it was futile to struggle. In the grasp of the Greek and the Arab, Mauleverer—fiercely resisting, but overpowered—went staggering through the narrow door of the tomb.

Only a square apartment cut in the solid rock met his eyes as he stared round him in the glimmer of sunlight that came in at the narrow door.

There were signs of occupation, however. A bed of rugs lay in a corner, and there was a lamp; utensils of various sorts, and canned food and fruit. It was evident that the lost tomb was used at times as a retreat and a den by some thief of the desert. Mauly had heard that dwellings in old tombs were not unknown in Egypt. On the farther side of the rock-room steps led downward into utter darkness.

"That is your way, my lord," said Kalizelos, pointing to the steps.

Mauleverer repressed a shudder.

All signs of burial of the dead had been removed from the rock-room in which he stood. But he had no doubt that below, all was left as in ancient days—sarcophagi and mummies.

"Descend!" grinned Kalizelos. "Unless your lordship will write——"

"Go and eat coke!"

Lord Mauleverer descended the dark steps without waiting to be handled again. At the foot he stood in darkness.

Above he heard a muttering in Arabic, then a thud as the great block of limestone at the door of the tomb was closed.

The sound struck him like a knell.

Even if he could have reached it to make the attempt, he knew that he could not have moved that huge block. Yussef, who had twice his strength, had had to exert every ounce of it. Mauleverer could not have stirred it an inch.

Not that he could have made the attempt, with the Arab on guard. In the upper chamber of the tomb remained Yussef. There was the camp of the hawk-faced Arab. He had light, food, drink—all he needed—and no doubt he was well paid for his services by the Greek. Mauleverer heard him moving about, and presently caught the scent of tobacco as the Arab lighted his Turkish pipe and smoked.

To ascend the steps and enter into a conflict with an armed and powerful ruffian was futile. Mauleverer's courage did not falter, but his face was grave and a little pale as he peered about him in the darkness of the lower tomb and groped in the gloom.

His hand came into contact with cold stone; he felt over the top of an ancient sarcophagus, from which the stone lid was gone. His hand touched something else, and he knew that it was a mummified body resting where it had rested for uncounted centuries. He jerked his hand away, shuddering.

"Good gad!" murmured Mauleverer.

He sat down at last on the lowest step. Escape was impossible; rescue seemed scarcely possible; there was no hope.

The Golden Scarab, which was said—and believed by Kalizelos—to be the clue to the treasure of Osiris, had led him to his death among the long-forgotten dead! Only the surrender of the scarab of A-Menah to the plotting Greek could save him! What would be his answer to the cunning Greek after a night and a day in that dim recess of shadows and death? Lord Mauleverer set his teeth as he asked himself that question. Konstantinos Kalizelos could do his worst, but he would never surrender.

THE ELEVENTH CHAPTER.

Missing!

HILMI MAROUDI, the rich Egyptian of Cairo, smiled.

Snore!

The sound was not musical.

And Billy Bunter, as he sprawled in the low chair in the shade of the tree, with his fat little legs stretched out, his eyes shut, and his mouth open, could not have been considered an object of beauty.

But Hilmi Maroudi smiled; while Sir Reginald Brooke gave a slight grunt. The plump Egyptian gentleman, and the stiff old English baronet, stood looking at Billy Bunter. Under the shade of the tree near Mena House, in sight of the towering Pyramids, Billy Bunter was enjoying his sojourn in Egypt in his own way.

Sunset glowed on the Pyramids and the Sphinx—the glorious sunset of Egypt. The radiance of gold in the sky was like the glow of burnished metal. It was quite lost on William George Bunter, who probably would not have wasted a blink on it had he been awake.

And he was fast asleep. He had wakened for tea—and he had disposed of a tea that made the waiters open their eyes. After which, as the other fellows had not yet returned, Bunter went to sleep again. Bunter could do with a great deal of sleep. He could do with more than usual, in the hot climate of Egypt. Fellows who wanted to root about mouldy old temples and tombs, could root about mouldy old temples and tombs—Billy Bunter preferred a long, cane chair, and a nap in the shade. Unconscious of the passage of time, Bunter snored on cheerily, and the two men, brown and white, stood looking at him, one smiling, the other grunting.

"This, I think, is our little fat friend," said Hilmi Maroudi.

"It is Bunter!" grunted Sir Reginald. "But he seems to be alone here—where are the others?"

There was a slight shade of anxiety on the old baronet's brow.

It had been arranged for the party at the Pyramids to return to Cairo before sunset. Hassan, the dragoman, had been specially instructed, and hitherto Hassan had been absolutely exemplary in carrying out his instructions. But the party had not returned.

Sir Reginald had spent a very pleasant day at the house of Maroudi in Cairo, while his youthful charges were seeing the sights of Egypt in the care of the faithful Hassan. He had visited the rich Egyptian's collection of antiquities, and discussed with him farming in the Fayyum—in which fertile district the old baronet had an estate adjoining Maroudi's. The Egyptian gentleman had driven back with him to his hotel to dine with him and the Greyfriars party. And there they found that Hassan and the juniors had not come back.

Maroudi, whom the juniors had met on the boat coming out to Alexandria, was a plump and good-natured gentleman, and he had taken a liking to the cheery party of schoolboys—especially Harry Wharton, whom he had saved from being washed overboard in the squall on the Mediterranean. His servant Ali had attempted to purloin the Golden Scarab, and endangered Wharton's life; for which reason, Mr. Maroudi seemed to consider that it was up to him to do everything in his power for the Greyfriars fellows. They had met him several times in Cairo, and found him very agreeable, and he was tolerant even of Billy Bunter, though that fat and fatuous youth hardly concealed the fact that he looked on the wealthy Egyptian gentleman as a "nigger"—merely that, and nothing more. Bunter, no doubt, would have been indignant had he known that the nigger found him very amusing.

As the juniors had not returned to Cairo, Mr. Maroudi proposed driving out to the Pyramids to pick them up; and on the way Sir Reginald had looked out rather anxiously for the juniors' car.

But it had not been seen; and on arriving at Mena House, they found that the car was still parked there, and that Hassan and the juniors were still absent on an excursion.

They learned, however, that one member of the party was in the garden, and went to look for him. Now they had found him. From quite a distance Billy Bunter's hefty snore guided them to the spot.

"I suppose they left Bunter here—he is a very lazy boy," said Sir Reginald. "But, where are they?"

"Perhaps Bunter can tell us," suggested Mr. Maroudi.

"I am feeling a little uneasy," said Sir Reginald. "The boys, of course, are safe with the dragoman—he was well recommended. But——"

"You are thinking of the Greek, Kalizelos?"

"Well, yes," said Sir Reginald. "The rascal has fled from Cairo to escape arrest, and I have no doubt that he is at a safe distance, and there is nothing now to fear from him. Nevertheless——"

The old gentleman broke off with a worried look. Since Kalizelos had disappeared from Cairo, he had concluded that the rascally Greek was done with. But he was feeling uneasy now.

Snore!

Bunter was going strong.

"The fact is, the hotel manager informed me that some hotel thief entered my nephew's room this morning while I was absent," said Sir Reginald. "It may be a trivial matter, but—in view of the fact that the boys have not returned——"

He stooped over Bunter, grasped him by a fat shoulder, and shook him.

"Beast!" murmured Bunter.

Shake.

"Urrrggh! Lemme alone! 'Tain't rising-bell, you rotter!" mumbled Bunter. "I'm not getting up yet, and you can tell Quelch so, blow him!"

Shake! Shake!

Billy Bunter's little round eyes opened at last, behind his big round spectacles. He blinked peevishly.

"Can't you let a fellow sleep?" he growled.

"Bunter!" rapped Sir Reginald. "Wake up at once!"

"Oh! It's you?" grunted Bunter. He blinked at Mauly's uncle, and then at Mr. Maroudi. "Have they come back? It must be time for dinner—I'm getting hungry." Bunter removed his spectacles, rubbed his sleepy eyes, and replaced the spectacles on his fat little nose, and grunted again. He had not awakened in a good temper. Two or three lunches, with two or three teas added, "peeved" the fat junior a little. "Just like the rotters—clearing off, and leaving a fellow on his own! After all I've done for them——"

"Where are my nephew and his friends, Bunter?"

"How should I know?" grunted Bunter. "They refused to wait for me—I told them I should keep them only a couple of hours, but they refused to wait! Blow 'em! I've no doubt they've run into some trouble, like they always do when I'm not looking after them. I dare say that beast Yussef has got after them. Serve them right!"

"Yussef! Who is Yussef?" snapped Sir Reginald.

"That Arab beast who got after Mauly this morning in the hotel," grunted Bunter. "The beast who wanted to pinch that rotten, silly scarab."

Mr. Hilmi Maroudi's face became very grave. Sir Reginald started.

"Tell me at once what happened to my nephew this morning, Bunter!" he snapped. "I have heard that a thief entered his room; that is all."

Bunter grunted it out.

"Then—there is no doubt that it was another attempt to steal the scarab," exclaimed Sir Reginald, when the fat Owl had finished. "Have you seen the man since, Bunter?"

"I spotted him," said Bunter. "The other fellows never noticed him, of course—they never see anything. I spotted him talking to Hassan, and told them—but they let him get away! Just like them!"

"He was talking to Hassan, the dragoman?" asked Mr. Maroudi.

"Yes; in that idiotic, jaw-cracking language they speak in this country," grunted Bunter. "Hassan said he was named Yussef, and was a donkey-man—and wanted us to hire his donkeys! But he cleared off jolly fast when I spotted him and gave the fellows the tip."

Sir Reginald compressed his lips.

"If some rascal employed by Kalizelos is in this vicinity, the boys may be in danger!" he said. "Do you know where they went, Bunter?"

"They went to the Sphinx, and to see some putrid tombs, or something," answered Bunter. "They said they'd be back in a couple of hours." He blinked at his watch. "That was more than four hours ago! Lot they care about leaving a chap on his own all this time—fat lot!"

"Yet, there could scarcely be danger, among so many tourists and guides, and other natives," said Sir Reginald slowly. "And I gave Hassan the most careful instructions not to take the boys into any lonely place."

Mr. Maroudi looked at him. He seemed about to speak, but checked himself.

"I say, are you going back to Cairo?" asked Bunter.

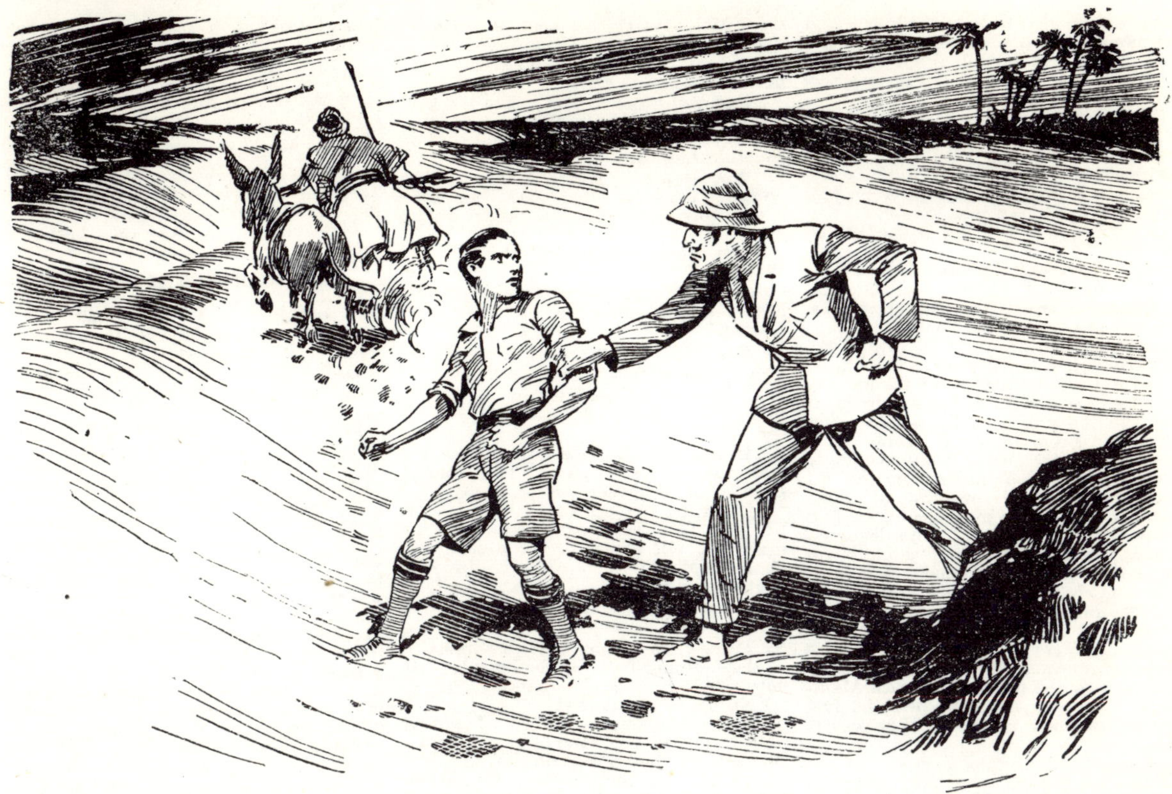

Kalizelos suddenly leaped out from a hollow in the sand, dragged at Mauleverer's arm, and wrenched him from the saddle. The next moment the hoofbeats of the donkey were dying away in the distance !

"We can scarcely go without my nephew and his friends, Bunter."

"But we shall be late for dinner at the hotel."

"That matters very little."

"Eh?" Bunter blinked at him. "But I'm hungry! Didn't you hear me say that I'm hungry?"

"Nonsense!"

"They can follow, I suppose?" said Bunter, with a grunt. "If they've lost themselves, what can they expect—going off without me? If that beast Yussef is after them, they've jolly well asked for it. I think——"

Sir Reginald did not appear to be interested in what Bunter thought. He made the fat junior a gesture to be silent. With a troubled brow he stood looking past the Pyramids towards the desert. The sunset was deepening to dark — tourists, guides, backsheesh-hunting Arabs, were coming in, but the Greyfriars fellows were not to be seen among them. A silver glimmer of the moon crept up over the Nile.

Leaving Bunter grunting, and wondering when on earth he was going to get any dinner, Sir Reginald and Mr. Maroudi walked down the road towards the Pyramids. That was the way the Greyfriars juniors would come when they came, and if they came. They passed the Great Pyramid and the Sphinx, glimmering strangely in the moonlight. Sir Reginald, with knitted brows, was thinking of Hassan the dragoman's carelessness, in having allowed his charges to wander from the beaten track. Mr. Hilmi Maroudi was also thinking of Hassan—but not of his carelessness. He was thinking of the circumstance that Yussef, the agent of Kalizelos, had been in talk with the dragoman on the Great Pyramid, as he had learned from Billy Bunter. And there were thoughts in the Egyptian's mind that he did not communicate to his companion.

Clatter! Clatter! Clatter!

It was a thudding of donkeys' hoofs on the road from the desert, and a bunch of riders came dimly in sight in the moonlight.

Sir Reginald uttered an exclamation of relief.

"They are coming!"

Hilmi Maroudi did not speak.

THE TWELFTH CHAPTER.

Lost!

"MAULY!"

"Mauleverer, old man!"

"Mauly!"

Harry Wharton & Co. shouted, and shouted again, and their voices rang and echoed among the sand dunes.

For an hour or more the Famous Five had ridden as fast as the donkeys could go on the track of Mohammed and the white donkey.

The sticks of the donkey-boys whacked and whacked, and cracked and cracked, and the juniors uttered no word of remonstrance now—they were too anxious to come up with their lost comrade.

Hassan, the dragoman, with the golden tassel of his red tarboosh dancing, kept pace with the donkeys.

For many miles it was easy to see which way the white donkey had gone. But not once did the juniors catch sight of it.

Round about them lay many hard, rocky tracts, where the footprints of donkey and donkey-boy might easily have been lost. But Mohammed and the white donkey seemed specially to have kept where the sand was soft, and left an unmistakable trail.

It was a trail that there was not the slightest difficulty in following—even at a gallop twice as fast as that of which the Cairo donkeys were capable.

It did not occur to the juniors that Mohammed had intentionally picked the soft sand to leave that trail and lead them farther and farther away from the comrade they sought.

What had happened was a mystery to them—they had seen nothing of Mauleverer or the donkey-boy or of the donkey since the three had vanished from sight beyond a ridge of sand—and they knew that there was no chance of overtaking the powerful white donkey on their own inferior mounts unless its rider chose.

But it was impossible to imagine that Mauleverer was deliberately leading them a dance. They remembered how Mohammed had grasped the rein and led the donkey out of their sight. And the suspicion was strong in their minds that Mohammed, the donkey-boy, was leading Mauleverer away into the desert for his own reasons—from which it did not take long to reach the conclusion that the brown-faced rascal was in the pay of Kalizelos. It was rather perplexing that Mauleverer went quietly, and they wondered whether a blow from the donkey-boy's stick had stunned him and put it out of his power to resist. But they did not suspect that Mauleverer was no longer on the white donkey, and that every stride of their steeds took them farther and farther away from him.

It was at a distance of four miles from the lost tombs that the trail failed at last. Not once had they sighted Mohammed—he had kept out of sight among the dunes all the time, till he reached the low range of hills in the west. There, still unseen, he was lost to all knowledge; on the hard rock there was no sign to be picked up. And the juniors came to a halt in dismay, and shouted and shouted again the name of Mauleverer till the rocks rang and echoed round them.

But only the echoes replied.

The weary donkeys were glad enough to halt, and the donkey-boys also. Both lay down to rest when the juniors dismounted to attempt to pick up some sign of their missing comrade.

But there was no sign to be picked up.

The hard rocks left no trace.

Mohammed and the white donkey had disappeared into the rocky, sandy hills, and the juniors had no doubt that Lord Mauleverer had disappeared with them. The Greek had laid his plans cunningly.

There would be search for the missing schoolboy—search in which hundreds, if not thousands of Arabs would join, tempted by the offer of liberal backsheesh. But the search would begin in the rocky hills, four miles from the lost tombs, where Mauleverer was a hidden prisoner. Thus far the juniors had followed the trail of Mauleverer's mount, and there the search would begin and go farther and farther. Who was to dream that all the time the missing boy was hidden in a tomb within sight of the summit of the Pyramid of Cheops? Certainly Harry Wharton & Co. did not dream of guessing it—they had seen only Mohammed, the donkey-boy with Mauleverer, and had no doubt that he had led his prisoner away into the desert hills.

"Mauly!"

Bob Cherry gave a last ringing shout, that rolled back in a thousand echoes from the hollows of the hills.

But it was clear now that Mauleverer was not within hearing, or that if he was within hearing he could not speak.

Round the juniors were a thousand rocky nooks and recesses in which the missing boy and his kidnapper might have been hidden.

Harry Wharton set his teeth.

"We've lost him!" he muttered. "There's one comfort—we made him leave the scarab behind—the scoundrels haven't got hold of that. But—but poor old Mauly——"

"Oh, my lordly gentlemen!" murmured Hassan, beating his breast. "What shall I say? What shall I do? The lordly one is lost, and the magnificent gentleman Brooke will say it is the fault of Hassan! Woe is me!"

"You're not to blame, Hassan," said Bob Cherry kindly. "I suppose you couldn't be expected to guess that that villain of a donkey-boy was put up to this."

"The blamefulness of the estemed Hassan is not terrific," agreed Hurree Jamset Ram Singh.

Hassan beat his breast and almost wept.

"If my honourable lords forgive me, can I forgive myself?" he wailed. "I Hassan, the son of Suleiman, have lost a noble lord who was in my charge? I am a dog, and the son of a dog, and the grandfather of pigs! I am ruined—for who will trust Hassan again? Woe is upon me!"

And the faithful Hassan bowed his head, tore off his tarboosh, and sprinkled dust upon his greasy hair.

The donkey-boys watched him stolidly. The juniors, even in their deep anxiety for Mauleverer, could not help feeling sorry for the dragoman. They could not see that Hassan was to blame. He had engaged donkeys and donkey-boys for the ride, as was his dragoman duty, Mohammed with the rest. The rest had done their service faithfully enough; only Mohammed had been a traitor—and no dragoman could be expected to guess that one of the donkey-boys had been bribed to treachery.

"Buck up, old bean!" said Nugent comfortingly. "We don't blame you—and Sir Reginald Brooke won't! You couldn't help it."

"Woe is me!" wailed Hassan dolorously. "I am covered with shame as with a garment! I am a ruined dragoman."

"The question is to find Mauly," said Wharton. "We've lost him—and we can do no more here. You've no idea where Mohammed would be making for, Hassan?"

"Yes, lord!" answered Hassan. "He go into the desert, many, many miles—only far away in the desert will he be safe—far, far away in the Libyan Desert, my noble lord!"

"It was unlucky that Mauly was the best mounted in the party," said Johnny Bull. "But for that——"

"Can't be helped now," said Harry. "I suppose Hassan's right, and the scoundrel will make for the desert with poor old Mauly. I dare say Kalizelos is waiting for him there, miles away."

Hassan started a little at the mention of the Greek's name.

"There's no doubt that Kalizelos is at the bottom of it," said Nugent. "He must have bribed the donkey-boy——"

"No doubt about that!"

Harry Wharton stared round almost desperately at the sand and the rocks. The sun was low now, and darkness was at hand. Further search for Mauleverer was obviously hopeless; but it was bitter to turn back and leave him in the hands of his enemies. Yet clearly the only thing to be done was to get back to Mena House, and to report the kidnapping to the Egyptian police officer on duty at the Pyramids. That was the first step; and then to hurry back to Cairo and inform Sir Reginald Brooke. Bitter as it was to turn back, it was useless to lose more time.

"Let's get back!" said Harry at last. "The sooner the search begins, the better—and we're losing time."

With heavy hearts the juniors returned to the donkeys and mounted. The donkey-boys dragged themselves to their feet, and the sticks whacked and cracked again.

It was a weary ride back to the Pyramids. The moon came up over the desert, sailing bright and clear over the Nile. In other circumstances, a moonlight ride in the desert, with the Pyramids looming ghost-like in the silvery glimmer, would have been enjoyable. But the chums of the Remove were thinking now only of their missing comrade. They pictured him, bound to Mohammed's donkey, carried farther and farther into the trackless desert, and that mental picture was a torment. If it was a comfort to know that the villain who had kidnapped him had not been able to lay hands on the Golden Scarab, it was very little comfort. They would have given all the treasures in ancient Egypt, thrice told, for the sight of Mauleverer safe and sound.

Bitter as their anxiety was, the juniors were silent as they rode. But Hassan was not silent. His lamentations and self-reproaches were incessant. He repeated again and again that the noble lord was far, far away, in the untrodden desert, far away in the trackless sands. It did not occur to the juniors that the faithful Hassan might have any reason for impressing that belief on their minds. There was dust on Hassan's head, and deep grief and sorrow in his brown face, and his lamentations made an incessant accompaniment to the thudding of the donkeys' hoofs.

The Sphinx came in sight—towering, shadowy, eerily majestic in the moonlight. Bob Cherry gave a sudden shout at the sight of two figures on the road.

"Hallo, hallo, hallo!"

"What——"

"Mauly's uncle—and who's that with him—Mr. Maroudi! Hold on!"

The donkeys clattered to a halt.

THE THIRTEENTH CHAPTER.

The Knocking on the Tomb!

LORD MAULEVERER rose to his feet wearily.

Darkness and silence encircled him—the darkness and silence of the tomb.

For hours—how many hours he could not guess—he had moved about his stony prison; groping, seeking in the darkness. There was little chance that there was another outlet, beside the one guarded by Yussef, the Arab; but anything was better than inaction, and Mauleverer groped and searched in the thick darkness till his limbs were weary.

Stone walls met his hands when he groped; stone walls on all sides. If he found an opening it proved to be only a recess, a niche in the rock-wall where a sarcophagus lay; and more than once his shivering fingers touched a mummy, or the fragment of a mummy, in the clinging gloom. If there had been another outlet it was blocked up now; and he gave it up at last, and sat down on the steps to rest, weary in body and mind. Whether it was still day or night he could not tell; but it seemed to him that a long, long time had passed.

In the rock-chamber at the head of the stone stair there was a glimmer of lamplight; hardly a ray of which penetrated to Lord Mauleverer's prison. But, as he sat silent and weary, there came to his ears a sound from above—the unmistakable sound of someone snoring. And it dawned on him that Yussef was sleeping.

He stood by the stone steps, listening. At length, without a sound, treading on tiptoe, he mounted the steps and looked into the upper rock-room of the tomb.

The lamp burned there, and the air was heavy and stuffy. Yussef lay on the rugs, his hawk-eyes closed in sleep.

Mauleverer's heart beat.

His glance passed Yussef to the narrow portal of the tomb; blocked by the great mass of squared limestone.

He could not move that huge block; he remembered how the muscular Arab had been forced to exert his strength to move it. Whether the watcher slumbered or wakened, Mauleverer was a prisoner in the lost tomb. But hopeless as the attempt seemed, he resolved to make it. Softly he stepped from the stone stair into the upper room, giving the sleeping Arab as wide a berth as he could.

He reached the portal; and a glance back at Yussef showed the hawk-faced Arab still asleep.

Mauleverer put his shoulder to the block, and braced himself to exert all his strength.

It did not stir.

With set teeth and straining muscles he drove at it. But it was in vain. His muscles were strained almost to cracking, the perspiration poured down him in streams. But the massive stone did not move.

It came back into his mind how, when Kalizelos had shut him in the sarcophagus in the Catacombs of Alexandria, he had striven to lift the stone lid—in vain! His prison was not so narrow now—but it was as secure! Then, his comrades had found and saved him—now, they could not find him; they could not save him. Unless he could save himself, he was doomed! And again and again he strove.

Lord Mauleverer was considered a slacker at Greyfriars; a fellow almost too lazy to live! No one would have thought him a slacker now, as he strained his muscles at the stone.

But it was in vain; and he desisted at last and stood leaning on the stone he had failed to move—hot, aching, his head almost spinning. He stood and leaned, and breathed in gulps.

His eyes turned on the Arab again. Yussef was still sleeping—the wretch could sleep, knowing that there was no escape for the prisoner. The schoolboy's eyes wandered round the rock-chamber in the glimmering light of the lamp. An iron-shod staff, of some heavy Eastern wood, stood in a corner, and the schoolboy earl, with a new idea working in his mind, stepped to it quickly and grasped it. If he could use the long, heavy staff as a lever, there was a chance yet.

He gave Yussef a last look—the Arab had not stirred. Then he bent to his task at the portal. Carefully, and as silently as he could, he prodded at the base of the rock with the pointed end of the staff. And at last he found a spot where, under the block of limestone, was not rock but sand.

His eyes gleamed with hope and his heart beat as he drove the staff under the great rock. Then he threw his weight on the end.

"By gad!" breathed Mauleverer, as he felt the great block shift.

What he could not have done with his hands he was affecting by leverage. The task was hard and heavy; but he felt the great stone move. If he had the strength to topple it over—— There was a grinding sound as the limestone block lifted at its inner edge.

"Bismillah!"

Lord Mauleverer could have groaned as he heard that exclamation behind him. The sound of the stirring rock, slight as it was, had awakened the Arab.

He turned his head as he heard Yussef spring up from the rugs. The hawk-faced ruffian came across the rock-chamber at him with the spring of a tiger.

Mauleverer tore the iron-shod staff out from under the stone and swept it in the air with both hands.

"Stand back, you scoundrel!" he panted.

"Wahyat-en-nabi!" snarled Yussef, and he came on, springing.

There was a yell from the Arab as Mauleverer struck, and the heavy staff crashed on his dingy turban. Yussef reeled back yelling. But before Mauleverer could recover the staff to strike again, the Arab was upon him and grasping him, and he went down heavily on the floor of the tomb.

He struggled fiercely.

"Dog of an unbeliever!" snarled the Arab. He realised that the prisoner would have escaped, had he not awakened, and his black eyes blazed with rage. Holding the struggling schoolboy down, he caught up a rope and bound his wrists together with cruel and ruthless tightness. Then Mauleverer's ankles were bound; and the Arab rose to his feet and stood staring down at him, muttering curses in Arabic as he rubbed his bruised head.

"Dog of a kafir!" hissed Yussef. "You will not escape now."

He grasped the schoolboy earl and rolled him roughly towards the steps. With a brutal shove, he sent him rolling down, bound as he was. Mauleverer bumped from step to step till he reached the lower tomb.

There, dazed by his fall, panting for breath, he lay helpless in his bonds. The Arab stared down after him, and a cruel laugh echoed down the gloomy stair.

"Lie there, dog of an unbeliever!" snarled the Arab.

And Mauleverer heard him throw himself on the rugs again.

Mauleverer suppressed a groan.

The game was up now, and there was despair in his heart. The ropes knotted cruelly on wrists and ankles cut into his flesh; he could hardly stir a limb. He could only lie where he had fallen, helpless; in darkness and despair. How long he lay in the dead silence he never knew; but suddenly, through the brooding silence, there came a sound.

Knock!

Mauleverer started.

Knock, knock!

The knocking came from the blocked doorway of the tomb above. He heard the Arab scramble to his feet, with a startled exclamation in his own tongue.

"Bismillah!"

Knock, knock, knock!

Surely it could not be Kalizelos returning yet! Still more surely it could

(Continued on next page.)

not be help and rescue! But as Mauleverer lay in the darkness and listened, the sound brought a throb of hope to his heart.

Knock, knock, knock!

THE FOURTEENTH CHAPTER.
Hilmi Maroudi Takes a Hand!

"HERBERT!" exclaimed Sir Reginald Brooke.

In the moonlight that glimmered on the Sphinx and the ghostly Pyramids, the old baronet peered eagerly at the donkey-riders as they clattered to a halt.

It was the Greyfriars party, returning from the desert, and for the moment Mauly's uncle did not observe that there were only five of them.

But Herbert Mauleverer's voice did not answer him.

"Herbert! What—— Wharton, where is Mauleverer?" exclaimed Sir Reginald. "Hassan, where is my nephew?"

"O lordly sar!" wailed Hassan. "A donkey-boy—the son of a thousand pigs—has led the noble and magnificent one into the desert, and now he is far away in the Libyan sands——"

"Good heavens!"

Hilmi Maroudi stood silent. His eyes were on the dragoman, who was beating his breast. He did not speak, but with his keen Egyptian eyes he watched, and his thoughts were busy.

"Wharton, tell me——"

"We've searched for him—hunted for him, sir!" panted Wharton. "That's why we're late——"

"My nephew is missing?"

"Yes. In the desert——"

"You should not have gone into the desert! You——"

"We followed Mauleverer there, sir," said Bob Cherry. "We couldn't leave him to it."

"What do you mean? Do you mean that my nephew deliberately rode into the desert, or what?" exclaimed Sir Reginald.

"He got ahead of us," explained Wharton. "We were going to some tombs on the edge of the desert, and Mauly got ahead, and——"

"Why?" snapped the baronet.

"He had a good donkey, sir, and we had rather poor ones; and I'm afraid the donkey-boy must have been bribed by that scoundrel Kalizelos. He drove him on ahead quite suddenly, and refused to stop when we shouted, and—and Mauly being well mounted, we couldn't catch up with him——"

"Then where are they now?"

"In the desert, sir! We followed the track of the donkey at least four miles—as far as the hills—and lost it there."

Sir Reginald Brooke groaned. He had feared a mischance when the juniors failed to return; but at the sight of the riders on the road to the Sphinx he had been relieved. Now he learned that matters were even worse than he had feared. The five juniors returning without Mauleverer. The sands of the desert had swallowed his nephew.

"Kalizelos!" he muttered "That scoundrel—— You have seen nothing of him?"

"Nothing, sir! But it's pretty clear——"

"I fear so! I fear so! If the donkey-boy deliberately led him away into the desert, he can have had only one reason."

Sir Reginald clenched his hands hard. He stared past the juniors, at the moonlit road winding past temples and pyramids, to the Libyan Desert. In that endless, tractless waste his nephew was lost, and his heart was heavy with the fear that he would never see him again in life. But it was no time for grief; it was the time for action.

"You had better ride on to Mena House," he said. "I will go to the Pyramids Police Station at once, and then——"

"One word, my good friend," broke in the quiet, soft voice of Hilmi Maroudi. "Perhaps I may be able to help."

"Oh, sir," exclaimed Harry Wharton, with a break in his voice, "if you could help us get Mauleverer back, sir——"

"The noble gentleman, he is lost in a desert!" wailed Hassan. "I throw dust on unworthy head! I am unworthy to look my noble gentlemen in the face! I, Hassan, the son of Suleiman, have lost my noble lord!"

The plump Egyptian gentleman gave him a searching glance. Then he turned to the juniors again.

"Surely, Mr. Maroudi, the first step is to notify the police," said Sir Reginald, "and then to set every Arab in Cairo on the trail. Even in the desert that villain may be run down!"

"We can guide them to the place where we lost the trail," said Nugent. "The sand may have covered the trail by this time; but we can find the place again. Hassan can, anyhow!"

"Truly, my lord!" said the dragoman. "You trust Hassan! He is your dragoman!"

"Then that is what must be done immediately," said Sir Reginald; but he looked inquiringly at Hilmi Maroudi.

The Egyptian's dark face was grave and thoughtful.

"My good friend, you have a proverb in your language that the more haste is the less speed!" said Maroudi quietly. "Let us learn first precisely what has happened. My little friend." He addressed Harry Wharton. "It appears that the young lord left you, because he was better mounted than any of the others."

"That was it," said Harry. "Mohammed's donkey was a big, strong, swift animal, worth twice as much as ours in a run."

"The villain picked him out, of course, intending to get away with poor old Mauly all the time!" said Bob.

"No doubt," said Maroudi, with a faint smie. "But he did not pick out the others, and it was very singular and unfortunate that all the other donkeys were so inferior. But for that you would have overtaken the young lord when Mohammed carried him off."

"That's so," said Bob. "You may be sure we rode as hard as we could. But these donkeys had no chance against Mohammed's."

Hassan, the dragoman, was still beating his breast and lamenting. But his dark eyes were fixed on Hilmi Maroudi now, with a strange gleam in their depths. Something in the Egyptian's face or in his words had startled the faithful Hassan.

Maroudi stood for some moments in reflection. The juniors waited, wondering what he was thinking of; hoping against hope that Maroudi, a native of the country, had some plan in his head for dealing with the situation which had not occurred to them.

Sir Reginald Brooke watched him, with suppressed impatience. The baronet was eager to get to action; to lose not a single moment in starting a general search. "Backsheesh" would set hundreds of Arabs scouring the desert, and the juniors could lead them to the place where the trail had been lost, to begin with. It seemed to the old baronet that there was nothing else to be done.

"My dear sir!" he said at length.

"My good friend," said Maroudi, "I understand your impatience. But I beg you to give me a few moments. I am not wasting time. It is in my mind that the young lord may not be so far away as you believe." His eyes, fixed on Hassan, did not lose the dragoman's start, and he smiled grimly. "I think, my dear sir, that the young lord may be found—I think that your dragoman may be able to find him. With your permission, sir, I will speak to Hassan, and point out to him some thoughts that have entered my mind. Will you allow me?"

Sir Reginald made a gesture of assent, and the juniors could only look on in wonder. Hassan, so far as they could see, was as helpless as themselves in the matter.

Maroudi made an imperious sign to the dragoman, and stepped aside, out of hearing of the staring donkey-boys. Hassan followed him, slowly and reluctantly, a strange expression on his brown face.

When Maroudi spoke to the dragoman, he spoke in Arabic, of which the juniors would have understood nothing, and Mauleverer's uncle little, if they had heard. But his quiet voice was out of their hearing, and out of hearing of the donkey-boys. Certainly the Greyfriars fellows would have been astonished had they known what the Egyptian gentleman was saying to their faithful Hassan.

"False dog, and son of unclean pariah dogs!" said Hilmi Maroudi, his dark eyes glinting at the dragoman. "What has Kalizelos paid you to betray the young lord into his hands?"

"By the beard of the Prophet," said Hassan huskily, in the same tongue. "By the holy trousers of Mahomet, I swear——"

"Silence, kafir!" interrupted Maroudi. "Have you no fear of Allah, that you swear falsely in the name of the Prophet? Dog of a dragoman, you know me, Hilmi Maroudi! When I tell you that you shall die under blows of the kourbash in my palace in Cairo, do you believe that I will make my words good?"

Hassan bowed his head.

"I am your slave!" he said. "But I swear——"

"Listen, kafir!" said Maroudi quietly. "You have served the English lords for backsheesh faithfully until this day. This day Yussef, the son of Hamid,

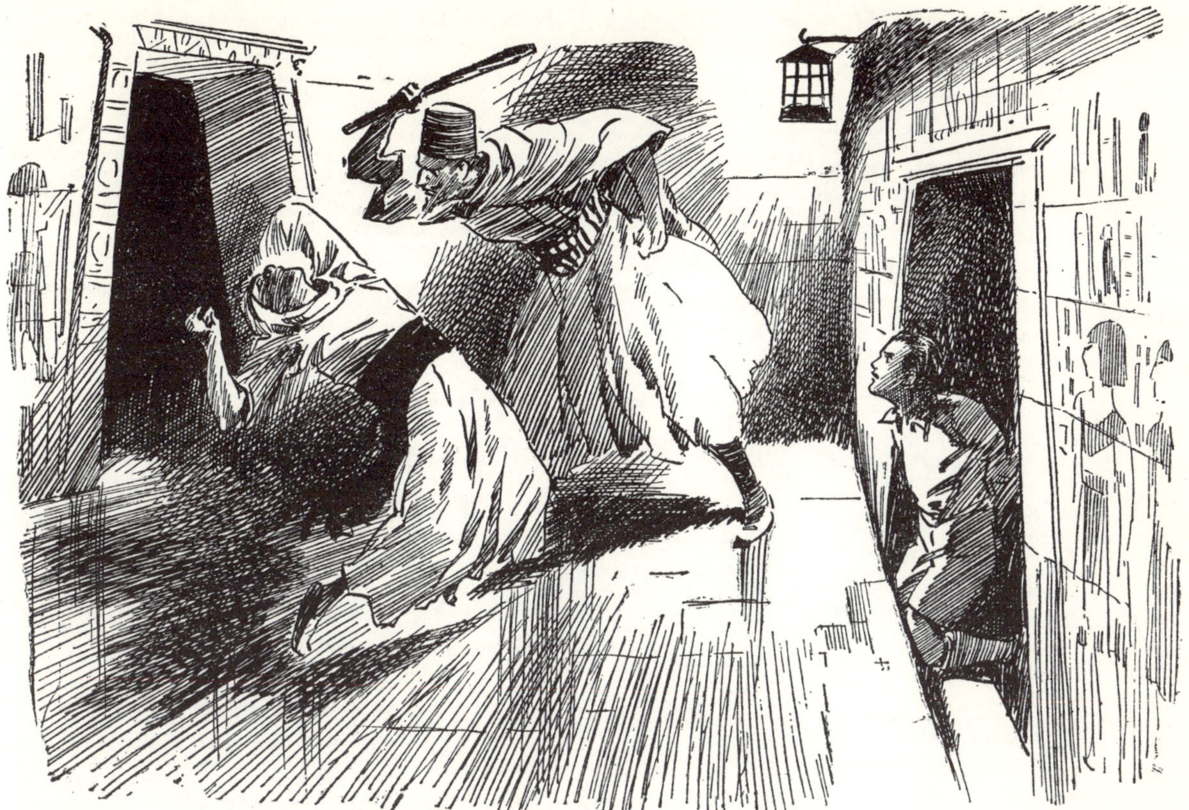

As Yussef stretched out a brown hand to take the paper, Hassan's right hand flew up, taking the ruffian completely off his guard. The next second the stick crashed on the head of Yussef, and he fell senseless at the feet of the dragoman. "Oh gad!" gasped Lord Mauleverer.

talked with you on the Pyramid of Cheops. Do not tell me that he talked of the hire of donkeys. Am I a simple Faringhee to believe you? Dog of a dragoman, he brought you word from Kalizelos, the Greek, and the offer of backsheesh, much backsheesh, to betray the young lord into his hands!"

"Lord of life and death, I swear——" groaned the dragoman.

"Give me ear, son of pariah dogs that howl in the ruins! Grandfather of unclean animals, listen! The proof is this—the young lord was placed on a powerful donkey to outpace all the others! Why, O lying kafir, did you see so carefully that his friends should not be able to overtake him when Mohammed led him into the desert? It was you, dragoman, who selected the beasts—and you selected them well for your purpose, O treacherous and unbelieving follower of the Prophet! Give me ear, Hassan, the son of Suleiman. Will the law and the judges protect you from my vengeance?"

"Lord of life and death," groaned the dragoman, "did this wretched Hassan know that your greatness concerned himself about unbelieving Faringhees? Is not the slaying of an unbeliever a good deed in the eyes of the Prophet? Have not the Ulemas said so, O master?"

"These young lords are my friends," said Hilmi Maroudi. "I am concerned for them to such a length that any man who lifts a hand against them shall feel my vengeance, even to death. If the young lord is slain, you shall die under the kourbash, and my ears shall listen to your crying during days of torment, O son of Suleiman."

"He is not slain!" interrupted Hassan eagerly. "O master, he is safe, but a captive! It is for some strange scar b—some miserable relic, that the Greek has taken him. He is to be ransomed by that which Kalizelos seeks!"

"That also is known to me," said Maroudi. "But he will not be ransomed, dragoman—he will be set free, and given back to his friends, and on your head be it! Give me ear, son of dogs! Here I will wait, in the shadow of the Sphinx, till you shall return with the young lord! Bring him safely to me, and you shall have twice what the Greek offered, whatever the sum—fail to bring him and you shall die by torture under the kourbash!"

Hassan's eyes snapped.

"Lord, the Greek, whom may the dogs devour for displeasing your greatness, offered the sum of five hundred Egyptian pounds, which, in piastres, is an immense fortune."

"Twice five hundred Egyptian pounds shall be yours, son of Suleiman, when the young lord is safe with his friends!"

"On my head be it!" said the dragoman. "But yet one thing I will ask, O master of death and life! Let not these foolish Faringhees know what is known to your greatness, or I am a ruined dragoman."

Maroudi made a gesture of contempt.

"Listen, kafir!" he said. "You shall serve my friends as a dragoman while they remain in my country, and you shall serve them faithfully! The eye of Maroudi will be upon you! Take from them all the backsheesh they will give, for it is your trade; but serve them faithfully, and protect them from dangers. Be this on your head, son of Suleiman. Fail in your trust, and you shall surely die!"

"I will be faithful to the Faringhees, lord, now that I know what is your will," said the dragoman submissively. "What am I but as the dust under your feet, O great Maroudi?"

"You shall be rewarded," said Maroudi; "but keep it in your memory that eyes will watch you, and that if you are false, you die under the kourbash. Now we have talked enough. Begone."

"On my head be it!" said Hassan.

Maroudi walked to the group with the donkeys, the dragoman following him, almost cringing.

"My good friends," said Maroudi gravely, "I have talked with Hassan, and put new thoughts into his mind, and it is Hassan's belief that he can find the young lord. Let him take a donkey and go."

"But——" said Sir Reginald, perplexed.

"Oh, sar, you trust Hassan!" exclaimed the dragoman. "Hassan knows all things! It has entered my thoughts that there is a hidden tomb, where it is my strong belief that the noble young lord has been taken, and this place is well known to me. Give me time, lordly gentlemen, to search the place of which I speak."

"If you advise this, Mr. Maroudi——"

"I advise it, my good friend," said Hilmi Maroudi, "and if you will wait on this spot, be it on my head that Hassan will return with the young lord."

Hassan had already picked out the best of the five donkeys. He mounted, waved the donkey-boy back, and disappeared at a trot into the dimness of the moonlight. Harry Wharton & Co. stared after him, and then looked at Maroudi, lost in wonder. So far as they could gather, the Egyptian had made some suggestion, which gave the dragoman hope of finding their lost comrade. Sir Reginald fidgeted. He was as perplexed as the schoolboys, and his anxiety was deep.

"My friend," said Maroudi gravely,

"I have said, on my head be it! Let us wait, and you shall be satisfied."

"If—if you feel sure——"

"I am sure!"

"Then we will wait," said Sir Reginald.

And they sat down to rest on the stone platform before the Sphinx, and waited. The hoof-beats of Hassan's donkey died away towards the desert, and there was silence.

THE FIFTEENTH CHAPTER.

Rescue!

KNOCK, knock, knock!

Lord Mauleverer, lying bound in the darkness of the lost tomb, lifted his head, listening with painful intentness.

Knock, knock!

Who was knocking at the stone that blocked the door of the tomb? It could not mean help and rescue—it could not! If the searchers were already at work they would be following the track of Mohammed's donkey into the desert, as the cunning Greek had planned.

Yet there was hope in Mauleverer's heart as he listened; his heart beat fast. He could hear the movements and muttering voice of Yussef, and though he could not understand the Arabic, the tones told him that Yussef was surprised and perturbed by that sudden summons at the door of the hidden tomb.

The man grunted angrily, and Mauleverer heard him move to the blocked portal; but he did not call out. Apparently he was listening. Yussef evidently had expected no one. It could not be Kalizelos.

But there was a sound at last of the stone moving at the portal of the tomb, whether moved from without, or from within, Mauleverer did not know. He could hear the grinding sound as it stirred.

With an effort, the bound schoolboy dragged himself up the steps. His wrists were fastened together, and his ankles; but he could manage to crawl on his elbows and knees, and slowly, painfully, he crawled up the steps, and lifted his head far enough to look into the upper rock chamber of the tomb.

Yussef was standing with his back to him, at the portal, from which the great limestone block was rolling aside. The lamp was still burning, and in its glimmer he caught the gleam of a bared knife in the hawk-faced Arab's hand. Evidently Yussef was not expecting a friend, and was ready for a foe.

The great stone shifted, and a glimmer of bright moonlight came in at the portal. Framed in the opening, with the night behind him and the lamplight on his face, was Hassan, the dragoman.

Mauleverer stared at him across the rock chamber, amazed. Glad as he would have been to see Harry Wharton & Co., he was almost as glad to see the faithful Hassan. The dragoman had found him—found out where he was kept a prisoner—that was all that he could suppose—and had come to save him. The schoolboy earl's eyes danced. He panted out a shout to the dragoman, fearful of seeing Yussef leap with his knife.

"Look out, Hassan!"

But, to Mauleverer's surprise, though doubtless not to Hassan's, Yussef did not lift the knife.

As soon as he recognised Hassan he slipped the weapon back under his dingy djubbah.

Mauleverer could not see his face; but had he seen it he would have read there only astonishment, not hostility.

Yussef was the first of the two Arabs to speak; but as he spoke in his own tongue what he said had no meaning for the bound schoolboy.

"Wahyat rasak! It is you, Hassan! Why are you here?" grunted Yussef, in Arabic. "It is not time yet by many hours for the Greek to come, and you put me in fear by knocking! Bismillah, but it came into my thoughts that all was discovered."

"Yet you might have known that it was Hassan, for this secret place is known only to three, and was it not I who told the secret to the Greek?" said the dragoman, in the same language.

Looking past Yussef, he saw the face of Lord Mauleverer, peering from the dark stair.

He salaamed.

"Lordly gentleman, Hassan is here!" he said. "You trust Hassan! Hassan is your dragoman."

"By gad, I'm jolly glad to see you, old bean!" said Lord Mauleverer. "Look out for that scoundrel's knife!"

Yussef, his hawkish face amazed, and growing suspicious, stared from one to the other.

"What means this, son of Suleiman?" he asked, still speaking in Arabic.

"The meaning, O my friend, is that there is a change in the plan," answered Hassan. "He who has paid us fears that this tomb may be discovered, and he has sent me to take the Faringhee away into the desert, and for this purpose I have brought a donkey."

Yussef wrinkled his brows.

"Son of jackals," he answered savagely. "the Faringhee stays here, in my care, by my master's order. You speak with a false tongue."

"By the beard of the Prophet——"

"Enough!" growled the hawk-faced Arab. "I obey only the orders of the Greek. The Faringhee remains."

Hassan, the dragoman, breathed hard and deep, and his grasp closed hard on the heavy stick he carried in his hand. He had had little expectation that the ruffian would allow him to take the prisoner away. But Hassan, the son of Suleiman, was ready for other measures, if trickery failed.

"O doubting one," said Hassan, still in Arabic, satisfied that Mauleverer could not understand a word that was said. "I have a writing from the Greek that I will show thee in proof of what I say."

"Show me the writing," said Yussef. "Then I will believe."

Hassan groped under his gold-braided tunic with his left hand, and drew out a folded paper, which he extended to the hawk-faced Arab. Lord Mauleverer watched them in sheer amazement.

Yussef stretched out his brown hand to take the paper, half-convinced. And as he did so Hassan's right hand flew up, taking the ruffian completely off his guard, and the stick crashed on the head of Yussef, with a crash that rang far in the silence of the night.

One gasping groan came from the hawk-faced Arab, as he pitched over and fell senseless at the feet of the dragoman.

"Oh gad!" gasped Lord Mauleverer.

Hassan looked down at the fallen man. His face, which the junior had always seen good-natured and amiable, was changed now; it blazed with ferocity.

The heavy stick whirled up again, in the hand of the man who was no longer the smiling dragoman of Cairo, but a savage and ruthless Arab, as savage as any bedouin of the desert. Crash came the stick on the head of the fallen man a second time. Hassan's hand flew up for a third blow, and Lord Mauleverer shouted to him:

"Stop!"

Hassan paused. He lowered the stick and salaamed to the schoolboy earl, the cheery grin returning to his face.

"To hear is to obey, my noble gentleman!" he said. "Yet is it wise to make sure of this son of pigs!"

"You've jolly well stunned him!" said Lord Mauleverer. "He won't come to in a hurry, Hassan! You don't want to crack his skull."

Hassan bent over the senseless Arab. There was no doubt that Yussef was stunned; the first blow had been enough. It was likely to be a long time before the son of Hamid came to his senses again.

"My noble gentleman is right," said Hassan, grinning. "The son of a dog is as senseless as the stone upon which he lies! Let him lie!"

"Get me loose, old bean," said Lord Mauleverer, and swiftly Hassan produced a knife and cut the ropes that bound the schoolboy earl, and with eager hands helped him to his feet.

Lord Mauleverer stood a little unsteadily, leaning on the arm of the dragoman.

"My noble gentleman, the dogs have dared to place bonds on your magnificent limbs!" exclaimed Hassan indignantly.

"Yaas, and jolly tight, too!" said Mauleverer. "How the thump did you find me, Hassan? By gad, you're some dragoman, old bean!"

Hassan salaamed.

"My lordly gentleman, Hassan knows all things. Hassan is your faithful dragoman!" he said. "Lordly and noble one, I have a donkey waiting, and your admirable friends await you at a Sphinx! Will it please your magnificent lordship to come with your faithful Hassan?"

"Will it?" grinned Mauleverer. "Yaas, old bean, I rather think it will! Never so jolly pleased in my life!"

Yussef, the son of Hamid, lay stretched senseless as Lord Mauleverer followed the dragoman from the tomb. Outside, Hassan rolled the limestone block into its place, shutting the tomb.

Then he helped Lord Mauleverer to mount the donkey. Mauly's face was bright as he sat in the red saddle. Hassan's stick cracked on the donkey, and the animal started at a trot. Under the brilliant moon, with the cool night wind from the desert fanning him, Lord Mauleverer rode, almost like a fellow in a dream.

He had given up hope of rescue, hope of life—and now he was free and riding back to rejoin his friends. Hassan, trotting at his side, cracked his stick on the donkey, grinning.

Lord Mauleverer gave a chirrup of delight as the majestic Sphinx came in sight in the moonlight. From the shadows round that ancient monument there came a shout:

"Mauly!"

"Thank Heaven—Mauly!"

"Herbert, my boy!"

And, with a rush, the Greyfriars fellows were round Mauleverer and dragging him from the donkey.

THE SIXTEENTH CHAPTER.

All Serene!

HILMI MAROUDI looked on, smiling. The plump Egyptian gentleman's dark face was full of satisfaction. The chums of the Remove were almost wild with delight as they surrounded Mauleverer, shaking his hands, thumping him on the back, and digging him in his breathless ribs. Somehow, they had had faith in Maroudi; they had trusted to his assurance. Yet it seemed almost like a miracle to them to see Lord Mauleverer ride up to the Sphinx, safe and sound. Hassan, the dragoman, had found him, and brought him back. But they knew that it was somehow due to Maroudi, though they did not know how.

"Mauly, old bean——"

"My esteemed and ridiculous Mauly."

"Oh, isn't this jolly!"

"Yaas!" gasped Lord Mauleverer. "No end jolly, old things. But don't punch a fellow so hard—what? You men, you don't know how frightfully it bucks a fellow to see you all again. Nunky——"

"My dear, dear boy, said Sir Reginald, "I could scarcely believe Mr. Maroudi when he assured me that Hassan would find you!"

"Mr. Maroudi here! How do you do, sir?" Lord Mauleverer bowed politely to the Egyptian gentleman, who smiled and nodded. "I can't imagine how Hassan nosed me out. I tell you he's some dragoman! I was parked in a jolly old tomb—half-buried in sand—along with mummies and things! I own up to you fellows that I hate mummies at close quarters. All right in museums and places—but not nice at a fellow's elbow, especially in the dark! But it's all right now—right as rain!"

"We owe it to Mr. Maroudi," said Harry Wharton, with a grateful glance at the Egyptian gentleman. "I can't guess how—but he put Hassan up to finding you. Isn't that so, Hassan?"

"My noble and lordly gentleman, this is true," said Hassan. "The great Maroudi, with his wise words, put it in my mind!"

"Then I owe my liberty to you, sir," said Lord Mauleverer. "I'm not a great hand at talkin', Mr. Maroudi. But when I tell you that I was tied up like a turkey and chucked into a tomb, you'll know how I feel about it!"

"God bless you, Mr. Maroudi!" said Sir Reginald, in a deeply moved voice. "You have been a friend in need!"

"It was the will of Allah that I should serve you," said the Egyptian gravely. "To me this is a happy day. Let us return to Mena House, my friends!"

With happy faces, the Greyfriars fellows started for Mena House. When they came to the hotel by the Pyramids, Hilmi Maroudi stopped to speak to Hassan, in Arabic.

"Son of a dog, to-morrow you will come to my house in Cairo for your reward, of which you will say nothing to your masters. From this day you will serve them faithfully, and guard them from the Greek. And if you fail, think of the kourbash!"

"What am I but dust under your feet, O great Maroudi?" answered the dragoman. "To hear is to obey!"

"Upon your head be it!" said Maroudi.

"I say, you fellows——" came a fat squeak, as the juniors came up the road to the hotel.

"Hallo, hallo, hallo! Is that jolly old Bunter?" exclaimed Mauleverer. And in the exuberance of his spirits he greeted the Owl of the Remove with a terrific smack on a fat shoulder.

"Yaroooh!" roared Bunter.

"By gad, I'm glad to see even Bunter again!" chuckled Lord Mauleverer. "Fancy a fellow bein' glad to see you, Bunter, old fat bean—what?"

"Oh, really, Mauly——"

Billy Bunter blinked at the juniors. The hour was late, and Billy Bunter was frightfully hungry. He could see that the chums of the Remove seemed highly pleased and satisfied about something. So far as Billy Bunter could see, there was no cause for satisfaction. It was true that he had had several teas, but he was hours late for dinner. In the inner Bunter there was an aching void.

"I say, you fellows, I've been waiting for you!" he groaned. "I thought you'd never get back!"

"Mauly was bagged by an Arab!"

"Silly ass! Might have expected something of the sort when you went out without me," said Bunter. "But never mind Mauly. What about dinner?"

"Ha, ha, ha!"

"Blessed if I see anything to cackle at!" roared Bunter, in great indignation. "I can tell you that I'm frightfully hungry—famished, in fact. Keeping a fellow waiting for his grub——"

"Mauly's had a jolly narrow escape!"

"Yes, yes. But what about dinner?" asked Bunter anxiously. "I say, we shall be frightfully late back at Cairo! I can't hold out till then—I really can't, you know. You fellows got any toffee?"

"Ha, ha, ha!"

"Will you stop cackling when a fellow's hungry!" roared Bunter. "Look here! Where's old Brooke? Why can't he order the car? Lot he cares whether a fellow's perishing of hunger—about as much as you fellows do! Where's that old codger?"

"Bunter!"

"Oh! Ah! I—I—I wasn't calling you an old codger, sir! I—I—I——"

"As the hour is so late, my boys, we will stop at Mena House for supper and drive back to Cairo afterwards," said Sir Reginald, with a glare at Bunter.

"Oh!" gasped Bunter. "Good! Fine! I say, you fellows, come in! What are you hanging about for? For goodness' sake, get a move on! I've had nothing since tea but some Turkish Delight and a few cakes and some oranges and biscuits and a bunch or two of figs! Buck up!"

It was a cheery supper-party at the hotel by the Pyramids. Cheeriest of all was the fat face of Billy Bunter as he packed away the foodstuffs at a rate unequalled by the rest of the fellows put together. And after supper a happy party rolled back to Cairo in the car, under the bright moon of Egypt, merry and bright after their peril at the Pyramids.

THE END.

(Look out for another feast of thrills in "BILLY BUNTER'S BARGAIN!" the next yarn in this ripping holiday adventure series. You'll enjoy it no end, chums!)

COME INTO THE OFFICE, BOYS!

ALTHOUGH I've got very little space at my disposal this week, chums, I can't leave out this amusing joke, for which George Thomas, of "The Bungalow, Redbrook, near Mon, will receive one of our useful pocket-knives.

RHEUMATIC!

Traveller (to night-watchman): "Yours is a 'romantic' sort of job, isn't it?"
Night-watchman: "It is that, guv'nor; I gets it in me knee-joints, so that I can 'ardly 'obble 'ome!"

Finished laughing? Good!

The first letter on my desk this week comes from Harry Walsh, of Stoke Newington, who informs me, most emphatically, that the MAGNET ranks as the finest boys' paper on the market. You've sure said a bibful, chum! I feel sure my many thousands of readers heartily endorse Harry's statement. My correspondent, however, has one "grouse," if it may be termed as such. He declares he doesn't like the stories of St. Sam's displacing the "Greyfriars Herald" supplement, and states that there are a good many "Magnetites" who think the same as himself. Doubtless there are a few of my chums who would prefer to see the old "Greyfriars Herald" occupying the pages now being devoted to Dicky Nugent's "shockers," but I must say in all fairness, that the "complaints" I have received in this direction could be counted on the fingers of one hand. As I like to please my readers when possible, however, I am going to put it to the vote. Your opinions on this matter are wanted, please.

The next letter comes from Stan Whiley, of Huddersfield, whose praises regarding the MAGNET are, indeed, highly flattering. He writes how he wishes the Old Paper could be published three times a week, and then goes on to say: "I would never tire of reading stories of Harry Wharton & Co., at Greyfriars." I wonder if my chum is aware of the fact that a 65,000 words-story of these popular chums appears in the "Schoolboys' Own Library" every month? The issue now on sale contains one of Frank Richards' greatest yarns.

Fancy yourself as a "poet"? Yes. Then try your hand at writing a Greyfriars Limerick. A first-class prize will come your way if your effort catches the judge's eye. One of this week's splendid pocket wallets goes to: "A Loyal Reader," of 26, Reeves Road, King's Heath, Birmingham, who submitted the following winning effort:—

Said Skinner to Snoop: "For a lark,
We will roll Bunter into the Sark!"
But Wharton & Co.
Intruded, and so
What happened is better kept dark.

I'VE just got space to put you wise as to next week's programme. Topping the bill is:—

"BILLY BUNTER'S BARGAIN!"
By Frank Richards.

This is the next yarn in our grand holiday series, with Billy Bunter, the fat and fatuous Owl, in the limelight again. "Birchemall's Bennyfit" is the title of Dicky Nugent's "ticklish tail," and you'll laugh both loud and long when you read it. What do you think of our new serial. "The Red Falcon"?, Isn't it just great? Look out, then for further chapters of this grand story of the "good old days" next week.

Till then, cheerio,

YOUR EDITOR.

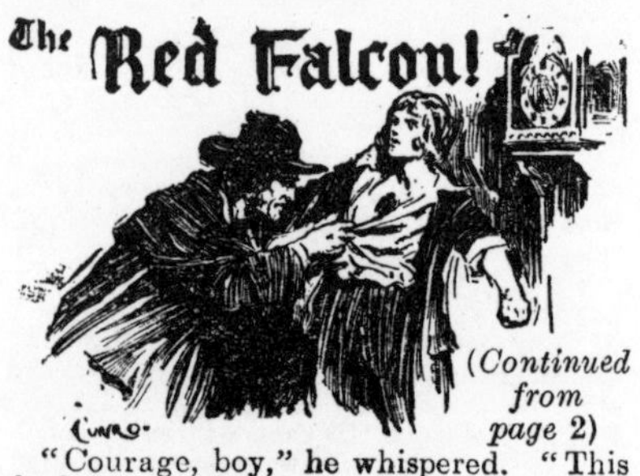

(*Continued from page* 2)

"Courage, boy," he whispered. "This foul den won't hold us for ever."

The mental torture and physical weariness went on every day. At last the Sessions opened, and, with other prisoners, Hal and Jerry were led along dark stone corridors and through doors which opened silently on well-oiled hinges, and ushered out into the bail dock of Newgate, where they found a sweep of blue sky above them.

The dock was walled in on two sides. On the third it led into the trial court, where the judge and jury sat and the public were admitted. The fourth side was enclosed by high, closed gates topped with unclimbable spikes. Beyond these gates, in the Old Bailey, sentries were stationed to prevent any of the prisoners from getting away.

The first day Hal and Jerry were taken into the yard nothing happened, and in the afternoon they were hustled back into the gaol again.

On the second day, however, after a long wait, they were taken into the court and ushered into the railed and spiked dock to stand their trial.

The Sentence!

HAL stared around with eager eyes taking in the rows of tightly packed spectators, the counsel and others in the well of the court, the judge on the bench, with the Sword of Justice behind him and the Royal Arms of his Most Gracious Majesty King George III. above his head.

Over in a corner Hal saw his father sitting. Samuel Lovett saw him, but turned his shifty eyes away as their glances met. And whilst Hal was searching the court he saw the Earl of Huntford, wearing a plum-coloured suit, stride gracefully to a seat among the bewigged barristers and drop languidly on to it.

The earl looked straight at the dock, eyed the prisoners scornfully, and then, taking a pinch of snuff out of a bejewelled box, made some remark to the man sitting next to him and laughed.

"That man's as dangerous as a rattlesnake, boy," said McLean, who had been watching the earl closely. "But if ever I get the chance, I'll make him do something else than smile!"

Hal nodded quickly, and glanced at the bail dock, into which the sunshine was streaming, and then beyond the high wall, into the street of Old Bailey, lined with sombre houses.

A sharp pluck at his sleeve and an order from one of the warders who sat in the dock with him bade him "pay attention to his Lordship."

Hal Lovett stood with shoulders squared whilst the charge against him was read aloud in the legal jargon that made it sound worse. Then followed the charge against McLean for conspiring with Hal to rob the Earl of Huntford, and "that he did, in an attempt to resist arrest and to rescue his fellow-prisoner, murderously assault the police."

McLean had borrowed from an old friend some money, with which he had secured the services of a counsel, but he knew and Hal knew, as they listened to the earl giving evidence and to Samuel Lovett heaping lie upon lie, that they stood very little chance of acquittal.

Samuel Lovett's lying evidence dovetailed so perfectly with that of the earl that the jury began to shift impatiently and to whisper to one another, as if they had already agreed upon their verdict.

The judge's questions and Lovett's replies as the trial neared its end decided the issue.

"The prisoner, Harry Lovett, is your son. He is charged with a very serious crime. Why is it that you have not been able to control the boy?" asked the judge.

"Never could do anything with him, me lord," answered Samuel Lovett, leaning on the ledge of the witness-box. "He's bin a sore trial to me ever since he was able to walk. I've thrashed the skin off him trying to show him the error of 'is ways, but it only made him worse."

"Did you know he was a thief?" asked the judge.

"He wuz always thieving, your lordship," answered Samuel Lovett, sucking at his teeth as was his habit. "He's thoroughly bad!"

"But you were with him, it seems, when the diamond star was snatched from the Earl of Huntford's breast?"

"I was there, me lord, because I went after the boy. We'd had a disagreement in the afternoon, and I was afraid Hal would stay out all night. I've a tender 'eart, I 'ave. I wanted to bring the boy 'ome, in spite of everything."

"Then you did not go with the prisoner to Drury Lane Theatre?"

"Never dreamt of doin' it, sir!" Lovett answered, piling lie upon lie. "I followed him there. It just 'appened by chance that I saw him with the other prisoner—Mr. McLean."

"H'm! What do you know about the prisoner—McLean?"

"Nothing that's any good, sir. I reckon he's partly responsible for leading my boy astray."

"May your soul frizzle in everlasting fire, you lying hypocrite!" came in McLean's clear, ringing tones from the dock, and the court echoed to the thrill of a new sensation.

"If the prisoner breaks silence again," said the Recorder, bending stern eyes upon the offender, who lolled nonchalantly in a corner of the dock, "have him removed!"

There was silence for a while, after which the Recorder continued:

"We have heard the evidence of the Earl of Huntford and various onlookers, now give me your version of the robbery, Mr. Lovett, in your own words."

Samuel Lovett, who had been in the witness-box for two hours, mopped the sweat from his forehead, and, after i n w a r d l y cursing cross-examining counsel and judge alike, said suavely:

"Your lordship, I told my boy to come home, but he wouldn't. This man McLean encouraged him in defying me. The audience had turned out, and, in the hustle and bustle, I saw the Earl of Huntford come out under the theatre porch. The moment my son saw the diamond star glittering on his lordship's breast he ran forward and snatched it. I was just behind him, and was able to seize him and hold him until the Runners arrived. They found the star in his pocket."

The jury almost rose in their eagerness to terminate the trial.

But there were counsel to be heard and the summing-up to be made.

McLean crossed his arms and smiled as he listened intently to his counsel pleading on his behalf and Hal's.

"Let the jury try to conceive the devilish situation. This young boy, charged with a crime that may cost him his life, had seen the Earl of Huntford enter Samuel Lovett's shop that afternoon. The earl was clad in rags, but his sound shoes, dirtied for the occasion, and a flashing diamond on his right hand, had betrayed him. The boy, Harry Lovett had seen the supposed beggar hand his father a purse of gold, and had heard the two plot something for that night at Drury Lane Theatre that concerned a diamond something—it might have been a star.

"From the moment the boy Lovett had left his father's house, after a bitter quarrel between them, intending, as he says, never to return, he had spent his time in the company of Jerry McLean. They had not gone to Drury Lane Theatre until the audience were leaving after the play, and there they had seen Samuel Lovett waiting. It was Samuel Lovett who tore the diamond star from the Earl of Huntford's breast and put it in his son's pocket. McLean had seen it, and was so enraged that he had tried to rescue the boy from the hands of the Bow Street Runners."

"And that," said McLean, from the dock, "is the solemn truth, as I hope for mercy!"

"Silence!" stormed the judge. "Restrain that man!"

His summing-up was like the knell of doom.

"Who could believe the mad story told by the prisoners? The jury had heard the clear-cut and unbiassed evidence of the Earl of Huntford, and they would know how to appreciate the evidence of the father, Samuel Lovett, who declared that his son had shown criminal tendencies almost from birth. If the wildly improbable tale concocted by the prisoners in their defence was untrue, then the jury could form their own conclusions as to the characters of the prisoners.

"The man McLean was known as a gambler and a bankrupt. A man who had once moved in high social circles, he had sunk to the level of the gutter. It was known that he was on the brink of starvation that night when he went to Drury Lane with the boy Lovett. What could be more probable in the circumstances than that they were lured by the flaming brilliance of the diamond star to snatch it from Lord Huntford's breast?

"They had heard the Earl of Huntford say that he had never in his life assumed the guise of a beggar. Whatever inducement could he have had to visit Samuel Lovett, who was an entire stranger? If the jury believed the story put up by the prisoners for their defence, then they must find them not guilty, but if, on the other hand, they looked upon that story as a string of lies, concocted with a view to hoodwinking the jury, then it would be their duty, nay double their duty, to find them—guilty."

The jury were absent from the court for exactly twenty minutes. When they filed back, looking immensely relieved and pleased and deliberately avoiding glancing at the dock, Hal and

Printed and published every Saturday by the Proprietors, The Amalgamated Press, Ltd., The Fleetway House, Farringdon Street, London, E.C.4. Advertisement offices: The Fleetway House, Farringdon Street, London, E.C.4. Registered for transmission by Canadian Magazine Post. Subscription rates: Inland and Abroad, 11s. per annum; 5s. 6d. for six months. Sole Agents for Australia and New Zealand: Messrs. Gordon & Gotch, Ltd., and for South Africa: Central News Agency, Ltd.—Saturday, August 27th, 1932.

Jerry McLean, who had just been **brought back to hear the verdict, knew** that the case had gone against them. A deep voice droned out the question:

"Gentlemen of the jury, have you considered your verdict?"

"We have."

"Then do you find the prisoners guilty or not guilty?"

"Guilty!"

Hal straightened himself up and clutched the spikes of the dock-rail. McLean's hand sought his and pressed it firmly.

Jerry's handsome face was wreathed in smiles.

"Courage, lad," he said in his usual cheery way.

The judge turned his cold, stern eyes upon them. His voice droned on in a monotonous chanting condemnation before he pronounced sentence, and here and there Hal caught a few words.

"It is to be hoped that in the time to come, you, Hal Lovett, will repent your evil doing. Seldom have I seen one so young convicted of such a crime. In spite of the stern, but just discipline administered by your father, you chose to leave your home and plunge into crime. And you, McLean, bankrupt and wastrel, can only be regarded as the ringleader who lured this wayward boy to destruction."

The droning voice quickened, grew colder, harder as, his sermon over, the judge sat back and drummed tapering fingers on the arm of his chair of justice.

"Much as it grieves me to send so young a boy to prison, I sentence you, Hal Lovett, to serve upon the hulks for a term of seven years—and you, McLean, for whose conduct I can find no words bad enough, will be transferred from Newgate Prison to the hulks, there to await shipment to Australia at the earliest opportunity. I sentence you to transportation for life!"

McLean started as if he had been struck. Every vestige of colour drained out of his cheeks to presently return in a warming flood.

For a moment he stood rigid, and the next he had thrown off the clutching hands of the warders and was leaning over the spiked rail of the dock, his rich voice ringing through the Old Bailey Court House like a trumpet.

"And what sentence shall I mete out to you, you miserable old sinner, if ever I manage to escape and meet you again? I may be a bankrupt, and a fool because I have run through more than one fortune, but it was my own money I spent. I have given away fortunes, but I've never robbed a man of a bronze farthing." McLean fought off the warders and held his ground, the dock shaking as strong arms strove to drag him clear. "Every word Hal Lovett said was true. Samuel Lovett stole the diamond star. The kid had it planted on him. I saw it, and that's why I fought the Runners—that's why—that's why—I ask for justice!"

"Take that man away," said the judge sternly.

A blow on the side of the head half-stunned McLean, whose hands relaxed their grip of the spiked rail. Strong arms dragged him away, though he fought furiously as they pulled him down into the well of the court.

The spectators, swaying in their excitement to see, added their shouts to the general uproar.

The Earl of Huntford, raising a gold-mounted glass to his eye, looked up at Hal Lovett as he neared the dock.

It was too much for the boy who had been framed. He tried to lean over the spiked rail.

"You were Mr. Who," shouted the boy in a frenzy. "It was you who played the beggar in my father's house. Why did you do it? Why?"

Four hands like steel grips seized the boy by the arms and tried to wrench him away.

"Come on out of this, you," snapped one of the warders who held him.

Hal began to struggle fiercely, and, as he did so, his shirt opened wide revealing the whole of his naked chest.

Through the crystal glass he held, the earl gazed upon the tattooed red falcon, jessed and belled and hooded, and the upturned smiling curve of his lips thinned into a hard, cruel, straight line.

"For the lying evidence your counsel made against me in court this afternoon, you gallows brat, I would have you hanged; but since the judge has been merciful I must see what I can do to ensure that you receive one hundred lashes with the cat."

Every word was uttered distinctly so that Hal heard even above the general uproar.

Then the warders tore him bodily away and cast him down the stairs of the dock. Below they shook him violently and struck him a blow on the side of the head which stunned him.

When Hal came to his senses again, he was lying in a cell with Jerry McLean beside him, and they were both handcuffed and set in double irons.

Hal looked up at Jerry McLean, whose face was bloodless and whose eyes glittered as if he had the ague. He forced a smile.

"And this is what they call justice, boy," said Jerry, with a sigh. "Me innocent, and you innocent. You for the hulks, and me to transportation for life!"

The Convict Hulk!

HAL LOVETT had lived all his young life in Wych Street, and had managed to retain some illusions and ideals in spite of the brutality of his father, Samuel Lovett, who had now betrayed him.

For years he had wandered barefooted about the neighbourhood of Covent Garden and Clare Market, and had seen almost every side of life, boy though he was.

In his boyish way he had, until the trial waned, believed that justice must prevail, and McLean and himself be given their liberty.

In Newgate that night, after his conviction, he threw himself down in his heavy irons beside McLean, and moved restlessly and miserably on the wretched mattress until a turnkey opened the door of their cell and told them roughly to "get up."

They were served with a miserable breakfast, and then marched to a vaulted room where their irons were removed. Fetters and handcuffs and strange and weird instruments of torture hung upon the walls. Hal was glad when they were taken from the place and led out into the prison yard where four other wretched convicts stood in line.

Here Jerry McLean and Hal Lovett were chained up with these four other convicts, the chain being run through a bracelet on each man's right arm.

A file of soldiers was drawn up in front of the convicts, and the governor of Newgate, having checked the names of the prisoners, handed them and their papers into the custody of the officer in charge of the detachment of guards.

Then out of the yard they marched, through gloomy passages whose walls

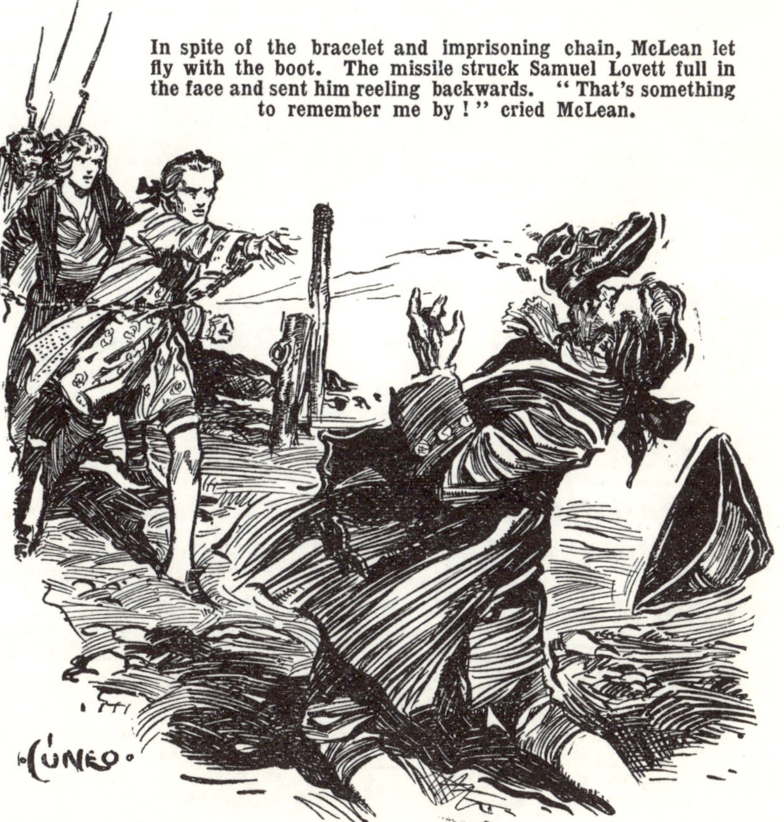

In spite of the bracelet and imprisoning chain, McLean let fly with the boot. The missile struck Samuel Lovett full in the face and sent him reeling backwards. "That's something to remember me by!" cried McLean.

were decorated with fetters and handcuffs and firearms of all sizes and dates.

To a thick, iron-studded door they were led, and through it to another half-door, beyond which was the street. The half-door was topped with pointed spikes, between which were set others, double-curled and half the length. Above the spikes was set an iron grid, like a ladder set horizontally, and at the left there hung a bell-pull.

The Old Bailey was enveloped in mist, and a slouching beggar, who dived down Sea Coal Lane, was the only person in sight when the escort of soldiers, with arms shouldered and long bayonets gleaming, marched the chain-gang down the hill to the steps at Blackfriars.

Here a big and cumbersome wherry was waiting, in charge of an officer from the convict hulk Ethalion.

A few loafers were hanging about, and the river showed up cold and grey in the veil of mist that hung over it.

The prisoners were handed over, and the papers delivered. Then the convicts were told roughly to get aboard.

They moved down to where the water lapped the thick coating of mud which lay upon the hidden stones.

It was as they were plashing through the water to the curses and jeers of the men in the wherry that Hal saw Samuel Lovett waiting just above the reach of the tide.

His feet were on sound gravel bottom. He had chosen a place where there was no mud. The sight of him infuriated the boy. This man was supposed to be his father; but he told himself, and not for the first time, that this man Lovett was not his father. It just could not be.

Hal touched the arm of McLean in front of him

"Look, Jerry!" he cried.

And Jerry McLean saw

Samuel Lovett had his coat tightly buttoned, and his hat drawn down over his eyes. His hands were set deep in his pockets, and his eyes glinted evilly, triumphantly, as he watched the chain-gang moving briskly to the waiting wherry.

"A good riddance to you, you gallows brat!" he called, as Hal went by. "I've kept and clothed and fed you, only for you to disgrace me! May you rot on the hulks, say I!"

Most certainly this inhuman brute could not be his father. Hal stopped, and the forward march of the convicts was checked.

"You ought to be where the boy is, you traitor!" cried McLean. "What compact had you with the earl? One of these days I'll be free, and then I'll find out!"

Samuel Lovett laughed derisively.

"You'll never be free!" he cried. "If you don't die during the voyage over in the convict ship, they'll lash the life out of you in Australia! You'll rot and die out there, Jerry McLean!"

His elation and his laugh maddened McLean who looked about him for a missile. In the mud to the right of him Jerry saw an old boot, washed up by the tide. It was covered thick with mud.

McLean reached down for it, and, in spite of the bracelet and the imprisoning chain, flung it full in the face of Samuel Lovett and sent him reeling.

"That's something to remember me by, at any rate!" cried McLean, as he went on with the chain gang and climbed into the wherry.

Samuel Lovett picked himself up, smothered from head to heels with a grey splodge of Thames mud. It dripped from his fingers as he shook his hands, and from his mouth as he cursed McLean.

Above, a sharp command rang out, and then, to tramping feet, the file of guards strode away.

A blow from a staff nearly felled McLean as he got into the boat, but he grinned at Hal Lovett as he dropped into the stern sheets with the rest of the gang.

"You'll get a hundred lashes," said the officer from the hulk Ethalion, as he glowered at McLean, "if you repeat that sort of thing!"

"And it would be worth it!" McLean replied impudently, as the boat swung out into a swift-running tide and moved down-river, hauled by three pairs of lusty arms.

They swept under London Bridge in a grey of fog, and passed through the Pool just as the sun shone and the mist began to rise.

As the Pool widened out, McLean bent to whisper in Hal's ear.

"Listen, pal," he said, "we shall be put to work in the dockyards or the Arsenal, at Woolwich, but there will be plenty of leisure aboard the Ethalion. We are allowed lights below deck after we are battened down, hal. There are from twelve to twenty men in each yard, and we sleep in hammocks, a lot of us together. We shan't wear irons unless we've done something bad."

"How can that help us?" asked the boy eagerly.

"A lot—when you've got brains, lad. Besides, I've got some pals aboard the Ethalion who know the ropes. I've been there before!"

Hal Lovett's blue eyes widened in dismay. He had held a great admiration for Jerry McLean ever since they had met by accident in the streets behind the Strand. Hal knew Jerry as a gentleman who had squandered more than one fortune, but he had never believed him to be a criminal.

"Have you been sentenced before, then, and escaped?" he asked.

McLean laughed softly.

"No, boy," he answered. "The only time I ever broke the law was when I tried to rescue you from the Bow Street Runners, and they gave me fourteen years for that. Fourteen years! Transportation for life! But I'm not in Australia yet!" Then his voice, which had hardened, grew soft again. "No, boy, I went on board the Ethalion as a visitor. I've a pal there, and if things pan out right we'll soon be free."

Just then McLean saw the officer in command of the boat looking hard at him, and he stopped speaking.

Half an hour later the convict hulks at Woolwich loomed up right ahead of them. They were anchored close in to the shore. There were four of them, three convict ships, and one hospital ship. Only one of them carried jury-masts. Hal and Jerry McLean could see gangways running zigzag down their sides. Two had a boom rigged out. A flag fluttered lazily from the stern of the nearest hulk. From amidships for'ard she carried a penthouse arrangement, which covered in her spar deck and forecastle deck. Her poop deck was enclosed by a high rail.

And as the burly watermen rowed the wherry nearer, Hal Lovett read the name of the ship sprawled in tarnished paint over the stern of her—"Ethalion." They had reached their destination!

(Hal and Jerry are booked for a rough time by the look of things! Boys, you'll be thrilled more than ever when you read next week's gripping chapters.)

"BILLY BUNTER'S BARGAIN!"

Thrilling holiday adventures of Harry Wharton & Co. in Egypt.

The MAGNET 2D

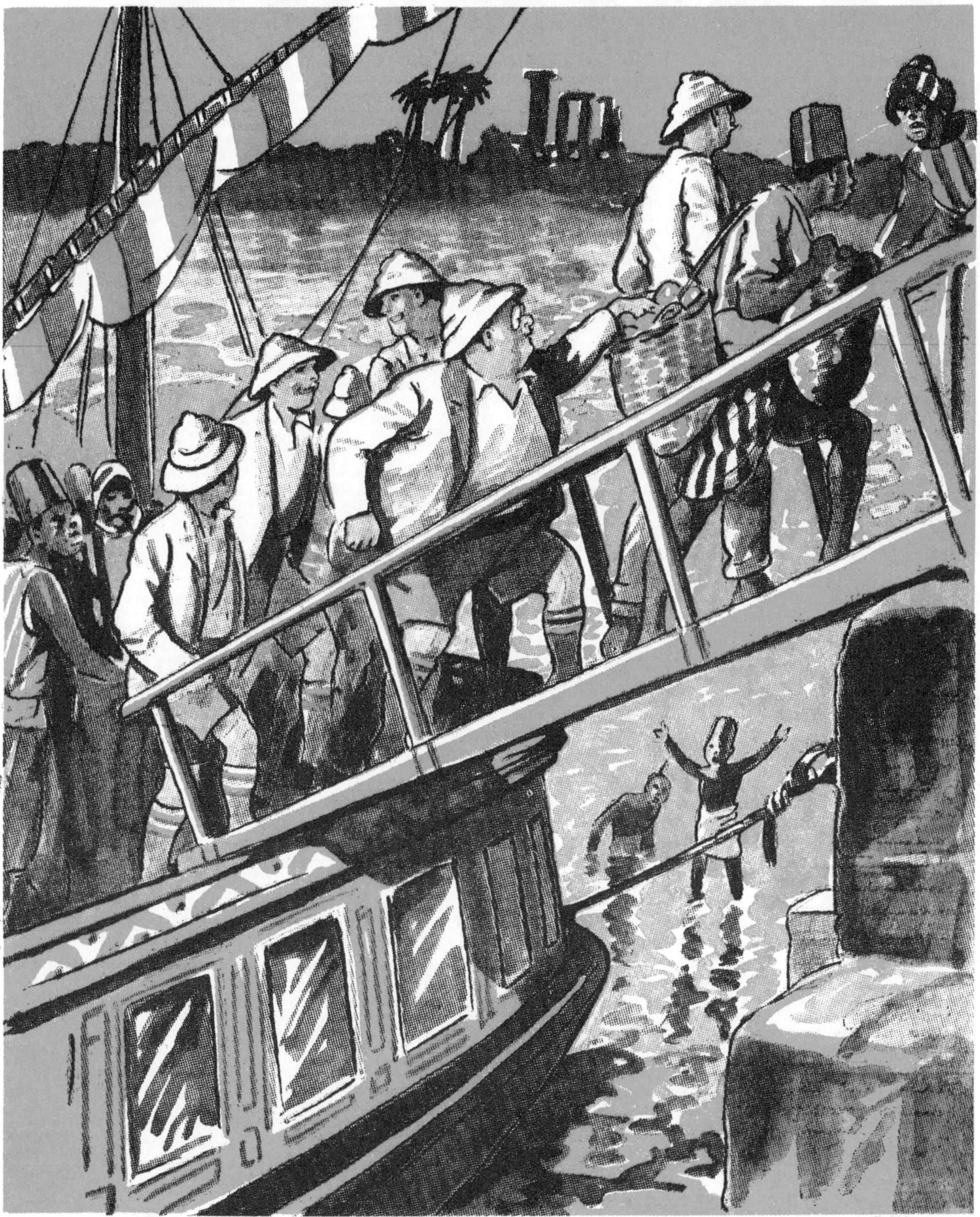

No. 1,281. Vol. XLII. EVERY SATURDAY. Week Ending September 3rd, 1932.

NEWS AND VIEWS FROM ALL QUARTERS.

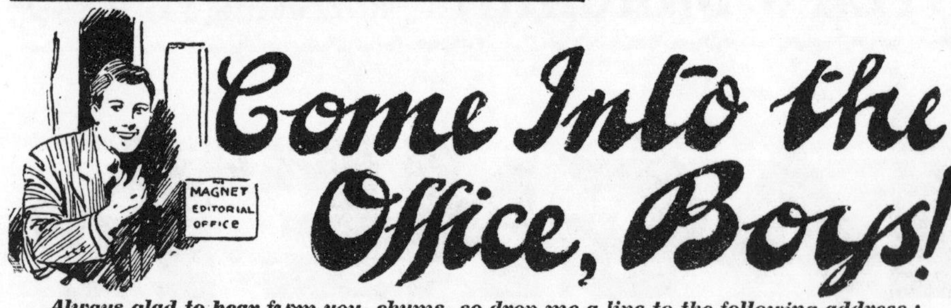

Always glad to hear from you, chums, so drop me a line to the following address: The Editor, The "Magnet" Library, The Amalgamated Press, Ltd., The Fleetway House, Farringdon Street, London, E.C.4.

GREAT NEWS! Glorious news! Stupendous news! This week I am permitting myself these expressive adjectives—and with good reason, for I am able to reveal to "Magnet" readers the first "hints" of what has hitherto been a closely guarded secret. As this number of the "Magnet" is going to press I am putting the finishing touches to a RECORD-BREAKING FREE GIFT SCHEME for all of you loyal boys and girls. This scheme will be starting very shortly, and I am convinced beforehand that all of you will vote it the finest you have ever experienced. Next Saturday I shall be able to reveal more about this colossal scheme, so a word of warning—DON'T MISS NEXT WEEK'S "MAGNET" WHATEVER YOU DO!

They make me merry, some of them. Others make me want to weep. Some set me scratching my head. Most of them, I am thankful to say, are real sensible. "What do—what are?" I can hear you exclaiming. I'm talking about readers' queries, of course.

Last week I had one from a fellow who wanted to be a tight-rope walker. I haven't answered him yet. But I hope to do so when I can get in personal touch with a real live rope-walker. You don't meet 'em every day, unfortunately. They're like sword-swallowers and red-hot-poker-eaters—a bit scarce.

The latest query to come to hand is from Maurice Burton, who forgot to include his address. He

WANTS TO JOIN THE ROYAL AIR FORCE.

Well, Maurice, there are different methods of enlisting in the various grades of the R.A.F., and you must first make up your mind whether you want to be a pilot, apprentice, or what not. It would take more than the space at my disposal to answer your question fully, so I advise you to get into touch at once with the Recruiting Officer, R.A.F., Gwydyr House, Whitehall, London, S.W.1.

That official will then send you, free of charge, the special pamphlets issued by the R.A.F. setting out all particulars of enlisting, terms of service, and so on. The pamphlets can also be obtained at any recruiting office.

Another reader wants to know about the *world's most famous screen mouse*, known to all the world as Mickey. "Where," he asks me, "does Mickey get his voice?"

Mickey's voice belongs to an Italian count, who has done all the speaking parts for Mickey Mouse ever since that celebrity featured on the "flickers." The count can also reproduce in an amazing way the exact sounds made by a frog, or a gnat, or any other living creature. In fact, the different sound-effects than can come from that wonderful human throat total no less than 2,000!

I WAS reading the other day a book that gives all sorts of startling and out-of-the-way facts, and thought these items worth passing on to my readers. The first concerned

1,632,000 Dozens of Tennis Balls!—That amazing number represents the total of tennis balls made in this country in 1932, their value being £634,000! In this country 14,000,000 of them were used, the others being exported.

Who's Lost a Pin?—Funny there's never a pin about just when you happen to want one. Yet in 1930 the value of the pins made in Britain totalled over £8,000! In the same period £69,000 worth of gramophone needles were made, and £340,000 worth of ordinary needles. Buttons and studs turned out by the factories in that year were 2,534,000,000 in number. Makes you gasp, doesn't it?

Making Two Cars a Minute.—I hear that the Ford motor-car factory which is starting work in Essex will shortly be turning out two fully completed, ready-for-the-road cars every minute. Fifteen thousand British workmen will be engaged in their production, and 800 tons of coal will be used there every single day!

READY for a laugh? Right, here goes! This rib-tickler comes from Eric G. Randall, of 62, Kingsdown Parade, Kingsdown, Bristol, who gets a splendid Sheffield steel penknife for it:

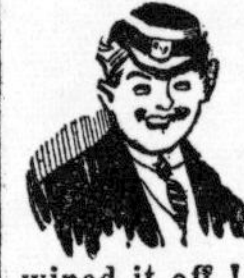

Diner: "Is there any tomato sauce on the menu, waiter?"

Waiter: "No, sir. I've just wiped it off!"

NEEDS SWALLOWING!

There are some facts that are not facts at all. I know plenty of 'em. But about these topical items of news there can be no manner of doubt!

Fish Up a Tree.—Show an ordinary fisherman a two-inch tiddler and he'll go home and tell folks he's just seen a hundred-foot whale. I wonder what he'd say to the sensational adventure of a well-known sportsman who recently SHOT a fish in a tree? The sportsman saw a big bird catch the fish—a bass—from a stream and fly up with it into the topmost branches of a tree. The man promptly aimed with his gun and shot—not the bird, but the fish!

Great Snakes.—A scientist in India says that one hundred people at least are killed every day in that country by snake-bite. The snakes account for more victims than all India's other wild animals put together!

Elephant versus Camera.—A government official in Kenya, Africa, the other day, met an elephant. The Jumbo was angry about something and started to "take it out of" the poor man. Jumbo rushed at him and gave him a wallop with one of its mighty tusks and hurled him into the branches of a tree. That tusk struck a small camera in the official's pocket and smashed it to splinters—but the tiny camera saved the man's life!

Tabby the Traveller.—We hear about old sea-dogs, but what about old sea-cats? Well, one has just been pensioned off from service in a White Star liner, and has been presented with a special collar to commemorate her sea travels of 360,000 miles! The cat was born in that liner and never left it until now, the liner being broken up in the shipbreaker's yard.

PITY THE FILM HERO!

It has just occurred to me that Maurice Burton, the reader whose query about joining the R.A.F. I have answered earlier, may like to know that he stands a far better chance of living to a good old age in the service of the Royal Air Force than if he became a flying-stunt merchant in the service of the films. I have by me a "schedule of prices" issued by the Hollywood screen magnates. I don't know if there is a revised tariff out since the one I have was published. If there isn't, there ought to be! Here are the prices for various "neck-risking" feats performed during the taking of special air films.

For changing planes in mid-air, £20. Changing from a plane to a train, £30. Parachute jump, £16. Fight on upper wing, one man knocked off, £45. Crashing a plane by flying it into a house, £240. Changing from one plane to another while upside-down in mid-air, £90. Blowing up a plane in mid-air, £300.

Now then, who's for a job of stunting out Hollywood way?

A splendid prize of a topping leather pocket wallet goes this week to Denis Fricker, of 80, London Road, Ipswich, Suffolk, in return for the following Greyfriars limerick:

At fisticuffs Cherry's renowned;
A Greyfriars champion uncrowned.
He'll take a bad biff
With only a sniff,
And come up smiling when he's "downed."

AND now for next week's bumper programme, chums. Topping the bill is:

"THE SHADOWED SCHOOLBOY!"
By Frank Richards,

which tells of the further exciting adventures of Harry Wharton & Co. on holiday in Egypt. It's hardly necessary for me to tell you what a topping yarn this is, because you know full well what Frank Richards can turn out in the way of first-class stories, but I will say that this one will take some beating. On no account should you miss it, then!

Still enjoying our new serial, "The Red Falcon"? It's a top-notcher, isn't it? Look out for further thrilling chapters of this stirring yarn of the "good old days" next week.

Now for Dicky Nugent's contribution! Here's a rib-tickler that will send you into fits of laughter: "BIRCHEMALL GOES WHALING!"—told in Dicky's inimitable style.

To complete this bumper programme there will be more jokes and limericks, and answers to several correspondents which have been crowded out this week.

Cheerio, chums,
YOUR EDITOR.

THRILLS, FUN AND ADVENTURE IN THIS GRAND HOLIDAY YARN.

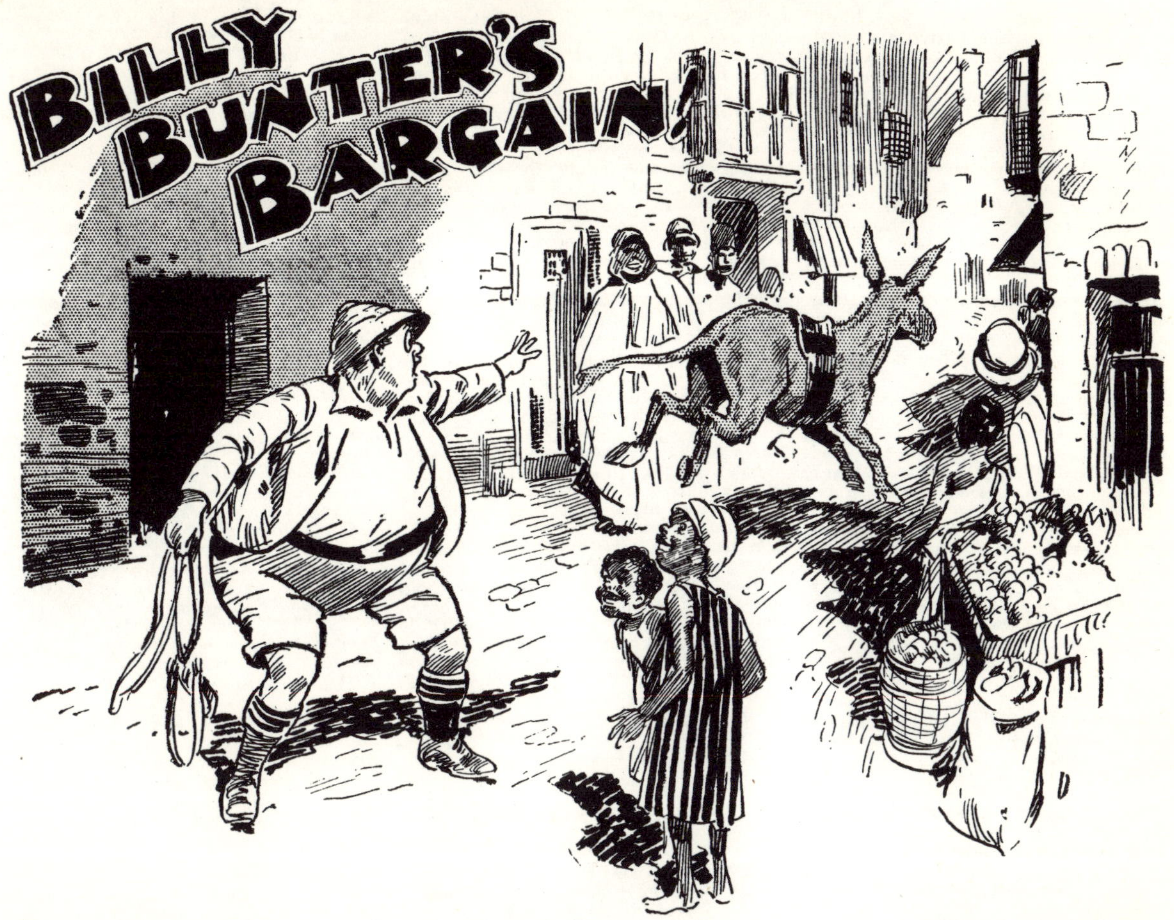

Featuring Harry Wharton & Co., the Cheery Chums of Greyfriars. By FRANK RICHARDS.

THE FIRST CHAPTER.
Cheap!

"DONKEY!"

"What?"

"Donkey!"

"You cheeky nigger!" snorted Billy Bunter.

"Donkey! Donkey!"

Billy Bunter of the Greyfriars Remove blinked at the brown-faced man in the tattered djubbah and turban through his big spectacles, with a devastating blink.

He was angry and indignant.

It was hot in the streets of Cairo. Heat and dust and flies had already annoyed Billy Bunter. Of all the Greyfriars party who were "doing" Egypt, only Hurree Jamset Ram Singh really enjoyed grilling under the African sun. But Harry Wharton & Co. were merry and bright. Bunter, on the other hand, was peeved. He was still more peeved when the brown gentleman marched up to him and called him—as he supposed, at least—a donkey!

Bunter had often been called an ass at Greyfriars School. But he did not like being called a donkey by a "nigger." He gave the brown man a blink that ought to have withered him on the spot.

Instead of being withered, however, the brown man only grinned, waved both his brown hands, and repeated:

"Yes, sar! Donkey! You—donkey!"

Harry Wharton & Co. were taking a walk in Cairo in the cool of the afternoon. But the "cool" of the afternoon was frightfully warm.

They had stopped at an Arab cafe for cooling liquid refreshment.

A bright-coloured awning stretched outside the cavernous-looking cafe sheltering them from the sun. On the "dekkas" under the awning, grave-faced Egyptians and Arabs were seated cross-legged, sipping sherbet or smoking long pipes. Lord Mauleverer, and the Famous Five of the Remove, sat in a row on one of the wooden benches, and Hassan, the dragoman, was talking in

When Billy Bunter buys a donkey he thinks it a rare bargain. Harry Wharton & Co., however, think Bunter a priceless ass—for he buys the same donkey on three separate occasions!

Arabic to the cafe-keeper, with a sound like the cracking of nuts, ordering cooling drinks for his "lordly gentlemen." Billy Bunter stood with Lord Mauleverer's best Panama hat pushed back from his streaming brow, mopping that streaming brow with one of Mauly's best handkerchiefs, when the native came up to him.

"Donkey, sar!" said the brown man. "Donkey! Yes! Donkey!"

There was a chuckle from the Famous Five, and a sleepy grin from Lord Mauleverer.

"Hallo, hallo, hallo!" yawned Bob Cherry. "I didn't know you had native friends in Cairo, Bunter."

"I haven't!" snapped Bunter.

"That man seems to know you!"

"Ha, ha, ha!"

"Blessed if I see anything to cackle at, in a blinking nigger's beastly cheek!" growled Bunter. "I've never seen the brown image before. What does he mean by calling me a donkey?"

"He guessed it in one!" said Frank Nugent.

"Well, really, it rather leaps to the eye, doesn't it?" remarked Johnny Bull. "After all, what else could he call you, if he calls you anything?"

"Donkey, sar! Yes! Donkey!"

"You sheer off, you cheeky nigger!" snapped Bunter. "I'll jolly well call a bobby, see?"

Billy Bunter glared at the brown man. The brown man grinned and gesticulated. Harry Wharton & Co. looked at him rather curiously. Had the native had a donkey with him, they would have supposed that he was a donkey-boy seeking a customer. But he had no donkey with him. Neither did he look like a donkey-boy. He looked like one of the innumerable native merchants who had been trying to sell things to the juniors ever since they had set foot in Egypt.

"Donkey, sar! You!" said the brown man. "Yes! Beautiful donkey!"

"He's got it wrong this time," said Harry Wharton gravely. "The noun's right—but not the adjective!"

"Oh, really, Wharton——"

"Fine big donkey, sar. You buy!" further elucidated the native merchant. "Me Abdullah, sar! Sell a donkey! Yes."

"Oh!" ejaculated Bunter.

Abdullah's English was evidently limited. But he had made his meaning clear at last. He was not calling Bunter a donkey! He was trying to sell him a donkey!

The variety of articles offered for sale in the streets and shops of Cairo was infinite. Natives had tried to sell the Greyfriars party all sorts of things, from "antiquities" made in Germany, to razors and hairbrushes, and even hairpins. But this was the first time that a donkey had been offered them.

Like all visitors to Cairo, the juniors rode on donkey-back. But they had never thought of buying donkeys. What the brown man supposed a schoolboy could want to buy a donkey for, was a mystery. Still, it was no more mysterious than the belief of native merchants that they were prepared to buy amber beads, powder-puffs, live doves, boxes of cosmetics, Turkish pipes, hairpins, razor-blades and the other surprising things that had been urged upon them.

"The silly ass!" grunted Bunter. "What the thump does he think I want to buy a donkey for? Silly ass!"

"Oh! No, sar!" exclaimed Abdullah. "No silly ass, sar—very clever ass, sar—fine clever good donkey, sar!"

"Ha, ha, ha!"

"You see a donkey!" said Abdullah persuasively. "I show you a donkey! Fifty piastres, sar! Yes."

"Oh, my hat!" said Bob. "That's a cheap line in donkeys! Let's see—a piastre is about twopence-halfpenny. That's about ten bob for the donkey. Never heard of a donkey going for ten bob."

"We'd take that for Bunter!" remarked Johnny Bull thoughtfully. "But any other donkey would be cheap at the price."

"Ha, ha, ha!"

"Yah!" snorted Bunter.

"Better close on that offer," chuckled Nugent. "It may turn out to be a long-lost brother."

"Ha, ha, ha!"

"Oh, don't be a funny idiot!" said Bunter. "I say, you fellows, I think I'll look at that donkey. I dare say we can put it up at the hotel. It sounds to me like a bargain."

"Fathead!" said Harry Wharton. "If the man offers a donkey for fifty piastres, that means that it can't be worth more than fifteen."

"The worthfulness is probably not terrific," agreed Hurree Jamset Ram Singh.

"I'm rather a judge of horseflesh," said Bunter. "We keep a lot of hunters at Bunter Court, you know. I can tell whether it's a good donkey or not. You can lend me fifty piastres, Mauly."

"Yaas!" yawned Lord Mauleverer.

"You see a donkey, sar!" urged Abdullah. "Fine splendid donkey, sar! You take two step, you see a donkey." He pointed along the street. "You come, sar! Yes! Donkey, sar! Donkey!"

He was pointing to a shady stone archway next to the cafe. Apparently the splendid donkey was there, waiting for a sale.

"I say, you fellows, let's step along and see it," said Bunter.

"Oh, all right!"

The juniors rose from the bench and followed Abdullah from under the awning.

Outside the awning was a blaze of burning sunshine. But they passed quickly into the cool shade of the stone archway. Billy Bunter was rather eager on the track of a bargain. The other fellows were grinning. They had no doubt that if the brown man was selling a donkey for ten shillings, it was a donkey that had seen better days, and seen the last of them long ago. Still, Bunter was not going to lose on the transaction, anyhow, as he was going to borrow the necessary piastres from Lord Mauleverer.

Abdullah waved them into the shady archway, with gesticulations of both brown hands.

"Donkey, sar! You see a donkey!"

"Oh, my hat!" exclaimed Bob Cherry, in astonishment.

There was a donkey tethered in the archway. But it was not the knock-kneed, broken-down relic of a donkey that the juniors expected to see. It was a big, powerful, handsome donkey; as fine a donkey as they had seen in Cairo. What its value might be they did not know; but it must have been worth hundreds of piastres at least.

Bunter blinked at it.

With all his experience of the hunters kept at Bunter Court, the fat Owl of the Remove did not know much about horseflesh, and he knew still less about donkey-flesh. But even Bunter could see that that donkey was a terrific bargain at fifty piastres. His eyes gleamed behind his big spectacles. He blinked at the brown merchant.

"Fifty piastres?"

"Yes, sar."

"I'll buy him!"

THE SECOND CHAPTER.

Parted Pals!

"FATHEAD!"

The Famous Five made that remark all at once.

The donkey was a bargain. There was no doubt about that. He was worth at least ten times as much as Abdullah asked for him. It was so extraordinary for a Cairo merchant to offer any article below its value that the juniors could not help suspecting that there was a "catch" in it somewhere. Still, they had to admit that they could not see where the catch came in. There was the donkey, and there was Abdullah, his owner, ready and eager to sell.

Nevertheless, that donkey, though evidently a valuable animal, was likely to prove rather a white elephant to the Greyfriars party. Donkeys had to be accommodated, fed, and looked after; and in a day or two the party were going up the Nile by water, and a donkey, howsoever valuable, would be superfluous on board a dahabiyeh.

"I say, you fellows——"

"Chuck it, Bunter," said Wharton. "You don't want to buy a donkey. What are you going to do with it?"

"Well, one of you fellows can lead it back to the hotel——"

"Oh, my hat!"

"And they'll look after it there, if they're paid. Mauly can arrange that, as he's paying the exes on this trip."

"Oh gad!"

"It's a topping donkey!" said Bunter. "Worth hundreds of piastres! Can't make out why the man's selling him so cheap! But I jolly well know I'm buying him. Why, I could sell him again and make a big profit if I liked!"

Billy Bunter patted the donkey's head. The animal looked round at him, opened his capacious mouth, and remarked:

"Hee-haw!"

"He knows Bunter!" said Bob. "He's talking to him in his own language already!"

"Ha, ha, ha!"

"You buy a donkey, sar?" exclaimed Abdullah eagerly. "Fine donkey, sar, you see. Yes! Fifty piastres—cheap price!"

"What's his name?" asked Bunter.

All donkeys in Cairo have names; sometimes the most extraordinary names. The juniors had ridden animals that rejoiced in such names as Queen Victoria, Lord Kitchener, Duke of York, and William Shakespeare.

Abdullah grinned at the fat Owl.

"You English, sar, or American?" he asked. "To the English his name is Prince of Wales. To American gentleman his name is George Washington. Yes."

"Ha, ha, ha!" roared the juniors.

"Well, I shall call him Quelch, after our Form master at Greyfriars," said Bunter. "He, he, he! I'm buying him! Lend me fifty piastres, Mauly."

Hassan, the dragoman, came along from the cafe. Hassan, gorgeous in his red tarboosh with a gold tassel, his gold-braided tunic, his sky-blue trousers, his crimson sash, and his yellow boots, looked rather like a tropical butterfly beside the donkey merchant.

"My lordly gentlemen, the sherbet is prepare!" exclaimed Hassan. "What you do here with a donkey, noble sars?"

"I'm buying that donkey," said Bunter.

Abdullah's dark eyes fixed uneasily and suspiciously on Hassan. Hassan's fixed suspiciously on Abdullah. The two natives were mutually suspicious and distrustful. Hassan, like a true dragoman, cheated his masters to the fullest possible extent. But it was his dragoman duty to see that others did not cheat them.

Only "backsheesh" slipped into his own greasy palm would have induced Hassan to let any other rogue rob his lordly gentlemen!

The dragoman addressed Abdullah in Arabic. The donkey dealer answered in the same tongue. Hassan replied, and the donkey dealer rejoined, and the volleys of Arabic went back and forth, not a single word comprehended by the Greyfriars fellows.

The argument sounded emphatic, and Harry Wharton & Co., though they did not understand the language, had learned enough of Egyptian ways to guess the purport. They had little doubt that Hassan was stipulating for "backsheesh" for himself as a condition of allowing the donkey to be sold to one of his lordly gentlemen. As they were thirsty, and the sherbet ready waiting next door at the cafe, the chums of the Remove were not disposed to wait for the end of the argument.

"Tell you what, you men," yawned Lord Mauleverer, "let's cut—what?"

"The cutfulness is the proper caper!" agreed Hurree Jamset Ram Singh.

"I say, you fellows——"

"Come on, fathead!"

"I'm buying that donkey!" hooted Bunter. "Lend me fifty piastres, Mauly. I'll settle up next term at Greyfriars. I believe I mentioned that I was expecting a postal order——"

"Oh gad!" said Lord Mauleverer. "Here you are, old fat bean. But don't buy the donkey. Two of you would be really too much, you know."

"Yah!" retorted Bunter.

Lord Mauleverer ambled away, the Famous Five following him, leaving Bunter to conclude his bargain, as he was evidently deaf to argument. Hassan remained with him, no doubt having a bargain to conclude also. If Hassan had allowed one of the party to buy anything without getting his "whack" from the seller, Hassan would probably have wept with grief.

The juniors sat down under the awning to sip their sherbet, which was grateful and comforting on a blazing hot Egyptian day. As they sipped they looked with interested eyes at the ever-moving crowd in the narrow, hot, somewhat scented street.

Water-sellers passed them—plenty of water-sellers of all sorts, for in Cairo on a hot day there was a great sale for that commodity. A big man dressed in red carried a huge jar slung to his belt, from which he sold liquorice water in a blue china bowl. Sherbet-sellers with great, green glass bottles; bread merchants with loaves and cakes made like rings and strung on sticks; pastry-cooks with baskets of sticky pastries balanced on their heads, at which sometimes a hawk came swooping down from nowhere—all had interest for the schoolboys from the far-off island in the North Sea.

"Hee-haw!"

Their attention was turned to Bunter again as the fat junior rejoined them, leading the big, handsome donkey by a halter George Washington, or the Prince of Wales, whichever he was, seemed quite content with his new master. Billy Bunter was more than content. He had made a tremendous bargain in "Quelch," as he had newly named the donkey, and there was no doubt that the handsome animal could have been sold again for a great deal more than fifty piastres, even by a stranger in the land. The Owl of the Remove felt that he had reason to be satisfied

"Hallo, hallo, hallo! Here come the twins!" said Bob Cherry.

"Ha, ha, ha!"

"Hold him, one of you fellows, while I have some sherbet," said Bunter. "I'm jolly thirsty! Here, hold him, Hassan."

"Yes, sar!" said the dragoman.

Hassan was smiling, as usual, and the juniors had no doubt that he had "touched" Mr. Abdullah for backsheesh.

But Mr. Abdullah's dealings were really perplexing. Anywhere in Cairo he could have sold that donkey for hundreds of piastres, yet he had sold it to Bunter for fifty, and out of the fifty he certainly had had to give Hassan at least ten. It really was mysterious, and the juniors felt more than ever that there was a catch in it somewhere.

Hassan held the donkey while Bunter absorbed sherbet and devoured sticky cakes. Bunter, apparently, was prepared to spend the rest of the afternoon at the Arab cafe, eating and drinking. But the other fellows had not come there to watch the fat Owl's gastronomic performances. They rose to their feet to move on. Hassan was conducting them to view the celebrated Mosque of El-Azhar, one of the sights of Cairo.

"I say, you fellows, what about chucking that mosque and getting back to the hotel?" asked Bunter. "I can't lead my donkey all over Cairo, you know."

"You should have thought of that before you bought him, fathead," answered Harry Wharton. "Come on, Mauly!"

"Well, look here. Let Hassan take him to the hotel," said Bunter. "We don't really want Hassan. I can tell you all about Cairo."

"My lordly gentlemen——" began Hassan.

"Well, one of you fellows lead him back to the hotel," said Bunter. "You can cut out the mosque, and I'll tell you all about it when I get back."

"Ha, ha, ha!"

"Blessed if I see anything to cackle at! Look here, that donkey's got to be taken home!" exclaimed Bunter warmly. "The question is, who's leading him home for me?"

"The whofulness is terrific!" chuckled Hurree Jamset Ram Singh.

"I say, you fellows——"

"My noble gentlemen will follow in my humble footsteps," said Hassan. "We go see great Mosque of El-Azhar, wonderful monument of Fatimid period—yes! Built in a tenth century——"

Harry Wharton & Co. followed the dragoman. Billy Bunter stood holding the halter of the donkey, and glaring after them through his big spectacles.

"I say, you fellows——" he bawled.

"Oh, come on, Bunter!"

"What about this donkey?" bawled Bunter.

"Oh, bother your relations!"

"Beast!"

Evidently, if anybody was going to lead Quelch, it was going to be Quelch's owner. Billy Bunter snorted with indignation. As he had bought Quelch, and Quelch was his property, Bunter might have been expected to take charge of him—by anybody but Bunter. But the fat Owl did not want the trouble. Trouble for anybody else was a lesser matter—in fact, a trifle light as air! But as Hassan and the juniors walked on Bunter realised that he had to lead the donkey himself, or else leave him where he was—so he led him.

But the difficulty was solved very

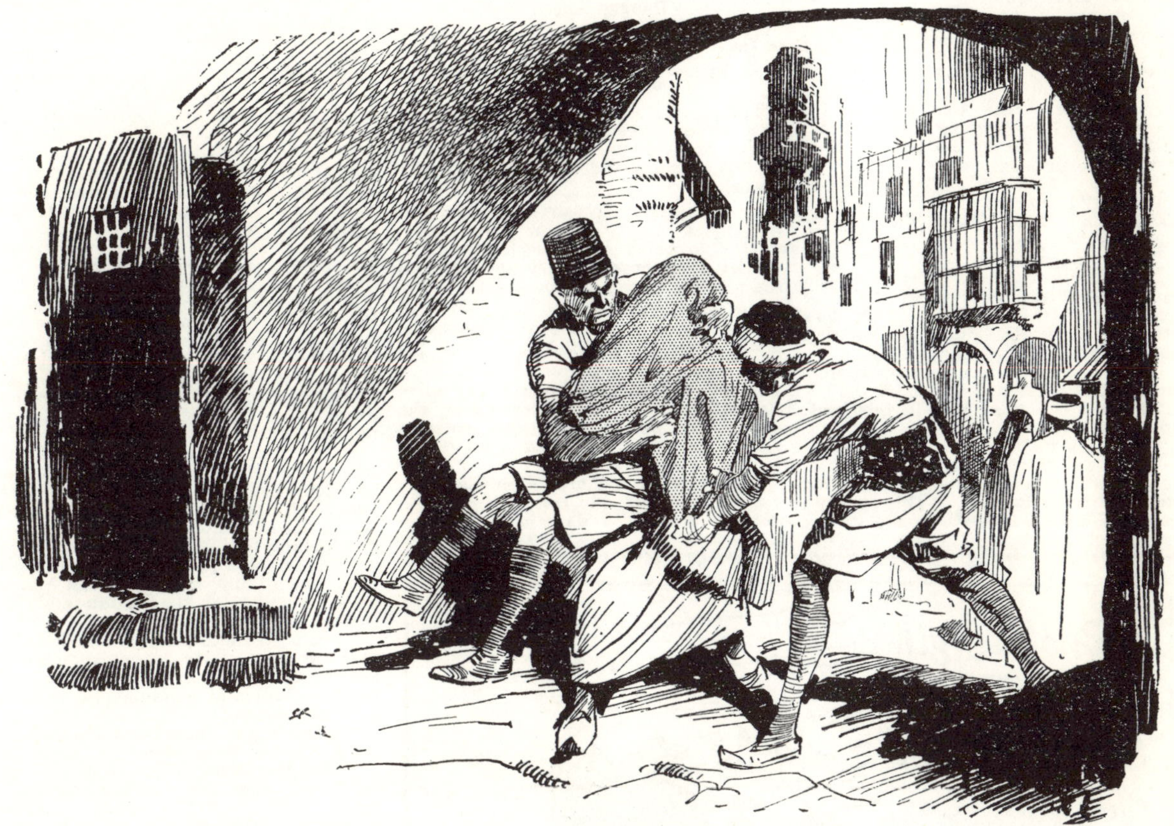

Maulеverer had stepped into the archway to fan himself with his hat when suddenly a dusty, evil-smelling sack was dropped over his head. The next moment he was whipped off his feet and rushed away!

quickly, and in a way that was rather unexpected.

Not more than a hundred yards from the donkey-dealer's archway Quelch suddenly slipped his shaggy head and his long ears out of the halter, and took to his heels.

Bunter, pulling him on by the halter, suddenly found the rope loose in his hand, and blinked round in surprise—in time to catch a farewell glimpse of Quelch's heels as he vanished in the crowded street.

"Oh crikey!" gasped Bunter.

Quelch was gone!

"I say, you fellows!" Bunter rushed after the juniors. "I say, that donkey's bolted! After him."

There was a chortle from the Greyfriars fellows. They could not see themselves chasing a runaway donkey through the hot and crowded streets of Cairo—not quite! Quelch was gone from Bunter's gaze like a beautiful dream—and he was going to stay gone, so to speak, so far as the Famous Five were concerned.

"I say, you fellows! Deaf?" hooted Bunter. "I say, get after that donkey! Catch him! After him! I'll wait for you here!"

"Ha, ha, ha!"

"You silly chumps, what are you cackling at?" roared Bunter. "I gave ten bob for that donkey! Now he's gone! Think I'm going to lose that donkey, you cackling chumps?"

"Well, get after him, old fat bean!" chuckled Bob Cherry.

"I can't run after him in this heat, you silly ass!"

"And can we?" bawled Johnny Bull.

"Yes, old chap! Don't be a slacker, you know! I say, you fellows, will you stop?" howled Bunter. "The donkey's gone the other way——"

"The stopfulness will not be terrific, my esteemed idiotic Bunter."

"Beasts!" roared Bunter.

The Greyfriars party walked cheerily on their way, and Billy Bunter rolled after them, snorting with indignation. And at the other end of the street a grinning brown gentleman of the name of Abdullah slipped a halter over Quelch's neck and led him away—with a view to selling him at a remarkably low price to some other tourist with an eye for a bargain in donkeys!

THE THIRD CHAPTER.

Danger Ahead!

"KALIZELOS!" breathed Harry Wharton.

"What——"

"Look—in the mirror!"

The juniors had stopped before a shop in a narrow street, where the projecting balconies above almost met in the middle, turning the street into a shady tunnel.

In the shop many articles were displayed, among them a large steel mirror, in which were reflected the faces of the schoolboys as they looked, and the passing figures in the street.

An olive-skinned face was reflected in the mirror—the face of a man who stood at a little distance behind the Greyfriars party.

It was a face they knew. The olive face of Kalizelos, the Greek dealer, the enemy who had dogged their footsteps all the days that they had spent in the land of the Pharaohs.

"My hat!" murmured Bob Cherry.

"Watching us, the rotter!" muttered Johnny Bull. "I dare say he's been following us, looking for a chance at Mauly and the scarab."

The Famous Five did not look round at the Greek. Evidently he was unaware that they had spotted him by catching his reflection in the mirror in the Cairo shop. Whenever they had seen him before Kalizelos had been dressed like a European; but now he wore the kaftan and turban of a native Egyptian, obviously for disguise. His olive face was dark enough to pass for an Egyptian's.

That he was following and watching them there was no doubt. Neither was there any doubt of his object.

The Golden Scarab—the sacred scarabeus of A-Menah—was what the Greek was after; and that scarab was in Lord Mauleverer's pocket.

Once a rich dealer in the city of Cairo, Kalizelos was now a fugitive, hunted by the Egyptian police. Twice Lord Mauleverer had narrowly escaped with his life at the hands of the Greek.

According to ancient tradition, that golden beetle was a clue to the treasure of Osiris, the wonderful diamond famed in the reign of Rameses the Second. The juniors did not believe it—it seemed a fable to them—but, amazing as it was, the Greek was prepared to risk his liberty and his life to obtain possession of the scarab, which proved that he, at least, was a firm believer in the tradition. The risks he had taken, and the losses he had sustained, showed how fierce was his desire to possess the mysterious scarab, how firmly he believed that it would lead him to an immense fortune.

Even now, in the crowded Cairo street, the Greek was running risks—as he shadowed the Greyfriars juniors. Doubtless, in his native dress, they would not have noticed him in passing; but looking at his face reflected in the mirror under their eyes, they had a good view of him, and they knew him at once, in spite of the kaftan and the turban.

"Don't give him the tip!" said Harry in a low voice. "He doesn't know we've spotted him. We may get a chance of bagging him and handing him over to a Cairo bobby."

"Good egg!" murmured Nugent.

"I say, you fellows——"

"Shut up, Bunter!"

"I say, what are you blinking at in that silly shop?" asked Bunter peevishly. "There's a pastrycook's next door. They've got some of those ripping cakes! Lend me twenty piastres—I can't see Mauly."

"Go and eat coke!"

"Beast!"

The olive-skinned face disappeared from the mirror. The juniors saw the reflection of the figure in the turban and the blue kaftan turn away. Then they turned from the shop and glanced after it. They could not see Kalizelos' face now—his back was turned—but they knew his figure in the crowd, and they followed on. He was not a dozen paces from them, and they glanced round, hoping to see an Egyptian policeman. Billy Bunter blinked after them.

"I say, you fellows——" he howled.

But the Famous Five did not heed Bunter. It was a chance of getting hold of the Greek and removing the danger that had haunted Lord Mauleverer ever since Kalizelos had discovered that he was the possessor of the Scarab of A-Menah. The man in the blue kaftan moved on, evidently unconscious that he, the watcher, was now watched; and the Famous Five drew closer and closer to him, with the intention of collaring him suddenly before he could dodge away in the crowd. They were hardly a yard behind the Greek when he turned suddenly into an arched doorway and disappeared from their eyes.

"My lordly gentlemen——" Hassan was hurrying after the juniors.

Harry Wharton & Co. stopped at the arched doorway. There was no door, and in the dusky interior they could see dimly a flight of stone steps. Harry turned to the dragoman.

"What place is this, Hassan?" he asked.

Hassan made a grimace.

"It is not suitable for my noble lords to enter," he said. "It is cheap place where poor persons lodge in great numbers. Once long ago it was great house of Mamelukes; now it go to pot, as you say in your noble language."

Three or four people came out of the arched doorway, and their looks bore out Hassan's statement; a half-clad negro, an Armenian pedlar, and a couple of beggars, who promptly demanded "backsheesh" as they saw the English faces. Hassan drove them off with a wave of his stick.

"My lordly masters, this is not a place to linger," said the dragoman. "Also and likewise, my magnificent gentlemen have not yet beheld the wonderful Mosque of El-Azhar——"

"Never mind the mosque now," said Harry Wharton.

Hassan opened his eyes wide.

"Oh, sar! That so wonderful mosque, which is builded in a tenth century, in the reign of the Caliph El-Muizz——"

"Yes, yes; never mind now! Look here, Hassan, we've just seen Kalizelos, that Greek scoundrel, and he has gone into this house."

"And we're after him," said Bob Cherry. "We're jolly well going to bag him. The mosque can wait."

"The bagfulness is going to be terrific, my esteemed and ridiculous Hassan," said Hurree Jamset Ram Singh.

"I say, you fellows——"

"For goodness' sake shut up, Bunter!"

"If you won't lend me twenty piastres, you stingy beasts, tell me where Mauly is! Mauly will lend an old pal a few piastres!" said Bunter warmly. "I can tell you, they've got some simply ripping cakes in that pastrycook's, and I can't see Mauly anywhere."

Harry Wharton started. In their keenness on "bagging" the Greek, the Famous Five had not noticed that Lord Mauleverer was not with them. They had supposed that he was at hand, probably looking into one of the dusky shops in the narrow street. But if Bunter could not find him, evidently he was not at hand.

"Hassan, where's Mauleverer?" exclaimed Wharton.

"I was of belief that noble lord was with my majestic gentlemen," said Hassan, staring round. "But perhaps he go entering into a shop."

The juniors exchanged a quick glance. It was possible that Lord Mauleverer had stepped into one of the cave-like, dusky shops out of sight. But they did not think so.

"I say, you fellows, I've been hunting for Mauly, and I can't see him. Look here, I can do with ten piastres——"

"If Kalizelos has got him——" breathed Johnny Bull.

Wharton set his lips. It seemed incredible that Mauleverer could have been seized and whipped out of sight in the crowded street. Yet, on the other hand, the swarm of jostling natives and foreigners might have given the kidnappers an opportunity, screening their movements; and it came into Wharton's mind that that was why Kalizelos had been watching them—watching to see that they did not intervene.

"Come on!" said Harry abruptly. "We're going in here; we're going to find that scoundrel Kalizelos——"

"My noble lords——" exclaimed Hassan.

"Come with us, Hassan," said Harry. "We've got to find Kalizelos. You can find him for us; he's in the house somewhere."

"To hear is to obey, my magnificent lord," answered the dragoman, but he looked very dubious.

Hassan entered the arched doorway, and the juniors followed him up a flight of dirty and evil-smelling stone steps. Natives were coming up or going down every minute; and the dragoman stopped to speak to several of them in Arabic. He turned to the anxious juniors with a smiling face.

"I hear of a Greek who stay in this beggarly house, sars," he said. "Perhaps he is Kalizelos. Yes, I think! We go to see him, and if he give a trouble, I, Hassan, will bash him, as you say in your noble language, with stick! Hassan is your dragoman. You trust Hassan."

And the juniors followed the dragoman up the evil-smelling stairs, their hearts beating fast.

THE FOURTH CHAPTER.

Pipped at the Post!

LORD MAULEVERER blinked.

He hardly knew what had happened.

While his companions were looking into the shops, Mauly had stepped into a shadowy archway out of the sun that streamed down into the narrow street, and there he fanned himself with his hat while he waited for the other fellows to come on.

Mauly was thinking of the heat and the flies, so far as his noble intellect was working at all. Certainly he was not thinking of danger. He was taken utterly by surprise when a dusty, evil-smelling sack was suddenly dropped over his head, and he was whipped off his feet and rushed up a staircase.

He heard a door open and shut.

Then the sack was jerked from his head, and the schoolboy earl of Greyfriars blinked round him dizzily.

He was in a bare, dingy, almost unfurnished room, with a narrow window that looked out on what had once been a garden, but was now rubbish-heaps. The door by which he had entered was closed, and with his back to it stood an Arab with an evil, grinning face and eyes like a hawk. Another Arab, with the scar of a knife-cut across his dark cheek, was in the room, and he was grinning, too. Mauleverer blinked at them.

He knew both by sight. The hawk-faced man was Yussef, who had guarded him in the lost tomb near the Pyramids, a week ago. The scarred man was the pickpocket who had shadowed him in the catacombs of Alexandria, two or three weeks since. Both of them, he knew, were rascals in the pay of Kalizelos, the Greek. It dawned on Mauleverer that he had fallen into the hands of his enemies, suddenly, unexpectedly, at a moment when he had not dreamed of danger.

"Oh gad!" gasped Mauly. He brushed the dust from his face—the sack had been very dusty. "Oh gad!"

"You will be silent, Faringhee," said Yussef. "One cry out, sar, and Hamza will knock you over your head."

The scarred Arab, Hamza, grinned and lifted a stick. Lord Mauleverer eyed it and decided not to call out.

"Well, you've got me, old beans," said his lordship calmly. "I suppose you've been watchin' for a chance like this."

Yussef chuckled.

"Yes, sar, we watch you step into a doorway," he grinned. "You choose to step into a doorway of house where we are. Bismillah!"

"Oh gad!" said Mauleverer.

He realised that the archway into which he had stepped for shade from the sun was the entrance of the building where these thieves of Cairo had their den. By sheer chance he had walked fairly into their hands.

His face set. The Golden Sarab was in his pocket. Mauleverer wished now that he had left it locked up in the manager's safe at the hotel.

He had taken it from that secure place to show it to Hilmi Maroudi, the Egyptian gentleman with whom the Greyfriars fellows had made friends. With his usual carelessness he had slipped it into his pocket afterwards and left it there. His captors, doubtless, were not aware of it, but a search would reveal it soon enough.

The two ruffians did not touch him, however. They seemed to be waiting, and Mauleverer could guess for whom they were waiting. He had no doubt that the Greek was at hand.

He was right. In a few minutes there came three taps at the door; evidently a known signal, for Yussef stepped away from it at once and allowed it to open from without. It was Kalizelos, the Greek, who entered, closing the door after him, and Yussef again put his brawny back to it.

Mauleverer stared at the Greek. For the moment he did not recognise him in the blue kaftan and turban. But he knew the olive-skinned, handsome face as he looked at it.

"We meet again, my lord!" said the Greek.

"Yaas," assented Mauleverer. "Can't say I'm glad to see you, old bean. It would be stretchin' politeness altogether too far."

"I have failed many times, my lord," said Kalizelos. "But the goddess of fortune has favoured me to-day; or perhaps it is Fate, as the Moslems would say—Kismet! Since I have become a fugitive, my lord, hunted in my own city by the police, this wretched building, which was once a palace of the Mamelukes, has been my hiding-place. It was obliging of you, my lord, to step into my humble doorway and place yourself in my hands." The Greek grinned.

"I'm an oblигin' chap," yawned Lord Mauleverer. "And I may as well remind you that my friends are quite close at hand, Mr. Kalizelos."

Kalizelos laughed.

"Quite; but your friends cannot see through stone walls," he answered. "I have been watching your friends, prepared to intervene if they should have followed you. But your friends are very interested in gazing into a shop, my lord, and I have left them so engaged. I do not think they will guess that you have disappeared into this house. Do you think they will, my lord?"

Mauleverer did not answer. Obviously Harry Wharton & Co. could guess nothing of the sort.

"Let us talk business, Lord Mauleverer," said the Greek. "At the

Pyramids you fell into my hands, but the scarab had been left in a safe place. Now you are in my hands again, and you will not escape as before. Where is the Golden Scarab of A-Menah?"

"Find out!" said Lord Mauleverer.

The Greek spoke in the native language to Hamza. The scarred Arab stepped towards Lord Mauleverer. Probably Kalizelos did not expect to find the scarab on the schoolboy earl, but he was not the man to leave anything to chance. Mauleverer was to be searched before other steps were taken. Bitterly at that moment the schoolboy earl repented of his carelessness. But it was too late for that to be of any use. He clenched his hands as the scarred man stepped to him.

Kalizelos' face lighted. That instinctive movement of resistance enlightened him; the scarab was on the schoolboy.

"Fortune has favoured me more than I supposed, my lord!" he grinned. "You have the scarab in your pocket! Me explettete! Eine dunation!" He dropped into his own language for a moment, and then went on in English: "Is it possible? My lord, I thank you from my heart; and you also may be thankful, for when the scarab is in my hands you will see me no more. I have lost my shop and my business in Cairo. But when I have sold the diamond of A-Menah, the Eye of Osiris, for a quarter of a million pounds, I shall make my peace. Oh, yes! With backsheesh one can do anything! Give me the scarab!"

He rapped out a word in Arabic, and the scarred man grasped Lord Mauleverer. It was futile to resist the brawny ruffian, and in that powerful grasp Mauleverer had to yield. The brown hands ran through his pockets, and there was a sudden gleam of gold in the shaft of sunlight from the narrow window.

The Greek gave a shout of delight. He bounded forward and grasped the golden beetle from the Arab's hand.

His black eyes danced.

The golden beetle lay in his olive palm. The prize he had so long sought was in his hand at last!

And even as that shout of triumph broke from the Greek, and the two Arabs, with curious eyes, drew nearer to stare at the gleaming golden beetle, the door of the room burst open, and Hassan, the dragoman, rushed in, with the Famous Five of Greyfriars at his heels.

THE FIFTH CHAPTER.
Turning the Tables!

CRASH!

Hassan's heavy stick struck as the Greek whirled round, and the blow caught Kalizelos fairly on the head.

He gave a gasping cry and lurched over, falling heavily, and the Golden Scarab shot from his hand and dropped in a corner of the dingy room.

"Go for 'em!" roared Bob Cherry. "Back up, Greyfriars!"

Yussef and Hamza jumped back from the rush of the juniors. Hamza dodged round the wall and darted out at the open doorway almost in a twinkling. His fleeing footsteps died away on the dingy stairs. Yussef flashed a knife from under his djubbah.

The dragoman flourished his stick.

But Yussef was not thinking of fighting. The game was up, and he knew it; the dragoman had only to call for help if he wanted it. Yussef brandished the knife to clear a way of escape, and the juniors, unarmed, had to jump back from the slashing, keen blade. Barely escaping a blow from Hassan's stick, the hawk-faced Arab darted out of the room and fled after his comrade.

Kalizelos lay where he had fallen, half-stunned.

"My lordly gentlemen, we have found our noble lord and rascally persons who lay hands on him!" exclaimed Hassan. "Yes! Hassan is your dragoman! You trust Hassan!"

"Mauly, old man——"

"Glad to see you fellows, by gad!" said Lord Mauleverer. "The jolly old Greek would have had the scarab this time, and no mistake!" His lordship lounged across to the corner where the golden beetle had fallen and picked it up. "This dashed old insect has had a narrow escape—what?"

"And we've got the Greek!" said Harry Wharton grimly. "Never mind the Arabs; they don't matter! We've got Kalizelos!"

"The gotfulness is terrific!" chuckled the Nabob of Bhanipur.

The Greek raised himself on his elbow, still dazed from the blow, and his jetty eyes glittered at the juniors.

In the very moment of triumph he had been defeated.

How the schoolboys had found their way to that room in the rabbit warren of a house was an utter mystery to him. But they were there, and he was a beaten man. His dusky hand slid under his kaftan and grasped a hidden weapon, and there was murder in his glittering eyes. Yussef and Hamza had fled promptly enough. But the Greek was desperate; even with the Cairo police at the door, he would not have yielded up the scarab without a struggle. From under the folds of the blue kaftan an automatic flashed out. But even as it came into sight Harry Wharton kicked it from his hand. It crashed on the floor, and Bob Cherry promptly caught it up.

"Collar him!" shouted Bob.

"Bag the rotter!" panted Johnny Bull.

The Greek bounded up. He made a spring towards the door, and Hassan leaped in the way with brandished stick. The chums of Greyfriars grasped at him on all sides, grasping the loose kaftan and dragging him down.

Kalizelos struggled furiously.

Five to one as they were, he was like a tiger in the hands of the Famous Five. They went to the floor in a scrambling, struggling heap, and then Kalizelos tore loose, leaving the long-flowing kaftan in the hands of the schoolboys. Hassan was rushing on him with uplifted stick, but the blow missed by an inch as the Greek bounded back. A second more, and he had plunged headlong through the narrow window.

"Collar him!"

"Oh, my hat!"

Harry Wharton & Co. scrambled to their feet, the empty kaftan in their hands. Kalizelos was vanishing, head-first, through the narrow window. Crash came Hassan's stick, and it struck the leg of the Greek as he went. Then he was gone.

"Inshallah!" gasped Hassan.

There was a crash below.

"Oh crumbs!" gasped Bob Cherry.

He stared down from the window.

Twenty feet below an evil-smelling rubbish heap rotted in the sun. From amid rotten vegetables and putrid bones, dust, and ashes, the Greek was struggling to his feet. He gained his feet, glared up at the faces in the window, and darted away and vanished in an instant into a dark and noisome alley.

"Gone!" said Bob. He whistled. "He might have broken his neck! No loss if he had! But he's gone!"

"The brute's got a nerve!" said Nugent. "Blessed if I should like to take a header from this window! But it was that or chokey!"

"Well, he's gone," said Harry. "But you've got the scarab all right, Mauly."

"Yaas."

"All serene, then!"

"I rather fancy that sportsman must be cracked," said Mauleverer. "He's takin' a fearful lot of risks to get hold of this jolly old beetle! I don't see it myself."

The juniors looked at the scarab in Mauly's hand.

The golden beetle, with the name and title of A-Menah inscribed on it in the picture-writing of ancient Egypt, was an interesting curio, all the more because it was known to be three thousand years old. But to the eyes of the schoolboys, at least, it was nothing more than that.

It seemed incredible to them that there could reside in the little golden object any power to lead its possessor to the discovery of the Eye of Osiris, the once-famous diamond of the reign of Rameses the Second. Yet the cool, cunning Greek believed it, and Kalizelos was a clear-headed, successful business man—anything but "cracked," as his lordship put it. The whole thing was a mystery to the chums of Greyfriars.

Hassan, the dragoman, eyed the Golden Scarab with curious eyes. It was evident that he knew it by sight. Many pictures of that famous scarab, with its inscription in picture-writing, were in existence.

"It is the Scarab of A-Menah," said Hassan. "That noble person was a great general of Rameses the Second, honourable sars. Ignorant persons believe that there is a magic in the scarab to lead to a treasure." Hassan shrugged his shoulders. "It is one fable; what you call piffle in your noble English language—what you call tommy-rot! Yes! I, Hassan, am a civilised Arab. I do not believe these ancient tales, sars. I am too civilised to believe anything, my lordly gentlemen."

"I say, you fellows"—Billy Bunter's spectacles gleamed in the doorway—"I say, I've found you, you silly asses! What the thump are you up to here? Buzzing off and leaving a fellow! Oh, here you are, Mauly! I've been looking for you everywhere, old chap! Lend me twenty piastres, old fellow!"

"Lordly gentlemen, let us proceed to see a mosque!" said Hassan. "This is not suitable place for my noble sars to linger!"

The Greyfriars fellows went down the dingy stairs. They turned to the right on reaching the street, which was the way to the Mosque of El-Azhar. Billy Bunter's voice was raised in indignant expostulation. The way to the pastry-cook's was to the left. Bunter was more interested in pastry-cooks than in mosques.

"I say, you fellows——"

"Come on, fatty!"

"I say, they've got some ripping cakes—almonds on top——" gasped Bunter. "Simply topping! Never mind that silly old mosque—let's go into the pastry-cooks and have a feed! See? I'll stand the feed—you needn't worry about that! You lend me some piastres, Mauly——"

But deaf ears were turned on Bunter. Hassan and his flock marched on, and Billy Bunter followed them, grunting and grousing, and the pastry-cook's shop and its delights were left behind.

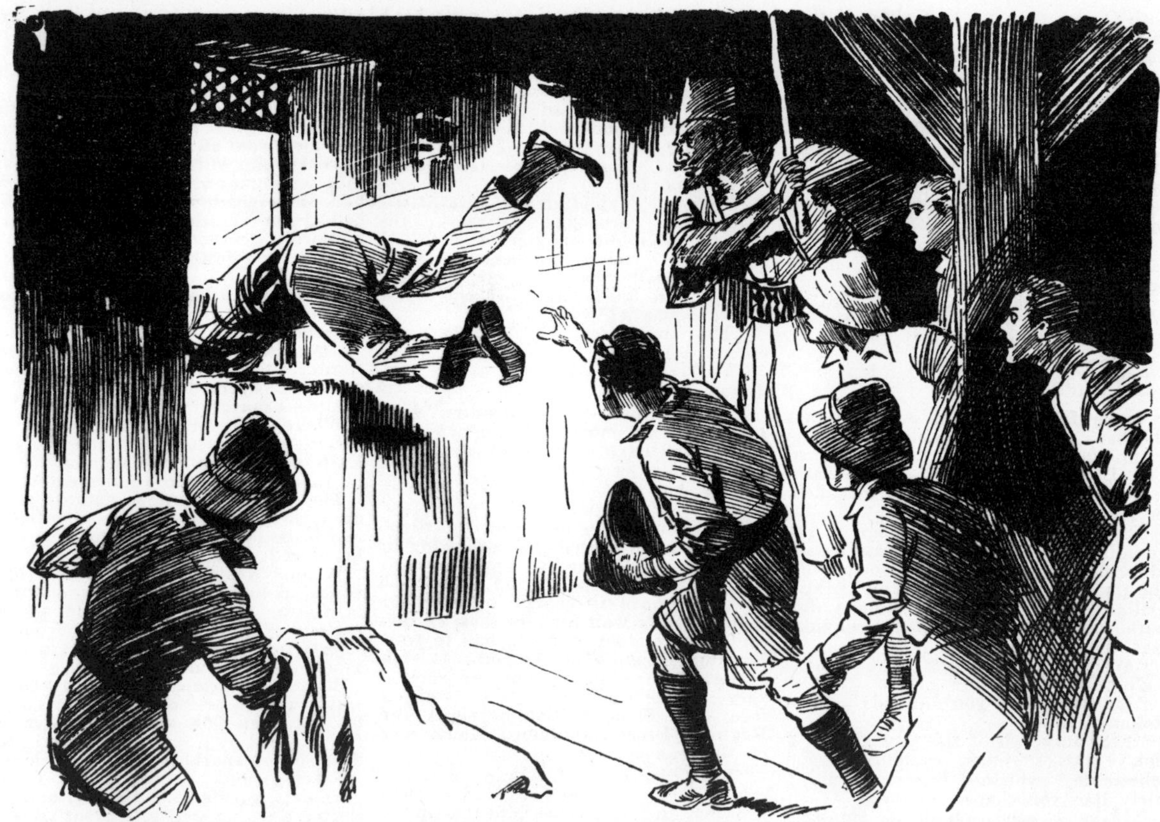

As Harry Wharton & Co. scrambled to their feet, the empty kaftan in their hands, Kalizelos was vanishing, head-first, through the narrow window. Hassan lashed out with his stick, and it struck the leg of the Greek as he went !

THE SIXTH CHAPTER.

A Tip for Bunter !

SIR REGINALD BROOKE jammed his eyeglass into his eye, and fixed it, and the eye, on William George Bunter.

It was the following afternoon. That day the Greyfriars party were to make a call on Mr. Hilmi Maroudi, their Egptian friend, at his house in Cairo. Billy Bunter had told the other fellows that he was not specially keen on calling on a "nigger." Still, he was not going to be left behind; moreover, nigger as Mr. Maroudi was, in Bunter's lofty estimation, it was certain that there would be refreshments, and that the refreshments would be ample and good.

That consideration weighed with Bunter very much. Indeed, there was no doubt that Bunter would have been willing to pay a friendly visit to a cannibal chief of Central Africa, if he had been sure that the grub would be good and ample.

The Greyfriars fellows were ready to start; and Mr. Maroudi had sent a big car to collect them. But there was grim disapproval in the frigid eye that Mauly's uncle fixed on William George Bunter.

Mr. Maroudi was a wealthy gentleman, and a very estimable gentleman, in the baronet's opinion; and all the party—excepting Bunter—had dressed themselves very nicely for the visit. Bunter hadn't! At Greyfriars School, Billy Bunter was not infrequently called over the coals by Mr. Quelch, his Form master, for slovenliness. More than once had Billy Bunter been sent out of the Form-room to wash his hands or put on a cleaner collar. But on vacation there was no gimlet-eyed Quelch to see that Bunter did not slack in such matters.

As a matter of taste, Bunter had never liked washing. Extravagant in many things, he exercised great economy in soap; and thrift in hot water. And if a fellow couldn't go easy on washing in the school holidays, Bunter would have liked to know what holidays were for.

"I say, you fellows, I'm ready," said Bunter, blinking down from the balcony at the waiting car. "Is that the nigger's car? Not a bad turn-out—pretty nearly as good as the Rolls at home, in fact. I say——"

"Bunter!" said Sir Reginald Brooke, in a deep voice.

"Eh?" Bunter blinked round.

"Have you washed to-day?"

"Wha-a-at?"

"Bunter washed the day we broke-up at Greyfriars," explained Bob Cherry. "He's making it last over the vac!"

"Oh, really, Cherry——"

"Bunter! There is something sticky on your face," said Sir Reginald.

"Oh, that's all right!" said Bunter. "Only jam!"

"Your collar is extremely soiled."

"Oh, really, sir——"

"Go, at once, and make yourself clean and tidy," said Sir Reginald. "Otherwise, I must leave you here."

Billy Bunter blinked at the stiff old gentleman in speechless indignation. Bunter really had washed that morning. Even Bunter washed of a morning. But in a hot climate—hot and dusty—a fellow who was scoffing sticky things all day long really needed more than one wash. Bunter's shining morning face grew grubbier and grubbier through the day, till by bed-time he might almost have been taken for a native.

Putting in an extra wash because he was going to call on a nigger, seemed quite absurd to Billy Bunter; and he could barely restrain his natural desire to tell Sir Reginald Brooke what he thought of him.

"Go at once!" said Sir Reginald.

Bunter, suppressing his wrath and indignation, went. Bob Cherry winked at his comrades, and they followed Bunter.

Billy Bunter could regard Mr. Maroudi as a nigger if he liked; but Harry Wharton & Co. had a great liking and respect for the Egyptian gentleman. The visit to Mr. Maroudi's house was, in their opinion, a rather important matter; and on such an important occasion they considered that Bunter ought to wash. And, as Bunter hated that kind of exertion with a deep and abiding hatred, they were prepared to lend him any necessary help.

"I say, you fellows, pretty thick, ain't it?" asked Billy Bunter, with a snort, on the stairs. "Making a lot of fuss of a nigger! I shan't stand much more cheek from that man Brooke! Making out that a fellow's face is dirty, you know! It's only jam and dust and some orange-juice and, perhaps, a bit of Turkish Delight! I'm clean, I hope!"

"Oh, my hat!" murmured Nugent. "He's got jam and dust and orange-juice and Turkish Delight plastered over his chivvy; and he hopes he's clean!"

"Hope springs infernal in the human chest, as the esteemed poet remarks," observed Hurree Jamset Ram Singh.

"Well, I'm jolly well not going to wash!" said Bunter. "I'll give my face a dab! Might as well be at Greyfriars, with Quelch snorting at a chap, if that interfering old ass is going to send a fellow up to wash! Jevver hear of such cheek!"

Each of the juniors had a room with a bath-room attached, in the big European hotel. Billy Bunter's bath-room never claimed much of his time. He did not intend to let it claim much now. But Bob Cherry kindly turned on the hot water for him, putting the plug in the bath.

"No need to plug the bath, old man," said Bunter. "Let it run! I shan't be a minute!"

Bob turned on the cold water, also.

"What's that for?" asked Bunter.

"You, old chap!"

"I don't want it."

"Well, you need it, at any rate!"

"Yah!"

Water from both taps streamed into the bath. Billy Bunter blinked at the grinning five. If these fellows fancied that Bunter was going to have a bath, these fellows were very much mistaken, in Billy Bunter's opinion.

The fat Owl dipped a sponge in the running water, and gave his face a dab. He could not venture to go down, with the jam, dust, orange-juice, and Turkish Delight still in evidence. But a dab with the sponge, in Bunter's opinion, was enough.

"Where's the towel?" he asked. "Gimme the towel!"

"My hat! Are you finished?" asked Johnny Bull.

"Certainly! Isn't the jam gone? I don't need so much washing as you fellows do," explained Bunter. "I'm not dirty like you chaps, you know."

"Make a good job of it, Bunter," urged Bob. "Give your ears a turn! Remember how it improved them when you washed them last term!"

"Ha, ha, ha!"

"And your neck!" said Harry Wharton. "Go it, Bunter!"

"I remember Bunter washed his neck when he was a fag in the Second Form," remarked Nugent. "Fellows hardly knew him afterwards."

"Ha, ha, ha!"

"Oh, really, Nugent——"

Bunter towelled his face, which had been slightly wetted by the sponge. His wash, apparently, was over. The Famous Five gazed at him. Bunter seemed to believe that he had finished. Harry Wharton & Co., on the other hand, were of opinion that he had hardly started.

"Is that the lot?" ejaculated Wharton.

"The lotfulness is not terrific!"

"Oh, don't jaw!" said Bunter peevishly. "If I've got to stand cheek from that old ass Brooke, I'm not standing cheek from you fellows, and I can tell you so. You can turn off those taps, Bob Cherry—you're filling the bath for nothing."

"Tumble in, old fat bean."

"Yah!"

"The esteemed bath is the proper caper, my idiotic Bunter," urged the Nabob of Bhanipur.

Bunter's fat lip curled.

"You niggers seem to think white men want as much washing as yourselves," he sneered. "Well, they don't! I'm going down."

"The bath's full, old bean," said Bob Cherry persuasively.

"You can have it if you like," jeered Bunter. "I dare say you need it. Thank goodness I'm not dirty like some fellows."

"Not going in?" asked Bob.

"No!" roared Bunter.

"Your mistake—you are!"

"Look here—leggo—oh, my hat! Yaroooh!" roared Bunter. "Yoop! Gerrrroooooogh! Gug-gug-gug!"

Splash!

Quite a water-spout rose from the bath as Billy Bunter tipped in. He disappeared for a moment and came up spluttering wildly.

"Urrrgh! Yug-yug-gug! Goooogh!"

"Ha, ha, ha!"

"Wooooch!" spluttered the fat Owl. "Ooooooch! Grooogh! Beasts! Oh crikey! Gug-gug-gug-gug!"

"Better strip," chuckled Bob. "You'll really have to change, old chap—you're quite wet! Wash while you're about it!"

"The wetfulness is terrific, my esteemed Bunter."

"Yurrrrrggh! Beasts! Gug-gug-groogh!"

"We'll wait for you downstairs," said Bob. "Don't mind us, Bunter! We don't often have to wait for you while you wash."

"Ha, ha, ha!"

"Beast!" roared Bunter.

The Famous Five departed, chortling, leaving the infuriated Owl wallowing in the bath. As Bunter had tipped in with his clothes on, there was no doubt that he would have to change. The other fellows had to wait for him; but, as Bob said, they seldom or never had to wait for Bunter while he washed. It was really worth while waiting, on such a very unique occasion. With smiling faces the Famous Five rejoined Sir Reginald Brooke and Lord Mauleverer on the balcony.

"Mind waiting a few minutes, sir?" asked Bob. "Bunter's decided to take a bath! In fact, I gave him the tip."

The juniors chuckled. The "tip" Bob had given Bunter was a tip over the side of the bath; but it was unnecessary to mention that detail.

"Very good!" said Sir Reginald.

It was a quarter of an hour before Billy Bunter reappeared. His fat face was full of wrath; but in other respects, there was no doubt that Bunter was much the better for the tip Bob had given him. Sir Reginald turned his eyeglass upon him and approved.

"That is better, Bunter," he said.

"Yah!" snorted Bunter.

"What?"

"I—I—I mean, all right! I'm ready!"

Sir Reginald gave him a glare.

"Come with me, my boys," he said. And the juniors followed the tall and stiff old gentleman down the steps to the waiting car. Billy Bunter gave the chums of the Remove a ferocious blink.

"I'll make you beasts sit up for that!" he hissed, "and as for that cheeky old fossil——"

Sir Reginald Brooke glanced round.

"Did you speak, Bunter?"

"Oh! No!" gasped Bunter. "Not a word! Never opened my lips! I only said what a—a—a nice old gentleman you are, sir!"

Grunt from Sir Reginald. And the Greyfriars party packed in the big car and started for the house of Hilmi Maroudi.

THE SEVENTH CHAPTER.

Tit for Tat!

"THAT it?" grunted Billy Bunter. The car stopped at the house of Hilmi Maroudi, near the Eskebiyeh Gardens of Cairo.

Billy Bunter blinked at the building disparagingly. Little was to be seen, but high walls and barred windows, with a great arched doorway. Mauly's uncle had visited the Egyptian gentleman several times, while the juniors were sight-seeing with their dragoman; but this was the first visit of Harry Wharton & Co. to the house, and they were rather curious to see the interior.

Hassan had told them much of the vast wealth and great power of Mr. Maroudi; and they were aware that the dragoman regarded him with fear and awe; though they were unaware that Hilmi Maroudi had intervened when the Greek had bribed the "Faithful Hassan" to betray his lordly gentlemen. Since that intervention, the faithful Hassan had been indeed faithful, for no bribe that Kalizelos could have offered would have tempted him to incur the anger of Maroudi.

"Don't think much of the show," said Bunter. "From what Hassan has been saying, I expected to see something like Bunter Court."

Whereat the juniors chuckled.

But the house of Maroudi, like most Eastern dwellings, was more attractive in the interior than in the exterior.

The Greyfriars fellows entered at the great arched doorway, on one side of which the doorkeeper sat cross-legged on his raised seat.

Within was a great entrance hall; which, as in most of the native mansions of Cairo, had a turning, to prevent curious eyes from looking in from the street—privacy being the great desideratum in Mohammedan countries.

Beyond, there was a vast courtyard, in which was an artificial lake, surrounded by trees and flowers and shady walks, the lake fed by a spraying fountain that flashed and sparkled in the sunshine.

Bowing dusky servants, in flowing garments, greeted the visitors, and conducted them onward to a great recess at the side of the court, the ceiling of which was adorned with gorgeous arabesques picked out with gold.

Here Mr. Hilmi Maroudi awaited his visitors.

Mr. Maroudi wore European costume, with the exception of the national headgear, the tarboosh. But he was cross-legged in the native way—which the juniors would have supposed to be rather difficult in trousers; but no doubt Mr. Maroudi was used to it.

He was on his feet with the swiftness of a Jack-in-the-box, as his guests were ushered in.

"Salamn aleikum!" said Mr. Maroudi gravely, salaaming to the visitors quite gracefully, in spite of his plumpness and the European trousers, and then he translated at once: "Peace be with you!"

"And with you be health, and God's mercy and blessing," answered Sir Reginald Brooke, in English—which in Arabic would have been "U'aleikum essalaam warahmet Allah wabarakatuh."

"Naharak said!" added Maroudi, with a smile to the juniors. "Thy days be happy, my little friends."

To which the polite answer would have been "Naharak said wemubarak," "Thy day be happy and blessed!" That answer, however, the juniors did not make, as their knowledge of Arabic was limited to the word "backsheesh"—a word which certainly was of no use on the present occasion.

The greeting of visitors is a ceremonious business in the East. "How do you do?" is extended into many flowing sentences. The host displays a deep concern for the health of his visitor—so far as words go, at all events; and the visitor replies with long-winded inquiries concerning the health of the host. But Mr. Maroudi had adopted many European ways, along with his European clothes, and he cut it short—for an Oriental.

Rather to the relief of the juniors, he had carried his European manners and customs so far as to have chairs, and they were not required to sit on prayer-mats, like Mr. Maroudi himself. Sitting cross-legged on rugs would have been rather a trial! Indeed, it would probably have been impossible for Billy Bunter, at least, without the sacrifice of a good many of his buttons.

The plump Egyptian gentleman, who spoke English perfectly, made himself very agreeable to the juniors, whom he evidently liked. The fact that he had saved Harry Wharton from going overboard, in the squall on the Mediterranean, seemed to have caused him to take a special liking to the captain of the Greyfriars Remove. Even to Billy Bunter he was kind and courteous; though doubtless he had his own opinion of that fat and fatuous youth, which politeness made him keep strictly to himself.

After a little conversation, Mr. Maroudi suggested that the schoolboys might like to look round on their own, a suggestion with which the juniors heartily agreed. Much as they liked the good-hearted Egyptian gentleman, they did not want to sit and manufacture conversation. Billy Bunter was keen for the refreshments to begin; but the refreshments were not yet due. The juniors walked out into the great courtyard, leaving Sir Reginald Brooke in conversation with Mr. Maroudi.

"Topping place," said Bob Cherry, as they strolled round the lake in the centre of the courtyard, in which the fountain played. "This is what Mr. Maroudi called his "poor house," when we met him on the steamer. More like a jolly old palace out of the Arabian Nights."

"The topfulness is terrific," agreed Hurree Jamset Ram Singh.

"I say, you fellows——"

"Is it up to Bunter Court, after all, old fat bean?" chuckled Bob Cherry.

"Well, hardly," said Bunter. "Still, it's a decent show! But look here—is that a goldfish?"

"Where?" asked Bob, joining the fat Owl at the edge of the mosaic pavement that bordered the lake.

There was a sly gleam in Billy Bunter's little round eyes, behind his big round spectacles.

Bob had already forgotten Bunter's enforced bath. Billy Bunter hadn't! A bath, from Billy Bunter's point of view, was one of those things which it is more blessed to give than to receive.

Billy Bunter was on the warpath. Thoughts of vengeance were in his fat and podgy mind.

Bob Cherry peered at the sunlit water, on which water-lilies floated, in search of the supposed goldfish. As he leaned over the edge, Billy Bunter gave him a sudden and unexpected shove in the back.

Splash!

"He, he, he!" gurgled Bunter.

"Ooooogh!" spluttered Bob.

Before he knew what was happening he was in the water. It was not more than three feet deep; but Bob, taken quite by surprise, went right under. He sprawled headlong in the pond, and as he scrambled up the falling stream of the fountain swamped over him and gave him a shower-bath.

"You silly owl!" roared Harry Wharton, running to the edge of the pond, as Bob Cherry spluttered and scrambled and struggled in the water. "You potty porpoise! What the thump—— Oh—ow—what—— Oh, my hat! Oooogh!"

Splash!

As Wharton reached out a hand to Bob the fat Owl gave him a shove behind, and he went in headlong.

"He, he, he!"

"Oooogh! Grooogh! Oh crikey! Ooooch!"

"He, he, he!"

"You fat lunatic!" shrieked Bob Cherry, standing up in the lake, drenched and streaming. "I'll—I'll burst you all over Cairo! I—I'll——"

"He, he, he! How do you like it yourself?" chortled Bunter.

Wharton and Bob Cherry came splashing to the side of the lake. Nugent and Hurree Singh and Johnny Bull ran to help them out, and Lord Mauleverer ambled up to lend them a hand.

Billy Bunter looked on and chortled. This, in Bunter's opinion, was tit for tat! But he ceased to chortle as Bob Cherry came scrambling out, drenched and dripping and infuriated. The expression on Bob's face was rather alarming.

Giving a fellow a much-needed bath at the hotel was one thing; tipping a fellow into a pond when he was on a visit was quite another. Bob looked as if he was going to make that distinction clear to William George Bunter, in a very drastic manner.

"Wait a tick, you fat maniac!" gasped Bob. "Just you wait a tick, and if I don't burst you into a million small pieces——"

Bunter did not wait a tick. He did not wait half a tick. Before Bob was fairly out of the pond, Bunter departed—on his highest gear.

"Come back, you fat villain!" roared Bob, as he crawled out, in a pool of water, streaming from head to foot.

"Beast!"

That reply floated back as the fat Owl vanished among the palms and shrubs and flower-beds.

Bob Cherry made a rush in pursuit. Lord Mauleverer, grinning, caught him by the arm.

"Hold on, old bean!" exclaimed Mauly.

"I'll burst him!" roared Bob.

"My esteemed chum——" exclaimed the Nabob of Bhanipur.

"I'll spiflicate him!"

"The spiflication is the proper caper, but not in the absurd mansion of the respected and ridiculous Maroudi!" said Hurree Jamset Ram Singh.

"Bunter will keep, old bean!" grinned Mauleverer. "You don't want to astonish the natives by bursting him all over Maroudi's house, old chap."

"I—I—I——"

Bob Cherry realised that it was not a time or place for giving Bunter his due. The fat Owl merited "spiflication," but the house of Mr. Maroudi was not the proper place for that hectic process.

"Let the fat idiot rip!" said Harry. "We'll kick him all round the hotel when we get back! Oh, my hat! I'm wet!"

"The wetfulness is terrific!"

"Here comes some of the jolly old retainers," said Lord Mauleverer.

Two or three Nubian servants came running up. They bowed, and spoke incomprehensible words; but the meaning was clear, and Wharton and Bob followed them into the house, to dry themselves—leaving a watery trail behind them as they went.

The other fellows continued to stroll round the sunny court, excepting Billy Bunter. That fat and fatuous youth considered it judicious to keep out of sight for the present, and he was not likely to be seen again until refreshments were due.

THE EIGHTH CHAPTER.

In Desperate Hands!

HILMI MAROUDI, sitting cross-legged on a Persian prayer-rug, smoked his hookah. Sir Reginald Brooke, in a long cane chair, smoked a cigar. They were talking of farming in the Fayyum, that fertile province of Egypt where the old baronet had an estate which adjoined Maroudi's.

A silent-footed Nubian came in, and stood waiting for his master to give him permission to speak.

For some minutes Mr. Maroudi did not seem to have observed him; then, politely excusing himself to Sir Reginald, he turned his eyes on the servant.

The Nubian spoke in Arabic, and Maroudi, with all his impassive Oriental calm, gave a slight start. Apparently the Nubian's communication had startled him. He answered the man in Arabic, and the servant went out as silently as he had entered.

Sir Reginald, who had been many times in Egypt, and had a smattering of Arabic. was aware that the Nubian had announced that a caller had come, and had been shown into the "mandarah," or guest-room, inside the house. And, to his amazement, he had caught the name of Kalizelos.

He looked very curiously at the Egyptian over his cigar. Kalizelos, the Greek, was charged with kidnapping and attempted murder, and was a fugitive from the police. It was amazing if he had ventured to show himself in public, and in the house of a friend of the Greyfriars party.

"My good friend," said Maroudi gravely, "Kalizelos, the Greek, has the audacity to come here and demand speech with me. If you will pardon me for leaving you for a few minutes, I will see the man."

"By all means," said Sir Reginald.

Maroudi rose from the prayer-rug, salaamed gravely to his guest, and left the colonnade by an inner door.

He traversed several passages, and entered the "mandarah"—a great apartment with many doors, one side of which was open to the court, with a perforated stone balustrade.

Kalizelos the Greek was there, alone.

He was seated on a low divan, but he rose to his feet as the Egyptian entered, and salaamed in the Eastern style—a greeting which Hilmi Maroudi did not return.

Kalizelos was dressed like a native, as the juniors had seen him the day before.

"Es-salamn aleikum!" he said as he salaamed.

"I have no greeting for you, Konstantinos Kalizelos!" said the Egyptian coldly. "Is my house a village of the Baggara, that a pariah dog dares to enter?"

"I come in peace, O Maroudi!" said the Greek, speaking in Arabic.

"Between us there is no peace, as you are the enemy of my friends," answered the Egyptian. "And the police of Cairo are seeking you."

The Greek shrugged his shoulders.

"But you will not call the police, Maroudi, for I have come trusting to your faith," he said. "And a good Moslem dare not violate the laws of hospitality."

"That is true," said Maroudi. "In my house you are safe, and you know it, or you would not have come. But I will have you driven from my door like a pariah dog, with blows of the kourbash."

"Let me speak first," said the Greek.

"Speak!"

"What I have to say is secret." Kalizelos glanced round the spacious mandara, to which there were many doorways, some of them covered only by latticed hangings.

"No ears will listen here," said Maroudi scornfully. "But be brief."

"I would speak of the Scarab of A-Menah," said Kalizelos, still in Arabic. "But for you, O Maroudi, this scarab would now be in my hands. I bribed the young lord's dragoman to betray him, and it was your intervention that forced Hassan to return to his faith, and save him from my hands. For some reason you have befriended these foreigners, who would be at my mercy in this land of Egypt, but for you."

"It is true!" said Maroudi. "And my protection will shield them so long as they remain in my country. Son of a dog, you bribed my servant, Ali, to rob them on the steamer, and the life of one boy was endangered. It was the will of Allah that I should save him. Ali has been punished by many blows, and sent to my plantations on the Upper Nile. And because peril came to these English lords through my servant, I am their protector."

"You are rich, and you are powerful, Maroudi," said the Greek. "Against you I am powerless. But listen! In an ancient papyrus, written by the scribe of A-Menah, three thousand years ago, I have learned the secret of the Golden Scarab!

"This papyrus is known only to me. It came into my hands by chance, in my shop in Cairo; it lay long neglected among many other papyri. But when I chanced to read it, Maroudi, I read the secret of the Scarab of A-Menah! And then I knew that the tradition was true, and that the possessor of the Golden Scarab holds in his hands the finding of the Eye of Osiris. Shall I tell you this secret?"

"That is as you choose!" answered Maroudi; but there was a glimmer of keen curiosity in his eyes.

"Listen again, O Maroudi! The great diamond, the Eye of Osiris, was famed in the reign of Rameses the Second, when the general A-Menah brought it back from the land of the Hittites, after the battle of Kadesh. It was known to be worth the ransom of many kings. In English money of the present day the value is a quarter of a million pounds."

"So I have heard it said!"

"Even you, Maroudi, rich as you are, will not despise such a sum," said the Greek. "As I have said, against you I am powerless. That is why I am here. Give these foreigners into my hands; withdraw your protection from them, that is all I ask. Let Hassan, the dragoman, learn that he need not fear your anger and vengeance, and he will betray them into my hands. They shall not be harmed—I seek only the scarab. And the half of its value shall be yours! Rich as you are, is not this worth your while, Maroudi?"

"Dog, and the son of a dog!" said the Egyptian, his eyes gleaming at Kalizelos. "If I were as poor as the beggars who ask alms at the doors of the mosques, do you think that all the treasures of the Pharaohs would tempt me to betray my friends?"

"Those are but words!" said the Greek coolly. "Listen, Maroudi! I have lost much in seeking the Golden Scarab. From a rich merchant of Cairo I have become a hunted fugitive. Only with a great fortune can I make my peace and pay the backsheesh that will turn from me the talons of the law. I am a desperate man now, Maroudi. Leave these foreigners to me, and take the half of the treasure to which the scarab will guide me."

"It is enough!" said Maroudi. "I will call my servants to drive you from my door!"

The Greek's eyes glittered.

"I have said that against you I am powerless, Maroudi," he said. "But there is too much at stake for me to retreat. There are many daggers and many desperate hands in this city, and even the powerful Maroudi is only mortal. If you should be taken to the Prophet, O Maroudi, who will protect these foreigners?"

Maroudi's lip curled.

"For that threat you shall receive blows from the kourbash when you have passed my door," he said. "Within my house no hand may be raised against you, as you came trusting to my faith. But in the street outside my walls you shall be beaten away like a jackal. Have you more to say, O son of pariah dogs, before I call my Nubians?"

The Greek gritted his teeth.

Maroudi stretched his hand towards a gong, to strike it, to summon the Nubians. But his dusky hand did not reach the gong.

With the spring of a tiger the supple Greek was upon him.

So swift, so sudden, was the spring—like that of a wild beast of the jungle—that the Egyptian was taken utterly by surprise. Not for a moment had it crossed his mind that Kalizelos would dare to attack him in his own mansion, with a hundred devoted servants within call.

The plump Egyptian went down on a rug, the Greek over him. A sinewy knee was planted on him, and two strong, sinuous hands gripped his throat.

Maroudi's starting eyes stared up at the Greek.

Plump as he was, the Egyptian was no weakling; but the Greek was twice as strong, and he was desperate and ruthless. The grip of his sinuous fingers choked Maroudi into silence. His black eyes blazed down at the suffocating man.

"Die, then!" hissed Kalizelos. "Die in your own palace, dog of a Moslem! The scarab shall be mine, in spite of you! When you have gone to your place, Moslem hound, the foreigners will be at my mercy! Powerful as you are, O Hilmi Maroudi, who shall save you now?"

The Egyptian could not speak. He struggled, but his struggles were futile. No servant would come to the mandara without his order, and the gong was out of his reach.

The fierce grip on his throat hardened and tightened, the savage face glaring down at him floated before his eyes, and Hilmi Maroudi knew that it was death, and that in a few moments more he would be crossing the bridge of a hairsbreadth to the paradise of the Prophet!

THE NINTH CHAPTER.

In the Nick of Time!

"THE fat idiot!"

"The podgy, piffling, potty porpoise!"

"Bother him!"

"Blow him!"

Harry Wharton and Bob Cherry were both speaking at once, and both speaking of William George Bunter.

A bowing Nubian showed the two drenched and dripping juniors into a room in the house of Maroudi, where there was a green marble bath sunk in the mosaic floor, bath-robes and towels in abundance.

With a grave black face—though probably the Nubian was inwardly smiling—he helped them to remove their drenched clothes, and handed them towels.

Another Nubian brought fresh garments to the room, evidently for the juniors to change into while their clothes were drying.

The garments were, of course, native: even in Mr. Maroudi's wealthy and well-appointed residence there was no supply of European clothes of boyish size at a moment's notice.

The juniors were glad, however, to get dry clothes to put on, though it was a little odd to think of dressing in djubbahs.

The Nubians carried away the wet clothes, making signs to indicate that the same were to be dried; and one of them pointed to a brass gong, evidently meaning that it was to be struck if anything more was wanted.

Then the schoolboys were left alone to towel themselves down; which they were very glad to do.

While they towelled they told one another what they thought of Billy Bunter.

Dry at last, they put on the Egyptian clothes, and grinned at their reflection in a spacious mirror.

"Two jolly Egyptians, except for the jolly old complexions," said Bob Cherry, laughing. "I say, these silky things are jolly comfy and cool in hot weather. I shall be glad to change back, though."

"Same here," agreed Wharton. "I wonder how long they will be drying our clobber! Can't stick indoors all the time. Let's get out.."

"So long as we can change before we leave, it's all right," said Bob. "Come on!"

He opened the door, and they left the

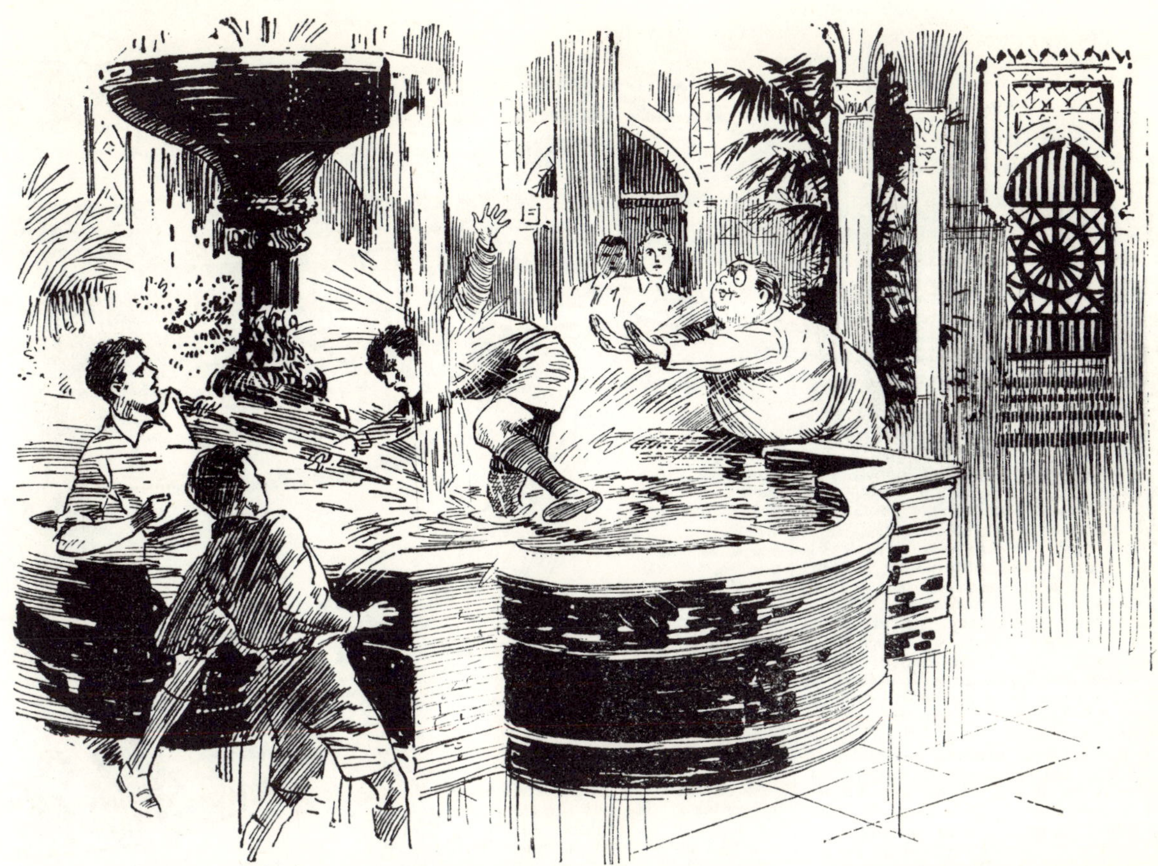

As Bob Cherry leaned over the edge of the ornamental lake, Billy Bunter gave him a sudden and unexpected shove in the back. There was a splash as Bob sprawled headlong in the water. "You potty porpoise!" roared Wharton, rushing to Bob's aid.

bath-room. It did not seem necessary to sound the gong to call the Nubians to show them out. But, as a matter of fact, they found that it was not easy to pick their way in the vast building.

They went down a corridor, and turned into another, under the impression that they were heading for the courtyard; but, instead of arriving at the court, they found their way barred by a latticed doorway.

The corridor led to some apartment; and though it would have been easy to push the lattice aside and pass through, they halted.

In an Eastern house one could not be too careful. If the room beyond the latticed doorway was one of the public apartments, all was well; but if it was a private apartment, they naturally did not want to enter it.

"I fancy it's all right," murmured Bob. "I'm certain we're heading in the direction of the courtyard. This would be one of the rooms looking on it, I think."

"Better make sure, though," said Harry, in the same low tone. "I think we ought really to have sounded the gong for a servant to take us out. Perhaps we'd better go back——"

"Well, we don't want to butt into the wrong shop," grinned Bob. "But——"

He broke off.

There was a sound in the apartment beyond the latticed doorway. It was a faint, low, but startling sound—a choking gurgle!

The two juniors started, and exchanged looks.

"What——" breathed Wharton.

"What the thump!" muttered Bob. "Dash it all, it sounds like somebody being strangled! What the jolly old thump have we dropped on?"

The juniors stood quite still for a moment.

They knew Mr. Maroudi as a polite and kind-hearted gentleman, who had been very civil and hospitable; but they knew, too, that the ways of the East were not the ways of the West. Life was cheap in the East; and they had heard of the bow-string! It was surely impossible that a dark Oriental deed was being done in the house of Maroudi; yet the sound from beyond the latticed doorway was undoubtedly, unmistakably that of some unhappy victim whose life was being choked out.

Wharton's face set.

"We're chipping in here, Bob, whatever it is," he said. "Come on!"

With a resolute hand Harry Wharton pulled the lattice aside, and stepped through the doorway, Bob at his heels.

The juniors found themselves in a vast apartment, with a lofty ceiling adorned with gilded arabesques, one side open to the courtyard, though screened by a high balustrade in graceful stonework. It was, if they had known it, the "mandarah," the guest-room of the mansion.

But they had no time for looking about them. They stared, with startled eyes, at the fearful scene that met them as they entered.

Stretched on his back on a prayer-rug was Hilmi Maroudi, and, bending over him, grasping his throat, and choking out his life, was Kalizelos, the Greek.

The sight was so astonishing that, for a brief second, they stood spellbound. Then they bounded forward.

"It's Kalizelos!" panted Wharton.

"Get hold of him!" gasped Bob.

Their grasp was on the Greek at once. They dragged him backwards by main force, and the Greek sprawled over on his back on the stone floor.

Maroudi lay gasping.

He had been near to death—very near to death—and his eyes were bulging, his brain swimming, and he lay powerless, as he gulped in the life-giving air when the cruel grip was gone from his throat. He could not speak, or lend aid—but the juniors did not need aid.

Strong and supple as the Greek was, they had him down, and they kept him down. He struggled like a wild beast, and contrived to get his hand under his kaftan and draw a knife; but Wharton had hold of his wrist in a flash, and twisted it savagely till he dropped the weapon.

"You!" panted the Greek, his olive face convulsed with rage. For a moment he had taken the juniors, in their native garb, for attendants of Maroudi; but now he recognised them.

"You scoundrel!" said Wharton, between his teeth.

"Hold him!" panted Bob.

Fiercely the juniors grasped the writhing, struggling rascal. But they had their hands full with Kalizelos. He was like a tiger in their grasp.

The three of them rolled on the floor, struggling, grasping, clutching, panting for breath; the Greek striving to escape, the juniors striving desperately to hold him and keep him a prisoner.

Maroudi sat up dizzily.

He could not rise, but he reached his knees, and crawled to the gong. He struck it, and a deep, booming sound rang through the building.

One boom of the gong was enough. There was a soft patter of feet, and a tall Nubian entered.

Maroudi panted a word in Arabic.

Instantly the Nubian's grasp was on

(*Continued on page* 16.)

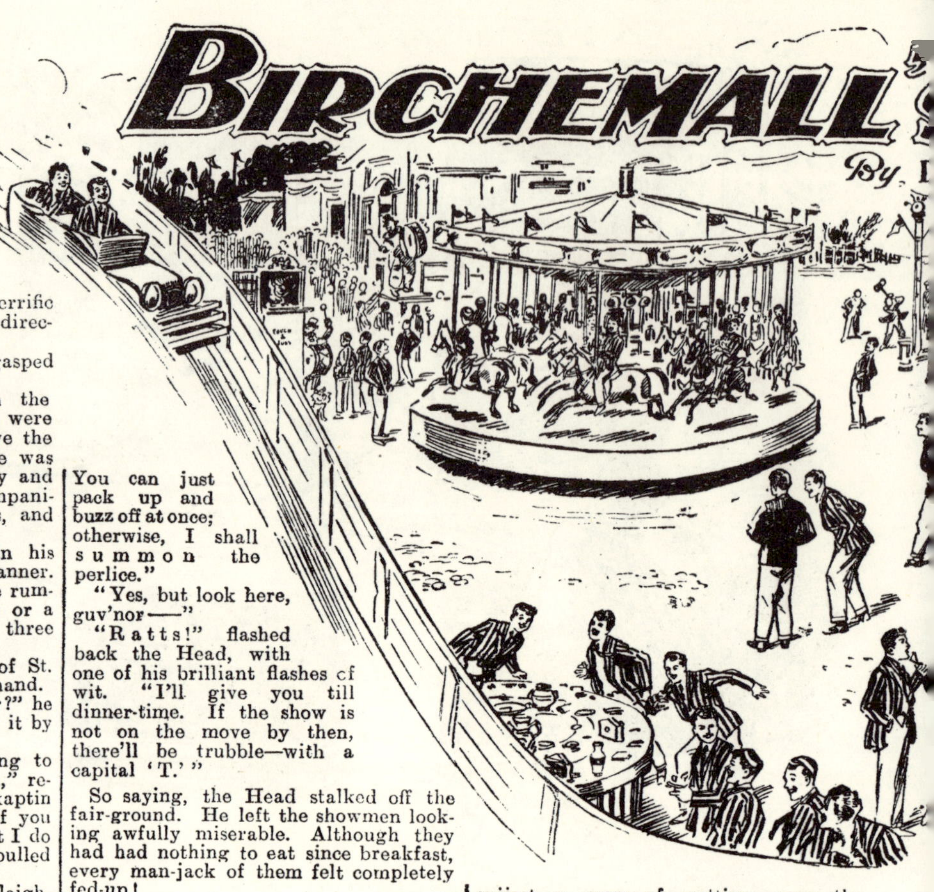

BIRCHEMALL

By

I.

A PLEZZURE-FAIR had been pitched on a field near St. Sam's, and all the juniors from Jack Jolly, the hero of the Fourth, to Midgett minor, the babe of the Second, were agog with eggsitement.

Unforchunitly, the proprietor of the fair had set up his swings and roundabouts without insulting the Head on the subject. So the first intimation Dr. Alfred Birchemall received was when a terrific din came floating across from the direction of the fair-ground.

“What the merry dickens——” gasped the Head.

As the hullabaloo arose from the showmen's pitch, mourning lessons were just starting. Dr. Birchemall gave the Sixth an awfully black look. He was not accustomed to teaching history and joggrafy and classix to an accompaniment of clanging bells, rifle shots, and harsh mewsick.

“Bust me!” he eggsclaimed, in his most refined and dignified manner. “What ever is the meaning of the rumpus, boys? Is it an earthquake or a cyclone or a hurrycane, or all three rolled into one?”

Burleigh, the hansum kaptin of St. Sam's, conscaled a smile with his hand.

“Haven't you herd the news, sir?” he asked. “I thought everyone knew it by now.”

“I trussed you are not referring to the deth of Queen Anne, Burleigh,” retorted the Head, eyeing the skool kaptin with a somewhat baleful eye. “If you are, I may as well inform you that I do not tollerate having my leg pulled during skool hours, Burleigh.”

“But I'm not, sir!” grinned Burleigh. “The news I am referring to consers that awful row that's going on outside. The fact is, sir, if you want to know, it's a fair.”

“A fair, eh? So that's it! A gang of common showmen have the dispertinence to set up their wretched tawdry show at our door without so much as a ‘By your leave!’ We'll soon see about that! Burleigh!”

“Yes, sir!”

“Kindly take charge of the Form during my absence. I am going to order the proprietor of this co-called fair to pack his traps and move on immejately—if not before that!”

“Okay with me, sir!” said Burleigh cheerfully.

“Shan't be a jiffy!” said Dr, Birchemall.

With that, the Head of St. Sam's stalked out of the Form-room, leaving the Sixth gleefully hoping that the showmen would give him a jolly good ruff-house.

There wasn't much chance of that, however, as a matter of fact. Tuff as they were, the fair proprietor and his assistants reckernised Class, and when Dr. Birchemall walked majestically into their midst they fairly cringed and fawned before him.

The Head went straight to the point.

“Now, then, what's all this here?” he asked, with his usual faultless grammar. “What do you think you're doing of, eh?”

“Please, guv'nor, we didn't think we were doing nobody no harm!” wined one of the showmen. “We just set up the show here hoping to earn an honnest copper or two.”

“Regardless of the fact that in so doing you are drowning the pearls of wisdom that fall from my lips as I teach the Sixth,” said the Head icily. “Well, you're not jolly well going to do it, see? You can just pack up and buzz off at once; otherwise, I shall summon the perlice.”

“Yes, but look here, guv'nor——”

“Ratts!” flashed back the Head, with one of his brilliant flashes of wit. “I'll give you till dinner-time. If the show is not on the move by then, there'll be trubble—with a capital ‘T.’ ”

So saying, the Head stalked off the fair-ground. He left the showmen looking awfully miserable. Although they had had nothing to eat since breakfast, every man-jack of them felt completely fed-up!

———

II.

“HAY-HO, come to the fair!” Jack Jolly, of the Fourth, sang out those words as he and a crowd of cheery Fourth-Formers swarmed down to the gates after mourning lessons.

The Fourth were feeling awfully bucked at the prospect of spending most of the dinner-break at the fair. But a shock was in store for them, for when they reached the fair-ground they found that the swings and roundabouts were being taken down and packed up as rapidly as possible.

“Grate pip! What are they doing that for?” asked Jack Jolly in serprize. “Why, it was only last night when they put them up.”

“Let's ask this johnny,” sujjested Frank Fearless. “He looks like the boss of the show.”

Frank promptly sawntered over to a fat jentleman in riding breeches and top-hat, and made the necessary inkwiries. The top-hatted jentleman's reply made the St. Sam's juniors prick up their ears.

“A lass, my young friend!” he cride. “The headmaster of that big skool over there has ordered us to pack up and move off. Failing that, he intends to call the perlice.”

“M-m-my hat! Then it's Dr. Birchemall that's put a stop to it!”

“Shame!” went up a cry from a score of juniors.

“ ‘Shame’ is the right word, young jentlemen—it's a blinking shame!” said the proprietor of the show. “Yet what can I do? I can't afford to get into trubble with the perlice.”

The juniors looked at him simperthetically; but nobody seemed able to sujjest a way of getting over the difficulty.

Then Jack Jolly's eyes began to gleem suddenly.

“I've got a wheeze that mite work!” he eggsclaimed. “But before I do anything, sir, would you be willing to give up a persentage of your prophets if you were allowed to stay on here?”

The top-hatted jentleman nodded eagerly.

“Certainly, young jentleman. I'd give up half of the prophets, if necessary, if I were allowed to carry on at a prophetable spot like this!”

“Good!” said Jack Jolly, with satisfaction. “In that case, I think there ought to be no difficulty in getting the Head to agree. What about going to him as a deputation, you chaps?”

“Oh crikey!”

“I'm willing to come along, for one!” said Frank Fearless fearlessly.

After a little hezzitation the rest also fell in with the skeem, and without wasting any more time, Jack Jolly led his deputation back to St. Sam's, leaving the fair proprietor looking a little more hopeful.

They went up to the Head's study and Jack Jolly tapped respectfully on the door.

Crash! Bang! Wallop!

“Trot in, idiot!” called out the Head, from within.

Jack Jolly marched in at the head of the deputation. The Head's eyes almost popped out of their sockits when he saw them.

“Bless my sole!” he gasped. “What do you call this game, Jolly? Follow me leader?”

“No, sir,” answered Jack Jolly quietly. “We're a deputation. We've come to ask whether you won't reconsider your decision about the fair, and allow it to stay on after all?”

Dr. Birchemall frowned.

BENNYFIT!

NUGENT

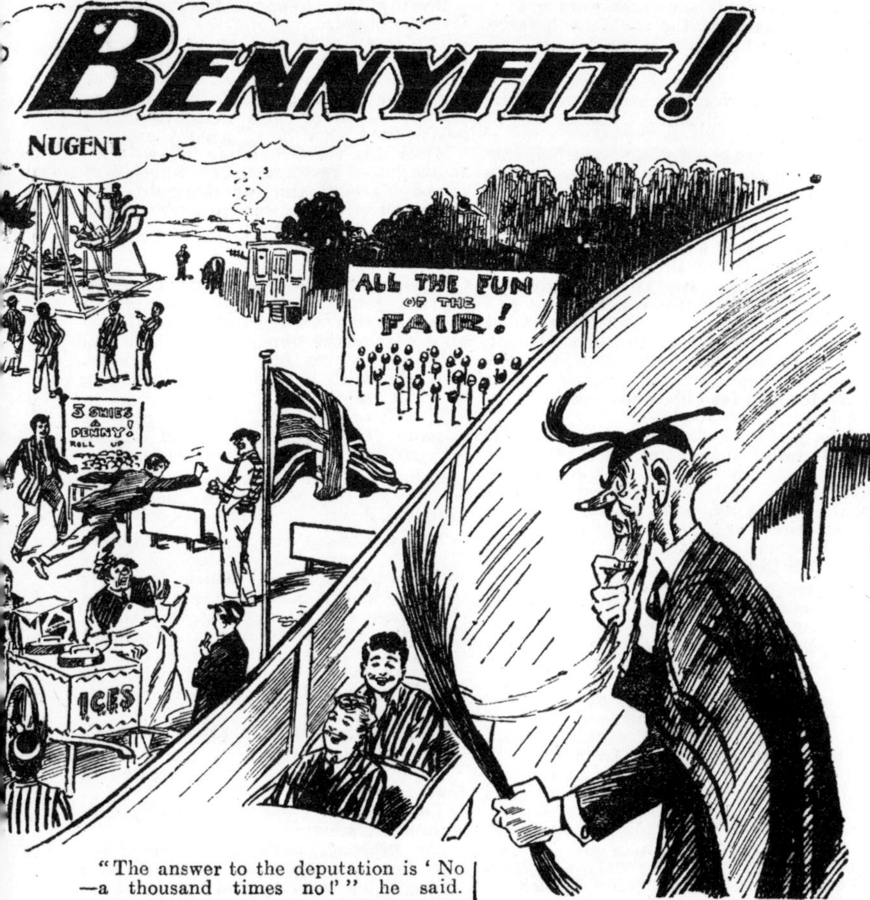

"The answer to the deputation is 'No—a thousand times no!'" he said.

"In that case, then," said Jack Jolly, "there's nothing to be said. But I feel I ought to mention that we've just seen the proprietor of the fair, and he's willing to give half of the prophets to charity if you'll let him stay on."

The Head's frown vanished, and a somewhat crafty, cunning eggspression took its place.

"Are your sure of this, Jolly?"

"Absolutely positive, sir!"

"Well, if that's the case, of corse—ahem!—it puts a different complexion on the matter. I should hate to do anything that would stop munny from going to charity. I will reconsider my decision. In fact, I will grant this showman the permission he wants here and now."

"Oh, thanks awfully, sir!" chirruped Jack Jolly & Co.

"I will do more than that," said Dr. Birchemall, in a sudden burst of jennerosity. "I will give the fair my harty support, and see to it that it acheeves a signal suxxess. Go down and tell them to get their swings and roundabouts and seenic railways going as soon as they can."

III.

AFTER dinner that day Dr. Birchemall stood up at his table.

"Boys!" he cride. "As many of you are no doubt aware already, I have come to the conclusion that my ban on the fair was unfair. I have therefore lifted the ban."

"Hooray!" roared the juniors of St. Sam's enthusiastically.

The Head smiled induljently.

"I'm glad you're glad, boys. But I have even more welcome news for you. The proprietor of this fair is giving half of his prophets to charity. I think it would be a good wheeze, therefore, if I gave the whole skool an extra half-hollerday to-day. so that one and all will have the chance of going to the fair. So you may consider it done."

Big Hall fairly echoed to the cheers of the delited skool. An extra half! It seemed almost unbeleevable that the Head could be so jennerous.

"One word before you dismiss," went on Dr. Birchemall, as the boys got ready to rise from their tables. "As the prophets are partly going to charity, I think it's up to everybody to patronise the sideshows extensively. I shall therefore eggspect every St. Sam's boy to spend a minnimum of two shillings before he leaves the fair. Remember the amount—two shillings. And woe betide the mean, stingy young rascal who tries to spend less! You may go, boys!"

Crowds of St. Sam's fellows were soon flocking to the fair. It was a jolly good fair, with swings and roundabouts and switchbacks and cokernut-shies, and by the time Dr. Birchemall arrived the fun was fast and furious.

Having interviewed the proprietor of the fair, Dr. Birchemall made a toor of inspection. Fellows gave him a wide berth when they saw that he was carrying a huge birch in his hand, but none escaped his pennytrating glarnse, nevertheless.

"Jolly!" he called out. "How much have you spent?"

"Half-a-crown sir," replied Jack Jolly.

"Poorhouse!" cride the Head soon after that. "How is it you're standing idly by instead of spending your munny on the amusements?"

"Sorry, sir!" said Poorhouse. "But the fact is I haven't a bean!"

Dr. Birchemall sniffed.

"Disgraceful! It's about time you went into the poorhouse, Poorhouse! However, I think I can soon solve your difficulty. Luker!"

"Yes, sir?" answered Luker, the young millionaire of the Fourth.

"Unless you lend Poorhouse a cupple of bob at once I shall thrash you till you shreek for mersy!"

"Oh, I'll lend him a cupple of bob with plezzure, sir," said Luker hastily. "Here you are, Poorhouse!"

"Good egg!" grinned the Head. "Now go and spend it as fast as you can, Poorhouse!"

A minnit later he came across Gasper and Grabbe hiding behind a caravan.

"Wretched youths!" he cride. "So you are making yourselves small so as to make your savings large and defrawd charity of its rightful dews! Bend over!"

Grasper and Grabbe obeyed, looking very sorry for themselves as they did so. They looked a good deal more sorry a little later, for the Head laid it on thick and hevvy.

"Now go and spend two shillings each before I sentence you to a birching every day for the rest of the term!" snorted Dr. Bichemall.

With the Head running round in this fashion, it was not to be wondered at that the takings mounted up and up till the proprietor of the fair was rubbing his hands with glee. Even after he had given half of his prophets away the remainder would still break all records! By tea-time Dr. Birchemall was sattisfied. He had another little interview with the proprietor, after which he addressed the crowd from the platform in front of one of the booths.

"Ladies and jentlemen and others!" he cride. "You will be glad to lern that my kindness and jennerosity in permitting this fair to be carried on has resulted in the large sum of ten pounds ten and tenpence being handed over to me to give to charity."

Loud cheers from the crowd greeted this announcement.

"As you may no doubt gess," went on the Head, "I have given a grate deal of thought to the problem of what eggsactly to do with this munny. Needless to say, I want to make sure that it goes to the most deserving charity. After careful consideration I have found what I think to be the most deserving charity of all."

"Name!" yelled a section of the crowd.

"With plezzure!" grinned the Head. "The name of the charity is the Distressed Headmasters' Fund, of which I happen to be the secretary and trezzurer. On behalf of the membership of this fund—by the way, I happen to be the only member—I thank you all for your very kind support. Good-afternoon. ladies and jentlemen!"

Dr. Birchemall then retired rather hurriedly. The crowd returned somewhat thoughtfully to the fun of the fair. They didn't like to say anything, of corse. But they couldn't help thinking that a better name for the "charity" would have been "Birchemall's Bennyfit!"

THE END.

*(Dicky Nugent contributes another winner next week: "**BIRCHEMALL GOES WHALING!**" It's a scream! If you miss it, chums, you'll regret it.)*

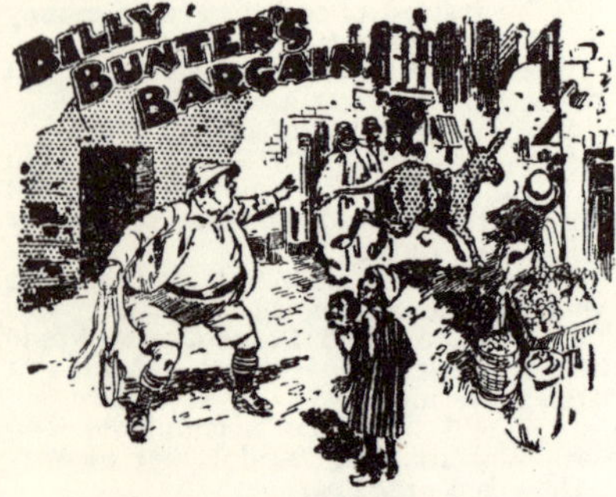

(*Continued from page* 13.)

Kalizelos. It was a much-needed relief to the Greyfriars fellows.

The powerful grasp of the Nubian finished the struggle. Kalizelos almost crumpled in it. He collapsed on his back, and a black, heavy knee was placed on his chest, pinning him down. One hand of the Nubian grasped him, the other jerked a dagger from some place of concealment under his loose garments, and the keen point was placed to the Greek's throat. The black man looked to his master for instructions, obviously prepared to drive the dagger home at a sign from Maroudi.

"Oh, my hat!" gasped Bob.

"Mr. Maroudi——" exclaimed Wharton.

To their relief, Maroudi made the Nubian a negative sign. Villain as the man was, it thrilled the juniors with horror to think of such summary justice executed under their eyes.

Maroudi smiled faintly at the juniors. He struck the gong again, twice, and four or five black servants entered. Maroudi spoke to them in Arabic, and the Greek, in the grasp of many hands, was led away.

THE TENTH CHAPTER.

Bunter is Satisfied!

HILMI MAROUDI stood silent for several minutes, his hand to his throat. Wharton and Nugent waited. But in a few minutes the Egyptian had recovered his accustomed calm.

"Marshallah!" he said. "My little friends, it was the will of Allah that you should save me from that son of ten thousand dogs. Already I could see the houris beckoning."

"Thank goodness we butted in, sir!" said Bob. "They've got Kalizelos safe at last!"

"He will go from this house to prison," said Maroudi. "Had he not lifted his hand against me, I should have had no choice but to allow him to depart in peace, for it is written that even the evildoer shall be safe in the house of his enemy. But since he has sought my life, he goes where justice awaits him. My servants will hand him over to the police of Cairo."

He paused, and eyed the juniors, in their strange garb, curiously.

"But how came you to enter this room so fortunately?" he asked, and when Wharton explained, the Egyptian nodded gravely.

"Kismet!" he said. "It is Fate! On the steamer, my little friend, I saved your life, and it was written that you should save me. All things are written in the book of Fate. Allah is great!"

Hilmi Maroudi and the juniors left the mandarah, the Egyptian returning to Sir Reginald Brooke, once more as calm and impassive as if nothing out of the ordinary had occurred, and the juniors rejoining their friends in the gardens in

the courtyard. Their faces were grave, and the faces of their chums became grave also when they learned what had happened.

"Well, that brute Kalizelos is safe now, at any rate," said Johnny Bull. "He won't be following us when we go up the Nile!"

"That's rather a relief," said Nugent.

"But—if that fat idiot, Bunter, hadn't ducked us!" said Bob. "If we hadn't butted in when we did—— Mr. Maroudi thinks it was all written in the jolly old book of Fate! But it was jolly lucky, anyhow! I think we had better not kick Bunter, after all." He glanced round. "Where is the fat frump now?"

"Keeping out of sight," grinned Nugent. "He's sure to turn up for grub. Hallo, there goes the jolly old gong! I suppose that means tiffin! Time for that fat villain to show up."

"I say, you fellows——"

The juniors looked round. That fat and familiar voice came from the other side of a high bank of glowing scarlet geraniums. Billy Bunter evidently had heard the gong, and guessed that it meant tiffin.

"Oh, there you are, you fat freak!" said Bob Cherry.

Bunter peered warily at the juniors over the tall geraniums.

"I say, you fellows, no larks," he said. "I hope you're not going to kick up a row here, Bob Cherry! There's such a thing as manners, you know! You're not in the Remove passage now."

"I've a jolly good mind——"

"You asked for that ducking," said Bunter, watching warily from the safe side of the geranium bank, and ready to bolt. "It served you jolly well right! I'm willing to let the whole matter drop. I'd give you a jolly good licking, only I've got some manners, if you haven't. Old Maroudi's only a nigger, of course, but I'm not going to kick up a shindy here. So——"

"It's all right, you fat freak! You can come out of cover," said Harry Wharton.

"Is it pax?" asked Bunter cautiously.

"Yes, ass!" grunted Bob.

"Oh, all right, then! I say, you fellows, you look rather guys in that rig," grinned Bunter, as he came down the bank and joined the chums of the Remove. "I suppose you were rather wet, what? He, he, he!" Bunter blinked curiously at the juniors. "What are you all looking so jolly solemn about? Don't you think we shall get good grub here?"

"Ha, ha, ha!"

Billy Bunter's question had the effect of banishing the gravity of the Famous Five.

"Blessed if I see anything to cackle at!" said the fat Owl, puzzled. "Nothing else to worry about, is there? My idea is that the grub will be good! Old Maroudi's jolly rich, and it stands to reason that he will stand us something decent. Don't you fellows think so?"

"Fathead!"

"Well, I think so," said Bunter. "I fancy the grub will be good, and plenty of it, too. Nothing to worry about that I can see. Come on! That gong means grub, and it's rather bad manners to be late. You fellows don't think much of manners, I know; but when you're with me, you ought to play up, you know."

"Oh gad!" murmured Lord Mauleverer.

Billy Bunter rolled off, with a look of happy anticipation on his fat face. He had little, if any, doubt that the grub would be good. He had given this important matter considerable thought, and was fairly satisfied that the grub would be all right. And if the grub was all right, everything, of course, was all right!

Bowing Nubians conducted the juniors into the house.

The ceremonial washing of hands before a meal struck Bunter as unnecessary and absurd; but it struck the other fellows as a custom that William George Bunter would do well to adopt in his native land when he returned there.

After this, the Greyfriars fellows were shown into a vast apartment, where they found Maroudi and Sir Reginald, and where refreshments were produced.

Billy Bunter found that his anticipations were well founded.

The grub was good.

Innumerable native servants waited on the juniors, and sweet strains of music came from a band of musicians on a dais at the upper end of the room.

In the centre of the room was a fountain, with a golden ball balancing in its jet of water.

The floor was of a rich, glowing mosaic. The ceiling, lofty and domed, was covered with gold arabesques.

Palms in tubs nodded against the walls, intermingled with banks of gorgeous flowers of every hue.

The musicians, in decorative native costumes, were half hidden by banks of flowers, through which glimpses could be had of their gorgeous garb and dark faces and strange instruments.

To the schoolboys it was all rather like a scene from the "Arabian Nights."

It was indeed a sight the chums of Greyfriars would remember for a long, long time.

Only Bunter gave no attention to his surroundings.

Bunter's attention was concentrated on the provender.

The fat Owl was soon happy and shiny and sticky.

Mr. Maroudi, showing no sign of the late terrible experience he had been through, was smiling and urbane, kind and attentive to all the juniors, not excepting Bunter.

Evidently the Egyptian gentleman was pleased to see the bright and cheery faces of the schoolboys round him, and his usually grave face beamed with smiles.

It was rather a lengthy meal, though by no means too lengthy for Bunter. Indeed, when it was over and the guests moved into the gardens in the court, Billy Bunter went with both hands full of sticky Turkish sweetmeats, and a supply of nuts stuffed with marzipan in his pockets—a proceeding to which Mr. Maroudi was politely blind.

In the falling dusk of the evening coloured lamps glimmered over the gardens, the lake, and the fountain, turning the scene almost into fairyland.

Music came from some hidden spot among the palms, and a troupe of dancers appeared from nowhere and performed a graceful Oriental dance for the entertainment of Mr. Maroudi's guests.

Mr. Maroudi smoked his hookah, and Sir Reginald a cigar, while the juniors looked on at the dancing, and Billy Bunter slowly and laboriously, but determinedly, travelled through his supply of sweetmeats and stuffed nuts.

After the dancers came a snake-charmer, whose weird exploits held the juniors spellbound. Then came a native conjurer, who made a palm-tree grow from a tub almost in the twinkling of an eye, who threw flowers into the air which—apparently, at least—never came down again, and who produced live, hissing snakes from an orange.

When the time came to depart, and the big car rolled away with the Greyfriars party, even Billy Bunter acknowledged that it had been a jolly good time.

"It was very fortunate," said Sir Reginald in the car, "that we paid our visit to Mr. Maroudi to-day——"

"Yes, wasn't it?" said Bunter heartily. "I told you fellows the grub would be good, and it jolly well was."

Sir Reginald gave the fat Owl a glare and went on:

"There is little doubt that Wharton and Cherry saved Mr. Maroudi's life. Now, my boys, Mr. Maroudi has offered to lend us his dahabiyeh for the trip up the Nile, and he was so insistent that I really had to accept the offer. It is a magnificent boat, much more commodious than any dahabiyeh I could have hired in Cairo. It is manned by Mr. Maroudi's own crew of Nubians, and the reis is a man in whom he has every confidence. In these circumstances, and now that that rascal Kalizelos is in the hands of the police, I shall be able to trust you on the Nile in the care of the dragoman while I go to the Fayyum to see to my business there. Mr. Maroudi is leaving for the Fayyum to-morrow, and I shall accompany him, and you boys will start up the Nile. I shall rely upon you, Wharton, to see that the party does not get into mischief."

"Leave it to me, sir," said Bunter. "It will be all right. I shall be there. I'm accustomed to looking after these fellows."

"Will you kindly hold your tongue, Bunter?" demanded Sir Reginald.

"Oh, really, sir——"

The car arrived at the hotel. A gold tassel on a tarboosh danced as Hassan, the dragoman, opened the door and salaamed to his lordly gentlemen. The juniors went to bed that night with great anticipations for the morrow.

THE ELEVENTH CHAPTER.

Bunter Bags Another Bargain!

"WALKING?"

"Yes."

"Rot!"

"The rotfulness is not terrific, my esteemed Bunter. The absurd distance is only a ridiculous mile."

"Think I'm going to walk a mile?"

"Are you ready, my boys?" called out Sir Reginald Brooke.

"Here we are, sir!"

The baggage was gone. Backsheesh had been duly distributed, and the Greyfriars fellows were going. It was early morning; not yet hot, but already bright and sunny. Every fellow in the party was quite keen on a last walk through the Cairo streets, even Mauly—but with the exception of William George Bunter. Bunter would not have walked from his bed-room to the dining-room if it had been possible to take a cab—so long, of course, as there was somebody else to pay for the cab.

On the trip to Egypt the "exes" were stood by Lord Mauleverer; therefore there was no reason why a car or an arabeyeh should not be taken on all occasions, so far as Bunter could see. The announcement that they were going to walk to the Kasr-el-Nil Bridge, where the boat was waiting, roused Bunter's deepest indignation.

"Come on, fatty!" said Bob Cherry. "It will shake down your breakfasts if you walk a bit. I suppose you want them to settle down?"

"Yah!"

"Bunter's got a lot of breakfasts to carry, though," remarked Johnny Bull. "Did you stack away six or seven, Bunter?"

"Beast!"

"Jolly mornin' for a walk," said Lord Mauleverer. "Come on. Can't keep nunky waitin'."

"But what the thump are we going to walk for?" demanded Bunter. "Has Mauly turned stingy, or what?"

"Oh gad!" said his lordship.

"If that's it," said Bunter, with deep scorn, "I'll pay for a car. You can leave that to me. Now, if I'm going to pay for the car, I suppose some of you will have the decency to lend me a few pounds——"

"My lordly gentlemen——"

"Shut up, Hassan! I don't like being interrupted by niggers! Now, look here, you fellows—— I say, don't walk away while I'm talking to you, you beasts!" roared Bunter.

But the chums of the Remove did walk away, and the fat Owl rolled after them, snorting. Lord Mauleverer marched ahead with his uncle, the Famous Five strolled after them, and Bunter grunted in the rear, with Hassan, the dragoman, hovering round the whole party, his brown face grinning cheerfully, and his stick poking away the common persons who got in the way of his lordly gentlemen.

Billy Bunter lagged behind.

A walk of a mile in the freshness of the morning was agreeable to all the other fellows, and really was not a martyrdom for Bunter. But the fat Owl had a sense of injury. Feeling quite certain that the other fellows would not sail up the Nile on Mr. Maroudi's dahabiyeh without him, Bunter took his time. Besides, Bunter had a lot to carry. He had distinguished himself, as usual, at breakfast, and astonished the waiters, for the last time, with the amount of foodstuffs he had packed away. He was not disposed to exertion, and he did not exert himself. Harry Wharton looked back and shouted to him:

"Buck up, Bunter!"

"Yah!"

"You'll get lost, fathead!" bawled Bob Cherry.

"Beast!"

Bunter did not buck up. At first it was obstinacy that made him lag. But after a half-mile he really was fatigued, owing to the cargo he had to carry. Six or seven breakfasts, one after another, weighed on him a little. He panted and perspired, and lagged more and more. He lost sight of the juniors, but the dancing gold tassel on Hassan's tarboosh guided him. Hassan was a tall dragoman, and his red tarboosh and golden tassel glowed over the crowd in the street.

"Donkey!"

Bunter blinked round.

"Donkey! You, sar! Donkey!"

For a moment Bunter had the impression, as he had had once before, that the brown man was calling him a donkey. But the brown man who spoke to him was leading a big, powerful donkey; so the fat Owl guessed that the animal was for hire or sale.

"Oh, good!" gasped Bunter. "Yes, I'll hire your donkey. Rather!"

A lift was exactly what Bunter wanted.

"Sell a donkey, sar!" said the brown man. "Me no donkey-boy, sar! No, sar. Me Hafiz, sar—me sell donkeys. Yes, sar. You buy a donkey. Me make a cheap price—sixty piastres, sar."

Bunter blinked at the man.

Hafiz grinned and salaamed.

"Fine big donkey, sar! Him name Queen Victoria, sar, to English gentleman. To American gentleman him name Abraham Lincoln. Yes, sar. Sixty piastres cheap price. What you say, sar? Buy a donkey?"

Bunter blinked at the donkey. It was a big, handsome animal, and very like Quelch to look at—the donkey Bunter had bought once before, and which had departed so soon after the purchase, and had not been seen since. Sixty piastres was an absurdly low price for such an animal. Once more Billy Bunter scented a bargain.

"Well, you see, I'm going on a boat—what you call a dahabiyeh in your silly language," he explained. "So——"

"Him donkey like go on dahabiyeh sar—very good donkey for dahabiyeh, sar—many times him go on dahabiyeh, sar——"

"Oh!" said Bunter thoughtfully.

He did not know whether there was accommodation for donkeys on board a dahabiyeh; but Hafiz, as a native, ought to know!

"You buy a donkey, sar," said Hafiz persuasively. "He carry you all over Egypt, sar—you look at a donkey, sar, you see him splendid fine animal, sar. Sixty piastres very cheap price, sar. What you say?"

"Saddle and all?" asked Bunter.

"Yes, sar—everything and all!" said Hafiz.

"Done!" said Bunter.

Sixty piastres was about twelve shillings, and such a donkey for twelve shillings was almost as big a bargain as Quelch for ten shillings. Billy Bunter felt that he could not afford to lose a chance like this. Even if he could not take the donkey on the dahabiyeh, he could hand it over to Hassan to dispose of, certainly for a larger sum than twelve shillings. Why Hafiz was selling a valuable donkey, saddle and trappings and bridle and all, for such a trivial sum, was as great a mystery as why Abdullah had sold a similar donkey at a similar ruinous price. But Billy Bunter, who had jumped at one bargain, now jumped at another.

(*Continued on next page.*)

"Help me up!" he said, making up his fat mind.

A big bargain, and a lift at the same moment, appealed to Bunter. Mounted on Queen Victoria, alias Abraham Lincoln, he would soon overtake the juniors, now far ahead. He rather fancied himself riding in style, on his own donkey, while the other fellows walked.

Hafiz assisted him to mount, the donkey standing quite still, looking as if butter would not melt in its capacious mouth. Bunter thought he had never seen a quieter or more good-tempered-looking donkey—except perhaps Quelch, who was possibly a relation; for there was undoubtedly a strong resemblance between Bunter's first bargain and Bunter's second bargain.

The fat junior counted out sixty piastres, and Hafiz salaamed, and salaamed again, and the donkey started. Even Bunter could ride a quiet, good-tempered donkey, so long as the donkey remained quiet and good-tempered. He trotted on cheerily, and with a clatter of hoofs, overtook the Greyfriars party.

"I say, you fellows——"

"Hallo, hallo, hallo! Bunter's found his twin!" exclaimed Bob Cherry.

"The twinfulness is terrific!" chuckled Hurree Jamset Ram Singh.

"Well, my hat!" said Harry Wharton, staring at Bunter's long-eared mount. "How on earth did you find him, Bunter?"

"Eh? I've just bought this donkey."

"You've bought him again?" yelled Wharton.

Bunter blinked at him.

"What the thump do you mean?" he demanded peevishly. "I've just bought him for sixty piastres. He's nearly as cheap as that donkey I bought the other day."

"It's the same donkey!" roared Bob.

"The samefulness is terrific."

"Oh, don't be silly asses, you know!" said Bunter. "This donkey is named Queen Victoria. The one I bought the other day was named George Washington. I'm going to name him Quelch, same as the other. He, he, he!"

"You fat owl, it's the same donkey!" exclaimed Frank Nugent. "Was it the same man sold him to you?"

"No, it wasn't, you ass—think I shouldn't know him again," snorted Bunter. "Think a nigger could take me in?"

"Well, whether it was the same man or not, it's the same donkey," said Harry Wharton, laughing.

"Rubbish!"

"Same donkey, sar," said Hassan, grinning. "Hassan know! Adullah he have many brothers, lordly gentlemen; very great rogues, sar; sell same donkey many times, always at cheap price. Yes. You trust Hassan. Hassan know everything."

"Ha, ha, ha!"

"Rot!" snorted Bunter. "I'd jolly well like to see the nigger that could take me in! I—— Oh! Help! Yooop! Hold him! Yarooooh!"

From somewhere in the crowded street came a long, shrill whistle. Apparently it was a signal to the donkey. Even as the whistle shrilled, the quietest looking donkey Bunter had ever seen suddenly turned into an infuriated buck-jumper.

George-Washington-Queen-Victoria threw down his head, threw up his hind legs, and cavorted frantically, and Billy Bunter, yelling wildly, sailed over the lowered head, and landed on one of the many heaps of garbage that adorn the streets of Cairo.

"Yoooooop!"

"Oh, my hat!"

"Ha, ha, ha!"

The instant Bunter was off his back the donkey vanished. There were other donkeys in the street, and camels, and a few buffaloes, and arabeyehs, and a crowd of early peasants going to market with their produce, and amid that assorted crowd, Queen Victoria-Abraham Lincoln vanished like a ghost at cock-crow.

Bunter sat on the garbage and roared.

"Yarooh! I'm killed! Yooop! Whooop!"

"Ha, ha, ha!" roared the juniors.

"I say, you fellows—— Yaroooh! Whoop! Help! I'm smashed—killed—dislocated. I say—— Whooop!"

The Famous Five dragged Bunter up, though they were laughing almost too much to help. Fragments of ancient vegetables clung lovingly to Bunter as he was rescued from the garbage-heap. He panted and gasped and spluttered. Fortunately he found that he was not killed, or smashed, or dislocated. But he was breathless.

"Where's my donkey?" he gasped.

"Gone!" chuckled bob Cherry. "You fat duffer, that donkey's trained to it. It's the same donkey——"

"'Tain't!" roared Bunter.

"I dare say he's been sold cheap to about a hundred tourists, or perhaps a thousand," chuckled Johnny Bull. "A different man and a different name every time——"

"And generally a different mug!" chortled Bob. "But in this case they caught the same mug again."

"Ha, ha, ha!"

"I say, you fellows, you go after that donkey—I gave sixty piastres for that donkey——" gasped Bunter.

"Sixty and fifty—that's a hundred and ten piastres altogether!" chuckled Bob. "If you buy him a few more times, you'll get up to quite a big figure—he'll be a dear donkey, in the long run."

"Ha, ha, ha!"

"You silly chump, it's not the same donkey——"

"Ha, ha, ha!"

The chums of the Remove walked on. Billy Bunter cast a last blink round through his big spectacles, in search of his second bargain. But his second bargain had vanished like his first; though Bunter was not willing to admit that it was the same bargain. He snorted, and rolled after the Famous Five—on foot. It was walking, after all, for William George Bunter.

THE TWELFTH CHAPTER.
Up the Nile!

MOUSSA, the reis, salaamed to the Greyfriars fellows, as they came on board the Cleopatra—that being the name of Mr. Maroudi's dahabiyeh. The Nubian boatmen salaamed also, in a swarm on the sailor's deck.

It was a huge houseboat; the largest and handsomest dahabiyeh that the juniors had seen. They had seen a good many on the Nile since they had arrived in Egypt; but nothing to equal the Cleopatra.

Obviously, Mr. Maroudi was a very wealthy gentleman indeed, to be the owner of this magnificent craft. Instructions had been given to the reis and the crew, and they greeted the Greyfriars tourists with great respect and attention.

The juniors looked about the great river-boat with delighted eyes. It was to be their floating home for many days to come, and they agreed that Mr. Maroudi was a real brick to lend them such a wonderful craft. They had looked forward to "doing" the Nile in a dahabiyeh; but a hired dahabiyeh would have been very different from this palatial boat. Even Billy Bunter admitted that it was "some boat," and even that it was nearly up to his pater's houseboat—an admission which made the juniors smile. Still, Bunter declared that he would have preferred a steamer.

"How do they get this thing along?" he demanded.

"Wind him blow big sail, sar!" said Hassan.

"Suppose the wind blows the other way?" asked Bunter.

"Most time wind him blow from the north, lordly sar, blow dahabiyeh up the Nile!" explained Hassan. "Wind he go up, current him come down, sar."

"Still, there isn't always a wind, I suppose," said Bunter.

"Wind him no blow, sailors push along with tremendous long pole," said Hassan. "Sometimes sailors run on bank, tow with tremendous big rope, sar. Suppose lordly gentlemen in pressed hurry, tow with a steamer."

At the stern of the dahabiyeh was a raised platform, where the reis, or pilot, stood, to steer with the huge helm.

Steps led down from the boatmen's deck into the cabins, and up from the boatmen's deck to the upper deck.

The juniors went down the three shallow steps to look at their quarters.

They passed through a wide doorway, over which was a gilded inscription from the Koran, though, as it was in Arabic, the juniors were unable to read it.

Within was a corridor on either side of which doors opened into the sleeping-apartments.

Passing the length of the corridor between the rows of bed-rooms, they arrived in a large room, which extended over the whole of the stern of the great boat.

Windows looked out on the balcony that ran round the stern outside, furnished with lattices in exquisite mushrabeyeh work, which could be closed as shutters. Three doors gave access to the outside balcony, which was sheltered from the sun by awnings.

The great cabin was furnished in the Oriental style, as was natural, as the boat belonged to a native. Embroidered divans in gorgeous colours were round the walls, with piles of cushions wonderfully soft to the touch and glowing with colour. Prayer-rugs covered the floor, which was of a hard, polished wood—prayer-rugs of every colour and design, and, as the juniors could see at a glance, extremely costly. But Mr. Maroudi had evidently made some preparations for the comfort of his European guests, for there were chairs and tables and several deep and comfortable armchairs. In the centre of the saloon was a sunken pool of marble, in which a tiny fountain played, surrounded by earth in which tiny dwarf palms grew. There was a faint musical murmur from the fountain, and the ceaseless jet of water gleamed and glistened in the sunlight that poured in at the windows and doors.

"Jolly!" said Bob Cherry.

"The jollifulness is terrific," declared the Nabob of Bhanipur.

"Beats the jolly old study in the Remove passage at Greyfriars, what?" said Nugent, with a grin.

"What-ho!" chuckled Johnny Bull.

"I think you boys will be comfortable here," said Sir Reginald, smiling.

"I fancy so, sir," said Harry. "It's simply ripping of Mr. Maroudi to lend us a magnificent boat like this."

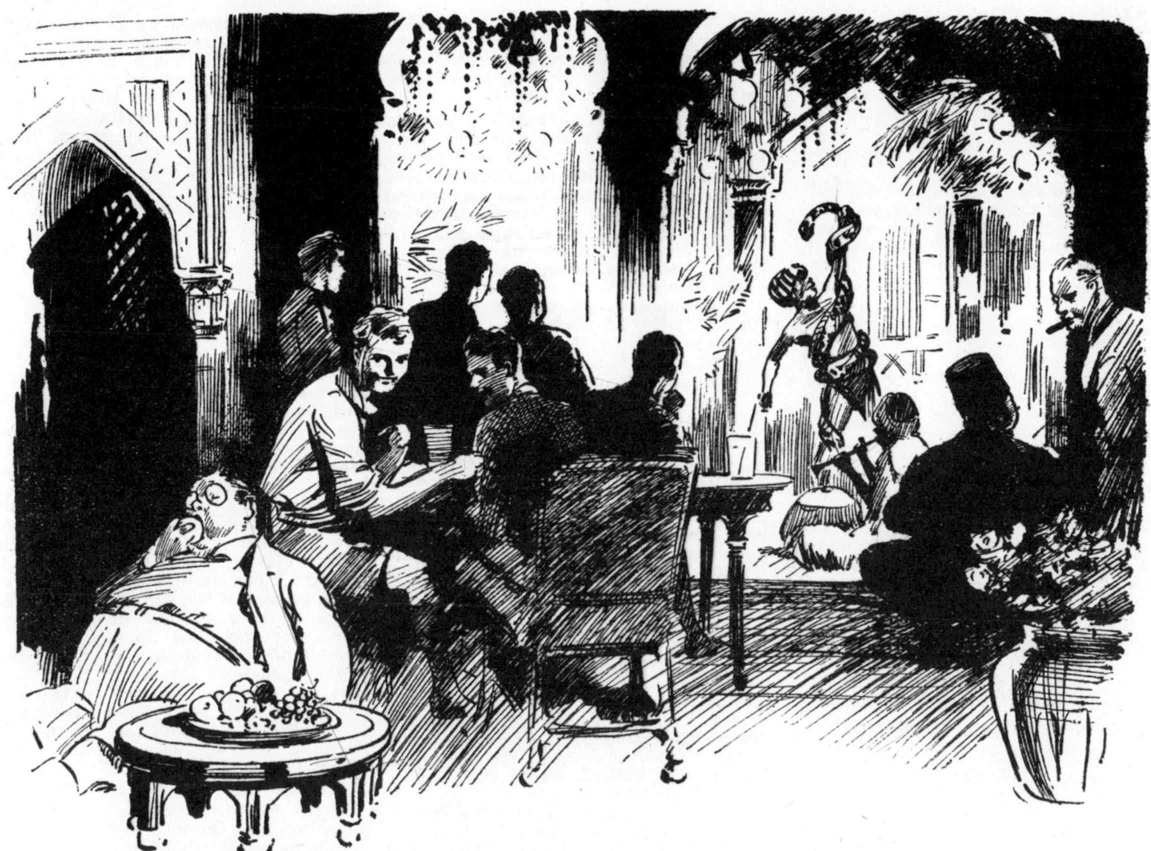

The weird exploits of the snake-charmer held Harry Wharton & Co. spellbound, while Billy Bunter, slowly and laboriously, but determinedly, travelled through his supply of sweetmeats and stuffed nuts !

"What about the grub?" asked Bunter.

"What?" barked Sir Reginald.

"Grub!" said Bunter firmly. "The boat ain't bad—but the grub's rather important, you know."

"Shut up, Bunter," said Bob.

"Oh, really, Cherry! Just like you fellows to be staring at fountains and paintings and carvings and things, and forgetting the grub!" said Bunter witheringly. "Lucky you've got somebody with you to think of it. If they haven't made proper arrangements about the grub——"

"Mr. Maroudi's cook is on board, my boys," said Sir Reginald, with a glare at Bunter. "Every arrangement has been made for your comfort. And——"

"I think we'd better look at the bedrooms," said Bunter. "I'm not going to sleep on a mat, I can jolly well tell you fellows."

"Shut up, Bunter!"

"Yah!"

The juniors looked into their rooms. They found that they were provided with European beds, and every bedroom had a recess in which was a marble bath, an armchair, and a tall mirror; the walls painted white, picked out with green. The baggage had already been deposited in the rooms. Billy Bunter was pleased to give a grunt of approval.

"Like your room, old fat man?" asked Bob.

"Not bad!" admitted Bunter.

"I hardly think it will suit you, though," said Bob, shaking his head as he looked into Bunter's room.

"Eh? Why not?"

"There's a bath in it."

"Ha, ha, ha!"

"Oh, really, Cherry——"

"And there's a lot of soap all ready," said Nugent. "Of course, Mr. Maroudi doesn't know Bunter as we do."

"Oh, really, Nugent——"

"Don't you worry, old fat man," said Johnny Bull. "You can drop the soap overboard as soon as we start, and put a screen round the bath so that it won't keep on reminding you that you want a wash——"

"Oh, really, Bull——"

The juniors returned to the deck. There Sir Reginald left them, with many parting instructions to the juniors, all of which they promised to remember; and to Hassan, which the dragoman received with endless salaams.

The old baronet went ashore, leaving the Greyfriars party to themselves. Now that Kalizelos, the Greek, was in prison, there was no doubt that the juniors would be safe on board Mr. Maroudi's dahabiyeh, in the care of the faithful Hassan, and it was an opportunity for Sir Reginald to attend to the business that had brought him to Egypt. And much as the juniors liked and respected the stiff old gentleman, they were by no means averse from the idea of going up the Nile "on their own."

Every comfort had been provided on the dahabiyeh by Mr. Maroudi's generous hospitality; and even if there had been danger ahead, the chums of the Remove were convinced of their ability to take care of themselves. But with their enemy in the hands of the Cairo police, it seemed that the danger was over, and that the Golden Scarab would no longer bring perils round them.

The Nubian sailors took in the gangway, and the dahabiyeh floated out into the Nile, the juniors on the upper deck waving their hands to the tall figure of the baronet ashore, Sir Reginald waving back.

"Now we're off," said Bob Cherry, "and we're going to have a gorgeous time, what?"

"The gorgeousness is going to be terrific, my esteemed Bob."

"My lordly gentlemen will see everything," said Hassan, beaming. "Tombs of the kings, tombs of innumerable and enormous numbers of dead persons. Denderah — Luxor — Edfou — Hassan knows all things, and will show them to his magnificent lords! Yes!"

The juniors gazed about them with keenly interested eyes, as the Cleopatra started on the long trip up the Nile.

The wind blew steadily from the north, and the great sail was set, filling with wind and driving the great boat up the river against the sluggish current. The reis stood like a bronze statue at the helm. The Nubian boatmen sang a song of the Nile in their own tongue as they went about their work. Hassan pointed out innumerable objects of interest on either bank.

After passing the Abbas II Bridge, old Cairo was on their left, backed by the Mokattam Hills; on their right, the Pyramids of Ghizeh. Both dropped out of sight as the dahabiyeh rolled on to the south. Other dahabiyehs and several steamers were to be seen on the Nile, as well as a crowd of feluccas. On the banks brown men looked at them as they passed, and every now and then from some hopeful brown man came faintly from the distance a cry of "Backsheesh!" From the shores at frequent intervals came the sing-song chant of the shaduf men.

"Isn't it ripping?" said Bob. "Think of jolly old Cheops floating along here 6,000 years ago!"

"And jolly old Rameses the Second, 3,000 years ago, coming back after his scrap with the giddy Hittites!" said Nugent.

"And the jolly old Ptolomies——" said Johnny Bull.

"And the merry old Pharaohs——"

"And the giddy Mamelukes——"

"Historical interest of celebrated river enormous and very large, my lordly gentlemen," said Hassan, beaming. "No country but Egypt contains such tremendous and gigantic numbers of dead persons."

"I say, you fellows——"

"Hallo, hallo, hallo! Enjoying life, old fat bean?" roared Bob, bestowing a hearty smack on Bunter's fat shoulder.

"Yarooooh!" Bunter dodged out of reach of the exuberant Bob. "I say, you fellows, I'm getting hungry!"

Whereat the chums of the Remove chuckled. Their thoughts had been on the past; but Billy Bunter's thoughts were on the present. Cheops and Rameses thhe Second and the Ptolomies, the Pharaohs, the Mamelukes and the Caliphs, did not fill so much space in Bunter's mind as lunch. And the fat Owl, leaving the other fellows to think of the immemorial past as long as they liked, went to look for provender.

THE THIRTEENTH CHAPTER.

Another Bargain for Bunter!

"MEMPHIS!"

"What's that?" yawned Billy Bunter.

"Memphis!" answered Bob Cherry, with a look of surprise.

"Oh, really, you ass——"

"Bunter," said Bob, adopting the manner of Mr. Quelch at Greyfriars, "you are not only the most backward boy in the Form—I mean on board the dahabiyeh—but you seem to have an absolute dislike to the acquisition of knowledge——"

"You silly ass!" said Bunter.

"I've a jolly good mind," said Bob severely, "to give you a detention, Bunter, and make you write a hundred times that Memphis was the ancient capital of Egypt—by the way, it was, wasn't it, you men?" asked Bob, breaking off in his instruction of Billy Bunter, to ask that rather pertinent question.

"Yes," said Harry Wharton, laughing.

"Tremendous vast city of ancient times, sar!" said Hassan. "Now in most interesting ruins, with innumerable dead persons; and suitable place for serious meditation on fall of human greatness and such things. Hassan show you all."

"It's the jolly old city where Rameses the Second used to roll about in his giddy chariot," went on Bob. "It's got a bit dilapidated, I believe, since the time of jolly old Rameses. We tie up the dahabiyeh at the bank, and go to the ruins of Memphis with the help of your relations, Bunter——"

"Eh? I haven't any relations in Egypt, that I know of," answered the Owl of the Remove.

"I mean on donkey-back," explained Bob Cherry.

"You silly chump!" roared Bunter.

The huge sail of the dahabiyeh had been lowered, and the Nubian sailors poled in to the western bank. The Pyramids of Sakkara stood out against the sky over the Libyan desert. All the fellows were interested in Memphis, the ancient capital—excepting Bunter, who was fed-up on ruins and tombs and mummies; and who did not agree with the dragoman that the chief attraction of Egypt was the "innumerable dead persons." Still, Bunter jerked himself out of his chair on the upper deck and blinked shoreward. He was not going to be left behind when the juniors rambled over Memphis.

"My donkey would have come in useful now," he remarked. "Both my donkeys, in fact. If you fellows had caught them——"

"Both your donkeys were the same donkey, fathead," said Bob. "They sold you the same donkey over twice, chump!"

"I tell you there were two donkeys!" hooted Bunter.

"Only you and the other."

"Beast!"

The gangway was run out to the shore. Harry Wharton & Co. and Lord Mauleverer crossed it, and Billy Bunter rolled after them, followed by Hassan, and a Nubian servant carrying a large basket of provisions for lunch in the ruins. Donkey-boys immediately surrounded them, eager for custom. Every donkey-boy shouted at once, urging the claims of his own special donkey, which, it appeared, was better than all the others put together. The dragoman proceeded to engage donkeys for the ride, while the juniors strolled on the banks of the Nile.

"Hallo, hallo, hallo!" ejaculated Bob Cherry suddenly. "I've seen that jolly old donkey before."

"Which?" asked Nugent.

"Look!"

A brown-faced man in a dingy djubbah and turban was leading a big, handsome donkey, which he was not offering for hire. He was looking round with keen black eyes, and as he sighted the Greyfriars fellows he came towards them with an ingratiating grin on his face. They had never seen the man before; but they had seen the donkey. They knew that donkey. It was the George Washington that Abdullah had sold to Bunter—likewise, it was the Queen Victoria that Hafiz had sold to Bunter! The juniors grinned. They could guess that the brown man was one more member of the donkey-dealing firm, with the same donkey to sell to some innocent tourist. No doubt that donkey had been sold so often in Cairo that the firm had decided to trot him out to Memphis for further business.

"Donkey, sar!" said the brown man, grinning with a flash of white teeth. "You buy a donkey, sar?"

"Oh, my hat!" said Harry Wharton.

There was no doubt about George Washington - Queen Victoria! Undoubtedly and indubitably, it was the same donkey. But as a new member of the firm was in charge of him, he naturally did not know the Greyfriars fellows by sight, and was unaware that they were well-acquainted with George Washington-Queen Victoria.

"Fine big donkey at very cheap price, sar!" said the brown man. "Me, sar, me Osman, sar, very honest donkey dealer, sar! Sell a donkey! Yes! Sell a donkey for price of forty piastres, sar."

"Cheaper than ever!" chuckled Bob. "The cheapfulness is terrific!"

"You buy a donkey, sar?" asked Osman. "You ride to Memphis on a donkey, sar. Buy a donkey forty piastres, sar! Cheap donkey, sar! Yes." He grinned and salaamed. "You like this donkey, sar! Saddle and all things, sar, all forty piastres! Noble lords buy a donkey?"

"I say, you fellows, that looks a decent donkey!" said Billy Bunter, blinking at the animal through his big spectacles. "He's rather like the one I bought the other day——"

"Ha, ha, ha!"

"Blessed if I see anything to cackle at! I say, you fellows, that donkey's jolly cheap at forty piastres."

"It's the same donkey!" roared Bob.

"Eh, what?" Billy Bunter blinked at the donkey again. "Rot, old chap! It's a different man with him. I say, you, what's that donkey's name?"

"You English, sar, him name King Edward," said Osman agreeably. "You American, him name President Hoover, sar."

"Ha, ha, ha!" shrieked the juniors.

"I say, Mauly, lend me forty piastres!" said Bunter. "I'm not losing a chance like this!"

"But it's the same donkey, dear man!" said Mauly.

"Don't be an ass, old chap!" said Bunter. "I know one donkey from another, I suppose! Lend me forty piastres, there's a good chap. Why, the saddle alone's worth that."

"You buy a donkey, sar?" said Hafiz, fixing his attention on Billy Bunter now. "You know one good donkey, sar—you buy a donkey."

"Yes, rather!" said Bunter. "Lend me—I say, Mauly, where are you going? Don't walk away while a fellow's talking to you, you beast! Mauly! Deaf, you ass! What's that silly chump Mauly walking off for, you fellows, when I want to speak to him?"

"Ha, ha, ha!"

"Lend me forty piastres, Wharton, old chap——"

"Can't you spend your own piastres?" asked the captain of the Remove.

"Oh, really, Wharton!" That resource, apparently, had not occurred to Bunter. "I say, don't walk away—beast! Bob, old man—beast! I say, Nugent, lend me forty piastres."

"You've bought that donkey twice!" roared Johnny Bull.

"Yah! Will you lend me—— Beast!" hooted Bunter, as the chums of the Remove followed Lord Mauleverer.

He was left alone with the donkey-dealer. Osman regarded him rather uneasily. He had caught some of the juniors' words, and realised that they had seen King Edward-President Hoover before. But he need not have worried. Billy Bunter was keen on a bargain; and Billy Bunter's obtuseness was an armour of proof that no instruction could penetrate. All the more because the other fellows declared that it was the same donkey, Billy Bunter was convinced that it was not the same donkey. Donkeys were much alike, anyhow; and Bunter was short-sighted as well as obtuse. He had not recognised it as the same donkey; and he was not going to be convinced.

But he had to dip into his own financial resources for the forty piastres. This was rather disagreeable; still, the donkey was obviously worth at least ten times as much.

"You buy a donkey, sar?" asked Osman, rather dubiously.

"Yes, rather!" answered Bunter.

Osman's brown face brightened again. He had come across many "mugs" in his career as a member of a donkey-dealing firm; but he had never struck such a "mug" as this before! People were not often glad to meet Bunter; but Osman undoubtedly was glad to meet him, and he would have been glad to meet whole tribes of Bunters.

The fat Owl counted out forty piastres, and slipped the reins of the donkey over a fat arm.

"You ride a donkey, sar?" said Osman, having tucked away the piastres under his dingy djubbah. "You like ride a donkey, sar?" No doubt Osman was anxious to see Bunter in the saddle—from which he would speedily have been tossed by King Edward - President Hoover.

"That's all right," said Bunter, and he led the donkey away with a fat arm through the reins, after the juniors.

Bunter did not believe that it was the same donkey; but he remembered his bad luck with George Washington and Queen Victoria; and he was going to be careful this time.

Osman stared after him. He did not depart. If he was to whistle that donkey back, he had to keep the tourists in sight till an opportunity came. So long as Bunter had an arm through the reins, even that well-trained and sagacious ass could not get away from him. Osman had some shadowing to do.

"I say, you fellows——"

"Here are donkeys, sars!" said Hassan. "You trust Hassan to find you some very fine and magnificent donkeys——"

"I've got my mount, Hassan," said Bunter. "You needn't hire a donkey for me."

The dragoman gave quite a jump when he looked at Bunter's mount.

"Oh, sar!" he ejaculated. "You find Abdullah's donkey one more time, sar!"

"Don't be a silly ass!" said Bunter peevishly. "This is a new donkey. I've just bought him from a man named Osman. What are you grinning at, you cheeky nigger?"

"Oh, sar!"

"Shut up!" snapped Bunter. "If you fellows are ready, we'll start! Look here! The basket of grub can be put on my donkey, and I'll keep an eye on it, see? That nigger can lead my donkey. Not that he's likely to bolt, you know—I fancy I can ride a donkey—still, that nigger may as well lead him! Gimme that basket!"

Harry Wharton & Co. were already mounted on the hired donkeys. Bunter, being in possession of his own steed, refused a hired donkey. The Nubian servant who carried the basket of provisions stared as Billy Bunter jerked it away from him. Bunter preferred to keep that important cargo under his own eyes; likewise, he felt that it was probable that he would be in need of a snack or two before lunch.

The Nubian looked to Hassan for instructions. The dragoman, with a shrug of the shoulders, spoke to him in Arabic, and the Nubian took the reins of King Edward-President Hoover to lead him. Billy Bunter clambered into the saddle, and took the basket of provisions on the donkey. And the Greyfriars party, turning their backs on the Nile, rode towards the ruins of Memphis. And behind them, with a rather anxious expression on his brown face, crept Osman—with an eye on Bunter's donkey.

———

THE FOURTEENTH CHAPTER.

A Famine in Egypt!

"ENORMOUS and gigantic statue of Rameses the Second——" Hassan, the dragoman, was going strong in the ruins of Memphis.

With a shouting of donkey-boys and a cracking of sticks, the Greyfriars fellows arrived at the spot where the gigantic statue of King Rameses lay on its back amid the ruins of the great city over which Rameses had reigned three thousand years ago.

Harry Wharton & Co. dismounted. Billy Bunter did not dismount. He was not very keen on Rameses the Second; but he was very keen indeed on the contents of the big wicker basket. He sat in the saddle, helping himself to bunches of figs from the basket, while the other fellows "did" Rameses the Second.

Billy Bunter had soon tired of holding the basket, and the Nubian had tied it securely on the donkey's back—with the lid within convenient reach of Bunter's fat hand.

This suited Bunter nicely.

It also suited the other fellows, for so long as Billy Bunter was munching figs and dates and sweetmeats, he was not talking. When Bunter was not eating, his conversation resembled the little brook in the poem, which went on for ever. And as it was a large basket, with an enormous supply of provender, even Bunter had to leave enough for the other fellows' lunch. Which was a rather important consideration, as provisions were unobtainable at the ruins, and had to be brought from a distance.

"Length of enormous statue, twenty-six feet English," said Hassan. "Crown, which is now absent, was six feet, also English! This gigantic and immense statue being of huge historical interest. Next we see alabaster sphinx close at hand, but here we wait if my lordly gentlemen desire to meditate solemnly on fallen greatness of magnificent, but now debilitated royalty."

Bob Cherry chuckled.

"Anybody going in for solemn meditation?" he asked. "Or shall we move on to the giddy sphinx? May as well see it—though I've given up counting the sphinxes we've seen."

The juniors remounted the donkeys and moved on. The Nubian led Bunter's donkey after them. So far the Nubian had not let go the reins of King Edward-President Hoover—which was no doubt the reason why Bunter was still mounted on that steed of many names. Now, as the donkey jerked into motion again, Bunter dropped a bunch of figs that he had just extracted from the provision basket.

"Here, pick that up!" snapped Bunter to the black man.

"Yes, sar!" said the Nubian obediently.

He stooped to pick up the fallen bunch of figs. To do so, he released the reins of King Edward-President Hoover.

From somewhere among the rambling ruins of Memphis, it seemed that a keen eye was upon them, for the moment the Nubian released the donkey, a shrill whistle sounded from amid a thicket of acacias close at hand.

Hitherto, King Edward-President Hoover had been as quiet and orderly a donkey as even a rider like Bunter could desire.

But at the sound of the signal whistle, King Edward-President Hoover developed on the spot the buck-jumping proclivities of Queen Victoria-Abraham Lincoln.

It happened so suddenly that Bunter was taken quite off his guard.

The donkey's head went down, and his heels flew up.

Before the fat Owl knew what was happening, he was shooting over the donkey's head and sprawling in the ruins of Memphis.

"Yaroooh!" roared Bunter, as he landed.

"Hallo, hallo, hallo!"

The Greyfriars fellows looked back.

They saw Billy Bunter sprawling headlong, they saw King Edward-President Hoover galloping off, and they saw the Nubian, with a bunch of figs in his black hand, clutch at him too late.

The donkey, going strong, vanished behind the acacias, leaving the Nubian staring, and Billy Bunter sprawling and roaring.

"Ha, ha, ha!" roared Bob. "He's gone again!"

"The gonefulness is terrific!"

"Him donkey go back to him masters, sars!" said Hassan, grinning. "Small fat lord no see him donkey again! No, sar!"

"Yarooh! Help! I say, you fellows —— Wow!"

"Ha, ha, ha!"

Billy Bunter sat up.

He blinked round him through his big spectacles. The other fellows reined in, chuckling. The donkey-boys grinned. Bunter did not grin. He had had a severe bump, and he had lost his donkey once more. He blinked round in vain for a sign of King Edward-President Hoover. The many-named steed had disappeared, and from a distance came back an echo of galloping hoofs. That was all.

"I say, you fellows! Where's my donkey?" gasped Bunter.

"Gone, old fat bean!" chortled Bob. "What did you expect? I dare say you will be able to buy him again farther up the river."

"Ha, ha, ha!"

"You silly ass!" yelled Bunter. "I tell you it wasn't the same donkey! Look here, you ride after him and catch him, see?"

"No takers!" grinned Johnny Bull.

"I say, you fellows——"

"My dear idiot, we've come here to see Memphis, not for a donkey race," said Harry Wharton, "and I fancy it wouldn't be easy to catch that donkey, either. Osman will take care of that."

Billy Bunter scrambled to his feet.

"Here, you nigger, you go after that donkey!" he shouted to the Nubian. "Go after him and catch him, see? Run! What are you standing there like a black image for, you dummy? Run after that donkey!"

"Yes, sar!" gasped the Nubian.

"I'll give you ten piastres if you catch him, and I'll jolly well kick you if you don't, see? Don't come back without him!" hooted Bunter.

"Yes, sar!"

The Nubian started at a run, and disappeared behind the thicket of acacias. As all the fellows but Bunter realised, there was not the remotest chance of catching that elusive donkey. His master was already on its back, putting on speed for parts unknown. The Nubian was as well aware of that as Harry Wharton & Co., and as soon as the acacias hid him from sight, he gave up the chase, and sat down to rest among the trees.

The Nubian had no objection to taking a rest, and quite possibly he had had enough of Billy Bunter. With a cheerful black face he went to sleep under the acacias, what time Osman and King Edward-President Hoover vanished into space.

"Well, let's get on," said Bob Cherry.

"I say, you fellows, we shall have to wait here!" exclaimed the Owl of the Remove. "I've not got a donkey! I can't walk, I suppose."

"Suppose again!" suggested Bob. "Come on, you men!"

The donkey-boys' sticks cracked again, and the party proceeded. Billy Bunter rolled after them, panting and gasping. He overtook them, while they were looking at the alabaster sphinx, which was quite close at hand.

"I say, you fellows——"

"Shut up, Bunter!"

"You silly asses!" roared Bunter. "I say, the grub was tied on that donkey! There won't be any lunch!"

"Oh, my hat!"

"We'd better chuck this, and go straight back to the dahabiyeh," said Bunter. "Buck up! We shall be jolly hungry by the time we get there!"

"Go and eat coke!"

"Oh, really, Cherry——"

"You fat chump!" exclaimed Harry Wharton, in great exasperation. "We told you it was the same donkey, and you might have known——"

"Beast!"

"Well, we're not going back," said Harry. "I suppose we shall have to cut it short, as there's no grub; but we're jolly well going to do Memphis while we're here. What do you fellows say?"

"Yes, rather!"

"The ratherfulness is terrific!"

"Come on!" said Harry. "There's another jolly old colossus to see somewhere——"

"I say, you fellows, are you mad?" roared Bunter. "How can we possibly stay out for the day without grub? Why, we shall be famished by the time we get back, if we start now? Have a little sense!"

"Rats!"

"I'm getting hungry already——"

"Fathead!"

"Look here, you beasts——" roared Bunter, in wrath and consternation. "I can't go back alone. I don't know the way. Look here——"

"Dry up!"

"I tell you there isn't any grub!" shrieked Bunter.

"Well, that's worse for us than for you," said Bob. "You can live on your own fat, like a polar bear. You've got enough to last you a week, at least."

"You silly chump!" yelled Bunter. "I tell you——"

"Better save your breath, old top! You'll need it, doing the jolly old ruins of Memphis on foot!"

"Beast!" howled Bunter.

The party moved on. Billy Bunter rolled after them, hot and panting and perspiring. But he was silent now, save for his gasps and pants. He needed his breath to keep up with the donkeys.

The juniors stopped to view the second colossal statue of Rameses the Second, clambering up the wooden platform that had been built for tourists to make their inspection. Bunter did not follow them up, however. He sat down on a rock and panted for breath. Whatever interest Bunter might have had in that ancient king of Egypt was gone now. Bunter was thinking of the lunch that had vanished with King Edward-President Hoover—and which Osman, probably, was disposing of internally, in some secluded nook.

The Nubian had not returned with that elusive donkey, and his return with it was highly improbable, as the black man was fast asleep in the acacias a mile away.

Even Bunter realised that he was not likely to see that donkey again—unless, indeed, the excellent animal was offered for sale once more at another stopping-place along the Nile. But that was not the worst—the worst was that the provisions had gone with King Edward-President Hoover, and there was no lunch for Bunter.

There was no lunch for the other fellows, either; but that did not worry Bunter. His concern, as usual, was wholly for W. G. B.

"Next we see celebrated Step Pyramid——" chanted Hassan, as the juniors came down after viewing Rameses the Second.

"I say, you fellows——"

"Oh, get on my donkey, you fat frump!" said Bob Cherry. "I'll walk! Get on and shut up!"

"We shall have to go back for lunch, you beast——"

"Shut up!" roared Bob.

"Beast!" groaned Bunter.

Hassan helped him into the saddle of Bob's donkey. That was a relief, as far as it went. But Bunter was thinking of lunch. It was getting near time for feeding. And there was no grub! Not only was there no grub, but this rotten sight-seeing was to go on for hours before the party turned back, and then it was a good distance back to the dahabiyeh—and grub! Obviously, it was more than flesh and blood could stand! Nevertheless, Billy Bunter had to stand it. He emitted a series of dismal groans as the party went on.

Afterwards, when Bunter thought of that excursion to the ruins of Memphis, it seemed like a nightmare to him.

He was hungry, and getting hungrier!

He felt that he understood now, as never before, the feelings of shipwrecked people in open boats at sea, and of famished travellers lost in the sandy wastes of the desert! And the the other fellows looked at such things as statues, tombs, and sphinxes, just as if lunch did not matter for once. When lunch was an hour overdue Bunter felt that he could bear no more.

"I say, you fellows——" he moaned.

"Shut up, Bunter!"

"I—I'm feeling awfully ill——"

"Too many breakfasts?" asked Nugent.

"Beast! I—I think I'm dying——" moaned Bunter.

"No such luck!" said Bob, shaking his head. "Anyhow, it doesn't matter; lots of tombs handy!"

"Ha, ha, ha!"

"Beast!" howled Bunter.

And the party went on, heedless of Bunter's awful sufferings. Minutes that seemed hours; hours that seemed centuries, passed; and Billy Bunter wondered dismally and drearily whether he would survive that awful day!

THE FIFTEENTH CHAPTER.

The "Sudden Death" of Billy Bunter!

"HELP!"

"What——"

It was a sudden yelp from Billy Bunter.

The Greyfriars sightseers had stopped in the shade of a tall, wide-spreading sycamore-tree for a few minutes' rest from the sun. They were, as a matter of fact, considering the idea of turning back to the Nile, and "chucking" the remainder of the lengthy programme that Hassan had marked out for them. Although not blessed with the unearthly appetite of William George Bunter, the Famous Five had healthy appetites of their own, and they were not quite indifferent to the claims of meal-times.

Certainly Bunter deserved it all. It was his own obstinacy that had caused the loss of the provision-basket, and caused the explorers to lose time by proceeding at a walking pace. As Bob remarked, so long as it was only Bunter it did not matter; but he admitted that things took on a different complexion when the Co. got hungry themselves.

Bunter, by this time, was in a state of desperation. Anyone might have supposed that Bunter was the least hungry of the party, as he had scoffed quite a large number of bunches of figs and dates before the basket vanished with King Edward-President Hoover. But anyone who had supposed that would not have known Bunter. Bunter was not only the hungriest of the party, but he was in a state of famine that was positively alarming.

Famine was one of the ancient plagues of Egypt, and Bunter realised now, with fearful clearness, what the

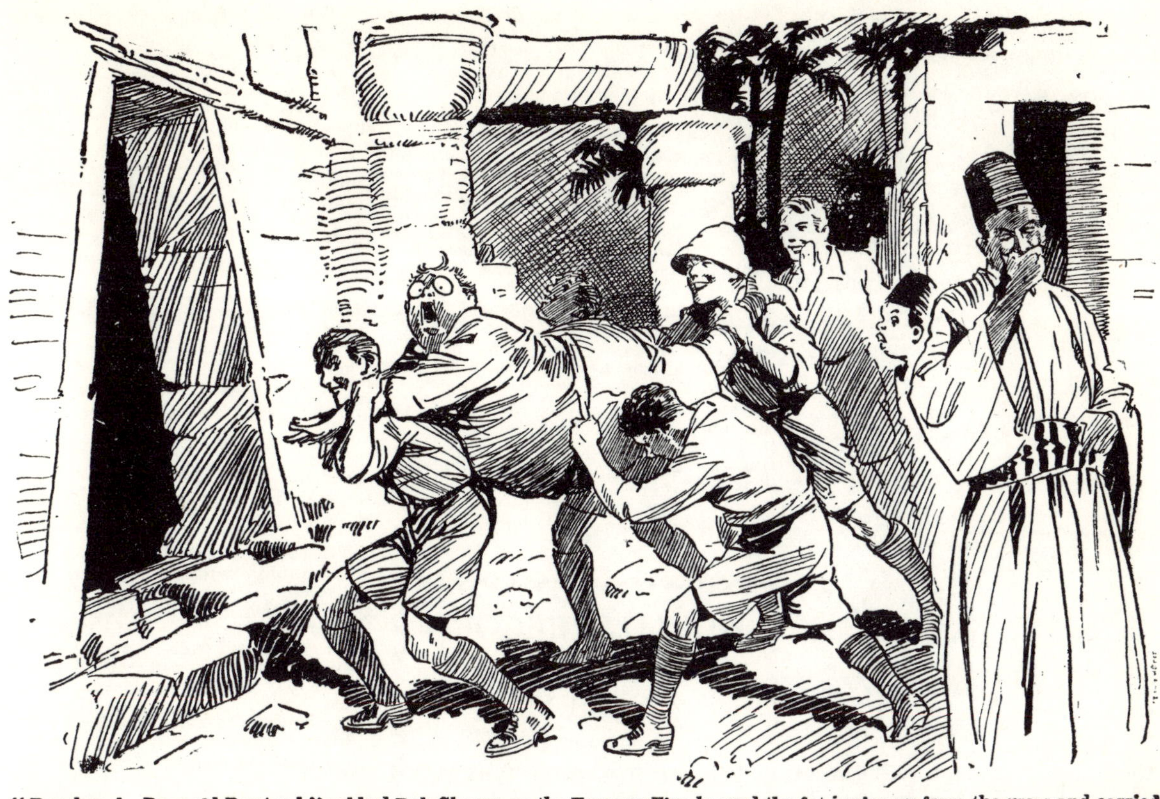

"Boo-hoo! Poor old Bunter!" sobbed Bob Cherry, as the Famous Five heaved the fat junior up from the grass and carried him to the nearest tomb. "No need to carry him down, he's too heavy. Just drop him in, and then we can cover him up with rocks!" "Beasts!" roared "dead" Bunter, coming to life!

Egyptians had felt like in the seven lean years.

So Bunter had resolved on desperate measures. Yelping suddenly for help, the fat junior slipped from the saddle and fell to the earth.

If the utter beasts saw him fall from the donkey from sheer weakness, even those unspeakable beasts would feel something like remorse—Bunter hoped so, at least.

"What the thump——" exclaimed Wharton, as the fat junior went down.

Probably the juniors would have been concerned had Bunter crashed to the ground, as he really ought to have done, when he was falling from weakness brought on by hunger!

But a crash on the ground was a painful prospect, and Bunter did not like the idea. So, although he fell to the earth, he fell carefully, picking a soft, grassy spot, and falling on it with care. Which rather spoiled the effect, so far as the beasts were concerned.

Instead of rushing to him with exclamations of horror and heartfelt sympathy, they only stared at him from where they stood.

"Hallo, hallo, hallo! What's the game?" asked Bob Cherry.

Groan!

"Bunter going in for acrobatics?" asked Nugent.

Groan!

"Bunter, old fat bean——"

Groan!

Hassan, the dragoman, stared at the sprawling fat junior in the grass under the tall sycamore. The donkey-boys stared and grinned. Billy Bunter emitted deep groans, which might have moved the stony heart of Rameses the Second.

"I say, you fellows, I—I—I'm ill!" groaned Bunter. "I—I think I'm dying! Leave me here! I can't move!"

"Poor old Bunter!" said Bob. "You feel as if you're dying, old chap?"

"Ow! Yes! Ow!"

"Then I dare say you'd like to die quietly. Come on, you fellows—let's get off, and leave Bunter to perish in peace."

"The perishfulness in esteemed peace is a wheezy good idea," agreed Hurree Jamset Ram Singh. "Let us bunkfully proceed!"

"Good-bye, Bunter!"

Groan!

"Any last request?" asked Bob considerately. "Any message to the fellows at Greyfriars when we get back?"

Groan!

"Any instructions what we're to do with your postal order if it's arrived while you were away, old chap?"

"Ha, ha, ha!"

Groan!

"I'll take the donkey again," said Bob. "Bunter won't need it any more as he's pegging out. We can get on a bit quicker now. Come to think of it, it's rather considerate of Bunter to peg out like this—it will save a lot of time. I suggest a vote of thanks."

"Hear, hear!"

Groan!

"Well, good-bye, old fat man! When you're finished there's a lot of tombs close to you, and you can take your choice. Come on!"

Bob mounted the donkey, and the juniors went onward. Hassan stared at them, and grinned. The dragoman understood that the small fat lord's podgy leg was being pulled. Bunter, lying full length in the grass under the sycamore, could hardly believe that even these utter beasts were going to desert him in this awful extremity. He lifted his head, and blinked after them through his big spectacles. They were going—going—and leaving him on his own!

"Beasts!" hissed Bunter.

He half-rose—and then lay down again. Billy Bunter was not a bright youth, but he was bright enough to realise that the chums of the Remove would not really depart and leave him to be lost in the ruins of Memphis. They fancied that he was spoofing, and they fully expected him to recover and follow on. So he decided that he would jolly well show them! He stretched out in the grass again, and remained there.

The donkeys clattered away—farther and farther.

The fat Owl felt a twinge of uneasiness. If the awful rotters were really going——

The clattering hoofs stopped.

Bunter grinned in the grass.

They weren't going, after all; as he jolly well knew. And as he heard the sound of the donkeys returning he gave a long, deep, horrible groan, and lay quite still in the grass, with his eyes closed behind his spectacles. He was going to give these unspeakable beasts a shock that would wring their hearts with horror and remorse.

The party halted again under the sycamore.

"Hallo, hallo, hallo! Still dying, Bunter?" inquired Bob Cherry.

No answer.

"Not dead yet, old fat bean?"

Silence!

Lord Mauleverer and the Famous Five stared down at him. Hassan stared. The donkey-boys stared. Bunter did not stir. He lay quite still, with his eyes shut, apparently insensible. In the dusky shadow of the sycamore he had a still and lifeless look.

Bob Cherry closed one eye at his comrades.

"Poor old Bunter!" he said. "This is rather sad, you fellows! I didn't believe he really was dying—but this looks——"

"By gad, it really looks——" said Lord Mauleverer, catching on the game, as it were.

"He can't be quite dead!" said Johnny Bull, in a hushed voice.

"The deadfulness of the esteemed Bunter seems to be terrific!" said Hurree Jamset Ram Singh sorrowfully.

"I say, this is rather awful, you know!" said Nugent. "Surely he can't be quite—quite——" He checked himself, as if unable to utter the terrible word.

"Poor old Bunter!" said Harry Wharton, with a break in his voice. "After all, you fellows, he wasn't a bad chap, in his way."

"In his way!" agreed Johnny Bull.

Bob Cherry dismounted, and approached Bunter. He bent over him, and pressed his hand to a well-filled waistcoat.

"Feel the heart beating?" asked Lord Mauleverer anxiously.

"No!" gasped Bob.

As Bob was feeling on the wrong side, it was not surprising, perhaps, that he failed to detect heart-beats! He rose to his feet, and took out his handkerchief.

"Boo-hoo! P-p-poor old Bunter!" he sobbed. "He-he's gone! We—we shall never hear him talking about his postal order again! P-p-poor old Bunter! We—we—we've lost him!"

There were sorrowful exclamations from the other fellows. Remorse, as Bunter had hoped, had smitten them—hard! They gathered round the fat Owl with solemn and serious faces. Billy Bunter, at that moment, had hard work not to chuckle. This was what the beasts deserved—and it served them right! Silent, lifeless, still, the fat Owl sprawled in the grass, in the midst of the sorrowing circle—heartlessly leaving them to the torments of horror and remorse!

THE SIXTEENTH CHAPTER.
Not a Funeral!

BOB CHERRY was the first to recover from that outburst of grief. He wiped his eyes, and put away his handkerchief. He addressed his comrades in broken tones.

"After this, you fellows, we can hardly go on sight-seeing! It would be unfeeling—in the circumstances!"

"Oh, quite!" agreed Harry Wharton.

"We'd better get back to the dahabiyeh at once——"

"Yes, rather!"

"Better not lose a moment!" said Johnny Bull.

Billy Bunter tried hard not to grin. But he could not help it—he grinned. Fortunately, the juniors did not seem to observe it. Had they observed it, no doubt they would have been surprised to see a lifeless fat Owl grinning. But they seemed to see nothing.

"Sooner we're back the better," said Lord Mauleverer, with a nod.

"Only we can't, of course, carry the body!" said Bob.

"Oh, no; quite impossible!"

"You see, we haven't a donkey for Bunter—and we can't expect him to walk, in the circumstances. Hassan!"

"Yes, sar!" said the staring dragoman.

"Show us the way to the nearest tomb. We've got to bury Bunter!"

"Oh, sar!" gasped the dragoman.

"Lucky there's a lot of empty tombs here," said Bob. "It couldn't have happened better, so far as that goes."

"The luckfulness is terrific!"

"No need to say anything about this afterwards, you men," went on Bob. "An inquest won't do Bunter any good now, poor old chap! And as we're on holiday, we don't want to be bothered with inquests—if they have them in Egypt! The simplest way is to bury him on the spot in one of these old tombs! Take his feet, Wharton!"

Bob Cherry stooped and took the lifeless form by its fat shoulders. Harry Wharton took it by its feet. Johnny Bull and Hurree Singh came to lend aid—which they needed. Billy Bunter was heaved up from the grass.

Hassan led the way to the nearest of the innumerable rock tombs. The four juniors staggered after him with Billy Bunter. Hassan was grinning, and the donkey-boys staring. But the Greyfriars fellows were serious and solemn.

"Here is tomb, my lordly gentlemen!" grinned the dragoman. "Here is opening over steep stair, which is difficult to descend."

"No need to go down," said Bob, gasping. "My hat! He's a weight! Just drop him in—it won't hurt him now! Then we can cover him up with rocks—the donkey-boys can chuck rocks in on him——"

"Beast!" roared Bunter.

Wringing these fellows' hard hearts with remorse was all very well; but obviously it had to stop short before Bunter was dropped into the rock-tomb in ancient Memphis, and covered with a pile of rocks. It was time for Bunter to come to life again, and he came to life quite suddenly.

"Come on!" said Bob. "Only a few steps more——"

"I say, you fellows——"

"Get on with it!" gasped Wharton. "I can't stand this weight much longer. Keep still, Bunter! What the thump are you wriggling about for like an eel when you're dead?"

"You beast, I'm not dead!" yelled Bunter, wriggling frantically. "Don't you drop me into that black hole, you beast—— Yaroooh!"

"Rot!" said Johnny Bull decidedly. "You were dead five minutes ago—so it stands to reason you're dead now! Chuck him in!"

"Yarooooh!"

"The chuckfulness is the proper caper!"

"Help!"

"For goodness' sake, Bunter, be quiet!" exclaimed Bob Cherry. "Don't you know that dead people have to be quiet? It's the thing."

"Beast! Leggo!"

"This is most unseemly, in the circumstances, Bunter," said Wharton. "I think you ought to chuck it."

"Help! Fire! Murder! Yarooop!" roared Bunter. "Keep away from that hole, you awful beasts! I might fall in! Whooop!"

"Get some rocks ready, Hassan! We'll fill it right up when Bunter's in. Ready, Bunter?"

"Oh, you beast! Leggo! Will you leggo, you rotters?" shrieked Bunter. "I'm not dead—you know jolly well that I'm not dead! I'm only hungry! Yarooh!"

"Lay him down on the edge, and then roll him in," said Bob. "For goodness' sake stop that row, Bunter—you ought to know better than to kick up a row at a funeral! It's in the worst of taste!"

"Beast!" howled Bunter.

The juniors laid down the fat Owl on the edge of the yawning gap. He sprawled there and roared.

"Now, all together!" said Bob. "One good shove, and over he goes—— Keep still, Bunter! We can't spend the rest of the day over your blessed funeral. What the thump are you getting up for, when you're dead, you fat ass?"

Bunter bounded up.

He bounded away.

"Collar him!" roared Bob. "The cheeky ass, making out he's not dead when we've taken all this trouble over his funeral——"

"Ha, ha, ha!"

There was a roar of laughter that awakened most of the echoes of the ancient city of Memphis. Billy Bunter—from a safe distance—blinked at the Famous Five, and glared at them with a glare that almost cracked his spectacles.

It dawned upon his fat brain, at last, that the juniors had been aware all the time that he was "spoofing." Their hard hearts had not been wrung with remorse, after all! And they had not really been going to bury him in the rock-tomb of Memphis! They had only been pulling his fat leg!

"You — you — you beasts!" gasped Bunter. "You knew all the time——"

"Ha, ha, ha!" roared the juniors.

"I—I've a jolly good mind to whop you all round——"

"Ha, ha, ha!"

"And I would, if—if it wasn't so jolly hot——"

"Ha, ha, ha!"

"Beasts!"

"Now Bunter's done his funny turn let's get on!" chuckled Bob Cherry.

And they got on!

Billy Bunter's fat brow was dark with wrath. But it cleared as he discerned that the party were proceeding in the direction of the Nile. The brown banks and the glimmering water came in sight again at last, and the dahabiyeh tied up to the bank.

Billy Bunter tottered across the gangway to the dahabiyeh. He tottered down to the dining-saloon. He howled to the Coptic cook. After which there was a sound of steady munching, and Bunter began to feel that life was worth living again.

THE END.

(The next yarn in this exciting holiday series is entitled: "THE SHADOWED SCHOOLBOY!" Make sure you read it chums, by ordering your copy WELL IN ADVANCE!)

OUR STIRRING STORY OF THE "GOOD OLD DAYS."

The Red Falcon!

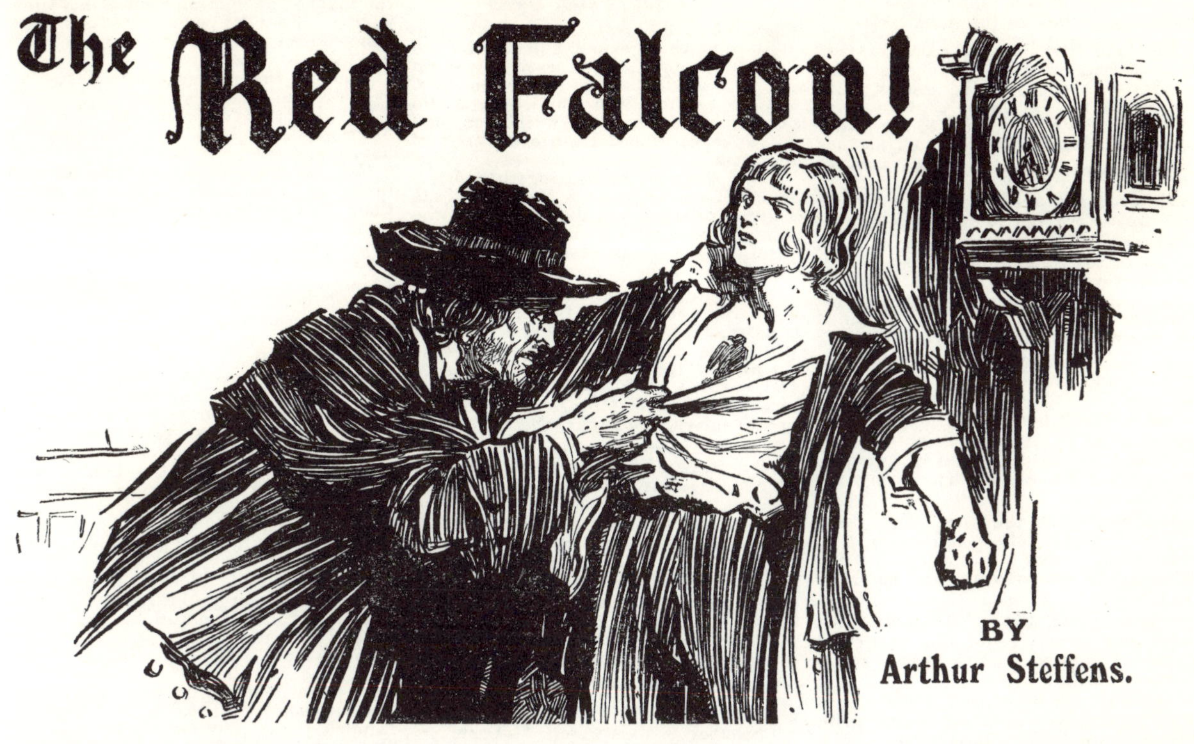

BY
Arthur Steffens.

READ THIS FIRST.

HAL LOVETT RUNS AWAY FROM HOME AND IS BEFRIENDED BY JERRY McLEAN, A ONE-TIME DANDY. HAL AND JERRY ARE OUTSIDE THE DRURY LANE THEATRE, WHEN THEY ARE BOTH ARRESTED FOR CONSPIRING TO ROB THE EARL OF HUNTFORD OF A DIAMOND STAR. HAL IS SENTENCED TO SERVE UPON THE HULKS FOR SEVEN YEARS AND JERRY TO TRANSPORTATION FOR LIFE. CHAINED TOGETHER WITH A FILE OF CONVICTS, THEY ARE CONVEYED TO THE CONVICT HULK ETHALION, ANCHORED AT WOOLWICH.

The Convict Hulk !

"GET along, the lot of you! More smartly now! Do you want a taste of the cat?"

The string of convicts, chained together, climbed out of the wherry which had brought them down-river from the steps at Blackfriars and clambered up the gangway which ran zigzag to the spar deck of the convict hulk Ethalion.

As they did so, Jerry McLean fancied he saw the boy, Hal Lovett, in front of him, falter. Instantly he stretched out a steadying hand.

"Stick it, kid!" he said. "We're home!"

The boy smiled as he flashed a keen glance at his friend. He was not funking.

A keen wind was blowing up the river, beating up lapping waves as the tide raced out. On the deck a pacing sentry came to a halt, grounded the butt of his rifle, and leered at the new arrivals. Some of the convicts who were lolling on the bulwarks grinned, and one of them, waving his hand, greeted them with a coarse joke.

Hal could see other convict hulks anchored near, and, at a distance, farther out in the river, lay a hospital hulk, a tattered red flag fluttering out over her stern.

The boy's eyes swept the wide and lonely river, then drifted ashore where he could see men in brown working on the construction of a new building. They were convicts from the hulks.

Suddenly a broad-shouldered, round-bodied man with a red face, came stalking towards them.

He was Mr. Bibery, the master of the Ethalion. At his heels strode some of the under-officers, or wardsmen. The officer who had been in charge of the wherry handed the master his papers and surrendered the prisoners.

The master, having read the names, and scanned the convicts, made them answer to their names. Then he addressed them briefly.

"Men," he said, in a rasping voice, though his blue eyes beamed on them not unkindly, "as long as you behave yourselves aboard my ship I'll treat you decently. But if you disobey orders or cause me any trouble, either on board or ashore, there's the black hole or double irons or the cat-o'-nine-tails to teach you manners!"

He then gave orders for the chains to be removed.

Hal gave a sigh of relief as the bracelet dropped away from his right wrist. He had hated being chained to the file of convicts. Mr. Bibery ordered him to step forward. His keen eyes seemed to burn into Hal's as the boy looked up.

"H'm! And so you're the boy Lovett who robbed the Earl of Huntford of his diamond star?" he said.

"That's what I've been sentenced for!" said Hal indignantly. "But I'm innocent."

"So innocent," said Mr. Bibery, tapping the delivery paper, "that you've been marked down here as dangerous. Well, I know a way to break your spirit if you try any tricks on me!"

He next called to McLean, whom he eyed critically. Mr. Bibery seemed a little taken aback by McLean's handsome face and smart appearance. Jerry's clothes were the faded finery of a gentleman.

"You come to me with a bad record, McLean," said the master of the Ethalion. "You are marked down for transportation, but as I don't know when the next convict ship sails you'll have to work ashore. You fought a dozen Bow Street Runners, but if I find you fighting here I'll have you triced up and flogged."

The men were ushered below where a brown suit of coarse material was doled out to each of them, together with a cap, a pair of boots, and a pair of roughly knitted socks. Then they were hurried down a gangway to a lower deck where they were shown their sleeping quarters.

Hal was given a hammock in a sleeping-berth which he was to share with seven other men. McLean's quarters were some distance for'ard.

The new arrivals were ordered to strip, and then taken up again to the upper deck where they were told to wash. Here they donned their new clothes, and were then allowed to stay on deck till the work gangs came back from Woolwich.

Some of the older convicts tried to chum up with them, but McLean was in no mood for talking. He answered brusquely, and drew Hal away.

Leaning on the bulwark beside Hal, he saw the convicts ashore marching to the wherries which were to bring them back to the hulks. The brown-clad figures tumbled into the boats, dropped into their places, and stout-armed wherrymen rowed the boats out and across the tide, handling them cleverly, so that they at last bumped the tarred hulks right close to the gangways.

Boatload after boatload came. Out of the wherries, and up the zigzag gangways to the decks of the convict ships scrambled the figures in brown. Some of their faces were tanned to the colour of their clothes. They shouted as they came. Some of them sang. Lots of them paid no heed to the orders of their overseers until they were told to line up. Then the uproar ceased.

There seemed to be hundreds of them on board the Ethalion. They were kept in divisions of seventy-five, with a wardsman or overseer in charge of each division. The men who had remained on board were sick men.

As they answered the roll-call they winked and grinned at Hal and Jerry McLean.

"Hal," said Jerry, in a low whisper, gripping his chum by the arm, "see that big man in the second row, number seven from the end? That's my pal —John Pryse."

Hal looked at the man, and John Pryse drew his left eyelid down in a slow and very significant wink. Already he was waving his hand to McLean.

"Order there, Pryse!" thundered the wardsman in charge of this particular batch of convicts. "Do you want a hundred lashes?"

"Haw! No!" droned Pryse, in a way that made the whole gang grin. "You wouldn't beat me, Mr. Haggerty."

Discipline on board these hulks was not very strictly enforced, Hal was soon to learn, in spite of the master's warnings and threats.

After the evening's meal had been disposed of, and they had all been shut up below hatches, the wildest scenes and orgies took place 'tween decks. With the few pence they earned by their labour at the docks and in the building operations at Woolwich, most of the convicts bought tobacco. Some of them bought drink. Although they were supposed to keep to their quarters they frequently defied orders, some of them even breaking down bulkheads to enable their party to join the others.

They sang and danced and cursed and fought at times, and the ship was turned into an absolute pandemonium.

On the day of Hal's arrival on board there was very nearly a riot. As soon as the convicts were dismissed they swarmed downstairs and surged into the mess-room, which had once been the middle gun deck of the old man-o'-war. Here they ate greedily the coarse meal of gruel, and stewed meat, and oaten bread. After this they were all ushered to their quarters, and the hatches were shut down, each one guarded by a sentry. Some of these guards were convicts, "selected" men.

Every quarter of an hour the ship's bell was struck, and Hal found himself listening for the sound after a while.

He found it stifling in the lower deck, though the ports were open. On the deck guards kept watch. Sometimes a boat rowed round the ship, seated in which was an officer who spied and listened.

Hal was one of the last to pass the door in the iron railings which formed a sort of pen at the bottom of the gangway. He looked sharply back and felt like an animal in a cage.

The Fight 'Tween Decks!

THE hold was lit by oil-lamps which gave out a feeble sort of glimmer. Soon even this light was dimmed by dense clouds of tobacco smoke. The convicts who did not smoke began to chew tobacco, and coarse songs echoed from every part of the hulk.

"I'm sorry we're not together, boy," said McLean, as he drew Hal aside from a group of stamping, dancing men, who seemed suddenly to have gone mad. "But maybe we'll be able to change that soon."

"Change it soon, change it now," said a hearty voice in McLean's ear, and turning, Jerry saw John Pryse standing with hand outstretched.

Hal saw that the hand was cracked and covered with corns. Pryse's coat was open at the throat, revealing a great, heavy, muscular chest.

He was a giant of a man, with coarse, good-natured features which wore a perpetual grin. Pryse had been lashed for that grin of his before the officers of the convict hulk had discovered that it was natural and not assumed.

"Never you mind where the guards have put the kid, Mr. McLean," said Pryse, as Jerry took the outstretched hand, "you bring him along to your berth if you've a mind."

"But it's full," answered McLean.

"Full, is it? Then turn one of the men out. What's the number of your berth?"

"Number 9," answered McLean.

John Pryse laughed.

"Number 9! Number 9! Did you hear that, boys?" Pryse swung round on the convicts, who had just stopped their mad dance for sheer want of breath. "Our new pal wants the boy in Number 9. That's where Big Jim is, isn't it?"

"You ought to know, since you put him there," answered one of the men.

"Put him there, did I?" said John Pryse carelessly. "Well, if I put him there, I can put him out again, can't I?" He turned again to Jerry McLean, and his perpetual grin broadened. "Big Jim's coming out and your pal's going in No. 9 Berth, sir," he said.

With that, Pryse strolled away. A crowd of men, clothed in ugly brown, followed him. Hal joined them. Stanchions and great wooden beams showed up dimly in the feeble light. Between the berths sat or lounged men drinking, smoking, gambling, cursing. It was a squalid scene, though Hal thought it lacked the filthy sordidness of Newgate prison.

Pryse soon came to No. 9 Berth. It was walled off from other parts of the hold by stout wooden bulkheads. As Hal joined the convicts, who stretched to peer over one another's shoulders, he saw that the hammocks in it had already been slung for the night. They were put up and taken down every day.

In one of these hammocks a man was stretched out asleep. John Pryse did not stand on ceremony, but, unlashing the hammock, let one end of it down. The man in it crashed heavily to the teak floor.

For a moment he lay glowering up at his tormentor, then looked at the line of laughing faces. The coarse laughter of his fellow convicts maddened him, and he got up to launch a smashing punch at Pryse.

Pryse, standing square with fists raised on a level with his chin and held close together and elbows crooked after the manner of fighting men of his time, parried the blow and gave one back which knocked the other man clean off his feet.

Instantly the hold echoed to deafening cat-calls and frantic shouts.

"A fight! It's John and Big Jim Jeffries. A fight! Let 'em fight it out!"

Hal was swept aside by a surge of men in brown, who hustled Pryse to where there was enough room. After them came another batch of convicts, who pushed Big Jim on with them.

Big Jim found Pryse waiting coolly, stripped to the buff, and garbed in a pair of shorts, the clumsy boots he wore showing up grotesquely.

"I'll kill you for what you did!" snarled Big Jim.

Hal elbowed his way to the front of the ring and looked at Big Jim, whose face showed in the yellow glare of a lantern held up by one of the men. The boy had never seen such a vicious-looking brute. He was a bigger man than even the giant Pryse. McLean, who weighed eleven stone, was a dwarf beside him.

Pryse was still smiling. He could not help it.

"Jim," he said, "I cut you down because my pal Jerry McLean wants your hammock for a friend of his. You can go and doss in Number 15."

"Not me," said Big Jim, with an oath.

"You're going to do what I tell you, you sneaking, treacherous hound," taunted Pryse. "Your tale-bearing got Ben Lyall a hundred lashes yesterday. I owe you another one for that. Jim, I'll fight you for whether you go or stay in Number 9."

Scarcely had he uttered the words when the battle began.

Hal had never seen such fighting. Big Jim began it with a lunging kick which would have broken Pryse's jaw had he not dodged away. Jim was wearing his thick-soled boots, and his foot crashed down on the wood floor like a hammer stroke. Then he shot a left arm swing just past Pryse's bobbing head and met the smaller man as he came in with a drive of his right fist.

Pryse did not attempt to dodge the blow, but taking it, sent both his fists driving into the bigger man's mid-section. The next moment they were in holds and wrestling desperately for the mastery.

Big Jim levered Pryse over and back-heeled him down, intending to crack his enemy's head on the deck as he fell and then drop on top of him.

In falling, however, Pryse, who was the quicker witted and more active man, managed to twist his opponent sideways, and it was Big Jim who hit the teak undermost and took the full drive of Pryse's weight on top of him.

Pryse rose, and Big Jim drove an upward kick at him which would have lamed John had he not backed away in time.

The two were at it again the next moment amid a deafening uproar which shook the ship.

Down they went again, Hal listening breathlessly to the dull thud of the blows as their fists drove home. They rose once more and Pryse, after being bent double by a savage kick, joined in the kicking, too. Fists weaved in and out and boots hurtled in deadly drives.

The convicts hemmed them in, leaving them scarcely enough room in which to move. The shouting grew louder. John Pryse's face was streaming, and

Printed and published every Saturday by the Proprietors, The Amalgamated Press, Ltd., The Fleetway House, Farringdon Street, London, E.C.4. Advertisement offices: The Fleetway House, Farringdon Street, London, E.C.4. Registered for transmission by Canadian Magazine Post. Subscription rates: Inland and Abroad, 11s. per annum; 5s. 6d. for six months. Sole Agents for Australia and New Zealand: Messrs. Gordon & Gotch, Ltd., and for South Africa: Central News Agency, Ltd.—Saturday, September 3rd 1932.

Big Jim's eyes were closing fast, his lips badly puffed.

The end came suddenly, unexpectedly. Jeffries, thinking that he had Pryse at his mercy, drove a savage kick at him.

But Pryse had read his intention and backed away, leaning hard against Jerry McLean, who was in front of the surging mass of men in brown.

As Jeffries' heavy-soled boot shot out, Pryse seized his foot and jerked it up. The next moment Big Jim's head hit the deck with a sickening thud. He lay still, like a corpse, and the ring of brown-clad figures opened out in sudden deathly silence.

Jeffries rose to his feet after a while, wiped his streaming face, and moved slowly to his berth. He reappeared, carrying something which he held behind his back. Hal saw that it was a heavy sledgehammer.

Big Jim began to swing it, intending to smash in Pryse's skull from behind.

"Look out!" shouted the boy, and Pryse instinctively leapt aside.

He was only just in time. The iron head of the hammer fairly whistled as it came down where his head had been a second ago and, as it crashed against the teak floor, its stout shaft splintered like a twig.

"Get out of here! Go to berth 15!" shouted Pryse, as he pointed aft. "You're moving out of No. 9, Big Jim!"

And Big Jim Jeffries went without a word.

"So you've got sledgehammers down in the hold, John," said McLean, when the crowd of convicts had gone back to their smoking and their singing and their gambling and he and Pryse and Hal were alone.

"Smuggled 'em in at night," answered Pryse, with a grin. "We're nearly ripe for a break-out, sir."

"Did you hear I was coming on board?" asked McLean, urged by an unsatisfied curiosity.

"Thought you might," answered Pryse. "I'd heard of your trial and conviction. Knew about the boy Lovett, too."

McLean frowned.

"The boy was innocent, Pryse," he said. "His own father, Samuel Lovett and the Earl of Huntford framed him. Why, we'll have to learn after we get out. I got a life sentence for trying to rescue him from the police."

Pryse looked straight into McLean's eyes, his face spread in its perpetual grin, though he winced with pain from his hurts.

"Well, you'll not stay here long if I can help it," he said. "I haven't forgotten how you helped me when I was down and out, McLean. You tried to save me from gaol. I owe you a lot. And John Pryse is not the man to let a bully pal down!"

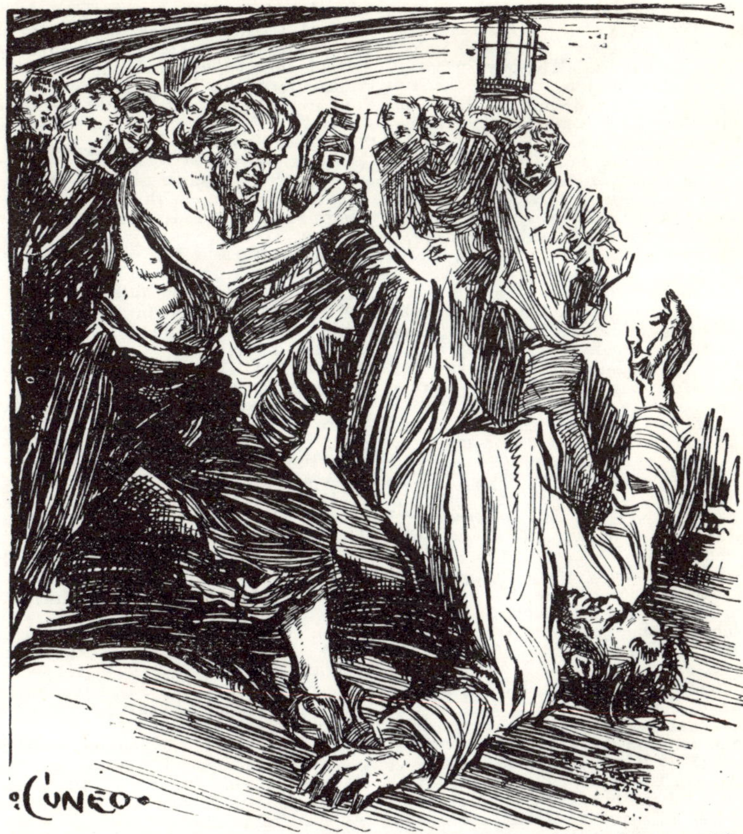

As Jeffries kicked out savagely, Pryse seized his foot and jerked it up. The next moment Big Jim's head hit the deck with a sickening thud!

The Escape!

THREE days after they had arrived on board the hulk Ethalion, Hal and McLean joined the work gangs on shore. Jerry McLean was taken to join the bricklayers and builders.

Here the convicts worked almost side by side with the ordinary workmen, who envied the "lags" because they were housed and boarded free of charge on board the hulks.

McLean found the work light, and the supervision not over keen.

Hal was drafted to the docks. There he had to shoulder a strap and help to haul a timber wagon from the barges to the sheds.

With half a dozen men he strained at the harness during the hours of enforced labour, and he had for an overseer a wardsman named Curtis.

Curtis was a brute of a man who carried a whip. The wardsman loved to lash the whip across the stooping shoulders of any member of the team who might ease for a moment in his hauling.

Twice he cut Hal in this way, and the boy turned on him, feeling as though he could knife him. The wardsman's answer was a grin, another blow, and a growled threat of more if Hal "didn't smarten up."

One morning during Hal's third week on board the hulk, the boy was moving slowly on in line with a batch of convicts who were passing down the gangway to be rowed ashore. He was keeping in line, doing nothing to attract attention, when Curtis, who was standing by, watching, suddenly strode up to him and, without a word, dragged him out of the ranks.

"I'll teach you to laugh at me!" he shouted.

"I didn't——" Hal began, when the wardsman struck him savagely, hurling him backwards against the bulwarks.

Hal's head struck the stout wooden barrier and he knew no more. He did not know that Jerry McLean sprang out of the line and felled the wardsman with two mighty punches. He did not know that Jerry was seized and hurried below and clapped in double irons. He knew nothing until late that morning, when he woke up to find his head all bandaged up and throbbing violently.

He was stretched out in his hammock in Berth No. 9—alone.

Nobody came near him until after the convicts had come back, had eaten their rough supper, and had been battened down below hatches.

Then Pryse came suddenly to his side. Pryse was grinning, as usual, but his voice was solemn enough when he spoke.

"Better, kid?" he asked.

"I'm all right," answered Hal, sitting up and slinging a leg over the side of the hammock as he spoke and sliding to the floor. "I kept to my hammock because it was nice to lie there with nothing to do."

Pryse nodded approval and drew Hal away. In a quiet corner behind a stanchion he broke some startling news.

"Boy," he said, "the master has arranged to have Jerry McLean triced up on deck in the morning and given a hundred lashes. That's for slamming Curtis. I'm to be one of the floggers, and if I don't lay on heavy, there'll be a man waiting to lay it on me!"

Hal's blood began to race.

"You're never going to do it, John," he said.

Pryse shook his grotesque head, still grinning.

"No," he answered, "I'm never going to do it. Kid, we're going to break out to-night——"

The convict silenced Hal by placing his right forefinger to his lips.

"Listen. Hear those chaps singing? Know why? They've got Jerry out of the black hole. They burst it in. Now they're getting the double irons off him. They're singing to drown the noise of their work. When they stop, Jerry will be free."

On deck a bell rang clearly above the din.

"Boy," Pryse went on, "we're all

ready. We've got a key to the bottom gate. For weeks we've had skeleton-keys, which we made, which can unlock the between hatches. The boys on guard in the middle and top gun decks will down the sentries when they hear the signal. We plan to get the boat alongside and make away in her. We're going to take the ship. We'll shut the master and his wardsmen up in the hold and lower the ports. Most of us will get ashore even if we have to swim for it."

Hal's blood seemed suddenly on fire.

"Can we do it?" he asked in a hoarse whisper.

"We're going to do it. We had meant doing it next week, but," and John Pryse's lips tightened, "we're not going to let them lash Jerry McLean."

Pryse drew Hal back among the convicts. Most of them were sitting cross-legged on the deck droning out a monotonous chant. They looked questioningly at Pryse as he came up with the boy.

"The kid knows," said Pryse. "He's in with us."

Then all the heads of the brown clad figures began to nod, and the song swelled louder.

Suddenly, among them sprang Jerry McLean, free of his fetters, his handsome face set, his eyes shining.

"Thank you, boys, for freeing me," he said. "I'm ready when you are for the get-away."

"Then," said Pryse, taking a step forward, "let's get on with it."

Hal next saw the iron gate of the cage at the foot of the gangway swing inward. Past it poured moving figures in brown led by Pryse. Pryse fumbled at the lock of the hatch above. Hal heard the click of metal on metal. Then the hatch swung upward.

Passing through it, the convicts gained the middle deck. Here they were joined by a swarm of convicts berthed on this deck, who had got through their cage door. Brown figures blocked the gangway leading to the upper deck. There a man was fumbling at the keyhole of another hatch.

Suddenly the hatch was flung back, and upward swarmed the army of men in brown.

As the first of them showed on the deck, the sentry on guard there wheeled, brought the butt of his flintlock up to his shoulder, and fired. The bullet was still singing its way over the Thames when a swarm of men in brown hurled themselves at him, lifted him high above the bulwarks, and hurled him and his gun over into the onrushing tide.

As Hal clambered into the open with McLean and Pryse beside him, he saw men in brown rushing all over the deck.

Then wardsmen with drawn cutlasses came rushing amidships, cutting and slashing at the escaping convicts.

McLean hurried Hal to the gangway, up which the convicts climbed every day on their return to the hulk.

"It's everyone for himself, lad," he said. "Can you swim?"

"Like a fish!"

Ahead of them loomed a mighty figure. The gangway was choked with convicts trying to get away. The giant figure turned, and Hal recognised Big Jim.

At the same instant a figure clad in black came rushing up from behind.

"Back, all of you!" cried the man as he levelled a pistol at McLean's head. "I'll shoot the first man who disobeys."

It was Mr. Bibery, the master of the hulk.

But McLean was to quick for him. Darting in, he tore the pistol out of the master's hand, the weapon exploding as Jerry dragged it clear of the man's clinging finger.

Then Big Jim uttered a savage laugh.

"He's the one I wanted!" he cried. "Watch me brain him!"

Big Jim held a sledgehammer in his two mighty hands. He swung it like a blacksmith, intending to brain the master as Mr. Bibery stood stock still, too startled to move.

At that moment, however, another volley rang out, and a batch of convicts came rushing along the deck with wardsmen in pursuit.

A flicker of light shone through the open ports, and Hal caught a whiff of burning smoke. The convicts had fired the ship!

Now came a loud ringing of an alarm bell ashore, the sound of a bugle, the crack of a rifle.

The alarm was up. Soon boats full of soldiers would be rowed out to the Ethalion.

All this Hal saw and heard as Big Jim swung the deadly hammer. But the blow did not fall, for Pryse loomed up just then, and, gripping Big Jim round the middle, lifted him bodily.

John Pryse was as strong as iron. Swinging Big Jim like a flail, he hurled him and his sledgehammer clean over the bulwarks into the Thames.

Then Pryse leapt upon the woodwork and prepared to dive.

"The soldiers are coming! The boys have failed to get the arms-chest!" he cried. "Get away now, or you'll lose your chance, McLean!"

Then Pryse dived.

Looking over the side, Hal saw his body vanish, then his head rise, saw him go off downstream swimming boldly on the full flood of the tide.

McLean drew Hal up. Together they balanced themselves on the bulwark. It was a dive of thirty-five or forty feet down to the swift-flowing river.

"It's our turn, boy," said McLean. "Let's go—together."

The two plunged into the water, and a minute later they were swimming boldly out across the stream, breasting it pluckily.

Shots rang out behind them. Loud curses and groans of agony rang out from the convict hulk. The sky was lit up by a spreading glare. And in the dim light Hal saw the hulk of the hospital ship Dromedary loom up suddenly above him. Tethered to its gangway was a boat. With a few swift strokes Hal gained this, caught the gunwale and drew himself up and over into it. He released the painter, and, as the boat slid away on the tide, he picked up the bobbing head of McLean ahead of him.

Hal whipped out a pair of oars and began to row. He backed water as McLean came alongside, and, shipping the oars, helped his friend safely into the boat.

Then he began to row, row with all his power, urging the boat into the blackness of the night on the full flood of a racing tide.

(Fortune has certainly favoured Hal and Jerry so far. But will their luck hold good? Dont miss next week's gripping chapters, chums, they'll thrill you more than ever!)

GRAND FREE GIFTS COMING SOON! See Important Announcement INSIDE.

The MAGNET 2d

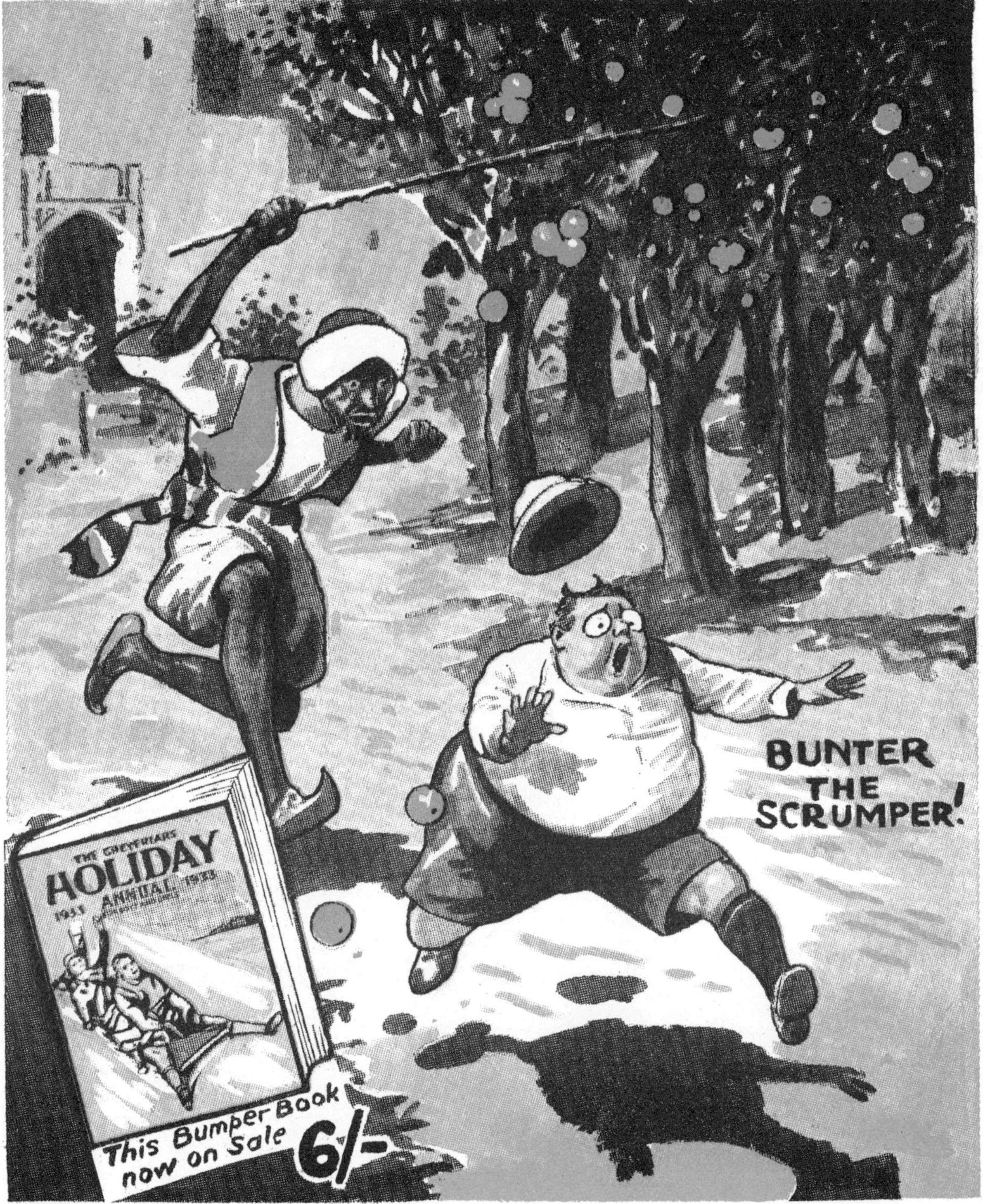

No. 1,282. Vol. XLII. EVERY SATURDAY Week Ending September 10th, 1932.

GREAT NEWS! SPLENDID TREAT IN STORE FOR ALL READERS!

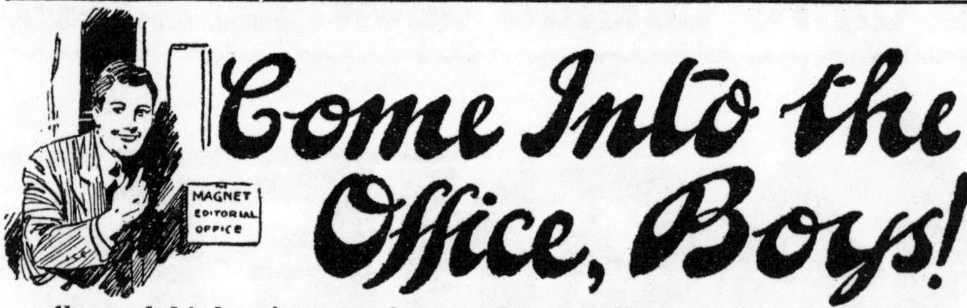

Always glad to hear from you, chums, so drop me a line to the following address: The Editor, The "Magnet" Library, The Amalgamated Press, Ltd., The Fleetway House, Farringdon Street, London, E.C.4.

"WHAT? When? How? Why?" I can hear my readers asking each other these questions and making all sorts of wild guesses as to the nature of this RECORD-BREAKING FREE GIFT SCHEME which I hinted at in last week's issue. Yes, you are all set now on

THE GREAT MYSTERY TRAIL!

You might guess a thousand times as to what this Stupendous Surprise is that I have in store for you, and then be nowhere near the mark! Because I want YOU to be right at the front when this BIG THING "comes off" I am going to warn you to

KEEP YOUR EYE ON THE "MAGNET."

The great secret will be revealed to you in a week or two. And that, I am afraid, is all I am allowed to tell you just now!

£10 FOR A WITCH!

A MAGNET reader who has just come over to this country on holiday from West Africa (lucky fellow!) tells me that a lot of the stuff we hear about the wonders of real Black Magic out there is all fudge. The West African natives, he tells me, are great at make-believe, and to disprove the so-called ability of the native witch-doctors, some white men out there have offered a prize of £10 to any witch-doctor who succeeds in any bit of magic—such as changing a human being into a fish! So far, my reader-friend says, no one has made any attempt to bag that tempting "tenner."

THIRTY TONS OF FLYING STEEL!

I wonder what one of those old fire-breathing dragons that we used to read about in story books would think of our modern "dragons" of the air—the monster flying-boats of to-day? The very latest British flying-boat to be launched not only weighs thirty tons, but can cleave the skies at 100 miles an hour, thanks to its mighty engines, which develop over 5,000 horse-power!

The only part of this monster flying-boat not made of metal is the fabric covering the wings. The part that lies under water when the thirty-tons flying-boat comes down in the sea is made of special stainless steel, and the enormous strange craft actually carries a spare engine which, by marvellously ingenious devices, could be brought into use almost at once. No wonder this flying-boat has been insured for £100,000!

DON'T MISS THESE!

A wonderful coincidence occurred this morning. I sat down, as usual, to read my big batch of letters from MAGNET readers, and the very first letter I picked up was from a chum named Harry Wharton. Now I call that really remarkable, because as I sat down at my desk this morning the thought was uppermost in my mind that I MUST tell you all that the new "HOLIDAY ANNUAL" is now on sale—and what would the "HOLIDAY ANNUAL" be without its magnificent long stories of the adventures of Harry Wharton & Co.? This great volume is better than ever it was, this year—and so is the POPULAR BOOK OF BOYS' STORIES!

Have you a birthday coming—or can you find some other excuse for persuading mother or father or uncle to buy you one (or perhaps both!) of these magnificent Annuals NOW? Don't wait until Christmas, because immensely popular books such as the two I have mentioned are likely to sell right out ANY day!

I FEEL remarkably bucked this morning! Probably it is because I've been reading a selection of jokes and Greyfriars limericks which have been sent in by you fellows. Here's a good yarn for which D. Turner, of 86, Coleridge Road, Cambridge, gets a pen-knife:

Boy: "Is it true, mother, that an apple a day keeps the doctor away?" Parent: "Yes, dear. Why?" Tommy: "Well, I've kept about ten doctors away this morning, but I'm afraid you'll have to call one in soon!"

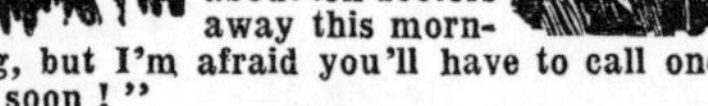

HARDLY BELIEVABLE!

I often think that some of the most startling bits of news in the daily papers are the items that are given only two or three lines of space. For example:

Carved on a Grain of Rice.—One of the commonest things in this world is a rice pudding, and I expect many of my readers regard rice pudding as pretty stodgy stuff. Nothing wonderful in it at all. But what would you think of a single grain of rice with a bust of the Pope carved on it? That was done by a Chinaman the other day, and that grain of rice, surely the most amazing in all the world, is now in the possession of the Pope himself.

Mischievous Elephants.—In East Africa a certain wild tract of jungle-land is being cleared to make farms, and so far 2,000 great elephants have been driven away from there so that the new crops shall not be interfered with!

Boy's Baboon Chums.—After searching among the Drakensburg (South Africa) mountains for four months for their lost son, the parents of a native boy found him living happily with a crowd of baboons—big hideous apes—that had accepted the small boy as their chum!

THAT TOOTHACHE!

I had a letter by the last post from a MAGNET reader who just had to tell me that he is overjoyed because he has lost something. That sounded queer to me, until I read on a bit farther and discovered the thing he has lost was an aching tooth! My reader tells me he had to walk five miles to the dentist's, as he lives in a very lonely part of the West Country. That reminded me of the amazing exploit of an Eskimo boy that came to my notice a few days ago. It's an almost unbelievable story of tremendous heroism.

THE CANADIAN MOUNTED POLICE

say that this twelve-years-old Eskimo's deed is one of the bravest they have ever heard of. And that's a lot for the famous "Mounties" to say, isn't it? The Eskimo boy was only ten when his father died, but he buckled-to—keeping the home going, hunting for food for his mother and baby brother. For two years this went on, and then the boy's hunting-luck changed. Meat-food became short and his mother became seriously ill. All their sledge-dogs but two died, and things became very serious indeed. Then the boy set out to travel

160 MILES TO THE NEAREST DOCTOR!

With his very-ill mother, his three-years-old brother, and a scant store of food in his sledge, the Eskimo boy set bravely out, helping his two remaining dogs to tug the heavy sledge over the snow and ice. For weeks and weeks they struggled on, through the terrific loneliness of the Frozen North, then food gave out completely, and for the last three days and nights of that nightmare journey none of the poor travellers had so much as a mouthful to eat. But they got to that doctor at last, and the mother's life was saved, though this splendid twelve-years-old Eskimo boy himself nearly died of exhaustion. Let's all raise our caps to him, you fellows!

THERE'S just space for a Greyfriars limerick before I go on to next week's list of features. This one comes from K. Waud, of 272, Fifth Avenue, Tang Hall, York, who is now the proud possessor of a MAGNET pocket wallet:

Old Gosling, the Greyfriars porter,
Drinks something that's stronger than water.
His bulbous red nose
A bright flaming rose,
Proves clear he has more than he ought-er!

Here's next week's programme. First and foremost:

"THE SECRET OF THE SCARAB!"
By Frank Richards.

It's a real corking yarn, this, dealing with the further adventures of Harry Wharton & Co.—a yarn that you will be reluctant to put down once you have started to read it. You'll find Frank R. in tip-top form, and you'll chuckle with delight at the adventures—and misadventures—of the ever-popular Billy Bunter.

Don't miss it—that's my advice!

Next comes another thrilling instalment of "The Red Falcon," which certainly puts Arthur Steffens on the pedestal of fame as a real boys' author.

Following this is another of Dicky Nugent's screamingly-funny effusions, entitled: "The Schoolboy Professional!" Laugh? I should just say you will! In addition to all this there will be the usual winning limericks and jokes, more answers to readers' queries, and more about OUR STUPENDOUS FREE GIFT SCHEME.

Cheerio, then,

YOUR EDITOR.

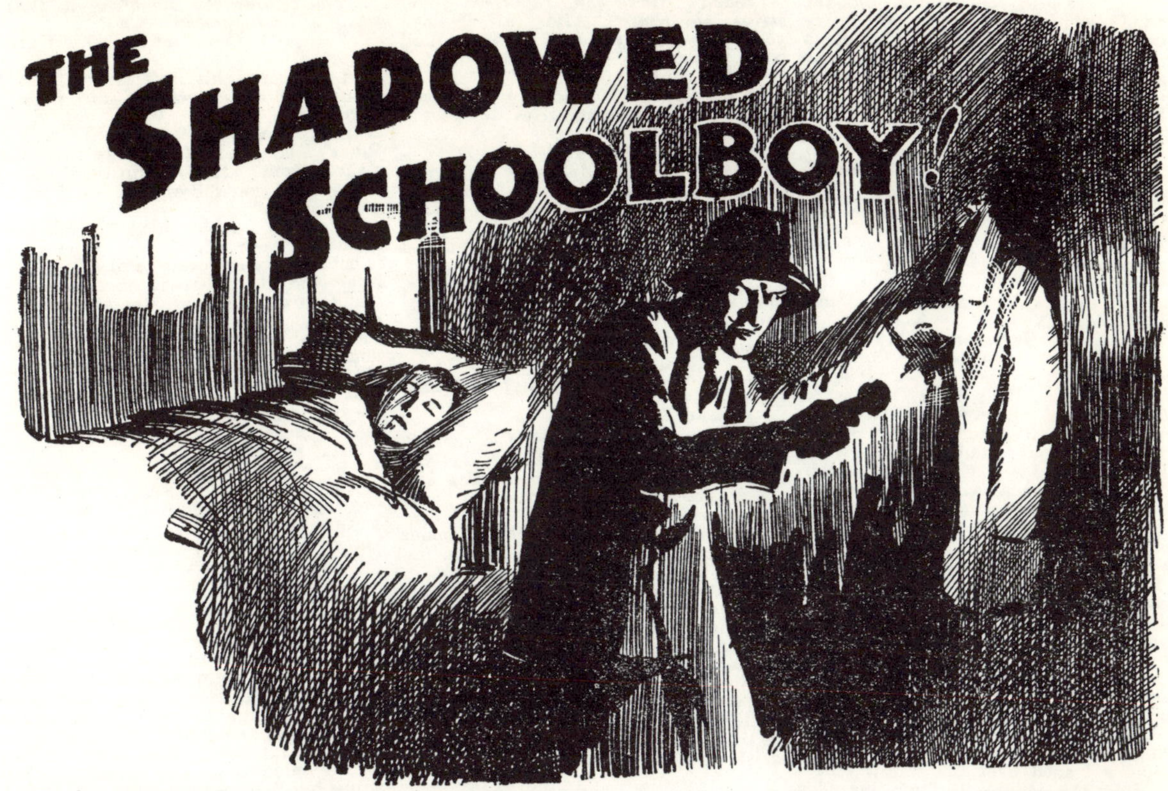

Featuring Harry Wharton & Co. and Lord Mauleverer, the Chums of Greyfriars. By FRANK RICHARDS.

THE FIRST CHAPTER.

Bunter's Treat!

BILLY BUNTER sat up and took notice.

It was hot on the Nile.

Under a sky of cloudless blue the dahabiyeh floated slowly up the great river of Egypt, a light wind from the north rustling the huge sail.

But the wind was very light, and the dahabiyeh moved very slowly. Some of the Nubian sailors were poling to help it along. The reis stood like a bronze statue at the tall helm.

Harry Wharton & Co. of the Greyfriars Remove sat under the awning in the balcony that surrounded the stern of the dahabiyeh. They were taking it easy, and watching lazily the gliding banks, and the craft on the river as they floated slowly onward to the south. Lord Mauleverer had nodded off to sleep.

Billy Bunter, sprawled in a big basket-chair, mopped the perspiration from his plump forehead, and dabbed at flies. There was a mosquito-net over the fat Owl as he sprawled, but the flies seemed to creep under it somehow. They seemed to like Bunter. Ever since he had been in Egypt the flies had shown a partiality for Bunter. One of the celebrated plagues of Egypt was a plague of flies, and Bunter's impression was that it was still going strong.

Bunter had requested the Famous Five, one after another, to fan the flies off him while he napped. One after another they had declined, with the selfishness Bunter was sadly accustomed to. Then he had told Hassan, the dragoman, to fan off the flies. Hassan had disappeared. Bunter had to smack at the flies himself, or leave them unsmacked. He smacked and smacked, and, like Samson of olden times, slew his thousands and tens of thousands. Every time he smacked, he shifted the mosquito-net, and the flies of Egypt seemed like those stout-hearted Scottish spearmen at the battle of Flodden:

"Each stepping where his comrade stood
The instant that he fell."

Bunter was tired of flies; but the flies were not tired of Bunter. Probably they were the only living creatures on board

Time and again has Kalizelos, the Greek, attempted to steal the age-old scarab—said to be the key to a fortune—which is in the possession of Lord Mauleverer. And not even aboard a large house-boat, surrounded by native servants, is Lord Mauleverer safe from his relentless shadower.

the dahabiyeh who were not tired of Bunter. With the Greyfriars fellows, with the dragoman, with the black servants and the Nubian sailors Bunter was not popular. But with the flies his popularity was unbounded. Bunter himself, perhaps, was not very attractive. But the traces of his last two or three snacks, smeared over his fat face, attracted winged things from near and far. Bunter liked sticky things, so did the flies.

But Billy Bunter forgot for a moment that plague of Egypt, and sat up and took notice as a native felucca glided behind the crawling dahabiyeh. The felucca's big lateen sail was down, and it was rowed by a couple of brown men. In the felucca was a huge stack of ripe, golden oranges. It was a fruit boat taking fruit to Luxor. But at sight of the foreign faces on the dahabiyeh the boatmen pulled round the stern, and a brown man in a dusty djubbah, who was sitting beside the mountain of oranges, rose to his feet, salaamed, and called out in Arabic. What he said in that strange tongue was a sealed mystery to the Greyfriars fellows. But they understood his signs. He pointed to the oranges and waved his brown hands, and grinned, with a flash of white teeth. He had oranges to sell, and the sight of English faces inspired him with a hope of selling them at ten times the price they would have fetched at Luxor.

"I say, you fellows, those oranges look good!" said Billy Bunter. "You fellows like some oranges?" He threw aside the mosquito-net, smacked several flies, and rose to his feet. "My treat, you chaps!"

"Who's going to lend Bunter some piastres to stand treat?" yawned Johnny Bull.

"Oh, really, Bull——"

"Wake up, Mauly!" grinned Frank Nugent. "Bunter's going to stand treat! Cough up some cash!"

"Yaw-aw-aw!" came sleepily from Lord Mauleverer.

"Oh, really, Nugent——"

"Might as well have some of these jolly oranges, as the man wants to sell," said Bob Cherry. "I think I've got some piastres."

"I've said that it's my treat, Cherry," said Billy Bunter, with a great deal of dignity. "Leave this to me!"

"Yes, I know your treats, old fat bean!" assented Bob, with a cheery grin. "You'll order twice as much as we want to pay for, and then remember that you've forgotten where you left your money."

"Ha, ha, ha!"

"If that's what you call gratitude when a fellow's standing treat——"

"You see, we know you, old fat man," said Harry Wharton, laughing. "But if you mean business for once, go ahead."

"Yah!" answered Bunter. "Look here, you beast!"

There was a golden glimmer as the fat Owl of the Remove drew a coin from his pocket.

"That's an Egyptian pound," said Bunter. "It's worth a hundred piastres. I got it when I changed some paper money at Beni Suef. You don't often see gold about. They call it a gineih in the silly language they speak here. But it's a pound."

Bunter waved a fat hand, with the gold coin between a fat finger and thumb, to the native in the boat.

The brown orange merchant salaamed and salaamed again. Gold was not often seen on the Nile, and the sight of a hundred-piastre piece evidently impressed the fruit seller.

The felucca hooked on to the dahabiyeh, the two oarsmen holding on to the stern. The fruit seller continued to salaam to Bunter, or to the golden coin, which probably impressed him more than Bunter did. Then he filled a large wicker basket with golden oranges, and lifted it.

Bunter leaned over the stern, blinking into the felucca through his big spectacles.

Harry Wharton & Co. watched him curiously.

Bunter was surprising them.

For Billy Bunter to stand treat, without borrowing the necessary cash from some other fellow, was rather a record.

But the fat Owl was evidently in earnest.

"How much?" asked Bunter, pointing to the basket of oranges.

"Feefty piastre, sar!"

"Shove it here, and give me change!" said Bunter.

"Yes, sar." The brown man salaamed again. "Speak English, sar! Me Mustapha, sar, very honest merchant, sar! All English lord say Mustapha very honest man, sar."

He heaved up the basket of oranges, and it was landed over the stern of the dahabiyeh, with help from Bob Cherry above.

There was a grunt from Johnny Bull.

"Oranges are cheap here," he said. "That lot's not worth more than twenty piastres, Bunter. You're being done."

"Oh, that's all right!" said Bunter. "I believe in being generous to niggers, you know."

"Oh, my hat!"

If Billy Bunter had surprised the chums of the Remove before, he astonished them now. Not only was Bunter standing treat with his own cash, which was unusual, but he was allowing himself to be recklessly overcharged, which was unprecedented. Really, the Greyfriars fellows could hardly believe their ears.

But evidently the fat Owl meant business. He tossed the gold piece down to Mustapha, and that honest merchant tossed up the change—fifty piastres. Then the felucca shoved off, and the two craft parted company.

"I say, you fellows!" Bunter selected a ripe, fat orange, and pushed his fat face into it, which was Bunter's elegant way of eating an orange. "I say, this is good! Have some? Help yourselves, old chaps! After this, I hope you won't make out that I never stand treat. Nothing mean about me, I hope."

"Well, my hat!" said Bob. "Some ass said the age of miracles was past!"

"Ha, ha, ha!"

"Oh, really, Cherry——"

"Wake up, Mauly, and have an orange," said Bob.

"Yaw-aw-aw!" came from his sleepy lordship.

"It's Bunter's treat, old bean," urged Bob. "An occasion worth waking up for. Are you going to eat this orange, or shall I squeeze it down the back of your neck?"

"Oh gad!" ejaculated Lord Mauleverer. He woke up quite suddenly.

"Like 'em, you fellows?" beamed Bunter.

"Fine!"

"The finefulness is terrific!"

As the dahabiyeh glided on the juniors sat under the stern awning and ate oranges. They were ripe and good, and very welcome on a hot day. There was general satisfaction. The Famous Five liked the oranges, and had an impression that Bunter was improving, so they were satisfied. Mustapha, the honest merchant, had sold his oranges for twice their value, so he was satisfied. And Billy Bunter had got rid of the bad gold piece that had been passed on him at Beni Suef, and received in exchange a basket of oranges and fifty good piastres, so Bunter was satisfied. So there was, for the present, at least, satisfaction all round.

THE SECOND CHAPTER.

Wrathy!

"LORDLY gentlemen!" It was the voice of Hassan, the dragoman.

Looking like a tropical beetle in his gold-braided jacket, sky-blue trousers, yellow shoes, and crimson sash, the dragoman came along the upper deck, the gold tassel on his tarboosh dancing and glancing in the sun.

He pulled aside the awning over the stern balcony to address the Greyfriars fellows below.

Hassan's dusky face was beaming. Hassan enjoyed showing the sights of Egypt to the Greyfriars tourists, and he never let them off a single sight if he could help it.

Harry Wharton & Co. had been a good many days coming up the Nile. Progress in a dahabiyeh was slow. Now, however, they were drawing near to Luxor, where they were to stop for a time. Luxor was a place that could not possibly be missed. Indeed, had the juniors thought of missing Karnak and Luxor, they would hardly have dared to tell Hassan so. The dragoman would have received too great a shock.

"Noble and gentlemanly lords," said Hassan, through the awning, "here you rise up on feet and look, for celebrated Temple of Karnak now bobs up on bank on Nile, and this is sight for sore eyes, as you say in your magnificent language."

The juniors smiled. Hassan was what he himself called a "speak-English dragoman." The juniors found his English quite as entertaining as what he told them in that language.

"Come on, you slackers!" said Bob Cherry. "Mustn't miss the jolly old sights! Wake up, Mauly, and get a move on!"

Lord Mauleverer yawned deeply. He was disinclined to move.

"You fellows tell me about it afterwards!" he suggested.

"Fathead! Come on!" said Harry Wharton.

"Look here, this isn't cricket!" said Mauleverer plaintively. "Hassan isn't playin' the game! We've got to do Karnak when we land at Luxor. What's the good of doin' it from the river as well? If we begin doin' things twice over, you fellows, we shall never get through."

"Oh, my noble lord," exclaimed Hassan, "view of Karnak from river is enormously imposing, and of gigantic interest! Also there is opportunity to meditate on fallen greatness of ancient kings, such meditation being easier in comfortable chair on dahabiyeh than on donkey back while visiting ruins."

"Oh gad!" said Mauleverer. "Well, look here, you men go up and do the viewing, and I'll sit here and meditate. That's whackin' it out fairly."

"Ha, ha, ha!"

"Poor old Mauly's too tired to move," said Bob. "But you fellows just watch him, and see him jump when I squeeze this orange down his neck. Hallo, hallo, hallo! He's up already!"

"Keep off, you dangerous ass!" gasped Mauleverer.

"Ha, ha, ha!"

The juniors went through one of the doorways, into the saloon, and through that apartment to the lower deck, whence there were steps to the upper deck. Billy Bunter rolled after them with an orange in each hand, and a considerable amount of orange-juice over his fat face. His escort of flies accompanied him. The flies of the Nile seemed to like orange-juice.

They mounted to the upper deck where Hassan, with his stick, pointed out the "view." Really it was worth looking at. Great limestone rocks and cliffs loomed against the blue sky on the western bank of the Nile. On the eastern bank the hills retreated, leaving a plain by the river.

Through masses of palm-trees the great pylons of the Temple of Karnak loomed into view. And as the dahabiyeh floated on there was a glimpse of Luxor in the distance.

But the attention of the Greyfriars fellows turned, all of a sudden, from the obelisks and pylons of Karnak to a felucca which was coming down the stream, with two brown men pulling at the huge oars, and a third brown man standing by a mountain of oranges.

"Hallo, hallo, hallo! That's the jolly old orange merchant coming back!" said Bob Cherry. "He seems to be excited about something."

Mustapha, the honest orange merchant, undoubtedly looked excited.

His brown face was infuriated, his black eyes glittered, and his brown hands sawed the air in wild gesticulations.

The juniors stared at him in astonishment.

The felucca had left the slow-moving dahabiyeh far behind, going on to Luxor, and they had not expected to see it again. But it was coming back, and it was clear that something was amiss.

Billy Bunter turned his big spectacles on the gesticulating Mustapha with an alarmed blink.

"I say, you fellows, is that the chap who sold me the oranges?" he exclaimed.

"That's the chap," said Johnny Bull. "What on earth's the matter with the man? What is he saying, Hassan?"

The felucca was still at a distance; but Mustapha's voice, shouting in Arabic, could be heard. Hassan gave a cough.

"My lordly master, I think I better not tell you what Mustapha he say," answered the dragoman. "Also it would be difficult hard for me, because I——"

"Because what?"

"Because, although I speak the noble English language like one native of your magnificent country, I have not learned the naughty words in that beautiful language."

"Wha-a-at?"

"To tell you what Mustapha he say, I must learn the naughty words in English," explained Hassan. "These words I do not know, sar."

"Oh, my hat!"

"Some very strong words I know, which I have heard English military the Arabic tongue. Very strong indeed, sars! I will tell the Nubians to drive him off."

The Nubian crew of the dahabiyeh were all staring at the boat, and even the grave reis at the tiller gave Mustapha curious looks. Some of the Nubians were handling poles to help the dahabiyeh through the shallows, and it would have been easy for them to keep the felucca off. But Harry Wharton stopped the dragoman as he was about to call out an order to the crew.

"Hold on!" he said. "Something's wrong, though I can't imagine what it is. Let him come nearer, and ask him what's the trouble."

"To hear is to obey, my noble gentleman!" answered Hassan.

surprising them, but Bunter surprised them still more. He was displaying a delicacy of which he had never been suspected before.

Mustapha's voice came more loudly as the felucca approached more closely to the dahabiyeh. The fury in his brown face was not to be mistaken. He shouted and raged. A torrent of Arabic poured and streamed from him, and both his brown hands waved in wild gesticulation.

The juniors saw a startled expression come over Hassan's face; and they discerned that the Nubian sailors were grinning. The natives, of course, understood the spate of Arabic, of which not a single syllable was comprehensible to the Greyfriars fellows. To the

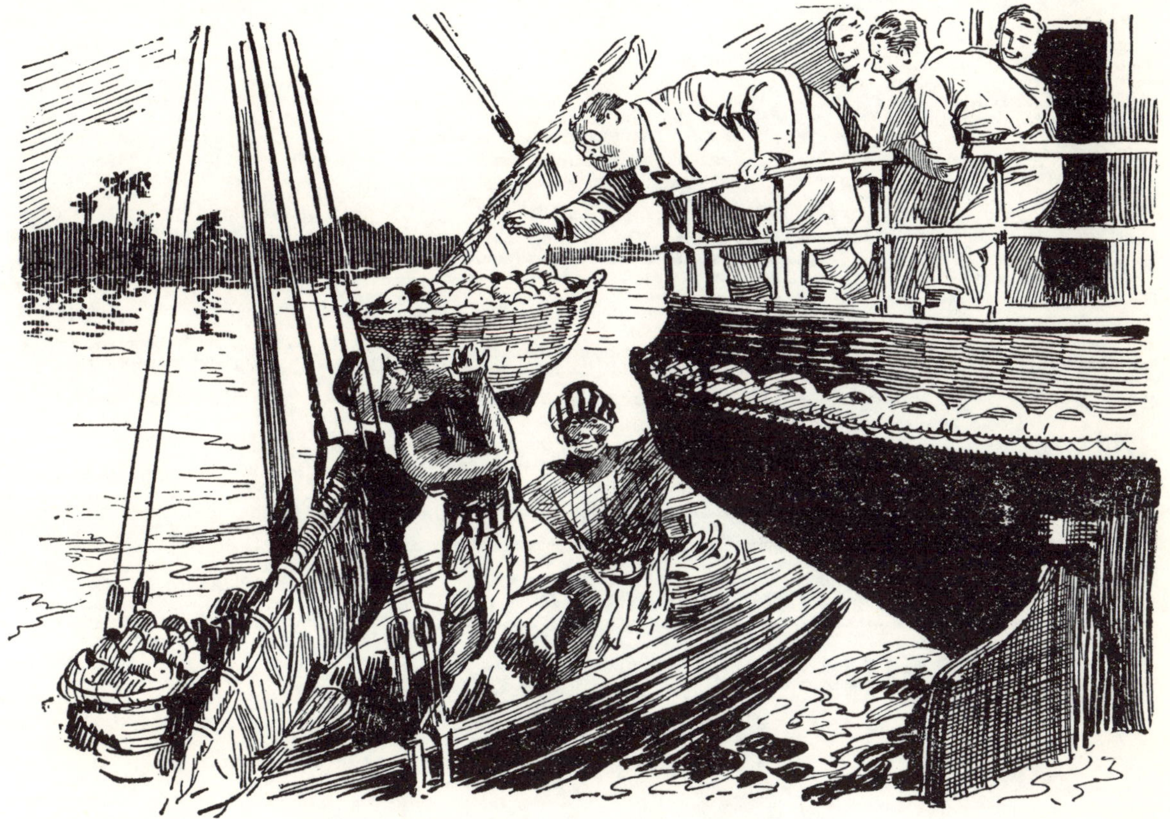

"My treat, you fellows!" Bunter waved a fat hand to the native in the boat. "How much for those?" he asked, pointing to the basket of oranges. "Feefty piastre, sar!" answered the fruit seller. "Right, I'll have them," said Bunter, handing down a gold coin. "Give me change for this!"

gentlemen speak to soldiers," said Hassan. "These words I will tell you——"

"You needn't trouble," said Harry Wharton hastily.

"Oh gad!" said Lord Mauleverer. "But what on earth's the matter with the man?"

"Goodness knows!"

"I say, you fellows!" Billy Bunter seemed uneasy, not merely surprised like the other fellows at Mustapha's antics. "I—I say, if—if that man's swearing, you know, I—I—I don't want to have anything to do with him. He's a bad character. Mauly's uncle told us to be careful not to get into bad company when he let us come up the Nile on our own. I—I think it's due to Sir Reginald Brooke to—to be rather careful, you know. Tell the sailors to keep that boat off with their poles."

"On my head be it!" said Hassan. "The son of several dogs and pigs is speaking words of the naughty kind, of which there are many very strong in

"I say, you fellows——"

"Shut up, Bunter!"

"Shan't!" roared Bunter. "If you fellows want to listen to a nigger blackguard, I jolly well don't, and I can tell you so! Make the sailors keep that brute off! I'm surprised at you, Wharton. In fact, I'm shocked."

"You silly ass!" exclaimed Wharton. "There's something the matter!"

"Rot! I expect the man's tipsy," said Bunter. "Well, if you're going to let him come alongside and use bad language, I'm going below. I'm a bit more particular than you are in such things."

"You howling ass!"

"Yah!"

Billy Bunter rolled down the steps from the upper deck, and went into the doorway from the lower deck to the cabins of the dahabiyeh. The juniors heard a slam below as he closed the door of his room.

They stared after him, and then looked at one another. Mustapha was

further surprise of the juniors, Mustapha held up a gold coin between a brown finger and thumb as his boat came alongside, and waved it in the air furiously. Apparently it was the Egyptian pound that Bunter had paid him for the oranges.

"Bismillah!" murmured Hassan.

"What's the matter with the man?" asked Harry. "Is it sunstroke?"

"My magnificent gentleman, he say——"

At this point, the orange-merchant broke into English. Brandishing the gold coin, and spitting with fury, he yelled up at the staring juniors.

"Bad! Naughty! This very naughty piece! Yes, sar! Too naughty! Bad! Faringhee teef! Yes, sar! Teef! Naughty gold!"

"Naughty!" repeated Wharton. "Is the man mad! What does he mean by saying that the quid is naughty?"

Hassan grinned.

"This common person, sar, speak not

pure and fine perfect English language like Hassan," he explained. "He mean to say gold piece not good."

"Oh!" exclaimed Wharton. "A bad sovereign—counterfeit! Is that it?"

"Yes, sar!"

"Oh, my hat!" gasped Bob Cherry.

The felucca bumped on the dahabiyeh. The two rowers held on, while Mustapha made a jump on board. He flourished the gold piece under the noses of the juniors and roared and spat.

"Bad! Naughty! Yes, sar, he naughty!" A torrent of Arabic followed, as Mustapha's English failed him.

Hassan volleyed back in the same language.

"Bunter!" roared Bob Cherry.

There was no reply from William George Bunter. The juniors understood now why the fat Owl had been so unwilling to meet Mustapha a second time. Evidently a counterfeit coin had been passed on Bunter, and he had passed it on to Mustapha. Bunter's treat was explained now. No doubt the fat Owl had been waiting for an opportunity to get rid of that "quid"; and the orange-boat on the Nile had given him his opportunity.

"The fat villain!" exclaimed Wharton, crimson with anger and vexation. "Bring him up here by his ears, Bob."

"You bet!" answered Bob.

He rushed down to the cabins.

Thump! Thump! Thump! There was a sound of energetic thumping at a door. Evidently the door was locked. The fat squeak of Billy Bunter was heard.

"Go away! Don't disturb me, you beast! I'm asleep!"

"Come on deck, you fat scoundrel!"

"Shan't!"

Arabic was volleying to and fro between Mustapha and Hassan. Mustapha was getting into a frenzy. Lord Mauleverer tapped the dragoman on his gold-braided arm, as Mustapha, with a furious gesture, hurled the gold piece on the deck.

"Is that quid really bad, Hassan?" he asked.

"Yes, sar," said Hassan, picking it up, and testing it with his teeth. "Plenty bad money in Egypt, sar."

"Give the man his hundred piastres, then."

"Yes, lordly sar."

Mustapha calmed down a little as he received a hundred piastres. But he did not seem satisfied.

"Backsheesh!" he howled.

All the juniors knew that word, at least! Nobody could travel in the East, even for a few days, without becoming acquainted with "backsheesh."

"Give him some backsheesh, Hassan," yawned Lord Mauleverer, "After all, he's had the trouble of coming back for his money. Give him fifty piastres."

"Yes, my gentlemanly lord."

Fifty more piastres were handed to the orange-merchant. Then Mustapha went back to his felucca, and the rowers pushed off. The felucca pulled away for Luxor once more, Mustapha standing up, staring back at the dahabiyeh, and making disrespectful and derisive gestures as he departed. But he was gone at last; and Harry Wharton & Co., with grim expressions on their faces, went below to talk to Bunter. And the faithful Hassan, with a cheery grin, slipped the counterfeit "quid" into his pocket, with the honest intention of passing it, in his turn, on some unwary tourist—all being grist that came to Hassan's mill.

THE THIRD CHAPTER.

Beastly for Bunter!

THUMP! Thump!

Bob Cherry banged on Bunter's door. Johnny Bull kicked at it. Frank Nugent shouted through the keyhole.

"I say, you fellows!" came a fat squeak from within the locked cabin. "I—I say, is he gone?"

"Open this door!" roared Bob.

"I—I've lost the key, old chap! Otherwise I'd let you in at once, with pleasure! I say, is that beastly Arab gone?"

"You fat rascal——"

"Oh, really, Wharton——"

"You've passed bad money on a native!" roared the captain of the Remove. "We're going to squash you as flat as a pancake!"

"How was I to know that it was bad?" demanded Bunter. "Of course, I never knew anything of the kind."

"What did you dodge below for, then, and lock yourself in?" roared Johnny Bull. "You podgy pirate, you knew you were swindling the man."

"Oh, really, Bull! What about the nigger who passed it on me, at Beni Suef, days and days ago?" exclaimed Bunter indignantly. "Think I've come to Egypt to collect bad money?"

"Then you did know it was bad?"

"No, I didn't! Hadn't the faintest idea there was anything the matter with it!" answered Bunter, through the door. "I hope I'm not the sort of fellow to pass bad money, especially on a nigger! I think that shows a rotten suspicious mind, Bull! That's you all over."

"You fat idiot, you've just said it was passed on you at Beni Suef——" roared Johnny Bull.

"So it was," retorted Bunter. "A beastly nigger changed a note for me and gave me that spoof quid among the other money. Of course, I was going to pass it on some other nigger! I can't afford to lose a hundred piastres! I mean, I can afford to, but I'm jolly well not going to, see? I'm jolly well not going to be done by niggers! Let 'em learn to be honest!"

"By gad! They won't learn that from you, Bunter!" ejaculated Lord Mauleverer.

"I say, you fellows, is that man gone? I want to have nothing to do with him—nothing whatever! He's not honest."

"Open this door, you fat scoundrel!"

"Shan't! Not till that nigger's gone. I say, you fellows, I don't think you ought to kick at the door like that! You're damaging Mr. Maroudi's property! Old Maroudi lent us this dahabiyeh, expecting us to take care of it. You fellows ought to remember that you're not in the Remove passage at Greyfriars now."

"Will you come out and be scragged?" roared Bob Cherry.

"Yah!"

"Lucky for you Mustapha didn't bring a bobby back with him. You might have been run in for passing bad money."

"Oh, really, Cherry! I keep on telling you it was a good quid—perfectly good! Besides, they wouldn't take a nigger's word against mine, I suppose? All you fellows are witnesses, too!"

"Wha-a-t?"

"Of course, I should expect you to stand by a pal," said Bunter. "If you all gave evidence that I never gave the beast that quid it would be all right! I'll do as much for you another time, of course."

"Ye gods!" gasped Bob Cherry.

"The real trouble is, that these niggers are not honest," said Bunter. "I can tell you, I'm fed-up with their dishonesty. It doesn't seem to shock you fellows as it does me! You're not so particular."

"I'm going to spiflicate him!" gasped Bob. "Bunter, you fat villain, open this door or we'll jolly well burst it in."

"If that's the way you're going to take care of the houseboat Mr. Maroudi lent us, Cherry, I can only say you're an ungrateful beast! I think you ought to be a bit decent when you're travelling with me. Your bad manners let a fellow down, you know."

"Will you open this door?" roared Bob.

"No, I jolly well won't!"

Bob Cherry bestowed a final thump on the door. But bursting it in was not to be thought of. The dahabiyeh belonged to Mr. Maroudi, the Egyptian gentleman of Cairo. With great kindness Mr. Maroudi had lent it to the Greyfriars party for the trip up the Nile. On board Mr. Maroudi's palatial houseboat manners and customs could not be so free-and-easy as in the old Remove passage at Greyfriars School. The door was not a stout one, and Bob Cherry could have driven it in with his shoulder. But the fat Owl was quite aware that he was safe from such drastic measures.

So long as Bunter kept the door locked there was nothing doing. But the Famous Five were determined that the fat Owl was going to have the lesson he so badly needed.

It was exasperating, no doubt, to receive bad money, but that was no excuse for passing it on to an innocent party. To Billy Bunter's fat mind, the fact that a native had "diddled" him at Beni Suef was a sufficient reason for "diddling" a native at Luxor. That sort of morality was not good enough for white men in an African country. Moreover, Bunter had run a serious risk of being tapped on the shoulder by an Egyptian policeman and taken before a native magistrate to explain himself—which was not the sort of thing the juniors wanted to happen on their trip up the Nile. Bunter had to be kicked—and kicked hard!

"You fat villain!" roared Bob. "We're going to kick you all round the dahabiyeh! Will you come out and be kicked?"

"Beast!"

"Well, it will keep! Come on, you men, let's go up."

The juniors returned to the upper deck. There they "viewed" Luxor in the distance as the dahabiyeh crawled slowly on up the golden Nile. Billy Bunter remained in his cabin, snorting with indignation.

But it was hot in the cabin, and there were more flies there than on deck. The fat Owl could hear the footsteps of the juniors overhead. A blink from the window assured him that the orange-boat and the obnoxious Mustapha were gone. He ventured at last out of the cabin and went along the lower deck and blinked up at the juniors.

What the beasts were so waxy about was rather a mystery to Bunter. He had explained that he had only passed on a bad coin that had been passed on him—with the further explanation that the coin was not bad at all, but a perfectly good one. This double-barrelled explanation ought to have satisfied any reasonable fellow, in Bunter's opinion, but he realised that these beasts were not reasonable. So he was ready to bolt as he hailed the juniors on the upper deck.

"I say, you fellows!"

"Hallo, hallo, hallo! Here he is!" roared Bob Cherry. "First kick to me!"

There was a thud as Bob jumped down from the upper deck.

But, quick as he was, he was not so quick as Billy Bunter.

Bunter fairly flew.

Slam! Click!

The fat Owl was locked in his cabin again.

"Come out, you fat snail!" roared Bob, thumping on the door.

"Yah!"

Bob Cherry grinned and returned to the deck. Billy Bunter was welcome to remain locked in his cabin as long as he liked. It was rather like an oven on a hot Egyptian afternoon.

"Oh crikey!" gasped Bunter.

He sat down on the bed, mopped his perspiring brow, and swatted flies. He did not venture to leave the cabin again. Often as Bunter had been kicked, he hated the process—and the prospect of being kicked all round the dahabiyeh had no appeal for him at all.

He crawled on the bed at last, arranged the mosquito-net, and went to sleep. Fortunately for Bunter, he could always sleep. The dahabiyeh rolled on, to an accompaniment of deep and steady snoring.

It was dark in the cabin when Bunter awoke. Night had fallen on the Nile.

Through the latticed window came a glimmer of the bright stars of Egypt. The dahabiyeh was still in motion; it had not tied up at Luxor yet. He could hear the Nubian sailors singing in their native tongue as they poled the heavy vessel slowly onward. From the dining-saloon along the passage under the upper deck came a cheery sound of voices, and a sound of knives and forks and plates. Billy Bunter snorted with indignation. The beasts had come down to supper and never even called him.

He unlocked the door and peered out into the passage through his big spectacles. The mushrabeyeh screens at the doorway of the dining-saloon were open, and he could see the Famous Five and Lord Mauleverer at supper in the lamplight.

"Hallo, hallo, hallo! There's Bunter!"

Bob Cherry laid down knife and fork and rushed into the passage. Like a fat rabbit dodging into its burrow, Billy Bunter popped back into his cabin and slammed and locked the door.

He was only in time.

Thump!

The door rattled under Bob Cherry's smite.

"Come out, Bunter!" roared Bob.

"I—I—I say, old chap!" gasped Bunter. "I say, are you going to make it pax, old fellow?"

"I'm going to kick you from one end of the dahabiyeh to the other! Come out and be kicked!"

"Beast!" roared Bunter. "Look here, I want my supper! I'm hungry!"

"Well, come out to supper," said Bob. "What's stopping you?"

"Beast!" groaned Bunter.

Bob Cherry went back to the dining-room. Billy Bunter remained in his cabin. He wanted his supper—and with every passing minute he wanted it more and more. But he did not want to be kicked. And it was evident that the kicking was going to precede the supper.

Harry Wharton & Co. finished their supper and went back to the deck. Bob Cherry tapped on Bunter's door as he passed.

"Still there, fatty?"

"Beast!"

"May as well come out and get it over!"

"Yah!"

Bunter did not come out. On the deck the chums of the Remove chatted as the dahabiyeh glided on to Luxor under the starlight, and the song of the Nubian sailors echoed on the shadowy river, and Hassan's tireless tongue ran on and on with a description of the wonders of Karnak and Luxor, both of which places had that irresistible attraction of "innumerable dead persons."

Twice Billy Bunter unlocked his door—and each time he heard Bob's heavy tread and locked it again.

By that time Billy Bunter was in a state of famine, but he dared not venture forth in quest of provender. The fat Owl was suffering for his sins—which, in the opinion of the Famous Five, was just and proper.

Bunter's door was still locked when there was a tramp of feet announcing that the Greyfriars fellows were coming down to turn in. There was a thump at the fat Owl's door.

"Hallo, hallo, hallo! Come out, Bunter! You've got to be kicked before we turn in!" bawled Bob Cherry.

"Beast!" roared Bunter.

And the juniors chuckled and went to their rooms.

Billy Bunter groaned. He was not merely hungry now, not merely famished—but ravenous! But he had to wait till the beasts were asleep before he turned out to search for grub.

Long, long minutes crawled by on leaden wings.

He heard a tramping of the Nubian sailors on deck, a calling of voices from the shore, and there was a bump of the dahabiyeh.

Luxor was reached at last, and the dahabiyeh was tying up at the bank.

Bunter waited till the noises had quieted down, and then cautiously opened his door.

All was dark!

On board the Cleopatra only one light burned—a lantern slung to the tall mast. Below the deck, where the juniors had their quarters, all were asleep, excepting Billy Bunter, and no light burned.

Bunter stepped out stealthily into the passage.

There was no sound from the adjoining cabins; the beasts were safe asleep at last. Bunter groped in his pockets for matches, and made the interesting discovery that he hadn't any. There were plenty of native servants on board in their rooms between the schoolboys' quarters and the sailors' deck, but Bunter did not think of calling any of them. He was painfully aware of what would happen if he woke Bob Cherry.

"Beasts!" he murmured under his breath.

And he groped his way along in the darkness.

He knew where to find matches in the dining-saloon, and he knew where to find provender—if only those beasts did not wake up. A professional burglar could not have been more cautious and stealthy than Billy Bunter as he crept and groped along the passage.

In the dining-room there was the faintest glimmer of starlight from a window that had been left uncurtained. The fat Owl blinked round him, and was about to grope across the room, when suddenly he stopped dead, his fat heart thumping.

In the darkness and silence there was a faint sound—the soft sound of a stealthy footstep entering the room from the other side.

Bunter stood quite still.

Someone, unseen in the darkness, was entering the room from the stern saloon. It could not be one of the juniors, who were all in bed; it could hardly be one of the servants creeping about in the dark at night. That stealthy tread in the deep gloom struck a thrill of terror to Bunter's fat heart. Someone—some native—some Arab thief—had climbed the balcony at the stern of the dahabiyeh, from the river, and gained an entrance! That flashed into Bunter's fat mind at once. He could see nothing, hear nothing, but the faintest of stealthy sounds. But his terrified mind pictured a desperado, knife in hand, and he stood where he was, chained to the floor by terror, scarcely breathing; and as he stood he felt the wind of a garment that almost brushed him as an unseen figure passed.

THE FOURTH CHAPTER.

The Enemy in the Night!

KALIZELOS, the Greek, stood in the shadow of the temple colonnade, by the landing-place at Luxor, on the Nile. His eyes were fixed on a light that burned from the mast of a dahabiyeh. Other vessels were tied up; two or three smaller dahabiyehs and a steamer and a crowd of feluccas. But it was on the riding-light of the Cleopatra that the Greek's eyes were fixed.

There were many dahabiyehs on the Nile, but the magnificent houseboat that belonged to Mr. Hilmi Maroudi, of Cairo, was not to be mistaken; it was as well known as the Egyptian millionaire himself, from the Delta to the Cataracts. The jetty-black eyes of the Greek glittered as he stood at the masthead light, and the shadowy shape of the dahabiyeh beneath it.

During the long sunny days and starry nights that they had journeyed up the Nile, Harry Wharton & Co. had given no thought to their enemy, and had, indeed, almost forgotten his existence.

They knew that Kalizelos had been taken by the police in Cairo to stand his trial for attempting the life of Mr. Maroudi; and they took it for granted that they were done with him. But for that, in fact, Sir Reginald Brooke would never have allowed his schoolboy charges out of his sight.

But the Cairo prison had not held the cunning Greek. Backsheesh works wonders in all Eastern lands; and the Greek had plenty of money, though his desperate quest of the Golden Scarab had made him a fugitive. No doubt liberal backsheesh had helped to open the prison doors for Kalizelos, and, after many days, he was once more on the track of Lord Mauleverer and the scarab that had belonged, in ancient days, to A-Menah, the Egyptian soldier of the reign of Rameses the Second.

No one looking at the Greek now would have known him. The handsome olive face was darkened to the brown of a desert Arab, and he wore the djubbah and turban of a native, and moustache and beard. His djubbah was dingy, his turban dingier, his shoes tattered. Anyone looking at him would never have dreamed that he was the handsome, properous Greek of Cairo; he looked like any one of the thousand native touts and hangers-on of the show-places on the Nile.

Long the Greek stood there, in the thickening shadows of the Egyptian night, staring at the dahabiyeh. On board that craft were the schoolboys from Greyfriars in far-off England, among them Lord Mauleverer, the possessor of the golden beetle—the mysterious Scarabeus of A-Menah.

Not for a moment did Mauly believe the strange old tale that the Golden Scarab could guide its possessor to the long-lost treasure of the reign of Rameses—the wonderful diamond called the Eye of Osiris, which A-Menah had brought home from Syria three thousand years ago.

But the Greek believed it.

If the mysterious scarab possessed such magical powers, certainly it had not exercised them while in Mauly's possession.

Many and many a time had Mauly and his friends examined the golden beetle, which, except that it appeared to be made of solid gold, was like thousands of other scarabs that had been picked up in the dead cities of Egypt. The inscription on it, in the ancient picture-writing, told that it had belonged to A-Menah, the soldier of Rameses, but it told nothing more.

The juniors knew that Kalizelos had read the secret of the scarab in an ancient papyrus that had come into his hands in his business as a curio dealer in Cairo. What the secret was, they could not begin to imagine, but, whatever it was, the Greek knew it, and it had caused him to risk liberty and life in seeking to lay hands on the scarab.

Kalizelos moved away from the colonnade at last, and went down to the bank of the river in the deep shadows. Under the bank lay a small boat, with two Arabs in it, evidently waiting for him. Had the juniors seen them, they would have recognised Yussef, the hawk-faced Arab, and Hamza, the man with the scarred face. Kalizelos muttered a word or two in Arabic, and stepped into the boat, and the two Arabs pushed off into the shadowy Nile.

Hardly a sound was made as they tooled the small, light skiff under the stern of the Cleopatra.

Yussef silently laid down his oar, and held on to the dahabiyeh. Kalizelos rose to his feet and looked up.

There were no lights to be seen. The balcony was deserted, dark under its awning, and there was no one on the upper deck. The Nubian sailors were forward on the lower deck, which at night was closed in by awnings. Kalizelos whispered in Arabic; and while Yussef held on, Hamza, the scarred man, gave the Greek a helping hand up.

Agile as a cat, the Greek climbed, with the help of the scarred Arab, from below.

In a few moments he disappeared over the stern of the dahabiyeh, and the Arabs waited in silence.

Standing in the balcony, the Greek bent his head and listened for a few moments. All was silent and still.

He stepped across the balcony to one of the doorways that gave access to the saloon of the dahabiyeh.

The doorway was closed by a latticed shutter, which was fastened, but it did not stop the Greek for long. In a couple of minutes the shutter was open, and the Greek stepped silently into the saloon.

Kalizelos knew the interior of the Cleopatra. Many times he had come aboard that dahabiyeh in former days to bring curios and antiquities for the inspection of Mr. Hilmi Maroudi, who had once been one of his best customers. With hardly a pause, the Greek groped his way across the saloon to the open doorway beyond, where a short passage led into the dining-room, beyond which were the sleeping-rooms.

Softly, stealthily, he stepped into the dining-room, and groped his way across it.

He paused suddenly.

There was only the palest glimmer of starlight, from one window where the shutter had not been closed. He could see nothing. But it seemed to him that he had caught a breath in the silence.

He listened intently.

But there was no sound, and he groped on—little dreaming that his dingy djubbah's lose folds almost brushed against a figure that stood rooted with terror in the darkness.

If the Greek had thought of Billy Bunter at all, he would have supposed that the fat schoolboy was fast asleep like the others.

But he was not thinking of Billy Bunter. He was thinking of Lord Mauleverer, and the Golden Scarab.

Softly and stealthily, he passed out into the passage beyond the dining-saloon, where the darkness was intense.

There he paused once more to listen.

No sound broke the stillness.

On the forward deck, the crew were sleeping under their awning; the black servants were in their rooms asleep; the schoolboys slumbered. The Greek's eyes glittered in the dark like a cat's. He had failed many times—at Greyfriars School far away, at Naples, at Alexandria, at Cairo, at the Pyramids—again and again he, who alone knew the secret of the scarab, had failed to seize it—but this time he would not fail. Success, at last, was within his grasp.

He moved again, softly, stealthily as a cat. He opened a door, and peered in. The steady breathing of a sleeper reached his ears. A tiny electric torch glimmered out from his hand, but it did not turn on the sleeper. It glimmered on a suitcase that bore the initials "H. W."; that was enough for him. He shut off the light, stepped back from the room, and closed the door as soundlessly as he had opened it.

Another door was softly opened; again he heard the steady breathing of a sleeper; again the tiny beam of light showed him that it was not Lord Mauleverer's room, and he closed the door without a sound.

A third door was opened, and the beam of light told a different tale. On the dressing-table a silver-backed brush

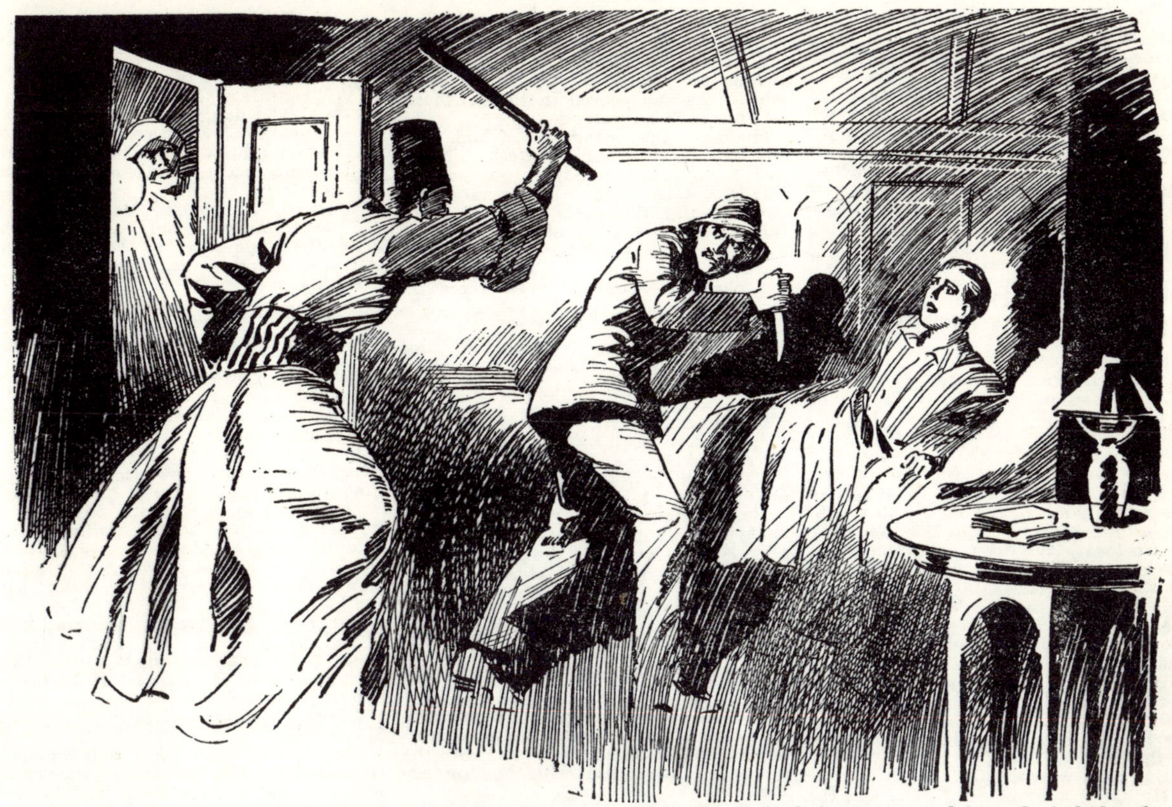

Hassan hurled the door suddenly open and leapt into the room. As he did so, Kalizelos spun round from the bedside, the dagger, which a moment before had been pressed to Mauleverer's throat, flashing in the light. "Oh gad!" murmured the schoolboy earl, while the Greek snarled.

glimmered in the beam, and showed the letter "M."

Kalizelos stepped into the room, and closed the door behind him. He stepped to the bedside.

The tiny gleam of light showed a sleeping face, that of Lord Mauleverer, fast asleep.

The Greek's black eyes glittered down at him.

Mauleverer slept soundly.

For several seconds the Greek stood watching him. Perhaps it was fortunate for Mauleverer that he slept soundly, and showed no sign of waking. The Greek, satisfied at last, turned away from him. Mauly's clothes lay where he had tossed them carelessly on a chair and a divan. At home, at Mauleverer Towers, Mauly's clothes were looked after by Mauly's "man," but on the trip to Egypt Mauly was travelling without his man, and his lordship was rather careless with his expensive garments. With the tiny torch glimmering in his hand, Kalizelos proceeded to search the pockets of Mauleverer's clothes—casting every now and then a cat-like glance of vigilance at the sleeping schoolboy.

But he did not find the Golden Scarab.

He had no doubt that it was in Lord Mauleverer's room on board the dahabiyeh. It was not likely that it had been left behind in Cairo. But after his several narrow escapes of losing the ancient amulet of A-Menah, no doubt Mauleverer had ceased to carry it in his pockets. Kalizelos threw the clothes aside at last, and began to search the cabin, his stealthy glances turning from moment to moment on the sleeper's calm and untroubled face.

The Greek's teeth set savagely.

There was a great deal of baggage in the cabin. Lord Mauleverer did not travel light. It was a long task to search the various bags and suitcases, and all the time the scarab might be under Mauleverer's pillow, or perhaps in the care of some other member of the party. Kalizelos knew that it had been in Wharton's keeping on the steamer, though Mauleverer had taken charge of it again after the attack on Wharton, which had almost cost him his life. He ceased the vain search at last, and stood beside the schoolboy earl's bed, and looked down at him with gleaming eyes. From under his dingy djubbah he drew a dagger and set the tiny electric torch on the dressing-table, placed for its beam to fall on the sleeper's face.

Then he touched the sleeping junior.

Lord Mauleverer awakened.

"Silence, my lord!" With a start of amazement, Mauleverer recognised the Greek's soft, musical voice in the darkness, and at the same moment he felt the keen point of the dagger at his throat. "Silence, Lord Mauleverer!"

"Oh gad!" breathed Mauleverer.

The beam of light on his face showed it startled and dismayed. But it showed no trace of fear there. After the first moment of amazement Mauleverer was calm, and cool as ice. But he made no movement. The point of the dagger almost pierced his skin, and he knew that there was a desperate hand behind it. He peered in the darkness at the shadowy figure of the Greek.

"I seem to know your voice." His tones were quite placid. "You're Kalizelos, I fancy. What?"

"You know me!" breathed the Greek. "Not a word above a whisper, my lord!"

"Oh, quite! What are you doin' out of chokey?" asked Mauleverer.

"Where is the scarab, Lord Mauleverer?" The dagger-point pressed a little harder. "The scarab—or death! This time you will not escape me. Your life is in my hands! Give me the scarab—or die!"

From the darkness the Greek's voice came like the hiss of a snake. Lord Mauleverer drew a long, deep breath, but he did not speak.

THE FIFTH CHAPTER.
Bunter Does His Best!

BILLY BUNTER forgot that he was hungry.

He stood rooted to the floor in the dining-saloon, his fat heart almost dying within him as the garments of the unseen intruder brushed by.

The unseen man might have touched him by stretching out a hand.

But he had passed on in stealthy silence, without knowing that the fat schoolboy was there.

Bunter did not stir.

He feared to make the slightest sound.

The unseen intruder had gone along to the sleeping-rooms, and Bunter dared not make a movement that might draw him back.

Minute followed minute. Cold perspiration trickled down Billy Bunter's podgy back. But the silence reassured him at last.

Who was it that had passed him in the darkness? Some Arab thief, in quest of loot on the millionaire's dahabiyeh? But the man had passed through the stern saloon, where there were many objects of great value, and had not stopped there. He had gone on to the bed-rooms, where there was risk of a sleeper awakening, and little in the way of loot. The fat Owl realised that it was not some thief of Luxor who had stolen on board the dahabiyeh.

It was the Golden Scarab that the unseen man was seeking. Kalizelos, the Greek, was in prison at Cairo when the Greyfriars party started on their voyage up the Nile. But he had many agents, and it was one of them who was now on board the Cleopatra. Or—the further thought flashed into Bunter's scared mind—perhaps the Greek was free again and it was Konstantinos Kalizelos himself who had brushed by in the darkness. That thought made Bunter shudder with dread, so deep was his terror of the Greek.

For the Golden Scarab Bunter did not care two straws. Indeed, more than once he had advised Mauly to let the Greek have it at the price he had offered. That, in Bunter's opinion, was the sensible thing to do. Certainly Bunter would not have run the slightest risk to save the Scarab of A-Menah from the hands of the man who sought it so desperately. But he was well aware that Mauly took a different view. As he stood there, shivering with funk, Bunter knew, as plainly as if he had seen him, that the stealthy intruder was seeking Lord Mauleverer's room, that sooner or later he would pick it out, and then——

Billy Bunter moved at last.

Death hung over Mauleverer in the darkness and silence, and he knew it. Even Billy Bunter could not leave it at that!

But what was he to do?

He dared not call out. If it was the Greek, or if it was Yussef or Hamza, whoever it was, the wretch would rate Billy Bunter's life no higher than a mosquito's. To call for help and draw the man's attention to himself was impossible—to Bunter, at least.

He thought of getting out on the stern balcony and climbing thence to the upper deck. But it immediately occurred to his fat mind that the intruder could hardly have come alone. He must have had assistance to clamber up over the stern. In that case his confederates were in a boat under the balcony; perhaps on the balcony itself. Bunter dared not take a step in that direction.

But the only other way to help lay by the passage—the way the unseen man had gone. Bunter dragged himself to the doorway and peered down the mid-way passage of the dahabiyeh.

It was dark, but there was a faint glimmer of stars from the open doorway at the other end, which opened on the lower deck. Bunter's eyes were accustomed to the dark by this time, and he could make out that the passage was empty. The stealthy intruder had gone into one of the rooms. Bunter did not need telling which! In those very moments Lord Mauleverer's life hung by a thread.

That thought spurred on the shuddering fat Owl. He took his courage in both hands, as it were, and tiptoed into the passage. With a thumping heart, but without a sound, he crept along, and as he came by the door of Lord Mauleverer's room he heard the faintest of sounds from within. Mauleverer, evidently, was still asleep, but someone was moving in the room. Bunter's heart gave a jump, and he tiptoed on.

His first thought had been to enter one of the rooms and wake Wharton or Bob Cherry. But he was too terrified to risk alarming the midnight intruder by making a sound.

He crept on to the end of the passage

There he tiptoed up the three shallow steps to the sailors' deck.

That deck was closed in by a canvas awning at night. Bunter pulled aside the canvas and peered in the darkness.

"Hassan!" he gasped.

Hassan, the dragoman, had his quarters on the sailors' deck. There was a murmur as Bunter gasped—or, rather, croaked. His voice came husky from his dry throat.

He heard a stirring of the sailors.

A faint light glimmered. Brown, startled faces peered at Bunter from the shadows — dark, grave faces of Nubians.

"Hassan!"

"Noble gentleman!" came the voice of the dragoman. Hassan came out of the shadows, staring at the fat schoolboy.

Bunter caught his arm.

The terror in his face made Hassan stare blankly.

"Mauleverer!" groaned Bunter. "Go and help him! Kalizelos——"

Hassan started.

"My lordly gentleman, that son of pigs is at Cairo, in the prison," he said. "Yes, sar. He is exceedingly safe in a prison!"

"There's somebody—in Mauleverer's room. Kalizelos, or one of his gang! Quick!" breathed Bunter.

"On my head be it, sar!" said Hassan.

He picked up his stick and went down the steps into the passage. At a murmured word in Arabic one of the Nubians followed him with the glimmering lamp.

Billy Bunter stood in the doorway, following them with his eyes—not with his fat person! Whether the man in Mauleverer's cabin was the Greek, or one of his gang, Bunter did not want to get to close quarters with him. That was up to Hassan, the son of Suleiman.

Hassan, the son of Suleiman, was a good deal of a rogue, but he was no coward. And Hassan had very particular reasons for seeing his noble master safe on the journey up the Nile. Although the juniors were not aware of it, Mr. Maroudi had taken measures to ensure Hassan's good faith. There was a great reward awaiting Hassan if he watched faithfully over the safety of the Greyfriars party, and grim vengeance if he failed in his trust.

The dragoman trod softly along the passage, the stick grasped in his hand. Behind him followed the silent-footed Nubian with the lamp.

Billy Bunter watched them, with a face like chalk.

Hassan reached Lord Mauleverer's door, and there paused to listen. Possibly he doubted whether Bunter might not have been the victim of a nightmare.

But as he listened his brown face hardened, and his eyes gleamed, and his sinewy fingers tightened on the heavy stick.

From within the cabin came a faint murmur of a voice—so low that even the dragoman's keen ears could not catch the words. But the tones of that voice were familiar to him, and he knew that it was the soft, musical voice of the Greek of Cairo.

"Bismillah!" breathed Hassan.

Kalizelos was in Lord Mauleverer's room. It was no surprise to Hassan to learn that the Greek was free again; he knew the power of "backsheesh."

Hassan's left hand turned silently the handle of the door. The Nubian held up the lamp behind him as he hurled the door suddenly open and leaped into the room.

THE SIXTH CHAPTER.

Mauly Means Business!

KALIZELOS spun round from the bedside.

The dagger, which a moment before had been pressed to Mauleverer's throat, flashed in the light of the lamp held by the Nubian outside the doorway.

"Oh gad!" murmured Mauleverer.

A snarl broke from the Greek—a snarl of savage rage, as the dragoman leaped at him with whirling stick.

With a sudden spring he escaped the blow, which barely missed him. Then, with another spring as swift, he hurled himself at Hassan, the dagger flashing aloft.

An upward sweep of the stick caught the Greek's arm as the blow descended, and the dagger shot from his hand and clattered on the floor.

In a fraction of a second Hassan struck again with the stick, and this time it crashed on the head of Kalizelos.

The Greek staggered and fell.

Hassan leaped at the fallen man. Another moment, and the heavy stick would have crashed down on the fallen man's head — probably cracking his skull.

But Lord Mauleverer, plunging out of bed, grasped the dragoman's arm in time, and turned the blow aside. The stick crashed on the parquet of the floor, a foot from the Greek.

"Draw it mild, old bean!" yawned Mauleverer.

The Greek, dazed and half-stunned, struggled to rise. Hassan jammed a foot on him and crushed him to the floor again.

"My noble gentleman, permit me that I give him exceedingly hard knock," said Hassan. "I will bash him, as you say in your beautiful language; I will give him what the English lords call kybosh. Yes!"

Lord Mauleverer grinned.

"Mustn't crack his coconut, old bean," he said. "Collar the brute; I'll lend you a hand!"

"As my lords wills!" said Hassan.

The Greek made another attempt to struggle up, his black eyes glittering like a wild beast's. Hassan and Mauleverer grasped him together, and he sprawled on the floor, struggling desperately.

"Come and lend a hand, you men!" shouted Mauleverer.

"Hallo, hallo, hallo!" came the voice of Bob Cherry.

The Famous Five had already been awakened by the crash of the Greek's fall. They crowded out of their rooms in startled amazement.

The Nubian with the lamp stood aside for them to pass, and they crowded into Mauleverer's room. They did not stop to ask questions. Five pairs of hands were laid on the struggling rascal, and he was quickly reduced to helplessness.

"Got him, whoever he is!" gasped Wharton. "But what—who——"

"It's jolly old Kalizelos!" yawned Lord Mauleverer.

"What?"

The juniors stared at the panting prisoner. They had taken him for an Arab. But now that they looked at him closely in the light they could make out the handsome, clear-cut features of the Greek under the brown stain.

"Kalizelos!" exclaimed Nugent blankly.

"Yaas!"

"Then he's out of chokey again!" exclaimed Johnny Bull.

"Looks like it, old bean!"

"Well, we've got him!"

"The gotfulness is terrific!"

Harry Wharton picked up the dagger.

He looked at it, looked at the writhing Greek, and at Lord Mauleverer.

Mauly was cool and collected, but the juniors knew now the fearful danger that had threatened him.

"The awful scoundrel!" muttered Bob Cherry.

"The esteemed and ridiculous rascal!" said Hurree Jamset Ram Singh.

"Mauly, old man——"

"All serene, old tops!" said Lord Mauleverer. "It was gettin' quite unpleasant, though, when Hassan butted in. I believe I've got a scratch on the neck. I can tell you fellows that that man Kalizelos is a sticker. He wants that jolly old scarab, and he won't be happy till he gets it. Hassan, old bean, I'm frightfully obliged to you; but how the merry thump did you know that the sportsman had called on business at this time of night?"

"The small fat lord called me, sar——"

"Bunter!" gasped Mauleverer.

"Yes, sar! And I came at once to save my lordly gentleman!" said Hassan. "With your noble permission, I will just give him what you English lords call a cosh, and the son of fifty thousand jackals may then be dropped overboard into the Nile, my estimable gentleman."

"Life's cheap in Egypt!" grinned Bob Cherry.

"I think we'll tie him up, instead," said Lord Mauleverer. "Find a rope somewhere, Hassan. We're goin' to make him safe this time."

"Yes, sar!"

Hassan called one of the Nubians, and a rope was brought. With scientific thoroughness, the dragoman proceeded to bind the writhing Greek hand and foot.

"It was Bunter who called Hassan!" said Bob Cherry, in amazement. "But what on earth was Bunter doing awake at this time of night?"

"Goodness knows!"

"It must be nearly midnight," said Harry. "How the thump did that fat duffer happen to be awake?"

"Oh, really, Wharton——"

Billy Bunter blinked in at the doorway through his big spectacles. His first blink was at the Greek.

"Got him safe?" he asked.

"Safe as houses, old fat bean!" said Bob. "But what the merry thump are you doing out of bed?"

"I'm hungry——"

"Wha-a-at?"

"I never had any supper, had I?" hooted Bunter.

"Oh, my hat!"

"Ha, ha, ha!"

"Ha, ha, ha!" roared Lord Mauleverer. "Bunter was up and rooting after grub—that's how it was."

"Oh, really, Mauly!" Bunter gave the infuriated Greek another blink. "Sure you've got him safe? Put in a few more knots, Hassan! You can't be too careful with a beast like that! I say, you fellows, is it Kalizelos? He looks like a nigger."

"It's Kalizelos," said Harry. "He must have got on board somehow without giving the alarm——"

"Lucky I was on the watch!" snorted Bunter.

"On the watch for grub, do you mean?"

"Ha, ha, ha!"

"No, I don't!" roared Bunter. "On the watch, looking after you fellows—saving Mauly and protecting him, which is all I joined this party for, as you know. And all you fellows can do is to keep a fellow without his supper and keep him frightfully hungry, because a nigger makes out that I gave him a bad quid! As if I'd give a nigger a bad quid! Besides, it was passed on me at Beni Suef, as you know perfectly well."

"That reminds me," said Bob. "We haven't kicked Bunter yet——"

"Why, you—you beast!" gasped Bunter, with a backward jump through the doorway. "You—you—you——"

"You're not goin' to be kicked, old fat man," said Lord Mauleverer. "You're goin' to have some supper. Hassan, if you've made that sportsman safe, will you be kind enough to see that Bunter has some supper? Wake up the cook—he won't mind, if you give him some backsheesh."

"On my head be it, noble lordship!" answered Hassan.

CRACK A JOKE
and
BAG A PENKNIFE!

One of this week's useful prizes goes to K. Clare, of 100, Ealing Park Gardens, South Ealing, W.5, who sent in the following rib-tickler.

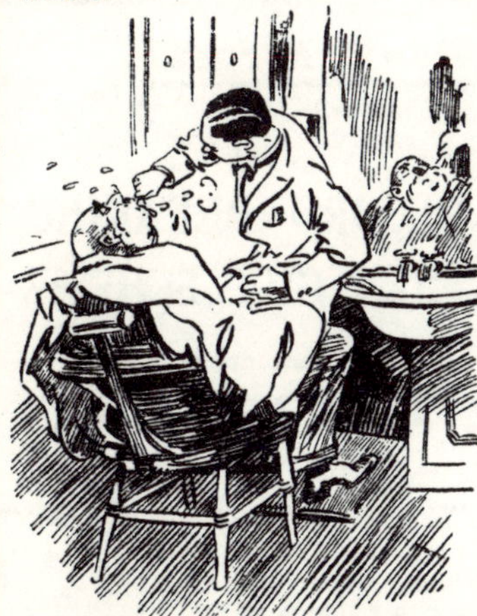

"What do you think of the soap, sir?" asked the over-vigorous barber, lathering his customer too generously.
"The — the best I've ever tasted!" choked the victim.

GET BUSY, BOYS!

"Better look round the boat," said Harry. "That rascal may not have come alone! Tell the sailors to search the dahabiyeh, Hassan."

"Yes, sar."

The search was prompt; but it did not reveal the Greek's confederates. At the first sound of alarm Yussef and Hamza had pushed off from the dahabiyeh, and the shadows of the Nile had swallowed them.

Lights gleamed on board the Cleopatra now. In the dining-saloon Billy Bunter sat at the table with a cheery grin on his fat face, and well-filled dishes within his reach. Now that the scare was over, Bunter remembered that he was hungry. The fat Owl had been frightened out of his fat wits; but his courage revived at a bound when there was no longer any danger. And Billy Bunter was quite pleased with the happenings of that wild night. He had escaped the kicking he deserved, and he was enjoying his supper all the more because of the delay. He tucked into the provender with immense satisfaction, and kept the cook busy for quite a long time.

Harry Wharton & Co. gathered again in Mauleverer's cabin where the Greek lay on the floor, bound hand and foot, and glaring up with eyes like a caged tiger.

"I suppose we'd better send Hassan ashore to call the police," said Harry. "Kalizelos will have to be handed over to them."

Lord Mauleverer shook his head.

His lordship had been doing some thinking, and he proceeded to astonish his friends with the result of it.

"Not at all," said Mauly. "The police have had him once, and let him slip. I don't know how it strikes you fellows, but I think this man Kalizelos is a jolly dangerous customer. Wakin' a fellow up at midnight, you know, with a jolly old dagger in his fist, like a johnny on the films! There's altogether too much of the film bizney about this man Kalizelos. I'm goin' to keep an eye on him."

"But you can't keep him here!" exclaimed Bob Cherry.

Lord Mauleverer raised his eyebrows.

"Why not?" he asked.

"Oh, my hat!"

"The whyfulness is terrific," chuckled the Nabob of Bhanipur.

"But——" exclaimed Harry Wharton.

"My dear men, I've thought it out," explained Lord Mauleverer. "This sportsman came aboard our craft without bein' asked. He can't possibly have fancied that we wanted him. Well, now he's here, I'm keepin' him. So long as he's after that scarab, he won't give a fellow any rest. And a fellow hates bein' woke up in the middle of the night, especially with a dagger pokin' at his neck. It's liable to get on a fellow's nerves in the long run."

"But what——" exclaimed Nugent.

"I've thought it all out," said Mauleverer cheerfully. "That sportsman is after the scarab, because he knows its secret, whatever it is. He hasn't the least respect for the right of property. Well, he's goin' to tell me the jolly old secret. What's sauce for the goose, is sauce for the gander. He's asked for this, and now he's gettin' it."

Mauleverer turned to the Greek.

"You catch on, old bean?" he asked. "I'm not lettin' you have the scarab. But there's another way of drawin' your teeth. Instead of you gettin' the scarab, I get the secret. What is it? Cough it up!"

Kalizelos glared at him savagely.

"Fool!" he snarled. "Do you dream that I will tell you a secret worth a quarter of a million English pounds?"

"Yaas."

"Fool!" snarled the Greek.

"Take your time," said Mauleverer placidly. "You've shoved yourself in here where you're not wanted, and now you're stayin'. I'm sorry I shall have to keep you tied up; you're a bit too dangerous to leave around loose, and I'm afraid I couldn't trust your parole. Hassan!"

"Yes, sar!"

"Bring some rugs and blankets for that johnny, and make him as comfortable as you can. Must be as comfortable as possible."

"Oh, sar!" gasped the dragoman.

"But, Mauly, old man——" exclaimed Wharton.

"My dear chap, leave this to me!"

"You're not going to sleep with that villain in your room!" roared Bob.

"Why not? He's tied up safe enough, isn't he, Hassan?"

"Yes, sar. Very exceeding and extremely safe," grinned the dragoman.

"He is safe as a house, as you say in English."

"That's all right, then. Good-night, you men!"

"Oh, my hat!" said Bob.

Lord Mauleverer went back to bed. The juniors stared at him. His eyes closed peacefully.

"After all, the man's safe," said Nugent, with a laugh.

And, having examined the Greek's bonds themselves, and made quite sure that there was no possibility of his getting loose, the chums of the Remove went back to bed.

THE SEVENTH CHAPTER.

The Prisoner of the Dahabiyeh!

"JOLLY old Thebes!" said Bob Cherry.

The Nile glimmered in the morning sunshine. The Greyfriars fellows were breakfasting, waited on by assiduous Nubians. Hassan hovered round like a highly coloured butterfly.

Bright and golden, the Nile flowed past the moored dahabiyeh. And on either side of the river of marvels, wide, fertile lands stretched away to ranges of hills, crowned by peaks. Luxor, with its temples and tall palms, glimmered in the sunshine from an unclouded sky of blue—the sky of Egypt—on the eastern bank.

Beyond the Nile on the western bank was the Necropolis of Thebes—tombs and tombs and tombs—"innumerable dead persons," as Hassan enthusiastically told his lordly gentlemen. Among which lay the tomb of Tutankhamen, discovered so recently as 1922, by English explorers, though it had been discovered and plundered by earlier explorers a thousand years before the beginning of the Christian era.

But it was towards Luxor that the juniors were glancing as they breakfasted under the awning on the balcony. Billy Bunter did not deign to give that ancient city a glance—his attention was wholly concentrated on his breakfast. But he blinked up through his big spectacles as Bob Cherry made his remark.

"Thebes!" repeated Bunter, blinking.

"Jolly old Thebes!" said Bob.

"You silly ass!" said Bunter witheringly. "Lot you know about geography! Thebes is in Greece!"

"Ha, ha, ha!" roared Bob.

And the Co. chortled.

"I say, you fellows, you are a lot of ignoramuses!" said Bunter scornfully. "Don't you know that Thebes is in Greece? Haven't you had it with old Quelch in class? Haven't you heard of Epaminondas, and the rest of the tosh? Fancy that silly ass thinking that Thebes is in Egypt!"

"Ha, ha, ha!"

"Blessed if I see anything to cackle at!" snorted Bunter. "The best thing you fellows can do is to listen to me and get some instruction, or you'll be as ignorant when you go back as when you started."

"You silly owl!" roared Bob. "That's Thebes!"

"Fathead!" said Bunter. "Here, Hassan!"

"Magnificent, sar!" answered the dragoman, salaaming.

Bunter jerked a fat thumb towards the city on the Nile bank.

"What's that show, Hassan?"

"Luxor, sar. Wonderful and atrociously interesting City of Luxor," answered Hassan. "On northern side adjacent is Karnak. Still more fearfully interesting."

"I told you so, Cherry. Now shut up, and don't display your ignorance!" said Bunter, with withering scorn.

"You howling ass!" said Bob. "Luxor's built on the site of ancient Thebes."

"Thebes is in Greece, you dummy!"

"There were two Thebes!" roared Bob. "This was the Egyptian Thebes."

"Rot!" said Bunter.

"I tell you, you fat chump——"

"No good telling me rot like that," said Bunter, shaking his head. "Think I don't know that Thebes was in Greece? Yah!"

"That was the other Thebes," said Harry Wharton, laughing.

"Bosh!" said Bunter.

"Much and enormous ruins of ancient Thebes remain here to be seen by an eye," said Hassan. "City was called Thebes by Grecian persons——"

"Rats!" said Bunter. "You can't gammon me that Thebes was in Egypt."

"My noble sar——"

"Bosh!"

Hassan gave it up. Billy Bunter snorted, and continued his breakfast. He was not to be convinced that the ruins of Thebes were to be found on the banks of the Nile.

However, there they were, and that morning the Greyfriars fellows were going to explore them.

The Famous Five and Lord Mauleverer finished breakfast, leaving Billy Bunter still going strong. What had happened in the night had made Bunter's peace; but perhaps he feared that there might be another period of famine, for he packed away the foodstuffs at a rate that made Mr. Maroudi's Nubian servants roll their eyes in wonder. Even some of the sailors made pretexts to come along the deck and look at the small fat lord, who was apparently trying to create another famine in Egypt.

Even Moussa, the reis, who was a grave man, with a face as expressionless as that of a bronze image, turned his dark eyes on the small fat lord in grave wonder. Perhaps the natives expected to see Bunter wind up by bursting on the balcony like a bomb.

The juniors went in from the balcony, the sound of the steady champing of Billy Bunter's jaws following them. Lord Mauleverer strolled along to his room. On the divan in that room sat Kalizelos, the Greek, bound hand and foot. Lord Mauleverer regarded him thoughtfully, and the Famous Five smiled. Mauly's wheeze of giving the scheming Greek "tit for tat" had surprised them, and it rather amused them. They were not disposed to raise objections. Besides, the easy-going Mauly could be obstinate when he liked, and it was clear that he had made up his noble mind on this subject.

Kalizelos looked at the juniors, his black eyes burning like coals of fire. But his murderous fury did not affect their cheery spirits in any way. The rascal's teeth were drawn now.

"Good-mornin', old bean!" said Lord Mauleverer politely. "I've called to hear that jolly old secret."

"Fool!" snarled Kalizelos.

"Now, be reasonable," urged his lordship amiably. "I never started this trouble. You'll admit that, Mr. Kalizelos?"

"Fool!"

"I can't say I like your manners," remarked Lord Mauleverer, while the chums of the Remove chuckled. "You're really not the sort of chap we want on board this boat, either. Let's come to business. You shut me up in a beastly old tomb, tryin' to get that scarab off me. One good turn deserves another. Accordin' to your own story, you've found out the secret of the scarab, and you won't be happy till you get it. Well, hand over the secret, my good man. If that jolly old scarab really can lead the way to the Eye of Osiris, as you seem to believe, cough it up! You can see for yourself that that's the only way of getting shut of you."

"Fool!"

"You're repeating yourself, Mr. Kalizelos," said Lord Mauleverer gently. "If we're to continue this conversation, I suggest that you put on a new record."

"Fool!"

"This gentleman's vocabulary seems to be limited," remarked Lord Mauleverer. "But I gather from his answers that he's not goin' to cough up that secret. Is that your impression, you fellows?"

"Sort of!" chuckled Bob Cherry.

"Well, we're goin' to give him time—all the time he wants," said Lord Mauleverer. "A judge ought to have given him time really——"

"Ha, ha, ha!"

"But here he is, on our hands, and we can't let him loose, so we'll give him time to think it over. Hassan!"

"Noble lord——"

"Is there a room on the boat where this fellow can be locked in safely?" asked Mauleverer. "Can't keep him tied up like this—it's cruelty to animals—and one must be kind even to wild animals."

"Perhaps better call policemans, sar——" suggested Hassan dubiously.

"Perhaps better do as you're told!" said Mauleverer gently.

"Oh! Yes, sar! To hear is to obey!" said Hassan, at once. "Here you are, lord, sar, by order of the great Maroudi! You give order, sar, and I execute him with the promptness of a dispatch, as you say in English, sar."

"Get on with it, then."

Hassan untied the Greek's legs and jerked him to his feet. He led the prisoner from the room, Kalizelos gritting his teeth with rage. The Greek had counted on possible failure, possible arrest, when he crept on board the dahabiyeh in the night. But he had not counted on this.

Handed over to the police, he had little doubt that backsheesh would see him through again. But it was very doubtful whether backsheesh would help him on board the Cleopatra, where all were devoted to the Greyfriars party, by the order of Mr. Hilmi Maroudi.

Hassan, the dragoman, had once taken his bribes, to betray his "lordly gentlemen"; but that was before Hassan was

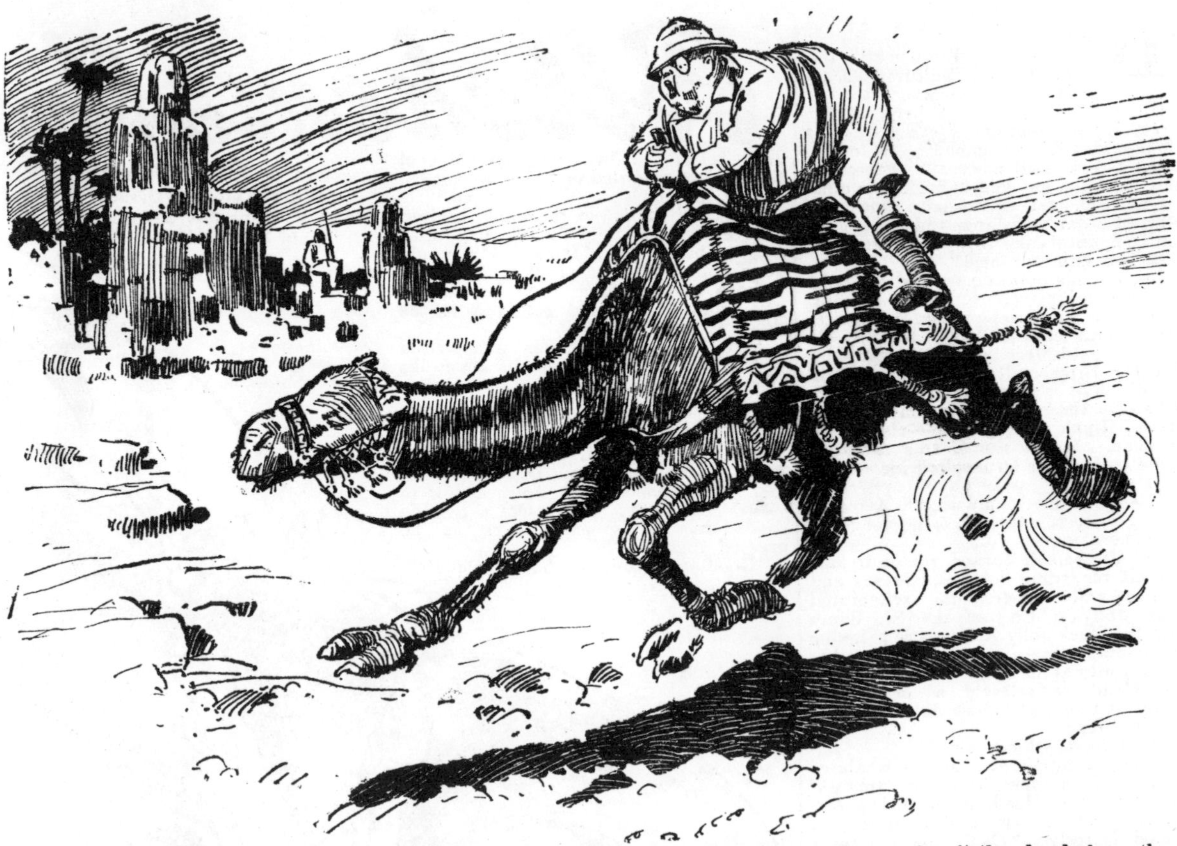

"Oh lor'! Help! Yarooop!" roared Bunter, swinging to and fro on the back of the camel as it thundered along the dusty track. "Stop, you beast!" Thud! Thud! Thud! The camel heeded him not, its hoofs beating an incessant tattoo as it thundered on.

aware that they were under the protection of Maroudi. Since he had been warned by the Egyptian millionaire, the "faithful Hassan" had become faithful indeed.

The juniors were aware that they were under many obligations to Mr. Maroudi—but they never dreamed of the extent of the Egyptian millionaire's power, or of how much they owed to it.

Hassan led the prisoner to a small room farther along the passage. With a rough shove, he sent him tottering in, and the Greek tripped and fell on the floor, panting with rage.

"Gently does it, Hassan!" said Lord Mauleverer. "Untie his hands."

"Yes, sar."

The Greek was released from his bonds. He turned towards the juniors with clenched hands, his eyes blazing. Hassan swished his stick in the air, and the Greek jumped back from it.

"Better take it quietly, Mr. Kalizelos," drawled Lord Mauleverer. "This isn't a luxurious cabin, but it's better than the tomb you shut me up in, by Jove! Look the shutter over the window, Hassan—can't have him yowling to his friends on the Nile. Tell the Nubians to bring him some food. The door's to be kept locked, and a man set to watch it. Got that?"

"On my head be it!" said Hassan.

The Greek panted.

"You will not keep me here—you dare not keep me a prisoner on this dahabiyeh——"

Lord Mauleverer raised his eyebrows.

"Why not?" he asked.

"My magnificent lord do as want," grinned Hassan. "Be silent, son of ten thousand pigs! Sar, all shall be as your greatness say! Ahmed shall watch this son of jackals, and he shall not escape! Never, sar! Here he is safe as Tutankhamen in his tomb!"

When the juniors prepared to go ashore, the Greek was safely locked in the prison-room, and Ahmed, a black Nubian, squatted on a mat outside the door to keep watch and ward.

Konstantinos Kalizelos was left pacing his confined quarters like a tiger in a cage. Whether Lord Mauleverer's method of dealing with the scoundrel was strictly in accordance with the law was rather doubtful; but undoubtedly it was the only way of keeping the schoolboys' enemy out of mischief. And as Mauly was impervious to argument on the subject, the Famous Five had to leave it at that.

They went ashore in Luxor in cheery spirits, and soon forgot all about the prisoner of the dahabiyeh.

THE EIGHTH CHAPTER.

An Ass and a Camel!

"WHAT about a car?"

"Nothing about a car."

"I'm not riding a donkey!"

Bunter spoke firmly. He felt that it was time to be firm. "I've had enough of these beastly Egyptian donkeys! The fact is, I don't like donkeys!"

"Let brotherly love continue, old chap!" urged Bob Cherry.

"You silly ass!" hooted Bunter. "I tell you, I won't ride a donkey, and that's flat! So there!"

"Fine and most excellent donkey, sar," said Hassan.

"You shut up!" snorted Bunter.

"Look here, you duffer——" said Harry Wharton.

"I hate donkeys!" roared Bunter.

Billy Bunter had reason to dislike that mode of conveyance, so general in the land of Egypt. He could hardly have counted the donkeys he had fallen off on the banks of the Nile.

"Oh dear!" said Bob. "This isn't the time to tell us about your family troubles, old fat man!"

"Ha, ha, ha!"

"I'll ride a camel if you like! I won't ride a donkey! You see," explained Bunter, "I'm a riding man! You fellows can't ride! You stick on those donkeys like so many sacks of coke. And, I can tell you, you look a dashed Bank Holiday crowd on your dashed donkeys! Get me a camel, Hassan."

"You'll fall off a camel, same as off a donkey—and it's farther to fall!" Harry Wharton pointed out.

"Yah!"

"Estimable lordly sar——" urged Hassan.

"Get me a camel!"

"Oh, get him a camel," said Lord Mauleverer. "Any old thing for a quiet life. We shall never get to Karnak at this rate."

It was easy enough to engage a camel. There were plenty of camels at Luxor. Hassan called in Arabic to an acquaintance—Hassan seemed acquainted with everybody along the Nile—and a camel was led up for Bunter.

Harry Wharton & Co. mounted on donkeys, like most tourists who rode out from Luxor to the ruins of Karnak. They were quite satisfied with donkeys.

(*Continued on page 16.*)

Birchemall G

A "Fishy Tail" of Jack Jolly & Co., the heroes of St. Sam's.

I.

"DRAT it!"

Thus Dr. Birchemall, the refined and cultured headmaster of St. Sam's.

He was sitting on the bank of the River Ripple, fishing. Fishing was one of the Head's pet hobbies, his others being Greek, Lattin, croaky, hopscotch, and wacking his long-suffering pupils.

Dr. Birchemall was usually considered a bit of a dab at fishing, and in Muggleton's annual fishing tornyment he rarely failed to gain a plaice.

But on this occasion he had sat holding his fishing-rod for several hours without a bite—except for the duzzen or so sandwiches he had eaten himself. Either the fish were taking a half-holiday like Dr. Birchemall himself, or else the Head's bait was not attractive enuff. Whatever the reasons, the finny denizens of the Ripple simply didn't rise to the occasion. Hence the Head's disgusted eggsclamation as he insulted his watch:

"Drat it!"

"Caught anything, sir?" asked a cheery voice behind him, as he got ready to make a move.

Dr. Birchemall turned round to find himself regarding Jolly and Merry and Bright and Fearless—the sellybrated Jack Jolly & Co., of the St. Sam's Fourth. Jack Jolly & Co. were grinning at the empty jam-jar which stood rather pathetically at his side. They "capped" the Head respectively as he glared round at them, and Jack Jolly repeated his question:

"Caught anything, sir?"

"Yes; a cupple of sharx, a whale or two, and a few tuns of tunny!" answered the Head, with biting sarkasm; then he altered his tone and added feercely: "Can't you tell by a meer glarnse at this jam-jar that I've caught nothing, fathead?"

"Well, now you mention it, sir," grinned Jack Jolly, "the fact that there are no fish in it does make it look a bit fishy, duzzent it?"

"Ha, ha, ha!" roared Merry and Bright and Fearless.

Dr. Birchemall snorted. Then his eye suddenly fell on the float of his fishing-tackle, which was bobbing up and down in the water, and he gave a sudden yell:

"Hurrah! A bite!"

"Good egg!" mermered Jack Jolly & Co.

Dr. Birchemall swooped down on his fishing-rod and began to wind in his line.

"Give me a hand, boys!" he cride. "By the feel of it, I have caught a really bewtiful spessimen—possibly a giant cuttle-fish or a man-eating octopus! My hat! It feels as if it weighs a ton!"

Jack Jolly & Co. "heaved" until the Head's fishing-line stretched vizzibly, and it seemed doubtful whether it would stand the strain. Then, suddenly, it shot out of the water—so suddenly that the Head and his youthful helpers were caught unawares and sent sprawling backwards, to land on the ground with a fearful bump.

Bump! Thud! Wallop!

"Ow-wow! Yaroooo!"

"Never mind, boys!" cride Dr. Birchemall, springing to his feet. "We've landed him at last, and—and—what the thump——"

The Head stared blankly at his "catch." He had quite eggspected to find a gigantic spessimen of fresh water life wriggling in its deth-throws on the towing-path. What he actually found was an old, tattered boot!

Jack Jolly & Co. looked at that boot. Then they yelled.

"Oh, my hat! Then it wasn't a fish!"

"Nothing like a giddy fish!" grinned Jack Jolly. "It was only an old boot that had got tangled up in the weeds!"

"Ha, ha, ha!"

"Well, if that's not the giddy limit!" gasped the Head. "I thought it mite be a sole; but I never imagined it would be a sole with a heel attached to it. Take a hundred lines each for larfing, you young idiots, and get back to the skool at once. Bust it!"

And the last two words summarised what Dr. Birchemall thought about his afternoon's fishing!

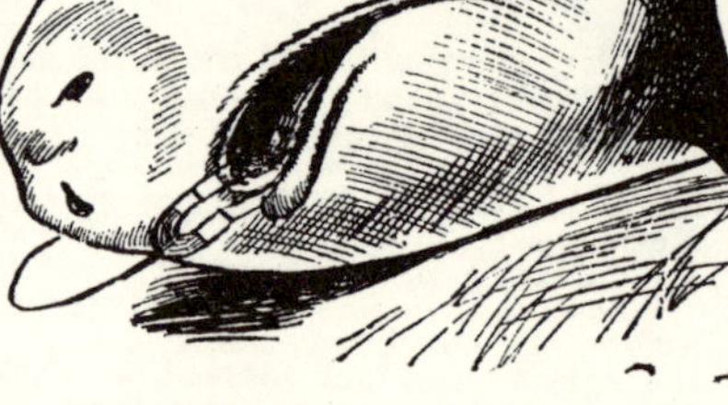

II.

THE following day, Dr. Birchemall summoned Jack Jolly & Co. to his study. There was a twinkle in his greenish eyes as he greeted them.

"Good afternoon, my boys! Squatty-voo and make yourselves at home. I've sent for you to discuss a somewhat confidential matter."

"Nothing doing, I'm afraid, sir!" said Jack Jolly, with a shake of his head. "We're hard up ourselves, as it happens!"

Dr. Birchemall cullered.

"It's not munny I want," he said hastily. "It's honner and glory—in the shape of the Muggleton Anglers' Gold Cup."

"You mean the gold cup they're awarding for the biggest fish caught in the Ripple to-morrow afternoon?" asked Frank Fearless.

"Eggsactly! And I think you boys can help me to win it!" said the Head. "In the first place, I want you to understand that there is nothing savouring of sharp praktiss in my little wheeze, though you mite think there was unless I eggsplained it to you. You see, you must understand that I am undoubtedly the best angler in the Muggleton district. That's agreed, of corse?"

"Oh, of corse, sir!" said Jack Jolly & Co. sollumly, winking at each other.

"Well, that being so, it's only right and proper that I should get the gold cup," eggsplained the Head. "Unforchunitly, however, by the terms of the contest, anyone who happens to catch a bigger fish than I catch wins the prize. So the only way I can secure justice for myself is to make sure beforehand that I shall land the biggest fish."

"And how can you do that, sir?" asked Jack Jolly.

Dr. Birchemall lowered his voice to a whisper.

"Mum's the word, of corse, boys," he said. "But I think my wheeze ought to work the oracle. There's a stuffed whale in the Muggleton Museum. What I want you to do is to borrow it—without permission—insert a powerful magnet in its mouth, and throw it into the river just above the seen of the Angling Contest!"

"Grate pip!"

"I shall have another powerful magnet hanging at the end of my line," went on the Head gleefully, "with the result that as soon as the stuffed whale drifts towards the competitors it will be attracted to my magnet and get hooked on to my line. I shall then proseed to land the monster and win the prize. Get the idea?"

"Grate pip! What a wheeze!" gasped Jack Jolly.

"It takes the whole giddy biskit factory, if you ask me!" said Frank Fearless. "Do you seriously eggspect us to pinch a stuffed whale, sir, just becawse you want to win a fishing championship?"

The Head raised his hands in horror.

"Goodness grashus, Fearless! What ever put such an idea into your noddle? I wouldn't dreem of asking you to pinch it. All I want you to do is to borrow it without permission!"

...es Whaling!

By Dicky Nugent.

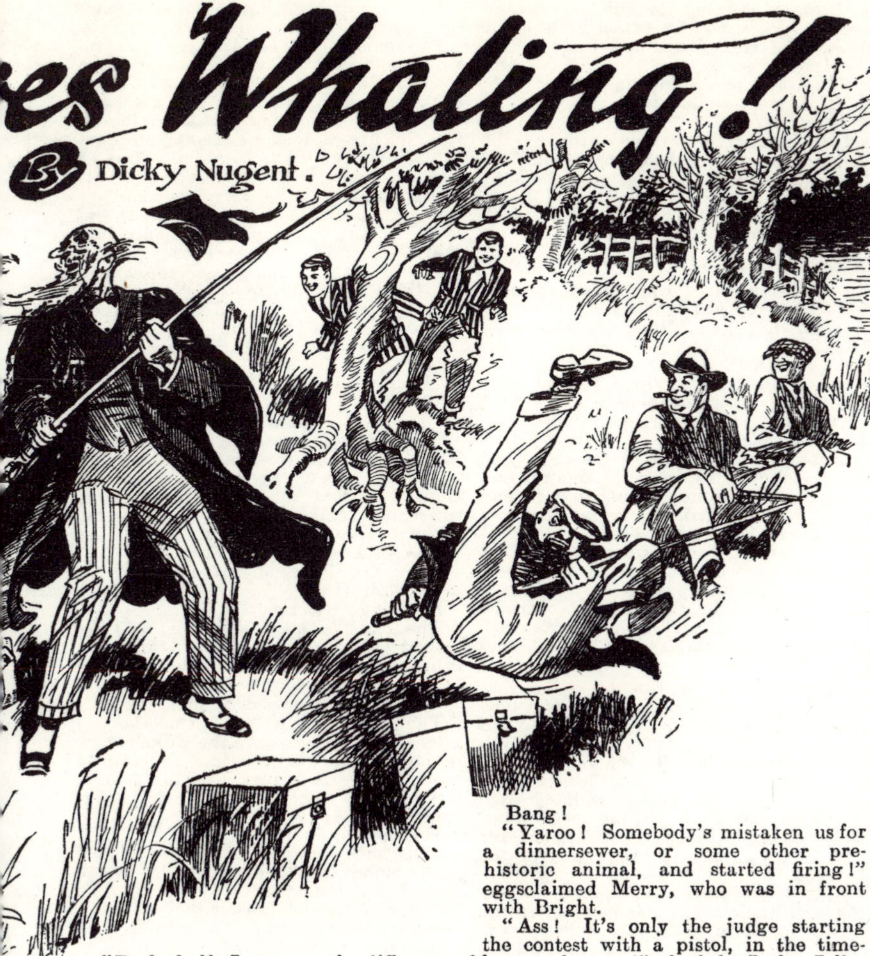

"Dashed if I see much difference, myself!" remarked Jack Jolly candidly. "However, if these are your orders, sir, we won't argew the toss. Rely on us to do our best!"

"Thanks, awfully, Jolly! Call and see me at this time to-morrow, then, and I will give you a powerful magnet for the purpose of fixing into the whale's mouth."

"It's as good as done already, sir!" grinned the kaptin of the Fourth. "You can leave it to us with perfect konfidence. Come on, chaps!"

The Co. then quitted the Head's study, leaving him rubbing his bony hands together in grate sattisfaction.

III.

THE following afternoon four juniors, wearing St. Sam's caps, sneaked steltbily into the museum at Muggleton. Five minnits later they staggered out past the sleeping porter at the front door, carrying between them the tremenjous karkase of a stuffed whale.

Luck was with them. Nobody spotted them coming out, and, though sevveral passers-by pawsed to glannse curiously at the unusual site of a whale in the villidge street, nobody trubbled to ask them where they were taking it.

At last they came in site of the gleeming River Ripple. Vast crowds of anglers and eggsited spectators had gathered at the spot selected for the fishing contest, but Jack Jolly & Co. approached the river from a spot a little higher up, where they could perform their fishy work undisturbed.

Bang!

"Yaroo! Somebody's mistaken us for a dinnersewer, or some other prehistoric animal, and started firing!" eggsclaimed Merry, who was in front with Bright.

"Ass! It's only the judge starting the contest with a pistol, in the time-honnered way!" larfed Jack Jolly. "Ease it up, you chaps, while I put the magnet in its mouth!"

"All sereen, old fellow!"

Fearless and Merry and Bright halted, and supported the stuffed whale between them while Jack Jolly fixed in the magnet. This little operation took him but a brace of shakes, after which Jolly glarnsed cawtiously through the trees to see that the time was ripe for doing the deed. He at once spotted Dr. Birchemall sitting in the long line of fishermen, glarnsing impatiently at his watch. The hour had evvidently arrived!

"All clear, I fansy!" he said, turning to his followers again. "Heave the giddy whale back into its natcheral element!"

Merry and Bright and Fearless were only too glad to obey. The grate stuffed fish slid gracefully off their sholders and glided into the water. In a few ticks it was drifting slowly down towards the fishermen.

"Now let's come and see the fun!" sujjested Frank Fearless.

All four hurried down the river to the seen of the grate fishing competition, keenly interested to see whether the Head's remarkable experiment would work. They found plenty of enthewsiasm prevailing. One competitor had already caught a fine kipper, and another, amid loud cheers, had brought up an unopened tin of sardines.

But these trivial catches were soon put in the shade. Almost as soon as Jack Jolly & Co. arrived, there was a sudden eggsited yell from Dr. Birchemall.

"Stand back, jentlemen! Here comes the catch of a lifetime!"

The Head then jumped to his feet, grinning all over his dial, and began pulling in his line for all he was worth. A great, dark mass arose from out of the water, and there was a roar from the crowd.

"It's a submarine!"

"No, it's not; it's a whale!"

"Hurrah!"

With a final teriffick effort the Head jerked the gigantic fish out of the water, so that it flew through the air and landed on the towpath with a deffening crash.

"There!" gasped the Head. "I fansy we can call the competition ended now. I've won in a canter, jentlemen, and it's all over bar shouting!"

"Half a mo! Where's the judge?" asked somebody.

For a time the judge was nowhere to be seen. But evenchally he crawled out, considerably flattened in appearance, from underneeth the whale itself!

"You—you silly ass!" he roared.

"Sorry!" grinned the Head. "I suppose my record catch must have nocked you over! Never mind; you're well enuff to announce me as the winner of the grate fishing contest!"

Dr. Birchemall was in for a bitter disappointment, however, for when the judge held up his hand for silence, it was not to announce the Head as the winner—far from it!

"Jentlemen!" he cried. "This impertinent raskal has had the cheek to nock the judge over in the middle of the contest. There is only one answer to such a serious breach of rules! Alfred Birchemall, you are disquallified!"

"Wha-a-at?" howled the Head, hardly able to beleeve his ears.

"You are disquallified!" repeeted the judge. "You are not allowed to take any further part in this contest! And if you want to escape even more serious consequences, I advise you to buzz off!"

"But you can't do this, sir," said Dr. Birchemall appeelingly. "I've landed the biggest fish and, according to the terms of the contest, I win the Gold Cup!"

"You'll win a thick ear if you don't vamooze!" roared the angry judge.

"M-m-my hat!"

Dr. Birchemall was almost parrilised with rage! After all the trubble he had gone to—after seeing his experiment suxxeed beyond his wildest hopes—he was disqualified! It was hartrending—maddening! For a moment the Head almost flung himself at the judge. Then he notissed that there were several others present who mite take a hand against him, and he decided otherwise.

With a silent gesture to Jack Jolly & Co. to pick up the whale and follow him, he turned his weery footprints in the direction of St. Sam's.

. . . . . .

It only remains to add that the insident didn't end up so badly from the Head's point of view, after all.

A reward of ten pounds was offered for the recovery of the missing spessimen, and this Dr. Birchemall had the nerve to claim. Although he didn't win the covveted Gold Cup for his fishing eggsploit, he was certainly well "in" on the day!

THE END.

(Look out for more fun and frolic in "THE SCHOOLBOY PROFESSIONAL!" next week's tip-top story of St. Sam's. You'll laugh loud and long when you read it, chums!)

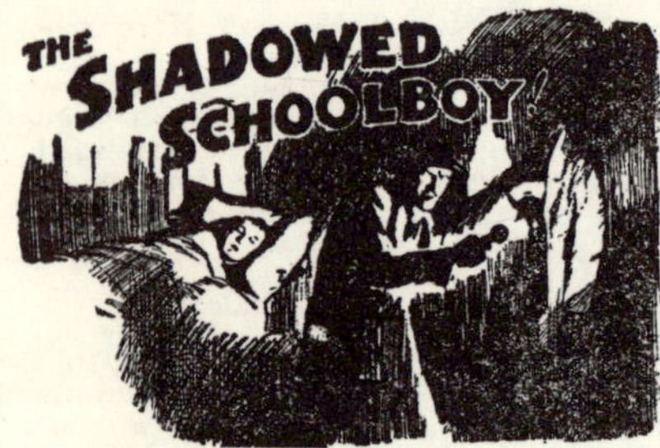

(*Continued from page* 13.)

No doubt that was due to the fact that they could ride them; whereas Bunter was likely to pitch over the head or the tail at a moment's notice.

The Egyptian donkey is a patient animal, and a long-suffering animal; but even the most patient of asses seemed rather worried when Bunter got on his back. Bunter was a rather uncommon weight, and when he was mounted his mount always seemed rather keen to drop him by the wayside at the first opportunity.

But even Billy Bunter's weight was nothing to a camel. And Bunter had no doubt that he could ride a camel. He never had any doubt that he could do anything, until he came to do it.

"Most good camel, sar," said a grinning fat Arab, leading up his tall, long-legged beast, in answer to the dragoman's call. "Oh, yes, sar! Me Ibrahim, sar, owner of finest trotting camel in Egypt, sar."

Bunter looked at the camel. The camel looked at Bunter, with a sneering expression. Really, it might have been supposed that that camel knew the kind of rider Bunter was, and was expressing his contempt in advance.

But that curious, sneering look was the habitual expression of a camel. The camel's sneer is well-known in the East, where it has an explanation which seems extraordinary enough to the West. Hassan had explained it to his lordly gentlemen, in simple good faith. Allah, he had told them, has a hundred names, of which only ninety-nine are known to men. The camel, in his wisdom, has found out the hundreth name, unknown to humans. Hense the scornful sneer of superiority with which the camel regards the human race.

This particular camel looked more sneering and scornful than most camels, and the Famous Five had an impression that he was rather a cross-tempered beast. Still, he was tall and strong, and equal to Bunter's uncommon avoirdupois, and really it was cruelty to animals to land Bunter on a small Egyptian donkey. So the fat Owl was allowed to have his own way.

At a word from Ibrahim, the camel knelt to receive his burden. Ibrahim and Hassan between them hoisted Bunter into the high saddle. The fat Owl settled down there quite comfortably.

He grinned at the donkey-riders.

"I say, you fellows, this is all right!" he declared. "You're welcome to your mokes! He, he, he!"

"This will make history in Egypt!" said Bob Cherry gravely. "First time it's happened, I fancy."

"Eh? Lots of people ride camels here," said Bunter.

"I mean, it's the first time a donkey has been seen riding a camel," explained Bob.

"Oh, don't be a silly ass!" roared Bunter. "Here, Hassan, make this beast get up! I suppose he's not going to stay kneeling all the morning."

Ibrahim grunted to the camel and flicked him with the camel-stick. The quadruped reared up, and there was a roar from Bunter.

"Ow! Help! Stop him! Yarooob!"

"Hold on!" yelled Bob.

"Ha, ha, ha!"

Billy Bunter flew backwards as the camel rose, and he held on for his life. Once the camel had started to rise it seemed to Bunter that he would never stop. He rose and rose and rose, with the fat junior clinging wildly to his hump.

"Oh crikey! Oh crumbs! Hold me!" howled Bunter. "I'm falling off—oh lor'! Oh, my hat! Whooooop!"

"Ha, ha, ha! Stick to him, old bean!"

"Yarooob!"

The camel, on all four feet at last, twisted round his long neck and stared at Bunter. His sneer was more pronounced than ever.

Ibrahim gave a jerk at the rope, and the camel ceased to stare at Bunter, and started. Billy Bunter swung to port, and swung to starboard, and swung fore and swung aft. He blinked with terror at the distance to the ground. At that moment he wished that he had been satisfied with the patient ass; it was a shorter fall if he tumbled off. But he was for it now, and he clung on with both hands, gasped and spluttered, and hoped for the best.

Rather to his surprise, he found that he did not roll off and hit Egypt. The camel's motion was decidedly jerky; and Bunter seemed to be playing at cup-and-ball in the saddle. But he remained in the saddle, at least; and there was no doubt that he was better mounted than the other fellows, so far as speed went. The Famous Five and Lord Mauleverer had to go all out to keep up with the trotting camel.

The donkey-boys ran behind, whacking with their sticks and howling to the donkeys. With a clatter of hoofs, the Greyfriars party went swinging down the road to Karnak.

Billy Bunter was ahead, with Ibrahim running and holding the camel-rope. Bunter's first thought had been to tell the camel-driver to sheer off and leave him to ride on his own. But now that he was aboard the camel, he decided to let Ibrahim go on leading him. Second thoughts were best. Perched high on the camel's hump, Bunter realised that he could no more control his mount than he could have controlled a runaway motor-car. But for Ibrahim's grip on the leading-rope, that camel might have carried Bunter off to the Red Sea or to the Arabian Desert, had the spirit moved him so to do.

Once settled in the saddle, however, and with Ibrahim leading, Bunter began to regain his confidence. Ibrahim was fat, and he panted and gasped as he ran, his brown face streaming with perspiration in the hot sun of Egypt. That, however, did not matter to Bunter. Consideration for others, or a concern for their troubles, had never been one of Bunter's weaknesses.

He blinked round at the donkey-riders behind.

"I say, you fellows! Buck up!" he called out. "I shall be leaving you behind on those mokes! He, he, he!"

Crack! Crack! Crack! rang the donkey-boys' sticks. In a merry bunch the Greyfriars fellows clattered on behind the tall camel.

"I'll wait for you at Karnak!" yelled Bunter. "He, he, he!"

"Don't get out of sight!" shouted Wharton.

"He, he, he!" chortled Bunter. "Can't hang about waiting for those mokes! He, he, he!"

Bunter was growing more and more confident.

The motion of the camel rather resembled that of a Channel steamer in a rough sea. But Bunter found that he could stick on. The camel looked rather a supercilious beast; but he was giving no trouble, except that he seemed to want to go faster than Ibrahim. Bunter fancied himself as a rider—and his experiences with the Egyptian donkeys had not cured him of that fancy! It was Bunter's way to jump, at a bound, into over-confidence. On second thoughts he had allowed Ibrahim to lead the camel. On third thoughts he decided that he was not going to be led along like a fellow who couldn't ride!

He blinked down at the panting fat Arab.

"You can let go!" he called out.

Ibrahim looked up at him.

"Let go!" rapped Bunter.

"Sar, me let go rope, camel he go fast——" gasped Ibrahim.

"That's what I want!" answered Bunter. "You can tell those fellows, when they come up, if they ever do—he, he, he—tell them I'll wait for them at Karnak. Let go my camel."

"Yes, sar!" gasped Ibrahim, relieved, but doubtful.

He let go the rope.

The camel's head shot up, and he looked round at his rider. Really, the camel did not seem to be able to believe in his own good luck!

"Gee up!" snapped Bunter.

The camel "gee'd" up! Once he was released by his master, the camel knew perfectly well that he had nothing to fear from the rider on his hump. Camels are sage animals; and that camel had taken Bunter's measure.

He shot into dizzy speed.

"Oh lor'!" gasped Bunter.

He clung to the high saddle, which rocked on the camel's hump with a horrible feeling of insecurity.

Bunter had intended to handle that camel in a masterly way. He intended to show Ibrahim, and the Greyfriars fellows, and all Luxor for that matter, that he could ride a camel! But a single second was all that was required, once the camel was released, for Bunter to realise that he couldn't!

"Help!" roared Bunter, after the lapse of that single second. "Gerrold of him! Hold him back! Stop him! Whooop!"

But Ibrahim hardly heard him—he was far behind. Anyhow, he could not have helped. The camel was going strong.

Ibrahim, mopping his perspiring brow with a fold of his dingy djubbah, gasped to a halt. The road to Karnak was once lined on both sides with hundreds of sphinxes, most of which have disappeared in the course of the centuries. But here and there a sphinx still crops up by the side of the ancient road.

Ibrahim gasped his way to the nearest, and sat on it and mopped his brow with the tail of his djubbah and blinked after Bunter. Ibrahim was well aware that that camel was an obstinate and bad-tempered camel; but it would have behaved itself so long as its master's hand was on the head-rope. But the master's hand was gone now, and the camel was left free to act according to the inwardness of its own nature. Its heels could hardly be seen for dust as it went up the road. Ibrahim sat on the sphinx and watched it disappear.

Bunter would have given much to do the same. But Bunter was on the camel; and everywhere that camel went, Bunter was sure to go! He rocked to and fro at a terrifying height from the ground, holding on for his fat life and yelling for help. Other passengers on the road stared at him. Arabs gave him grave stares; negroes cackled with laughter. An American tourist hurriedly snap-shotted him with a camera. Bunter hardly saw them as he raced by.

"Oh lor'! Help! Yarooop!" roared Bunter. "I say, you fellows—whooop!"

But Harry Wharton & Co. were out of sight behind. A motor-car whizzed by, with a loud honking, and the camel swerved and reared and snorted. He did not seem to like cars. Bunter swung to, and he swung fro; and nearly pitched off. Somehow he clung on, sprawling over the high saddle and clutching wildly at the camel's hairy neck.

A Good Samaritan on the road jumped at the camel to stop him. The camel swerved away and thundered into a dusty track that led away from the right of the road. Bunter had told the other fellows that he would wait for them at Karnak. But he was not heading for Karnak now. He was heading for the Red Sea—if he had only known it. Still, as the Red Sea was about seventy miles distant, it was to be hoped that Bunter would not arrive there.

Thud! Thud! Thud!

The camel's hoofs beat an incessant tattoo on the dusty road. Once off the main road, there was little traffic, and no help for Bunter.

"Stop, you beast!" shrieked Bunter.

The camel showed no sign of stopping.

Egyptian fellaheen, working in the fields, looked up at Billy Bunter, and stared after him as he flew past. Peasants carrying burdens on the road dodged out of the way of the camel, and turned to stare till it vanished. A village appeared in view, and dark-skinned children, ducks and geese and fowls scattered frantically out of Bunter's way. Brown men stared at him; brown women peered at him over their yashmaks. Bunter flew on. He flew through the village, and thundered on past an orange plantation.

Red, ripe oranges glistened in the sun on the trees, without getting a glance from Bunter. Even eatables had no appeal for him now. He rocked on along the rows of orange-trees. An Arab appeared in the road ahead, and shouted and brandished a stick at the camel. The camel did not stop. He swerved suddenly in a new direction.

That sudden swerve did it!

Bunter flew!

The camel, still going strong, thundered on without a rider. Billy Bunter crashed!

Branches broke his fall—and his fall broke the branches. He found himself sitting on the earth, with oranges showering down on him. And the roar he gave as he landed might have been heard almost from the Nile to the Red Sea.

"Yarooooooh!"

THE NINTH CHAPTER.

Where is Bunter?

"HALLO, hallo, hallo!"

"That's Bunter's keeper!"

"But where's Bunter?"

"And the jolly old camel?"

Harry Wharton & Co. reined in the donkeys. Sitting by the roadside, dusty and dismal, squatting on a damaged sphinx, was Ibrahim, the camel-owner. With the tail of his djubbah he was still mopping his dusty brow, wiping away great drops of perspiration, as the chums of Greyfriars came trotting up. The juniors, finding the camel-man there, looked round for the camel and its rider, but nothing was to be seen of either. They had doubted whether Bunter would have good luck on that camel. Now they no longer doubted.

Ibrahim crawled off the roadside sphinx and salaamed to the donkey-riders as they halted in a bunch. Hassan spoke to him in Arabic, and Ibrahim answered in that tongue at great length and with considerable emphasis. The camel-man was obviously excited about something.

"Gentlemanly lords," said the dragoman, "him say small, fat, lordly gentleman ride away on a camel at gigantic speed, and is seen no more."

"He must have gone on to Karnak," said Harry.

"Ibrahim think him lose," answered Hassan cheerfully. "Think him run away from a road and never come back at any time whatever. Think small, fat lord fall off a camel and break a neck. Yes, sar! Ibrahim want pay for a camel."

"Oh, my hat!"

The juniors stared up the road towards Karnak. A tall column showed against the sky, and round it masses of ruins, like a dismantled city of the dead. There were several passengers to be seen on the road, going to the ruins or coming away from them. But among them there was no Bunter. But at the speed at which Bunter had been going he could easily have reached Karnak long since, and the Removites hoped that he had done so.

Ibrahim waved excited hands, and talked Arabic. Evidently he was very anxious about his camel. Translated by Hassan, he explained, with voluble earnestness, that that camel was a very precious camel. Such a camel was not to be equalled among all the camels from the Red Sea to Morocco. It was his means of livelihood, his favourite and his pet, his father and his mother and sister and brother; in fact, all his family. It was a camel that he would not have lost for uncounted piastres. But now it was lost, and only backsheesh on a liberal scale could set the matter right.

Ten thousand piastres was, according to Ibrahim, a low estimate of the value of that precious camel, but, being a particularly honest man, and an example to all camel-drivers in that respect, he would only ask the English lords for that sum. This would reimburse him for the material loss, but leave his grief at the loss of the camel unassuaged. But his grief, it seemed, could be had free of charge.

Hassan translated all this, and more. Obviously, Ibrahim's concern was wholly for the camel. He was not thinking of Bunter.

"Ten thousand piastres is a hundred pounds," said Wharton. "Tell him to go to sleep and dream again, Hassan."

"Sar!" roared Ibrahim. "You pay for a camel! Yes! Fat person, sar, he tell me let go a camel. He take away a camel. I lose a camel. I am a ruin! Yes, sar, I am a ruin! You pay for one camel!"

"Tell him he's gone to find Bunter, Hassan, and never mind about the camel!" said Bob Cherry.

Hassan put this into Arabic, and the effect on the camel-driver was quite startling. He waved his hands, he shouted, he danced. The donkey-boys screeched with laughter.

"Ten to one Bunter's at Karnak," said Frank Nugent. "We've got to look for him, anyhow. Come on!"

Whack, whack, whack! went the donkey-sticks, and the party trotted on. After them whisked Ibrahim, still waving his hands and roaring. Whether that honest man really believed that his camel was lost the juniors did not know, but they thought it improbable. It was much more probable that he had scented wealth in the party, and wanted to annex some of it. Anyhow, the matter of the camel could be dealt with later. At present they were anxious about Bunter.

Shrieks in Arabic followed them from Ibrahim.

"What is he saying now, Hassan?" asked Harry.

Hassan grinned.

"He say he take five thousand piastres for that most excellent camel, sar, which is lose."

The price is coming down," grinned Bob Cherry. "Let him rip! By the time we get to Karnak it may be quite a cheap camel."

"Ha, ha, ha!"

The juniors trotted on cheerfully. Falling into the distance behind them, Ibrahim followed on, evidently determined not to lose sight of them. The juniors arrived at the ruins of Karnak, and halted near the Temple of Khons. Nothing was to be seen of Bunter.

"Now, where's that fat frump?" asked Johnny Bull.

"Goodness knows!"

"Must be somewhere about," said Bob. "It would be like Bunter to sit down in the shade somewhere and leave us to hunt for him."

"Just like him," grunted Johnny Bull. "He would think it funny to let us spend the morning rooting about after him while he was scoffing cakes and sherbet in some shady corner."

"Great and enormous Temple of Khons——" began Hassan. The dragoman was getting down to business. His lordly gentlemen had ridden out to Karnak to see the sights, not to discuss what had become of Bunter.

"Blessed if I know what to do," said Harry. "Ten to one he's somewhere about, and if he isn't, we don't know where to look for him. I think we'd better get on with it and give him a chance to turn up."

"Yaas," assented Lord Mauleverer.

"What do you think, Hassan?" asked Harry.

"Me, sar, me think him little fat gentleman fall off a camel, sar," said the dragoman. "Him walk to Karnak afterwards. Yes!"

"That's about it," said Harry.

And the juniors started to explore Karnak. They had no doubt that the camel had dropped Bunter somewhere between Luxor and the ruins, and that he would come rolling in on foot sooner or later. They decided to give him till lunch, anyhow. If Bunter did not turn up for lunch, certainly there would be grounds for alarm. Only something of a serious nature could possibly keep the Owl of the Remove away from a meal.

There was plenty to be seen at Karnak, and Hassan's sing-song voice never ceased as he pointed out its wonders: The great Temple of Khons, the Temple of Epet, the hippopotamus

(*Continued on next page.*)

goddess; the vast Temple of Amun, in which Hassan pointed out a gigantic relief of the Battle of Kedesh. This rather interested the juniors, as Lord Mauleverer's scarab had once been an amulet worn by the warrior A-Menah at that ancient battle in Syria. Then they visited the Temple of Ptah, and more temples and pylons than they could have counted, and by lunch-time, as Bob Cherry remarked, they had done a good morning's work.

But Bunter had not turned up!

If the camel had dropped him anywhere near Karnak, Bunter had had time to arrive, even at his usual snail's pace. And the juniors began to wonder whether, after all, there had been any accident.

At the same time they knew it was quite likely that Bunter had stopped somewhere to feed, especially as he had borrowed a handful of piastres from Lord Mauleverer that morning.

If he had stopped to feed, it was highly probable that he had stopped to nap after the feed. And they knew their Bunter too well to suppose that he would care two straws whether they were alarmed or not.

In these circumstances they did not feel disposed to be unduly alarmed. Lunch had been brought in a basket, and they sat down under a shady acacia-tree to dispose of it. Ibrahim hovered on the horizon; but whenever he came near, Hassan volleyed Arabic at him and drove him off again. Every now and then a shout from him reached the juniors:

"Pay for a camel! Yes, oh, yes! Pay for a camel! You pay 2,000 piastres for a camel that is lose!"

"Getting cheaper," grinned Bob Cherry. "We shall get that jolly old camel at a bargain in the long run."

The juniors lunched, and rested in the fiercest heat of the Egyptian day. When it was time to move again Hassan was keen to recommence on the wonders of Karnak, of which his lordly gentlemen had by no means seen all. But the juniors were getting worried about Bunter now.

"Better give Karnak a miss, and look for him," said Harry. "If the fat chump's got lost he's got to be found. Hassan can inquire along the road; lots of natives about, and anyone who has seen Bunter will remember him——"

"You bet!" grinned Bob. "They don't often see a circumference like Bunter's. Let's get after the howling ass!"

And the juniors, remounting the donkeys, rode back on the road towards Luxor, Hassan inquiring of innumerable natives for news of a small, fat Faringhee on a runaway camel—and very soon picking up news. Plenty of people had seen Bunter on his wild career—indeed, he seemed to have astonished all the natives between Luxor and Karnak.

Behind the juniors, as they trotted away, trotted Ibrahim, evidently determined not to lose sight of them. His voice formed a sort of accompaniment to the thudding of the donkeys' hoofs.

"You pay for a camel! Yes, sar! Oh, yes! Pay for one camel which is lose! Wahyat-en-nabi! Shall you not pay for a camel? You pay 1,000 piastres for a camel!"

"Cheaper and cheaper!" chuckled Bob Cherry. "Price still coming down, you fellows. He'll be giving us that camel at the finish!"

"Ha, ha, ha!"

The juniors had little doubt that the camel, after getting shut of its rider, would go home. Indeed, the fact that Ibrahim had brought the indemnity down to 1,000 piastres—which was only ten pounds—rather indicated that he did not really expect to lose that valuable camel. Anyhow, they were not bothering about the camel now; Bunter was enough to bother about. They trotted on, with Ibrahim trotting and perspiring behind, his voice coming plaintively every few minutes:

"You pay for a camel! O protectors of the poor, I think you pay for a camel! By the beard of the Prophet, you pay for a camel!"

THE TENTH CHAPTER.
The Way of the Transgressor!

PLOP, plop, plop, plop!

"Oooooogh!"

Billy Bunter liked oranges. But he liked them taken internally; now he was taking them externally, in a shower.

Bunter hardly knew what had happened. His parting with the runaway camel had been sudden and surprising. He found himself sitting on the earth, with broken branches of orange-trees trailing round him, and dislodged oranges falling on his head. He roared, he spluttered, and he gasped.

His first impression was that he had been smashed into several pieces. That impression proved to be unfounded. It dawned upon him that he was still in one piece, and that nothing had happened to him except a bump and a shaking. Slowly his breath came back, and he blinked round him, wondering dismally where he was. Obviously he was nowhere near Karnak; the camel had covered a considerable distance since leaving the road, following the dusty track that led away among maize-fields and plantations and irrigating canals. The camel was gone; there was no chance of remounting his fiery, untamed steed—not that Bunter would have remounted him at any price. Bunter did not like walking, but he would have walked miles and miles rather than have perched himself on that camel's hump again.

"Oh dear!" groaned Bunter.

He sat and gasped for breath for quite a long time. Oranges ceased to plop on him. They lay thickly around him on the earth. They were ripe, red oranges, and as soon as he realised that he was not hurt, and had recovered his wind, Bunter helped himself to the juicy fruit. The camel had hurled him into the orange plantation—and he might really have landed in less attractive quarters. There was solace in scoffing the oranges, and Billy Bunter was soon surrounded by pips and peel. He had to find his way back somehow. But there was plenty of time for that; he wanted a rest first. And the oranges were good.

Bunter was on his tenth orange, when a figure in turban and djubbah appeared in the plantation, coming along through the rows of orange-trees.

Bunter blinked at the newcomer.

It was a native—no doubt some "nigger" who worked on the plantation, or perhaps the proprietor. Bunter hoped that he would be able to speak English, and tell him where he was and how to get away.

The native spotted him under the trees and came quickly towards him. As he approached, something familiar in his aspect struck Bunter. He had seen that dark-skinned man before somewhere.

"Oh crikey!" gasped Bunter, as he recognised him.

It was the orange merchant of the Nile, to whom Bunter had handed that bad Egyptian "quid." Bunter had landed in the orange plantation belonging to Mustapha!

Mustapha stared down at him, evidently recognising the fat Faringhee with whom he had done business on the dahabiyeh. The expression that came over his dark face made Bunter shudder.

"You—teef!" said Mustapha, pointing a brown and somewhat dirty forefinger at the fat Owl. "You steal oranges! Yes!"

"Oh crumbs!" gasped Bunter.

He had "scoffed" the oranges that lay thick about him without giving a single thought to the fact that they were obviously private property. Mustapha really was not in the orange business for the purpose of supplying a fat Faringhee with oranges for nothing.

"Teef!" roared Mustapha.

Bunter scrambled up.

"I—I—I say——"

"You steal oranges!" roared Mustapha. "Yes! You give bad, naughty pound for oranges, and you come steal! Yes! Teef!"

"Oh, draw it mild!" gasped Bunter. "I'll pay for the blessed oranges! I say, I never came here; I fell off a camel——"

"You pay!" said Mustapha grimly. "Yes! I think! You pay backsheesh! Oh! Yes! By the beard of the Prophet, yes! I think!"

He turned his head and shouted to someone as yet unseen in the plantation. Bunter did not understand Arabic, but he fancied that he caught the word "kourbash." He was aware that kourbash implied a stick.

Evidently it was time for Bunter to go!

He made a strategic movement to depart while Mustapha's head was turned. But the orange-grower seemed to have eyes in the back of his head. He spun round, jumped at Bunter, and grasped him by the shoulder. The fat Owl gave a yell of terror.

"Ow! Leggo! I—I wasn't going to——"

"You stay on the spot!" grinned Mustapha. "Yes! You pay backsheesh, and you take stick! Oh! Yes!"

A dark-skinned "fellah" came through the trees with a stick in his hand. He handed the stick to Mustapha. Billy Bunter eyed it, with deep apprehension.

"I—I—I say——" he gasped.

"You pay backsheesh!"

Bunter fumbled in his pockets. Fortunately, he had borrowed a lot of piastres from the long-suffering Mauly that mornng. He was able to pay—and oranges were cheap on the Nile. A few pastres ought to have settled the matter. Bunter held out a fat hand with a dozen piastres in it.

"There you are!" he gasped.

Mustapha accepted the piastres, stared at them, sniffed contemptuously, and slipped them into some recess of his djubbah.

"More backsheesh!" he snapped.

"Look here, I've jolly well paid you!" howled Bunter indignantly. "I'm not going to pay you any more! See? Here, I say, keep that stick away, you cheeky nigger!" yelled Bunter.

"You pay more backsheesh!"

Billy Bunter fished out a dozen more piastres. They followed the others into the dingy djubbah, and the brown hand was held out for more.

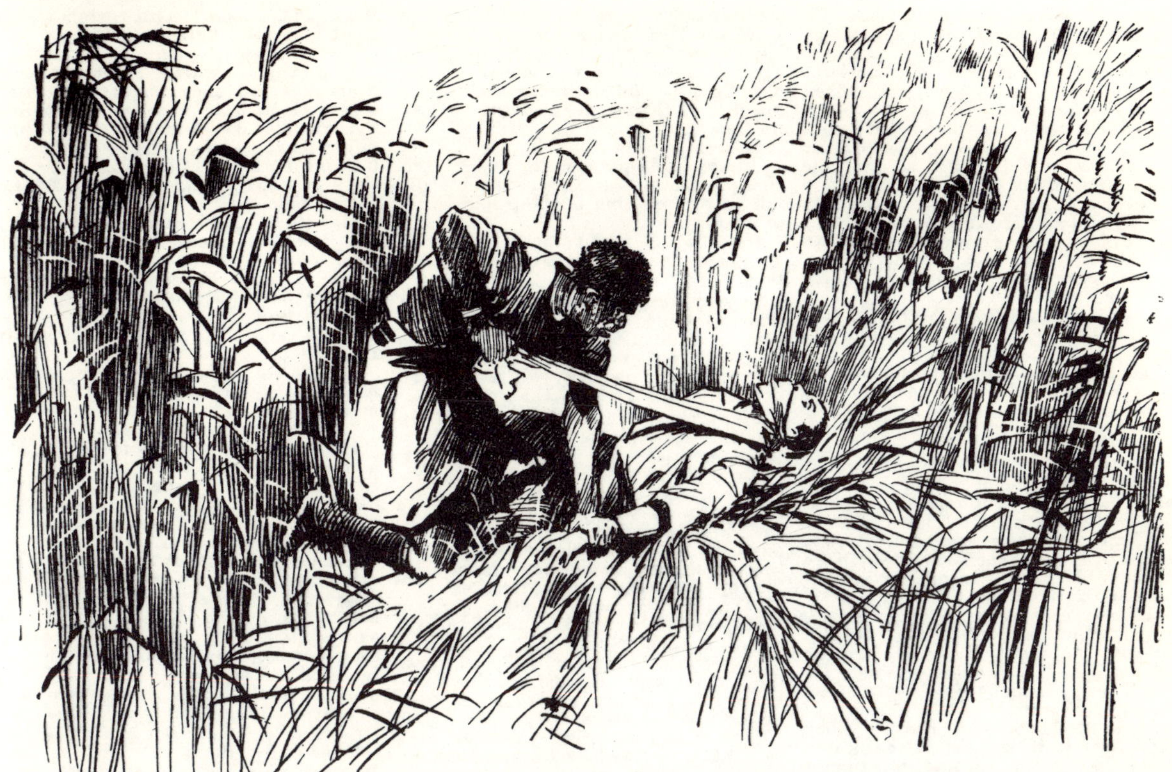

Lord Mauleverer sprawled in the crushed maize, the scarred Arab kneeling on him, gagging him with a strip of turban before he could utter a cry. Half-choked by the gag, only able to breathe through his nose, the Greyfriars junior stared dizzily at the face above him !

"Look here——" gasped Bunter, in dismay.

"You pay more backsheesh !" roared Mustapha. "You steal oranges ! Yes ! You teef ! You pay backsheesh !"

Mustapha held out his left hand for the backsheesh. He flourished the stick in his right.

"Oh lor' !" gasped Bunter.

There was no help for it. Evidently Mustapha had a very bitter recollection of that deal in oranges on the Nile. In any case, Mustapha would doubtless have extracted the uttermost backsheesh from any Faringhee whom he had discovered trespassing in his plantation and pinching the oranges. But in Bunter's case, he had an impression that he was dealing with an even bigger rogue than himself. Bunter had "done" him on the Nile—and Mustapha was accustomed to "doing" Faringhees, not to being done by them. This unexpected meeting was a sheer satisfaction to Mustapha. The satisfaction was all on his side !

Bunter handed over more piastres. The flourishing stick was not to be argued with.

"More backsheesh!" rapped Mustapha.

"Oh, you beast!" gasped Bunter. "Oranges ain't worth much here——"

"More backsheesh!" roared Mustapha.

"I've given you three hundred piastres, you awful beast!" yelled Bunter.

"More backsheesh !"

"Look here—— Yarooooh !"

The stick cracked on Bunter's fat shoulders.

"You give more backsheesh !" shouted Mustapha. "Yes ! You teef ! Yes !"

"Oh lor' !" groaned Bunter.

More piastres were handed over. It dawned on Bunter that the Arab merchant intended to take all he had about him. It was sheer robbery; but the hapless fat Owl had placed himself in the wrong. A fellow who passed bad money and was caught "pinching" oranges in a plantation had little sympathy to expect from the law if he laid a complaint at Luxor.

Bunter did not know how the law would regard the transaction; but he felt that he would be misunderstood, as usual. Anyhow, there was no law on the spot. Mustapha was on the spot with a big stick in his hand !

"More backsheesh!" hooted Mustapha.

Bunter groaned and went through his pockets. He had "touched" Mauly for a thousand piastres that morning. Exactly a thousand piastres passed over to Mustapha. Still he was not satisfied.

"More backsheesh !" he howled threateningly.

"Oh crikey ! I haven't any more !" wailed Bunter. "I've given you all I have, you beast !"

Mustapha scanned him keenly. He flourished the stick. He realised that he had taken all the fat Faringhee had.

As there was no more backsheesh to come, it was time for the stick to be featured in the programme.

Whack, whack !

"Yaroooh !" roared Bunter. "Oh crikey ! Keep off, you beast ! You beast ! You cheeky nigger—— Whoop !"

Whack, whack, whack !

"You teef !" grinned Mustapha. "You give naughty money—you steal oranges ! I, Mustapha, beat a teef with stick ! Yes !"

Whack, whack, whack ! Billy Bunter ran for his life.

After him plunged Mustapha, with the stick still whacking. Mustapha seemed to be quite enjoying himself.

Whack, whack !

"Yarooooooop !"

Bunter burst out of the plantation into the dusty lane. Mustapha followed on. Bunter ran—and Mustapha ran ! The stick whacked and whacked !

Mustapha seemed to fancy Bunter a donkey and himself a donkey-boy ! Bunter put on a burst of speed, panting and perspiring as he flew. Whack, whack, whack, whack, came the stick behind as he raced.

"Teef ! Yes ! I beat a teef !" chanted Mustapha, as he whacked. "Very naughty teef ! I beat a teef with stick ! Yes !"

Whack, whack, whack !

"Oh crikey ! Oh lor' ! Help ! Whoooooop !"

The hapless Owl of the Remove was suffering for his sins. The way of the transgressor was hard ! A licking from Mr. Quelch at Greyfriars was nothing to this !

Whack, whack, whack !

"Yow-ow-ow ! Stoppit ! Yooooop !"

Mustapha stopped at last. Probably it was only because he was out of breath. He grinned, tucked the stick under his arm, and walked back to his oranges.

Billy Bunter plugged desperately on, still yelling. But he realised at last that he was no longer pursued, and he threw himself down in the shade of a group of date-trees by the wayside, and gasped and groaned and groaned and gasped, as if he would never leave off gasping and groaning.

THE ELEVENTH CHAPTER.

Lost !

"OH lor' !" groaned Billy Bunter. He wiped the streaming perspiration from his face and swatted his millionth fly.

He wondered dismally where he was.

He was somewhere in Egypt! He knew that! But that was about all he knew.

After resting under the date-trees for an hour or so the fat Owl had started on his homeward way—or, at least, what he hoped was his homeward way. Karnak was somewhere, and Luxor was somewhere else, and so was the Nile! The sight of any of the three would have been welcome to Bunter. But he did not see any of them. He had a horrid misgiving that perhaps he was wandering away from them.

Tramping along a narrow dusty track, he did not know where it led, but he was fairly certain that it was not the same track by which Ibrahim's camel had carried him that morning.

Fields of maize, plantations of oranges, and other fruits, endless tiny canals, date-palms, and bunches of acacias, met his view as he plugged on; but Bunter had no use for them. From the bottom of his fat heart he repented him of having mounted that detestable camel to Luxor. But repentance, as is usually the case, came too late! Bunter was lost—hopelessly lost—and it was frightfully hot, and the flies were innumerable. He streamed with perspiration as he plugged dismally on.

It was useless to question the natives he spotted in his wanderings. They did not speak a word of English; and he did not speak a word of Arabic. He longed for the sight of a white face, but though there were plenty of tourists at Luxor and Karnak, they were apparently keeping to the beaten tracks, in the way of tourists; Bunter did not see any of them.

Matters would have been better if he had had money in his pockets. By holding up a handful of piastres and saying "Luxor," he might have found a guide. But the iniquitous Mustapha had taken care of that! Bunter had not a single piastre in his possession.

He had tried to ask his way once or twice, and one good-natured "fellah," comprehending that he wanted to get to Luxor, had pointed across the fields—which was not of much use to Bunter. A handful of piastres might have induced the man to leave his work and guide the fat Owl; but once more Bunter found himself up against the selfishness of human nature. The Egyptian fellaheen seemed to have business of their own to attend to, and no time to attend to Bunter's.

It was getting too hot for further exertions. Bunter was hungry by this time; but even the hope of lunch could not keep him going in the tropical heat of midday.

He blinked round through his big spectacles for a shelter from the sun, to take a rest.

At the corner of a field of waving dhurra, close by a wide-spreading acacia, he spotted a shed. It had a doorway, but no door, and Bunter limped into it, gasping with relief as he got out of the glare of the sun.

Big wicker baskets were stacked up one side of the shed. No doubt they were used for the packing of agricultural products; but they were empty now. Bunter blinked dismally round the shed. It was a shelter from the sun, but that was all. Had there been anything of an edible nature in the baskets Bunter would have been comforted. But they were empty.

"Oh lor'!" groaned Bunter.

He blinked out of the open doorway. There was no one in sight. A dusty donkey-track ran from the shed, past the acacias and the maize fields, probably in the direction of a road. But no one was to be seen.

There was cultivation—the close, rich cultivation of Egypt—all round Bunter; but he might as well have been in the desert, so far as human beings were concerned. Had there been a native at hand, Bunter could have announced that he was hungry by the language of signs. But there was no one at hand to whom he could make that important and pressing announcement.

Still, it was something to be out of the fierce glare of the sun. The fat Owl stretched himself on the earthen floor, pillowed his head on a fat arm, and went to sleep.

Bunter did not think much of Egypt and its customs; but there was one Eastern custom that appealed to him—the midday snooze! That custom struck Bunter as solid horse-sense!

He slept and snored.

Had any Egyptian fellaheen come near the shed they might have been surprised to hear a sound resembling the rumble of distant thunder, and might have fancied that a storm was brewing on the banks of the Nile. But the spot remained deserted, and Bunter snored unheard.

He might have snored on till sunset; but it was the inner Bunter that woke him. There was an aching void in Bunter. Since breakfast he had had nothing but Mustapha's oranges. The heat of the day was over when he awoke, and he awoke frightfully hungry!

He sat up, rubbed his sleepy eyes, set his spectacles straight on his fat little nose, swatted flies, and groaned.

"Oh lor'!" said Bunter.

He rose wearily to his feet. He was hungry—famished—ravenous! It was like his awful experience on the dahabiyeh over again! He rolled to the open doorway and blinked out.

"Beasts!" groaned Bunter.

The Greyfriars fellows, of course, were mooning about Karnak with the dragoman, staring at idiotic temples and tombs, instead of looking for Bunter as they ought to have been. Or if they were looking for him, they hadn't found him, which was just as bad. Not even a beastly nigger was to be seen.

That shed, no doubt, was used for something or other; but nobody seemed to be using it now! Nothing met Bunter's view but a dusty track, scattered acacias, and endless, moving maize.

The fierce heat of the day was over; but it was still hot—very hot! Bunter was extremely unwilling to recommence his wanderings, with yawning emptiness in his fat inside. But he had to get something to eat!

If only some beastly nigger would have turned up—— Bunter felt that even a bunch of dates would save his life!

"Oh, good!" he ejaculated suddenly.

A dingy turban showed over the waving maize. It was coming in the direction of the shed.

Bunter blinked at it eagerly. It was a "beastly nigger" at last—and the blackest nigger in Africa would have been welcome to Bunter just then. The man in the turban came in sight—and Bunter gave a convulsive jump, and backed farther into the shed. It was not one of the "fellaheen" who worked in the fields. It was an Arab who was coming towards the shed. It was an Arab that Bunter knew. Well he remembered that hard, hawkish face—the face of Yussef, the Arab desperado, in the service of Kalizelos, the Greek. Any other Arab—excepting Hamza—would have been welcome to Bunter's eyes. But the sight of the hawk-faced ruffian almost froze him with terror.

"Oh crikey!" gasped Bunter.

He fairly bounded away from the door. The ruffian had not seen him—and Bunter did not mean to be seen, if he could help it. This was the ruffian who had attacked Lord Mauleverer in the hotel at Cairo, weeks ago, and whom Bunter had smitten on the head with a stool. He did not expect Yussef to have forgotten that incident. The thought of being cornered by the ferocious rascal almost curdled his blood.

The man was coming to the shed! Bunter could hear his footsteps now. No doubt Yussef had been with Kalizelos when he crept on the dahabiyeh the previous night, and was hanging about the vicinity, probably wondering what had become of his master—perhaps spying on the Greyfriars party. If he entered the shed and found Bunter there—— Bunter remembered the dagger hidden under the ruffian's galabieh, and shuddered.

He backed out of sight behind the stack of baskets against the wall. There was plenty of cover. Certainly, Yussef was not likely to suspect that he was there if he did not see him.

Bunter palpitated and waited and listened.

The footsteps came nearer.

If they passed the shed——

But they did not pass the shed. They came in at the open doorway.

Billy Bunter suppressed his breathing.

Only the stack of wicker baskets stood between him and the savage Arab—a desperate outcast, to whom his life would have been no more than a mosquito's.

What did the beast want there? What could be his business in that lonely shed, far from all habitations? Evidently he had some business there, for he did not go.

Bunter heard him sit down, leaning back against the pile of baskets. The wicker baskets creaked as he leaned on them, and Bunter barely suppressed a gasp. A scent of smoke came to him.

The Arab was smoking cigarettes. From where he sat he faced the open doorway. It dawned on Bunter, at last, that the lonely shed was a place of appointment—that Yussef was waiting for someone to join him there—as likely as not the scarred ruffian Hamza. Perhaps the outcasts were camping in that shed, while they waited for news of their missing master.

Bunter could have groaned at the thought. But he did not dare to groan. He crouched in the shadowy recess behind the baskets, and stilled his breathing, while the hawk-faced Arab, little dreaming that he was there, sat and smoked, and watched the sunny, dusty track winding away among the maize fields.

——

THE TWELFTH CHAPTER.

Hunting Bunter!

"LORDLY sars, here we go turning on!" said Hassan, probably meaning "turning off."

The Greyfriars fellows had reached the spot where Bunter's camel had turned off the road that morning. Three or four dark-skinned fellaheen, working in the fields, answered Hassan's inquiries, bawled in Arabic. It had not been at all difficult to pick up news of Bunter, so far.

Billy Bunter rather prided himself on his distinguished appearance, and flattered himself that he was worth a second glance anywhere. Undoubtedly he was distinguished enough to draw a second, and even a third and fourth glance; but the other fellows believed that it was his width that did it! Anyhow, the juniors found that quite a lot of people had seen a fat Faringhee careering on a runaway camel.

Hassan pointed along the dusty way with his stick. The juniors looked along the narrow route among the maize fields.

"Him fat lord go this way on a camel!" said Hassan.

"What the thump did he turn off the road for?" grunted Johnny Bull. "What the dickens did even that fat ass want to do that for?"

"Him no want, sar; him camel want," said Hassan.

The juniors grinned. They had no doubt that it was the camel, not Bunter, that had decided to leave the road.

"Well, if the howling ass went that way, that's our way!" said Bob. "Come on. If Bunter hasn't snaffled any lunch, matters will be getting serious. Instead of seeing the ruins of Karnak, we shall see the ruins of Bunter!"

The donkey-riders turned off the road, and the hoofs knocked up dust on the track through the fields. Behind them Ibrahim came puffing and panting, his dusty djubbah blowing out behind him. His voice came plaintively from afar.

"You pay for a camel! O noble gentlemens, you pay for one lost camel! You pay five hundred piastres for one camel which is lose!"

The price of the lost camel was still coming down. Perhaps, now that the juniors were on Bunter's trail, Ibrahim feared that they might sight the lost camel. He was anxious to bag his backsheesh before such a disaster could happen. But the juniors gave no heed to the voice behind.

Again and again Hassan questioned natives in the fields, in incomprehensible Arabic. Sometimes they grinned as they answered—from which the juniors guessed that they had seen Bunter, and remembered him.

Never had there been so many clues to a lost article. The party kept on the trot, assured that they were drawing nearer to Bunter—feeling strongly inclined to kick him if he had had no serious accident, while prepared to sympathise if he had—which was rather a mixed state of feeling.

They passed through a village, where there was plenty of news of Bunter. The Egyptian villagers had not forgotten how he had scattered infants and ducks and fowls in his wild career.

They passed through the village, and trotted on beyond. They did not expect to find Bunter still on the camel, after all these hours; but evidently he must have stuck on for a considerable time before falling off. Where had he fallen off?—was the question.

"Hallo, hallo, hallo!" roared Bob Cherry suddenly.

"What——"

"The jolly old camel!" roared Bob.

"Oh, my hat!"

"Him camel!" grinned Hassan. "Him lose small fat gentleman! Yes, sar!"

Under an acacia by the wayside sprawled an ungainly form, which the juniors knew at once. It was the supercilious camel that had sneered at Bunter that morning. It sprawled on its stomach, its long neck extended, taking a rest in the shade of the acacia. No doubt it was waiting for the cool of the evening before it trotted home to Luxor.

"You pay for a camel!" Ibrahim was chanting in the rear, when he broke off suddenly at the sight of the animal under the tree, and ejaculated:

"Bismillah!"

Ibrahim's jaw dropped.

His misgivings had been well-founded! Here was the camel; and Ibrahim's hopes of an indemnity for a lost camel vanished on the spot. It was quite a dismaying encounter for the honest man.

The camel raised his head, and sneered at the donkey-riders. No doubt he recognised the party again; and perhaps he thought that his fat burden was to be landed on him once more.

He dragged himself on his long, ungainly legs, sneering more than ever, and looked inclined to take to his heels. Ibrahim came to a halt, at a distance behind. No doubt he considered that if the camel escaped, he might still claim to be indemnified for a lost camel.

"Catch him!" exclaimed Bob Cherry. "Spread out and surround the brute. We shall want him to stick Bunter on when we pick him up."

"Yaas, begad!" said Lord Mauleverer. "Catch his rope, somebody."

The head-rope was trailing from the camel. The donkey-riders spread out to cut off the camel's escape, and Hassan approached him with soothing gestures, to seize the trailing rope. But the camel declined to listen to the voice of the charmer. He backed, snorting, to the wayside, turned, and plunged into a field of tall, waving maize.

"After him!" shouted Wharton.

The donkey-riders plunged into the maize, leaving the donkey-boys on the road. The camel streaked across the maize field, but on the farther side was a canal, and he stopped and swung round. He rushed back towards the road again, snorting and squealing, with the juniors round him, and Hassan making frantic clutches at the trailing, whisking rope.

"Stop him!" roared Wharton to the donkey-boys.

Hassan yelled in Arabic.

The camel ran out into the road again and one of the Luxor donkey-boys grabbed the head-rope and swung him to a halt. A moment later, Hassan came panting up and grasped the rope, and his stick cracked on the camel, warning him that it was time to cease his antics. The camel evidently understood, for he was submissive at once.

"Got him!" gasped Bob.

"The gotfulness is terrific!"

"Keep him safe, Hassan!"

"Him safe, sar!" panted the dragoman. "Him camel safe as one house, as you say in English."

"You'd better ride him, till we find Bunter," said Wharton. "Come on! Where's Mauly? Mauly!"

"Mauly, you slacker!" roared Bob.

In the excitement of chasing the camel, the juniors had not missed Lord Mauleverer till that moment. Now they observed that his lordship was no longer with them. They stared round in surprise.

The maize was high; but it was not high enough to hide a rider. But there was nothing to be seen of Mauleverer.

"Has the duffer tumbled off his donkey?" exclaimed Nugent.

"Looks like it! Mauly!" roared Bob. "Mauly, you ass!"

"Mauly! Mauleverer! Mauly!"

"Hallo, hallo, hallo! Here comes the moke!"

The donkey-boy to whom Lord Mauleverer's mount belonged was calling and whistling. A riderless donkey dashed

out of the waving dhurra, and the donkey-boy caught him by the rein.

"Well, my hat!" exclaimed Nugent. "Mauly's the best rider of the lot of us, but he's let the donkey throw him off."

"Mauly!" roared Bob.

There was no answer from Lord Mauleverer. The juniors stared round them in astonishment. Even if Mauly had been thrown by the donkey, it was hardly to be supposed that he was injured—too severely injured to answer to his friends. Why he did not answer was a mystery.

"Him noble lord do not come!" said Hassan, puzzled. "Why do not a noble lord come? Mashallah! This I do not understand."

"My hat!" Wharton caught his breath. "If that villain Kalizelos was not a prisoner on the dahabiyeh, I should think——"

"Thank goodness Mauly left him safe on the boat," said Bob. "It can't be that! But what the thump's become of him?"

Harry Wharton set his lips hard. With the scheming Greek a safe prisoner on the dahabiyeh, the juniors had not dreamed of danger. But it was possible, at least, that the Greek's confederates had been watching them. What had happened to Mauleverer in the waving maize field?

"We've got to find him—and at once," said Wharton. "Bunter will have to wait! Hassan, we've got to find Mauleverer."

"Yes, sar! We find a noble lord!" said Hassan. "Oh, yes, sar! Hassan is your dragoman—you trust Hassan!"

Leaving the camel and the donkeys in charge of the donkey-boys, Hassan and the Famous Five plunged into the maize again to seek Lord Mauleverer. But they did not find him—and no answer came to their anxious calling.

THE THIRTEENTH CHAPTER.
Held by the Enemy!

HAMZA, the scarred Arab, grinned savagely. Crouching in the tall, thick maize, his knee was on the chest of the schoolboy earl, and he was winding a rag from his turban round and round Mauleverer's head, over his mouth. Lord Mauleverer blinked up at him with dazed eyes.

For some moments Mauly hardly knew what had happened. He had been riding through the maize, not three or four yards from the nearest of his friends, when a crouching figure leapt at him and dragged him suddenly from the donkey's back—grasping his leg and unhorsing him before he knew that he was being attacked. The donkey ran on with empty saddle, and Lord Mauleverer sprawled in crushed maize, the scarred Arab kneeling on him, gagging him with the strip of turban before he could utter a cry.

Half-choked by the gag, only able to breathe through his nose, Mauleverer stared dizzily at the savage, scarred face above him.

He could hear the movements of his friends; he heard them go chasing back to the road after the camel. They had not missed him yet. He struggled to throw off the Arab; but the muscular ruffian pinned him down helplessly. In the grip of sinewy hands, his wrists were dragged together and tied fast with another strip of dingy turban. Bound and gagged, he was powerless in the hands of the scarred ruffian; and he could only wonder what the scoundrel intended. The man could not rise to his feet without revealing his presence in the maize field; yet the fact that he had made Mauly a prisoner showed that it was his object to get him away, if he could.

Hamza lost no time. He was taking a desperate chance, and he had not a second to spare. Once Mauleverer was safely bound and silenced, the Arab moved away on his hands and knees through the maize, dragging the schoolboy earl after him by the collar.

It was hard going through the rugged maize roots; but the sinewy ruffian never paused a moment, and evidently he cared nothing for the bumping and bruising of the dragging prisoner.

From the direction of the road, shouting voices came to Lord Mauleverer's ears; his friends were calling to him. Even yet he was not fifty yards from them; but he could make no sound or sign in answer. But they would be searching for him through the field in a few minutes at the most—surely he could not be spirited away under the very eyes of his friends.

There was a glistening of water through the maize. It was one of the narrow irrigating canals that cover the cultivated land in Egypt like a network. Mauleverer felt himself pushed over the bank of brown earth, and for a moment he fancied that the scarred ruffian was dropping him into the water. But it was on timber that he fell; and he found himself sprawling in a small boat—a khiassa, as it was called. The scarred Arab plunged in after him, still keeping his head low, and kneeling in the khiassa, he seized a pole and drove it into the shallow water.

The khiassa shot away.

Mauleverer understood now. Either the Arab had the khiassa in readiness, or he knew where to find the boat belonging to the maize farmer. With swift, strong arms he poled the khiassa away, and it shot past the border of the maize field, into another canal that ran by the edge of a grove of date-palms. Swiftly, silently, the scarred Arab poled on, following canal after canal, Lord Mauleverer watching him helplessly. He had no hope that his friends would find him now. If they were still calling to him, their voices had died away far behind.

Several times from the high paths along the canals brown faces glanced down at the khiassa. The banks of the canals are the usual paths in the cultivated fields of Egypt; and Lord Mauleverer sighted more than a dozen fellaheen, as the khiassa was poled rapidly on But he could not call out to them; and they gave him no heed. The khiassa passed them so swiftly that they probably did not observe that the Faringhee was a prisoner in the boat; and in any case, the timid Egyptian fellaheen would have been very unlikely to look for trouble with the black-browed, savage-looking Arab, with his harsh face disfigured by a knife-cut.

The canal narrowed and shallowed, and there was no further way for the khiassa. Hamza leaped ashore at a point where a path opened in a field of date-trees, and dragged Lord Mauleverer after him.

Out of sight of the canal he threw his prisoner to the ground among the trees. He grinned down at him.

Still he did not speak. But kneeling beside the bound schoolboy, he began to search him.

He grinned with satisfaction as he took possession of a purse which was well supplied with money. But it was evidently not money of which he was in search, though he was glad to get his thievish fingers on it. Mauleverer knew that it was the scarab he was seeking; and he was glad that he had allowed his friends to persuade him not to carry it about with him. Since the day when the Greek had so nearly seized it in Cairo, the Famous Five had promised Mauly the ragging of his life if he carried it in his pocket again; and Mauly was glad now that he had yielded to that gentle persuasion.

It did not take the scarred man long to ascertain that the Golden Scarab was not to be found. He spoke at last, in English.

"Unbelieving son of a dog, where is the scarab?"

Mauleverer could not have answered if he had wished to. Hamza rose to his feet, stared round him, and listened for several minutes. Then he knelt by the schoolboy earl again, and unwound the rag from his mouth, at the same time pressing the edge of a knife to his throat as a warning.

"A curse on all unbelievers!" said Hamza. "Speak low, son of fifteen thousand dogs! One cry, and with this knife I will send you to Shaitan, who waits for all infidels! Where is the scarab?"

"Where you won't find it, you thief!" answered Lord Mauleverer, gasping.

"Listen, unbeliever! The Greek will give twenty thousand piastres for the Scarab of A-Menah! Is the life of a Faringhee worth half so much? Speak!"

The harsh, brown, disfigured face blazed with ferocity. But there was only cool scorn in Mauleverer's answering look.

"Did you leave the scarab on the dahabiyeh? Speak!"

"Yaas."

"Dog of an unbeliever!" The scarred ruffian was evidently savagely disappointed. "To me it is worth twenty thousand piastres, and with such a sum I could make the pilgrimage to Mecca. Son of dogs and pigs!" The ruffian broke into Arabic, and, without understanding what he said, Mauleverer could not fail to be aware that he was cursing in that language so fluent in curses. But he spoke again in English at last. "But you, at least, are in my hands, and the Greek will pay well for you, for it is his plan to ransom you with the scarab. You, dog of a kafir, will remain in a safe place till Kalizelos comes."

With the words he wound the strip of turban again over Mauleverer's mouth, gagging him. He dragged the schoolboy earl to his feet, and signed to him to walk.

Mauleverer hesitated a moment. A savage blow that made him reel put an end to his hesitation.

"Dog of a kafir, go!" snarled the scarred Arab.

Mauleverer's eyes glinted. But he was helpless, and he moved on, with the Arab's grip on his shoulder.

They wound a way among the date-palms, the Arab's eyes glancing to and fro, watchful as a cat's. It was evident that he knew the country well, and was avoiding roads and paths. Twice, at the sound of footsteps, he dragged Mauleverer into cover, and held him in a savage grip till the footsteps died away.

It was clear that he was heading for some definite object—some den,

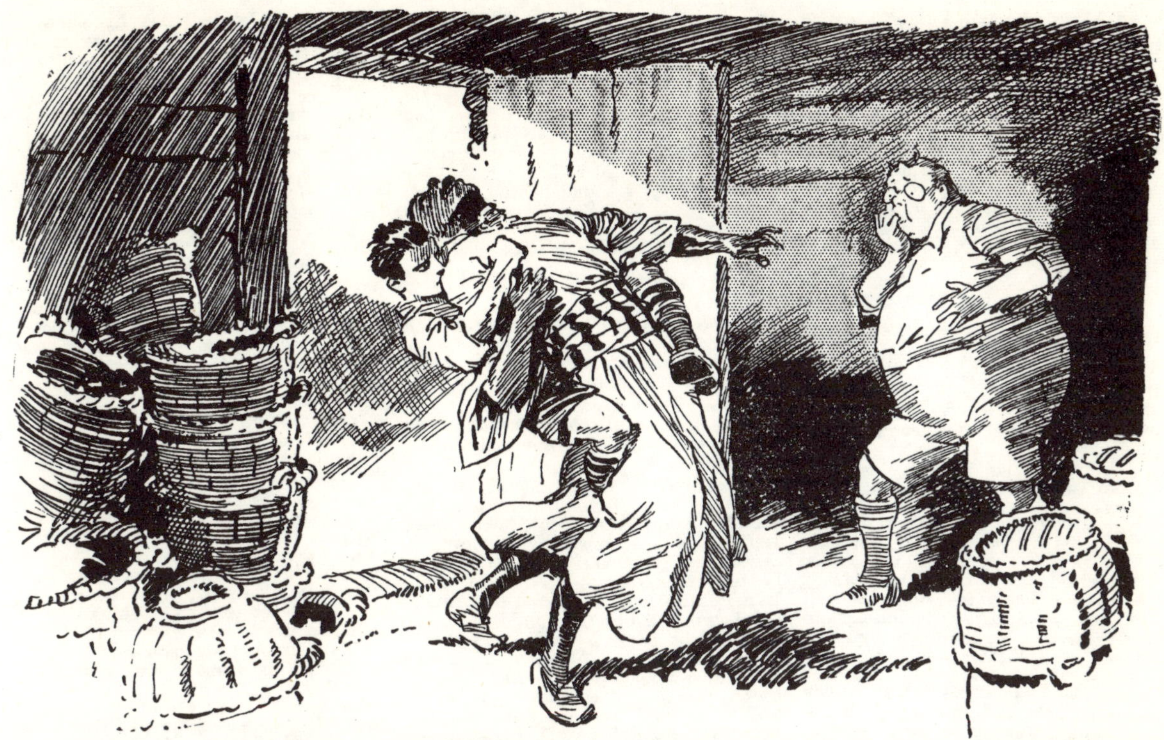

Hardly had Hamza stepped into the shed when Mauleverer was upon him with the spring of a tiger. "Buck up, Bunter!" he roared, as the Arab gave a startled howl and crashed backwards. "Oh crikey!" gasped the terrified Owl.

Mauleverer guessed, where the prisoner would be concealed in safety till he could be handed over to the Greek. It was a comfort to Mauly to reflect that the Greek was a prisoner on board the dahabiyeh, and was not likely to rejoin his confederates. If the scarred man intended to wait till Kalizelos came, he had a long wait ahead of him.

Hamza stopped at last under a shady acacia, and peered out at a path beyond the trees.

The sun was sinking over the Nile, and the gorgeous colours of the Egyptian sunset glowed over the fields. For several minutes the scarred Arab watched the path, then, satisfied at last that the coast was clear, he left the acacias, and dragged on his prisoner along the dusty track. Near the trees was a shed, with an open doorway, at the corner of a field, and Mauleverer could see dimly the shape of a man in a dinghy galabieh squatting inside.

"Faster!" snarled Hamza, dragging at him savagely.

He was anxious to get his prisoner out of the open.

Lord Mauleverer stumbled into the shed, dragged by the Arab's rough hand. The man who was leaning on the pile of baskets, smoking, sprang to his feet with an exclamation, staring at Mauleverer in astonishment.

Mauleverer's heart sank as he recognised Yussef, the hawk-faced Arab who had attacked him in the Cairo hotel, and who had kept him a prisoner in the lost tomb at the Pyramids. Yussef stared at him, evidently surprised to see him in the hands of his confederate.

The two Arabs spoke together rapidly in their own tongue. Yussef was grinning with satisfaction. Hamza's arrival with the prisoner had been a surprise, and evidently a pleasant surprise to him. Lord Mauleverer sat down on the earthen floor, and leaned back wearily against the baskets.

The Arabs continued to talk in animated tones, and several times Mauly caught the name of Kalizelos. He could make a guess at what they were discussing. Now that the owner of the Golden Scarab was a prisoner in their hands they were anxious to see their master, and receive their reward from him.

But it was fairly clear that they were in total ignorance of what had happened to the Greek. They had seen and heard nothing of him since they had pushed off from the dahabiyeh at the sound of alarm in the night. They could have ascertained easily enough that he had not been handed over to the police at Luxor; but they were not likely to guess that Mauleverer had taken the law into his own hands, and locked the rascal in a room on the dahabiyeh. There was little doubt that they supposed that the Greek had escaped from the dahabiyeh after the alarm, and were expecting to get into touch with him again.

The talk was long, incomprehensible to Mauleverer, though he thought he could guess its purport from the expressions on the Arabs' faces, and the frequent repetition of the name of Kalizelos. Many times the two brown-skinned rascals looked out of the shed as if half-expecting to see the Greek coming, at which Mauleverer smiled inwardly. The clatter of Arabic ceased at last, and Yussef left the shed, and Mauleverer watched him disappear in the distance along the dusty track in the sunset.

Hamza turned to him.

With a length of cord he bound the schoolboy's ankles. He grinned down at him savagely as he knotted the cord.

"Here you wait!" he grunted. "Yussef will find the Greek—he will find him at Luxor—and he will come. Here you wait for Kalizelos."

And Lord Mauleverer, from the bottom of his heart, was thankful that Konstantinos Kalizelos was a safe prisoner on board the dahabiyeh, under lock and key, and watch and ward.

THE FOURTEENTH CHAPTER.

Bunter on the Spot!

BILLY BUNTER squatted in his shadowy recess between the stacked wicker-baskets and the wall, breathing with care, and hardly daring to squash the enterprising flies that had followed him into his nook.

It seemed to William George Bunter of the Greyfriars Remove that this was the limit—the very outside edge. He was hungry—fearfully hungry—but he had almost forgotten it in his terror for his fat skin. It was hot and stuffy behind the baskets, and he hardly dared to stir as insects crawled over him. But heat and flies and beetles, even the aching void in his capacious inside mattered nothing in comparison with the danger from the Arabs.

Bunter had hoped that Yussef would go. Instead of that the scarred Arab had come. Bunter listened in terror to the voices in growling Arabic. He had an impression that there was a third party in the lonely shed; but he heard only two voices.

At last, to his intense relief, he heard Yussef depart, and hoped to hear the other beast follow. Once the coast was clear the fat Owl would not have lingered. But the other beast did not follow. Bunter heard a rustling, fumbling sound, but he did not know that the scarred Arab was binding a prisoner's feet. But he heard Hamza's words to Lord Mauleverer, and knew that there was a prisoner in the shed. It was a comfort to Bunter, as well as to Lord Mauleverer, to remember that Kalizelos was safe, and that Yussef, who had gone to seek him at Luxor, would certainly not find him there. There was no danger of the Greek arriving.

That was a comfort; but the scarred Arab obviously intended to remain and wait for Kalizelos with his prisoner. Yussef was gone, but the other beast was in his place, and Bunter groaned silently—he dared not groan aloud.

He guessed that the prisoner was Mauleverer, and no doubt he would have felt rather concerned about him had not all his concern been required for his own fat self. How was he going to get out of this? That was the pressing question that filled Bunter's fat thoughts.

Fortunately the Arabs had not suspected for a moment that anyone was hidden in the shed. Evidently it was their meeting-place, at a safe distance from the town—perhaps belonging to one of them, or hired from its owner for a few piastres.

It was not likely to occur to them that a fat and fatuous fellow who had lost his way had taken shelter there, and dodged out of sight behind the baskets. Which was fortunate for Bunter, for a single conspicuous glance behind the stack of wicker baskets would have revealed him.

Hamza had sat down, cross-legged, on the floor, and was waiting with the impassive patience of an Oriental for the return of his confederate. It was only a few miles to Luxor; but Bunter knew, if Hamza did not, that the hawk-faced Arab was not likely to return soon.

The sun was setting; crimson and gold streamed in at the open doorway. It looked as if Bunter was booked for the night—if he was not discovered sooner. Every now and then there was a creaking of the baskets as Lord Mauleverer, leaning wearily on them, stirred. Every creak sent a thrill of terror to Bunter's fat heart. If the baskets toppled over and revealed him——

Billy Bunter heard a movement from the Arab at last. Hamza rose from his crossed legs, and stepped out of the shed, and stood looking along the dusty track by the acacias. Billy Bunter's fat heart beat. If the beast was gone——

Bunter was getting desperate now. He stirred at last and shifted his position so that he could look from behind the piled baskets. If the Arab was gone, it was an opportunity not to be lost. He put his head round the stack of baskets as cautiously as a tortoise poking its head from its shell, and blinked across the shed.

"Oh lor'!" breathed Bunter, in despair.

The scarred Arab was standing outside the doorway, fortunately with his back to the shed. He was watching for his confederate to return from Luxor, little dreaming of the eyes, and the spectacles, that were fastened on the back of his dusty djubbah.

Bunter's head popped back again like a tortoise's.

He suppressed a groan.

The beast was not gone. He did not intend to go. He was only watching for the other beast.

There was a sound of footsteps—receding! Bunter hoped again! Again he peered out from cover.

Hamza was walking slowly down the dusty track, towards the road which it joined at a distance. Apparently, he was going to look up the road to see whether Yussef and the Greek were coming.

Bunter's heart thumped.

It was a chance—if only he could dodge out of the shed, and escape before the ruffian turned back.

Farther and farther went Hamza; without looking back once; there was nothing to look back for—so far as Hamza knew.

Billy Bunter took his courage in both hands—such as it was—and made up his fat mind. He had only to get to the doorway, dodge round the shed, and he would be out of sight, if the Arab did look back. A few moments——! In his deep concern for himself, the fat Owl had quite forgotten, for the moment, that there was a prisoner in the shed, and that it was most likely Mauleverer. He tiptoed from his hiding-place.

Lord Mauleverer, leaning on the baskets, heard a sound behind him, but did not heed it. But, as a fat figure stole out into his line of vision, Mauleverer stared at it with eyes opening wide.

Of all the dwellers in the land of Egypt, Billy Bunter was the last he would have expected to see at that moment. The sight of Mark Antony or Cleopatra could hardly have astonished him more.

He hardly believed his eyes as they fell on the well-known fat figure and podgy face and shining spectacles of the Owl of the Remove.

Bunter, his eyes fixed on the doorway and the Arab beyond, did not look round. Mauleverer could not speak. But he gave a convulsive wriggle to attract the fat Owl's attention, and the baskets creaked and swayed. Billy Bunter, startled, uttered a fat squeak of alarm, and blinked round.

"Oh!" he gasped. "Mauly!"

The gag silenced Mauleverer, but his look was eloquent. How Bunter was there, was an utter mystery; but he was there, and even Bunter—now that he was reminded of Mauly's unimportant existence—could hardly have scuttled off and leave him to it. For a second he blinked at Mauleverer in dismay and doubt; and then he rolled to him. Where Mauly sat was out of sight of the open doorway, so Bunter was now out of view of the Arab if he looked back at the shed.

Billy Bunter was trembling from head to foot. Every moment he dreaded to hear the returning footsteps of the Arab. But he saw that Mauleverer could not stir, and he fumbled for his pocket-knife. He fumbled in the wrong pockets first, as a matter of course, but he found the knife at last, and opened it. It was blunt—that was a matter of course, also. But he sawed desperately at Mauly's bonds with the blunt blade.

Mauly's hands came free, and he tore the gagging strip of turban from his mouth, and gasped in breath. He jerked the knife from Bunter, and cut his feet loose.

"By gad!" breathed Mauly.

"C-c-come on!" stuttered Bunter. "C-c-come on, q-q-quick! That b-b-beast may come back any minute."

Mauly rose to his feet, stretching his cramped limbs. Bunter clutched him frantically by the arm.

"C-c-come on!" he gasped.

"Keep cool, old fat bean," said Mauleverer. "There's two of us now, even if the brute comes back."

"You silly idiot! I'm going!"

Bunter rolled to the doorway, while Mauleverer stood rubbing his limbs where the bonds had been knotted. The fat Owl peered out cautiously, and popped back, almost fainting with terror.

"He—he—he's coming!"

"Yaas?" yawned Mauleverer.

"We—we're done! Oh lor'! Oh crikey! It's too late——"

"Keep cool!"

Hamza's footsteps could be heard on the dusty, sandy track. He had looked along the road, and failed to see a sign of Yussef returning, and he was coming back to the shed. Billy Bunter groaned in dispair. By staying to help Mauleverer he had lost his chance of dodging out of sight. Emerging from the shed now meant stepping into full view of the returning Arab.

"Keep cool, old bean," whispered Mauleverer. "We'll snaffle him as he comes in."

"Oh lor'!"

"Back up, Bunter! We've got to scrap now, to save our bacon!"

"Ooooogh!"

Bunter did not look much like scrapping. Mauleverer, cool as ice, stepped to the side of the open doorway. Bunter rolled behind him. The Arab was coming back, without the remotest suspicion that his prisoner was loose—never dreaming of an attack. Mauleverer's teeth were set, his eyes glinting. There was a chance of dealing with the ruffian, taken utterly by surprise as he would be. And the cool determination of the schoolboy earl helped the hapless Owl to screw up his courage.

The footsteps came closer; the shadow of the Arab fell into the doorway. The next moment he stepped in—and, as he came, Mauleverer was upon him with the spring of a tiger.

One startled howl broke from Hamza as he went over, crashing on the earthen floor.

Mauleverer was upon him.

"Back up, Bunter!" he roared.

"Oh crikey!"

Hamza, after the first shock of utter surprise, struggled like a wild beast. He had gone down on his back, and Mauly, grasping him fiercely, desperately crashed his head on the hard earth. The back of Hamza's head hit the earth hard, and the crash dazed him, but he struggled furiously.

"Bunter——" panted Mauleverer.

Crash!

A fat knee, with all Bunter's weight on it, landed on the stomach of the sprawling Arab.

Hamza's struggles ceased on the instant.

He gave one horrible, gasping groan, and lay writhing, with every ounce of wind knocked out of his carcass. His jaw dropped, his eyes bulged, and he gurgled hideously.

Mauleverer panted.

"Oh, good man! Hook it, old fat bean."

He grasped Bunter by a fat arm, and they dashed out from the shed. Behind them, groans and gasps and gurgles were all that came from Hamza, as he writhed on the floor in anguish. The scarred ruffian was hors de combat.

"Buck up, Bunter!"

Bunter did not need bidding. His fat little legs fairly flashed as he flew. Even the slim Mauly had to put it on to keep pace with the terrified Owl. In a couple of minutes they reached the end of the track where it joined the road. Lord Mauleverer gave one glance round him. The setting sun showed him the direction of the Nile—and in that direction lay Luxor—somewhere. He turned into the road, and ran on, with Bunter spluttering at his side. The crimson glare of the sunset was giving place to mauve twilight; and under the gathering shadows they ran and ran and ran.

THE FIFTEENTH CHAPTER.

Unexpected!

"LORDLY gentlemen, it is a game which is up, as you say in your noble language," said Hassan, the dragoman, somewhat dismally.

(*Continued on page* 28.)

THE RED FALCON!

By
ARTHUR STEFFENS

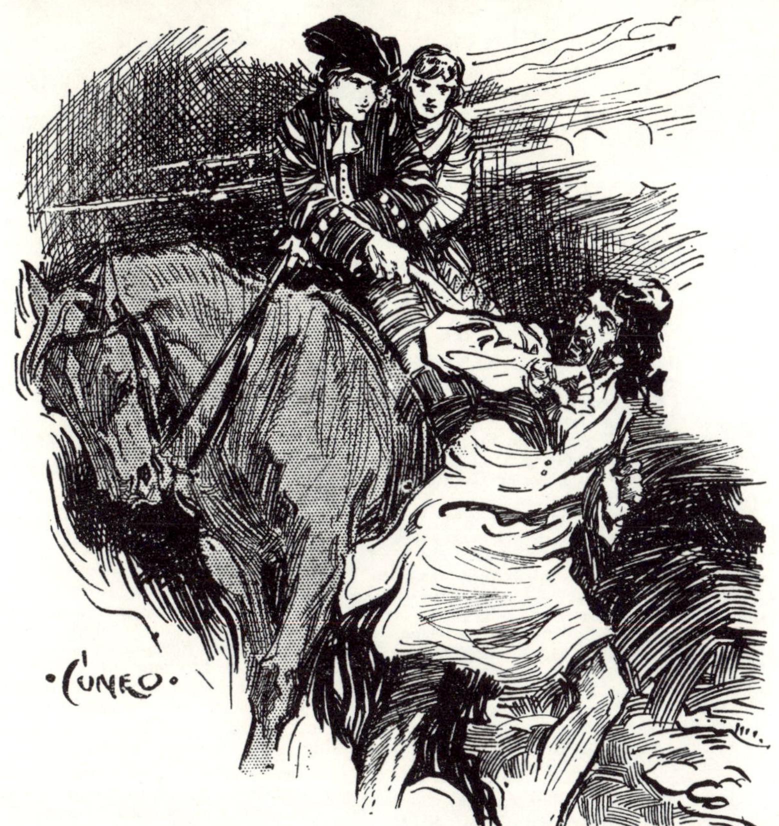

Down-River!

"STEADY, boy!"

As Jerry McLean spoke, he gave the tiller a pull which swung the wherry out into the full flood of the racing tide, and then looked at the boy.

Hal Lovett was pulling for all his worth at the oars, and his face was white and strained from the desperate work.

"No need to row like that now, lad; we're safe." Jerry rose and moved forward, his water-soaked, rough brown-cloth convict's clothes clinging to him, his heavy boots squelching river water as he stepped. "You take the tiller, lad. It's my turn."

From sheer exhaustion the boy obeyed. But as he took the oars and dropped upon the thwart Jerry did not immediately begin to row. Instead, he frowned into the darkness, focusing his eyes upon a bright red glow which came and went. Up-river, where the convict hulks lay beside the dockyard at Woolwich, a shot rang out, then another.

The racing tide bore wild shouts and cries of agony to the ears of man and boy. Suddenly the blaze grew brighter—so bright that Jerry and Hal could make out the anchored hulk, and above the brightening glare in her a pall of dense black smoke which drifted back to London town.

Hal turned his towzled head and stared aghast; then he dropped his head upon his folded arms and burst into a fit of sobbing which shook him violently. It was only for a little while, however. Soon he looked up, dashing the tears angrily from his blurred eyes.

"Jerry," he choked, "we ought to have gone back. It was cowardly to run. The convicts are fighting for their lives back there."

McLean's lips tightened.

"Ay," he said, "they are fighting for their lives. But as soon as the alarm-bell rang on shore, and the soldiers came racing to the boats, it was every man for himself, and we are lucky to have got where we are, boy."

"If only John Pryse were with us!" Hal thought hungrily of the big and plucky convict who had been the means of his and Jerry's deliverance.

"I wish he were, boy," Jerry agreed. "I lost sight of Jack after I saw him dive. It was useless waiting any longer. But I know Jack. There isn't a river that can drown him. I don't think he's dead. If he's alive we'll meet him again soon, unless——"

The boy looked at Jerry McLean questioningly.

"Unless he is taken, or the Runners capture us," explained Jerry, with a grin.

The boat was drifting onward at a rare speed. A bend in the river showed Hal and Jerry the convict hulk with all her ports aglow with fire. They could see boats, like walnut-shells, moving around her. More fiendish cries and a few more shots came to their ears. Then flames began to lick the jury mast of the Ethalion. The convict hulk which had been their prison was doomed!

McLean swung his back into a lusty stroke and urged the wherry on at a faster speed.

"No use waiting!" he cried.

Before they were aware of her approach they almost ran into the bows of a great barge which was sailing up-river. Only a swift turn of the tiller and a hard stroke from Jerry's right-hand oar carried them clear of the threatening stem, and Jerry was forced to ship the oar and fend the boat off the barge with his hand.

A coarse oath followed them into the darkness, and Jerry hauled the boat round.

"Let's get ashore!" he cried.

The Thames began to broaden out, and the tide was so swift that it took Jerry some hard rowing before the shore loomed up ahead.

A pebble strand ran up from the out-flowing river to a high bank. A few hefty strokes, and then Jerry McLean shipped his oars. The keel of the boat grated on the shingle, and Jerry vaulted over the side and held the boat fast. In a moment Hal joined him.

"It was no good going on, boy," whispered McLean. "We'd have been seen as soon as day broke. We've got to take our chance on shore."

"We haven't come far. They'll send out search parties," said Hal, who was shivering from the cold. "They're bound to catch us. We've got no friends and nowhere to go."

"I've got friends," McLean assured the boy through teeth which chattered violently. "We'll find a safe hiding-place before morning. Then we'll get some clothes—somehow. It's these cursed convict rags that may betray us."

"But we mustn't leave the boat here, Jerry; it would be seen."

"You're right, boy," said McLean, pushing the stolen wherry into deep water and wading knee-deep after it to give it a final thrust, which hurled it beyond the eddies into the racing tide. "There she goes—and may she be past the Nore before the 'busies' find her!"

Side by side the two waited until they saw the vanishing boat merge with the night; then they climbed up the bank and looked about them.

Above a bank of dense black cloud the moon began to peep, and they realised they were in an open meadow. Crossing this, they found themselves stopped by a high, overgrown hedge. By the side of this they went, searching for an opening. They could see cattle

READ THIS FIRST.

CONVICTED OF CONSPIRING TO ROB THE EARL OF HUNTFORD OF A DIAMOND STAR, HAL LOVETT AND HIS CHUM, JERRY McLEAN, ARE CONVEYED TO THE CONVICT HULK ETHALION, ANCHORED AT WOOLWICH—HAL TO SERVE A SENTENCE OF SEVEN YEARS, AND McLEAN TO AWAIT DEPORTATION. AS THE RESULT OF A PREARRANGED PLAN, ORGANISED BY A BURLY PRISONER NAMED PRYSE, WHOM McLEAN HAD PREVIOUSLY BEFRIENDED, THE CONVICTS FIRE THE SHIP, AND HAL AND JERRY GAIN POSSESSION OF A WHERRY AND MAKE GOOD THEIR ESCAPE IN THE BLACKNESS OF THE NIGHT.

lying on the dew-laden grass, and presently came to a high gate, over which they climbed.

Beyond the gate ran a narrow, muddy, rutted road, and, after emptying the water out of their thick-soled boots, they followed this until their chilled bodies steamed from the vigorous exercise.

The moon was up now, and by its aid they followed a footpath which led them to a farm. In order to gain the road beyond the farm they had to pass close to the farmhouse, and as they neared it a dog began a ferocious barking as it strained at its chain.

Hal stopped, hesitating.

"Never mind the dog, boy," said McLean, urging him on. "We've got to find shelter before the day breaks."

They paced on together, whilst the furious barking of the dog awakened other dogs in the neighbourhood, which joined in the canine chorus.

"This way!" cried McLean. "Through the farmyard! It's the nearest way to the road!"

They raced past the farmhouse, their hearts beating fast.

Suddenly a window rasped up.

Hal cast a glance back over his shoulder and saw a man in a nightshirt appear at the window. His round face was topped by a nightcap, the tassel of which bobbed ludicrously.

"Thieves!" roared the man, as he caught sight of the running figures. "I'll teach 'ee to rob my hen-roost!"

Hal slowed in his running. The sight of the nightcap fascinated him. Suddenly he saw a gleam of metal as the farmer swung a bell-mouthed weapon up to his shoulder and fired.

Bang!

The report of a blunderbuss echoed deafeningly in the night, and as Hal and Jerry pounded on, they heard the patter of bullets rip and tear the leaves of the trees and bushes near them.

"Come on, boy!" shouted McLean, as he swung back a five-barred gate and pelted out on to the road. "Let's find cover!"

Hunted!

HAL and Jerry followed the road for a mile or two before they came to a dense wood which invited confidence. Although the moon was up now, they did not meet a soul.

The hedge which fringed the wood was broken here and there, so that it was easy for them to scramble over a low bank of earth and dive among the trees. Here they waited till the day broke and they could see their way about.

Around them grew clumps of bushes and great, upstanding trees. The wood was of considerable extent, they discovered, as they penetrated into its depths.

Completely hidden by bushes, they threw themselves down, and, removing their boots, rested.

They were tired and hungry and footsore. Their heads nodded and their eyelids closed, but they dared not go to sleep for fear of being captured.

As the day lengthened Hal became so sick with hunger that his sleepiness passed away. If only they had some food!

In the afternoon they ventured farther afield, and, finding a stream running through the wood, lapped at the crystal clear water. It gave them new life.

They had no sooner slaked their thirst, however, than they heard the echo of voices close at hand.

McLean crouched, straining his ears to listen.

"It's no use combing this wood for escaped convicts," he heard a man saying. "How'd they get this way? You're much more like to find 'em round Blackheath, and they're shore to head Lunnon way."

McLean gripped Hal by the arm and pulled him down. They were ringed in with dense, close-growing rhododendron bushes, and it would have been impossible to detect them at ten yards' range.

It was just as well, for less than a minute later a ranger came along, with a stick under his arm. At his heels trailed a crowd of sportsmen belonging to the neighbourhood.

Hal held his breath as the party stopped within reach of the bush under which he was hiding.

"There's fine cover here for escaped convicts," said a stalwart young farmer.

"Sure there is," answered the ranger, "but they'd never come this way, I tell 'e. It only leads to Farmer Goodyer's farm and the river."

"Farmer Goodyer had a fright last night. Saw two men in his farmyard, and fired at 'em," returned the young farmer. "And they fired back, he says, and hit him. They must have been two of the convicts."

"Bah!" replied the ranger. "Convicts with a gun! I say Farmer Goodyer hit hisself. And he imagined seeing the two men. He'd bin drinking!"

"All the same," said the young farmer stubbornly, "seventeen of the convicts got away after setting fire to the Ethalion, and we're going to search this wood."

"Come on, then, let's search it," answered the ranger, with some heat. As he spoke, he turned and poked his stick deep into the rhododendron bush, the sharp, steel-capped point of it touching Hal where he lay. Then the man moved a step, and raised a great branch of the shrub up high. "Convicts in here!" he jeered. "Come on, let's find 'em!"

To Hal's intense relief, the whole lot moved away. Snapping twigs and rustling boughs marked their retreat, and, as the sounds grew fainter, McLean reached out a hand and touched Hal's.

"Pass a vote of thanks to our unknown pal, boy," he said. "I reckon he saved us."

But though the danger passed so quickly, it was not the end of the day's alarms.

Later that same afternoon McLean and Hal, who had left the shelter of the rhododendron bushes and climbed up high into the branches of a giant spreading oak, heard dogs baying as they scoured the undergrowth, and the deep-throated shouts of men who urged them on.

Sometimes the sounds almost died away, then they came again. Once they grew quite loud, and from their hiding-place in the tree the two convicts saw the hounds raking through the very clump of bushes under which they had recently hidden.

"You'd almost think someone was hiding there, to hear the dogs baying," came in a loud, deep voice. "But it's a false alarm. Let's go this way."

The hunters and their dogs moved off, and a little while later a mist began to rise among the trees.

Jerry Gets Some Clothes!

AS soon as night fell, Hal and McLean worked their way cautiously to the fringe of the wood. Hungry, and shivering with dampness, they waited, until the farm hands and cottagers went home and only a few belated travellers remained abroad.

Then they hurried along the lane in front of them and made their way to a main road. Along this they went until they came to a signpost that told them it was three and a quarter miles to Blackheath.

"Blackheath!" chuckled McLean. "Burn me, boy, but if I once get in that neighbourhood I'll know where I am and what to do."

They followed the direction of the signpost, trudging on side by side, their heavy boots beating out an echoing stamp at every stride, no matter how lightly they trod.

Whenever a cottage loomed up they scouted before taking a chance. If an inn came into view they reconnoitred before they dared to pass it.

It was pitch dark when Hal and Jerry at last reached the great bleak expanse of common. At once they left the road and began to cross the grass.

"Boy," said McLean, "I have more than one friend among the innkeepers around these parts, for I used to ride out or drive out here, and spend my money lavishly as long as I had it. But deuce take it, I shan't be able to take my bearings until the moon rises."

"I'm hungry," said Hal. "Shall we be able to get something to eat?"

"All we want, I hope," encouraged Jerry McLean. "And shelter and rest, too, unless my good friend fails me. If he does, why, then, boy, it will mean—the hulks—or worse, maybe. Already we must be condemned as escaped convicts, and mutineers, and——"

"It might mean the gallows, Jerry," said Hal, finishing McLean's unspoken thought.

"More than likely," said McLean.

They were moving stealthily and noiselessly up and down the hollows of the heath, making no sound. And now, as they went, McLean gripped Hal's arm.

"Look, lad!" he cried.

In the distance bobbed two dancing lights, like will-o'-the-wisps. They were advancing slowly. As they drew nearer, the convicts heard the crunching of wheels upon the flint road.

Then a man's voice raised in anger split the night. His oaths rolled across the heath, and the sharp crack of a whip accompanied them.

"Whoa, you black devil!" a voice cried. "I'll steady you—I'll make you do what I want!"

Crack, crack, crack!

Again came the crack of the whip.

The lights had stopped. On the road which topped a gentle rise stood a cart in black silhouette. The man who held the reins was reeling in his seat and lashing the horse until it reared up between the shafts. At the same time the man hauled at the reins, and his curses showed that he had been drinking.

It was a case of sheer brutality on the part of a drunken man towards an inoffensive horse, and Jerry McLean's blood boiled at the sight.

Printed and published every Saturday by the Proprietors, The Amalgamated Press, Ltd., The Fleetway House, Farringdon Street, London, E.C.4. Advertisement offices: The Fleetway House, Farringdon Street, London, E.C.4. Registered for transmission by Canadian Magazine Post. Subscription rates: Inland and Abroad, 11s. per annum; 5s. 6d. for six months. Sole Agents for Australia and New Zealand: Messrs. Gordon & Gotch, Ltd., and for South Africa: Central News Agency, Ltd.—Saturday, September 10th, 1932.

Jerry loved horses. At one time, as Hal Lovett knew, he used to own them. It was too much for him to see this poor beast ill-used by a drunken bully. Screwing up his convict's cap, which he pulled out of his pocket, he raced up on to the road and presented it at the astonished driver.

"Your money or your life, and all the clothes you're wearing, you gallows dog!" cried Jerry. "Out of that trap—sharp—and off with your clothes, or I'll slit your throat, and be hanged to you!"

The man stared down, and as he recognised the clothes of rusty brown Jerry was wearing, and saw the shadow of Hal behind, he gave a terrified scream and came hopping obediently to the ground.

Then, shaking with terror under the menace of a rolled-up convict's cap, he got out of his clothes as quickly as he was able.

Soon the man stood bared to his shirt, socks, and boots.

"What size boots are you wearing?" demanded Jerry savagely.

"Eig-eig-eights!" gasped the terrified traveller.

"Then off with 'em!" said McLean; "they're my size!"

The man squatted on the grass and removed his boots.

As soon as he had got out of his convict's clothes and donned the rather ill-fitting clothes he had "borrowed," and put on the man's boots, Jerry tossed the discarded things at his victim.

"There," he said, "if you're cold get into those, but don't blame me if they arrest you and put you aboard the hulks."

Jerry beckoned to Hal. The moon was rising, and they could see.

"Help me unharness the horse, Hal," he cried.

"No!" howled the traveller, in a frenzy. "How'm I to get home?"

"Thank your lucky stars I didn't put a bullet through your cowardly hide!" answered McLean. "You wouldn't have bothered about home then. Come, Hal, boy, help me release the horse!"

They soon had the horse free. Then Jerry vaulted on to its back, and, gathering up the long reins, looped them over his right forearm.

"Up behind me, boy!" he cried. "It's better to ride than to walk, and it's a long cry yet to our friends!"

"I'll see the pair of you hanged at Tyburn!" screamed the infuriated traveller.

"Do you want me to come back and blow your brains out?" said McLean, turning the horse about and once more presenting his rolled up convict's cap at the man's head.

The traveller did not reply. He started off at a run across the heath, and a string of threats and curses trailed along behind him.

Jerry McLean drove the horse along the road at a steady trot.

"Where are you taking me to, Jerry?" asked Hal, as he bumped up and down behind.

At every other step his teeth met together with a snap, and he had to cling on to Jerry desperately to save himself from being thrown.

"To the Swan With Two Necks, and mine host, Peter Davey," answered Jerry McLean.

The "Swan With Two Necks"!

THE Swan With Two Necks was not a coaching inn, but one of those smaller wayside taverns which, nevertheless, dispensed a splendid and bounteous hospitality in the reign of His Most Gracious Majesty King George III.

Picturesquely gabled with a coach-yard behind, and a long range of stables and outbuildings, it nestled in a bower of spreading trees and luxurious shrubs within a mile of the heath.

As they approached it, after having had much difficulty in finding the right road, McLean slowed the horse into a walk. Then he brought the beast to a standstill.

The sky was now deepest blue above, and aglow with the silver light of the moon. The winking stars shone pale.

"Hop down, boy!" said Jerry.

Hal obeyed. Then, following him, McLean gave the horse a smack on the flank, which sent it careering away into the night, the reins trailing out behind it in the dust.

"We'd best approach the inn on foot," said McLean, unwinding the rug he had wound about his body before riding the horse. "Drape this over your convict's clothes, and cross your fingers for luck, boy."

In this weird fashion, the rug falling almost to his ankles and concealing his convict's garb, Hal Lovett accompanied Jerry to the door of the inn.

Beside the road a signpost stood, and, as its board creaked in the gentle wind, Hal saw painted upon it a swan with two necks.

Before him stood the gabled inn itself, its half-timbered walls clustered with climbing roses and ivy.

Jerry McLean knocked loudly on the door. The diamond-paned windows were in darkness, and no light showed anywhere within.

Again and again Jerry knocked, the echoes dying away in the distance reluctantly. Jerry had almost given up hope of being heard when at last footsteps rang beyond the closed door, and then came the sound of bolts being drawn back, and a chain shot. Finally a key turned in the lock, and the door swung open.

A sleepy-looking man with tousled red hair stood in the doorway, peering at them suspiciously over the fluttering flame of a lighted candle. A glance told him that they were no gentlefolk, these.

"Who be you, and what do 'e warnt?" he asked gruffly.

"Bed and breakfast, and a word with Peter Davey," answered McLean cheerfully, making as if to enter the inn.

The man barred the way, however.

"Maister Davey's in bed, and we can't take you in!" snapped the man with the ginger hair.

He would have shut the door on them if Jerry had not thrust his foot in the way.

"Peter Davey would not drive us from his inn," said McLean. "This is scurvy treatment, fellow."

"I'll not take you in," snarled the man, looking suspiciously at Hal. "How do I know you're not them convicts that escaped from the hulks?"

A deep, ringing, heavy voice behind made the man suddenly leap back.

"Here, what's to do, Tom Kinch?"

"Travellers. Suspicious coves, who want bed and breakfast," growled Tom Kinch, who was the potman at the Swan With Two Necks.

"Travellers—eh?" grumbled the man with the deep voice, as he strode up to the door. "Hold that candle high so that I can see, Tom."

His eyes travelled to Hal, and he frowned. Then they switched to McLean's face, and he stared and gasped.

"Mr. McLe——" he began, but checked himself quickly. "Why, come in, sir, and bring your friend with you! I don't know what good luck brought you my way to-night, but come right in and make yourselves at home."

"Thank you, Peter Davey!" said McLean, as he stepped across the threshold.

Peter Davey, landlord of the Swan With Two Necks' Inn, winked. He was a broad-shouldered, deep-chested man with a red face, topped by a cluster of natural curls. Clean-shaven and hearty, he beamed at McLean before he sent Tom Kinch about his business.

"Stir up the fire in the coffee-room, Tom," he ordered, "and get ready Rooms Nos. 7 and 8. Use the warming-pan, and mind that the sheets are aired. I'll see to the supper."

Ten minutes later Hal and McLean were seated in a pew with cold roast beef and pickled walnuts, crisp bread-and-butter, and a bottle of liquid refreshment set in front of them.

A Cheshire cheese stood at the side of the table, and the landlord, after peering cautiously about him, dropped into the seat on the other side.

He looked grave, and his eyes searched McLean's face anxiously. Hal sat with the rug drawn close about him.

"Sir," said the landlord, in a hoarse whisper, "I'm glad you came to me. I'll save you, if I can. I'll never forget the generous way you treated me whenever you came out to the Swan With Two Necks. After you've eaten go upstairs and sleep without fear."

He crept to the end of the pew, looked round, then came back again.

"The hue and cry is out," he whispered. "I heard all about your escape from the hulks, sir. But there are some who think you are dead. And your friend?"

"Is Hal Lovett, Peter."

"The boy who stole the Earl of Huntford's star," said the landlord, darting a keen glance at Hal. "Well, if he's your friend, he is safe with me, too. I'll see about getting him some clothes to-morrow."

"That potman of yours, Peter. Tom Kinch, can he be trusted?" asked Jerry, leaning across the table. "I almost thought he suspected us just now."

"Tom—what Tom Kinch?" said the landlord heartily. "He's dour, but he's safe enough. His bark is worse than his bite. Besides he knows nothing."

Peter Davey, landlord of the Swan With Two Necks, would not have felt quite so sanguine could he have seen Tom Kinch at that very moment crouching down and spying in at the slightly opened door.

(Hal and Jerry have certainly found a friend in Peter Davey. But what of Tom Kinch? He looks like spilling the beans, doesn't he? Stand by for more exciting adventures next week, chums!)

The SHADOWED SCHOOLBOY.

(*Continued from page 24.*)

The Famous Five were reluctant to admit it, but it was evident that the dragoman was right.

Darkness was falling on the valley of the Nile. Not a sign had been found of Lord Mauleverer. For weary hour after hour the juniors and the dragoman had searched by fields and paths and canal banks, but it was in vain. The schoolboy earl had vanished as completely as if the earth had opened and swallowed him up, and there could no longer be any doubt that he had fallen into the hands of a lurking, watching enemy.

It was futile to continue the search after dark, and the Greyfriars fellows gathered in the road again in a dismal group, where the donkey-boys were waiting with the donkeys, and Ibrahim with the camel.

"I—I suppose there's nothing more doing," said Harry Wharton, clenching his hands. "They've got poor old Mauly——"

"We can't go back to Luxor without him," said Bob.

"My noble sars, we go back to Luxor and utter information to policemans," said Hassan. "Policemans find rascally persons who lay hands on noble lordship. Yes, sar! Egyptian policemans very good and top-hole policemans."

"We're not going," said Harry. "But I think we'd better send word to Luxor, and get the police on to it. Hassan can go——"

"Me go, sar, on a camel with a prompt dispatch," said the dragoman. "But you, sar, you come also on donkey, sar. What you do here in a dark?"

It was useless to linger, but the chums of the Remove could not make up their minds to return to the dahabiyeh without Mauleverer. They consulted in low tones while the dragoman and the donkey-boys waited. The shadows were falling more thickly, and stars coming out in a sky of dark velvet.

Through the thickening shadows came a sound of footsteps on the road. Many natives had passed, and Hassan questioned them in the native tongue, but without learning anything of Mauleverer. As for Bunter, the juniors had almost forgotten the lost Owl in their anxiety for Mauly.

Bob Cherry peered along the shadowy road in the direction of the approaching footsteps.

"Here comes somebody," he said. "Hassan may as well ask them. They may have seen something——"

Two shadowy figures loomed up in the gloom. Bob Cherry's voice evidently reached them. There was a fat, startled squeak.

"I say, you fellows——"

"Bismillah!" gasped Hassan. "It is the small fat lord!"

"Bunter!" yelled Johnny Bull.

"Thank goodness he's turned up!" said Harry. "But poor old Mauly—— Why, what—what—what—— Mauly! Is—is—is it you, Mauly?"

There was a chuckle.

"Yaas!"

"I say, you fellows——"

"Mauly!" roared the Famous Five, in utter wonder. They almost fancied that they must be dreaming.

"O day worthy to be marked with a white stone!" ejaculated Hassan. "We find him noble lordship! Yes! Him noble and magnificent lordship is of a return to sorrowing friends! Inshallah! Wahyat-en-nabi! Him lordship here!"

"Mauly!" gasped Wharton. "Is it you or your ghost, old man?"

Lord Mauleverer chuckled.

"Little me. And jolly glad to see you fellows," he said. "I fancied we were on the right road, and here we are. Sorry you've been bothered, as they say on the telephone. Not my fault, really."

"I say, you fellows——"

"But what—how—— Thank goodness you've turned up. But how——" gasped Nugent.

"I say, you fellows——"

"Mauly, old bean, we'll keep you on a chain after this!" exclaimed Bob. "But how the thump——"

"I say, you fellows——"

"Shut up, Bunter!"

"Shan't!" roared Bunter. "I'm hungry!"

"Ha, ha, ha!"

"Blessed if I see anything to cackle at! I'm famished—ravenous! I've had nothing to eat all day!" gasped Bunter. "Is this a time for jaw? Have you got any grub with you? Look here, let's get back to Luxor. Look here, I—I tell you, after I've shaved Mauly's wife—I mean, saved his life——"

"What?" yelled the juniors.

"Great Scott! Did Bunter——"

"Yaas," grinned Lord Mauleverer. "Bunter turned up—goodness knows how—always turnin' up, like a bad penny——"

"Oh, really, Mauly——"

"Let's get goin', dear men. Here's your camel, Bunter. Here's your jolly old camel and your jolly old camel-man——"

"I'm not going to ride that camel again!" roared Bunter. "Keep the beast away! I say, you fellows——"

"Well, this is luck!" said Bob Cherry. "Stick Bunter on my donkey, Hassan. I'll ride the camel. Sure you won't have him, Bunter?"

"Beast!"

It was a joyous party, after all, that rode back under the stars to Luxor.

. . . .

Kalizelos, the Greek, like a caged tiger in his locked cabin, heard the tramping of feet and the ringing of cheery voices as the Greyfriars party came on board the dahabiyeh. But Bunter's voice was not heard. Billy Bunter had scoffed the remains of the lunch on his way back to Luxor, but he was still ravenous when he arrived on the dahabiyeh, and Bunter made a bee-line for the supper table, and his podgy jaws were too busy for speech. For a solid hour Billy Bunter sat and ate and ate and ate, and kept the Nubians busy. Then he leaned back and smiled. Once more William George Bunter found life worth living.

THE END.

(Billy Bunter and the chums of Greyfriars meet with heaps more exciting adventures next week in "THE SECRET OF THE SCARAB!" Be sure and read this yarn, boys. You'll enjoy every line of it.)

GREAT AND GLORIOUS NEWS FOR READERS! (SEE... INSIDE.)

The MAGNET 2D

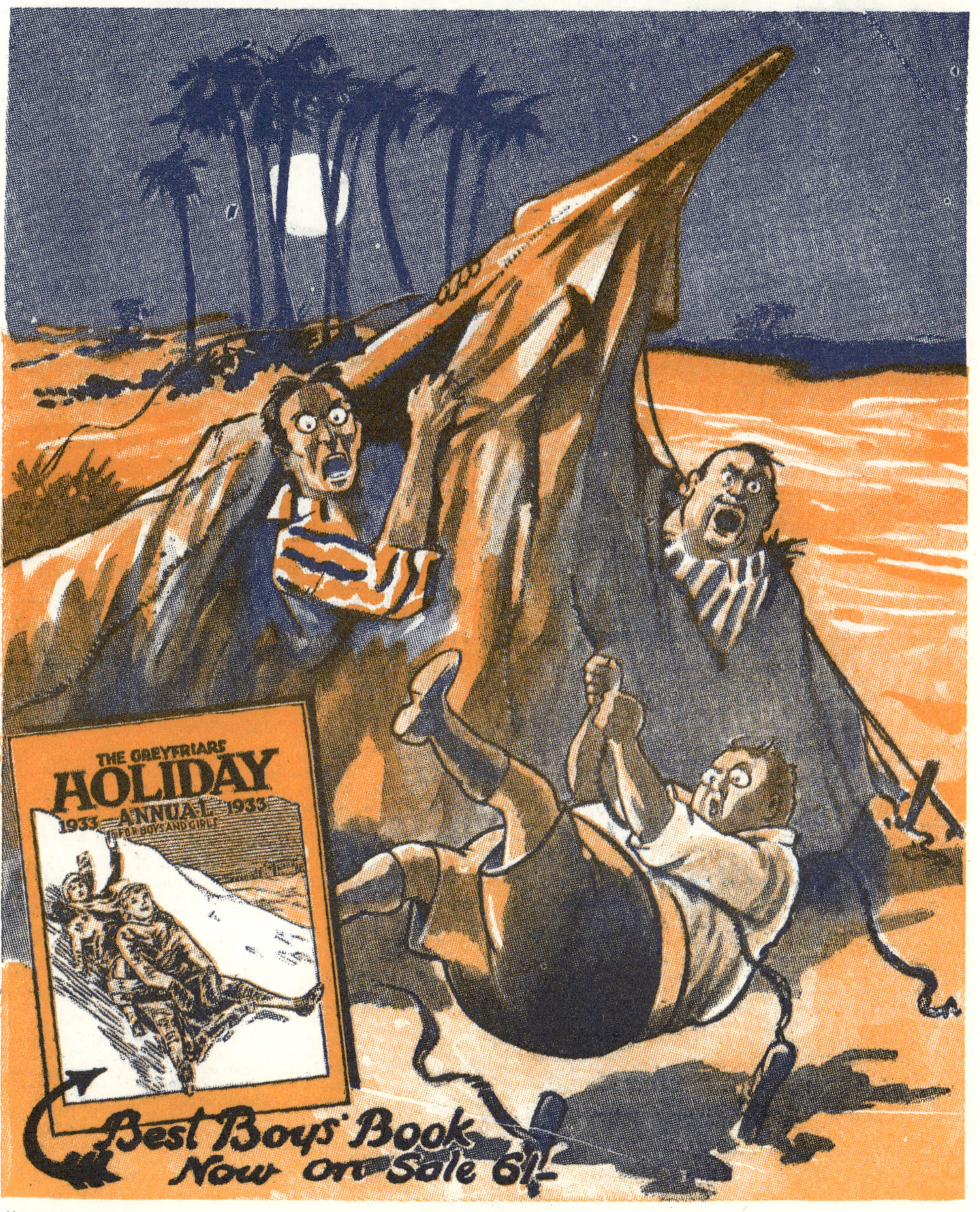

No. 1,283. Vol. XLII. EVERY SATURDAY. Week Ending September 17th, 1932.

ANOTHER GRAND STORY IN OUR NOVEL HOLIDAY SERIES!

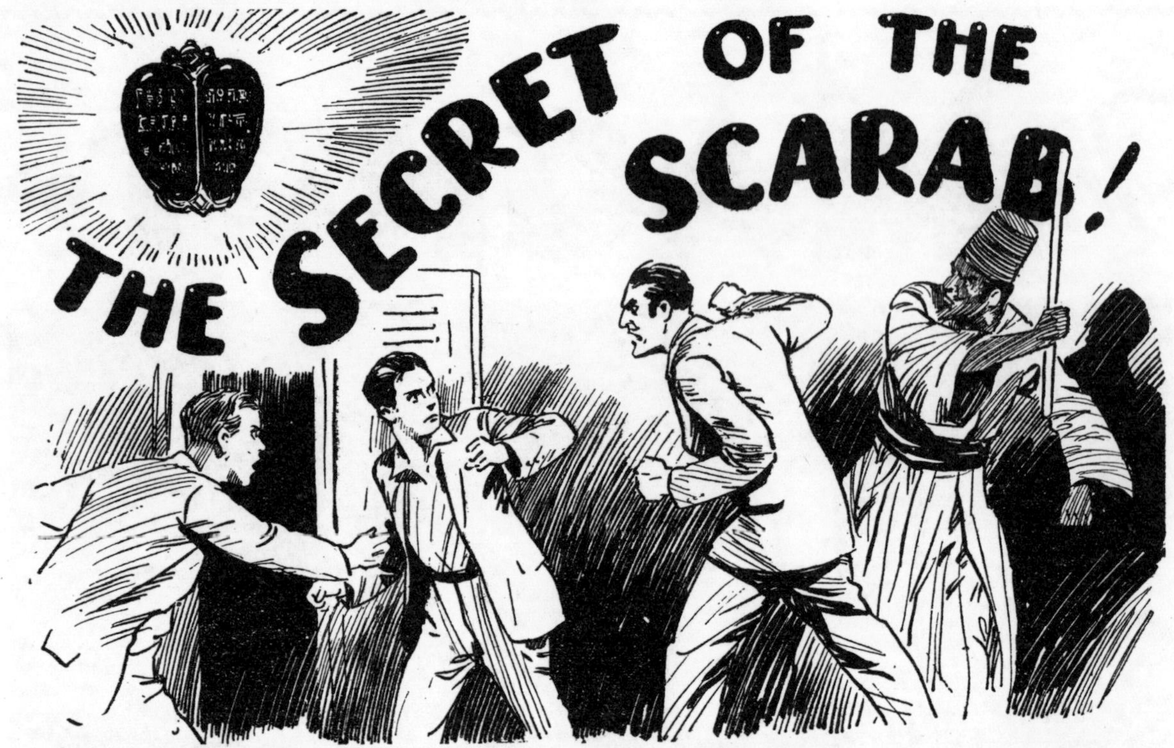

THE SECRET OF THE SCARAB!

Featuring Harry Wharton & Co.'s amazing adventures in the Mysterious East. By FRANK RICHARDS.

THE FIRST CHAPTER.
All Mauly's Money!

"SHEER off!"

"What?"

"I'm talking to Mauly!" said Billy Bunter, with dignity. "We don't want to be interrupted, do we, Mauly?"

"Yaas."

"Oh, really, you beast——"

Whereat the Famous Five of the Greyfriars Remove chuckled.

It was a warm day on the Nile. All the days on the Nile were warm. Sunshine, the clear, dry sunshine of Egypt, streamed down on the slow-rolling river, on the city of Luxor, and on the dahabiyeh tied up to the bank.

Harry Wharton & Co. had been ashore with Hassan, the dragoman, seeing the sights. Warm as the Nile valley was, the Famous Five did not seem to tire—in which they were very unlike Billy Bunter and Lord Mauleverer. Billy Bunter was fat and lazy. Lord Mauleverer was slim and lazy. Mauly liked to see the sights of Egypt from a long cane chair on the upper deck of the big Nile houseboat, with his legs resting on another chair, and his hands clasped behind his head. Billy Bunter did not care a lot for sights, anyhow, and he declared that he was fed-up on temples and tombs and mummies. Sitting under an awning, eating sticky Turkish sweetmeats had more appeal for Bunter. So the two slackers had been left on board the dahabiyeh while the energetic five "did" Denderah with Hassan.

Warm and dusty, but merry and bright, the chums of the Remove clattered back to Luxor on their donkeys, and came tramping cheerily across the gangway to the tied-up dahabiyeh. Lord Mauleverer gave them a sleepy grin and a tired nod as they tramped on the upper deck. Billy Bunter gave them an inimical glare through his big spectacles; and as the glare produced absolutely no effect on the five, he requested them to sheer off. Bunter, it seemed, did not want their company just then.

But what Bunter wanted, or did not want, was a trifle light as air to the cheery chums of the Remove. Black Nubian servants pulled out deckchairs for them, and they sat down, with smiling faces.

"I say, you fellows, I think you might sheer off!" said Bunter. "It's rather bad form to interrupt a private conversation!"

"Fathead!" said Bob Cherry politely.

"I'm talking to Mauly!" roared Bunter.

"Poor old Mauly!" said Frank Nugent, with deep sympathy.

"The poorfulness of the esteemed old Mauly is terrific!" remarked Hurree Jamset Ram Singh. "The interruptfulness is a boonful blessing, isn't it, my estimable idiotic Mauly?"

"Yaas!" yawned Lord Mauleverer.

"What's the jolly old secret?" asked Johnny Bull, with a glare at Bunter. "Are you expecting a postal order in Egypt, and asking Mauly to cash it in advance, you fat fraud?"

"Ha, ha, ha!"

"I don't think you fellows ought to be inquisitive," said Bunter. "If there's one thing I can't stand, it's inquisitiveness!"

"Oh, my only summer hat!"

"Butting in when a fellow's having a private talk with a pal!" said Billy Bunter indignantly. "Rotten bad form, you know! I say, Mauly, old man, come down to the balcony!"

"Can't!"

"Why not?" demanded Bunter.

"Tired!"

"You silly ass, you've been sitting in that chair for two hours! What's made you tired?"

"You!"

"Ha, ha, ha!"

Billy Bunter fixed his big spectacles on his noble pal with an expression that did not seem at all pally. But he controlled his wrath. He had an important matter to discuss with Lord Mauleverer—a very important matter indeed. It was not a time for telling the schoolboy earl what he thought of him.

"We've had no end of a time, Mauly!" said Harry Wharton. "You ought to have come! The Temple of Hathor at Denderah is a corker!"

"I'll take your word for it, old man!" said Mauly.

"And the Temple of Isis!" said Bob Cherry.

"I say, you fellows, shut up!" said Bunter. "If you haven't the good taste to sheer off while I'm talking to my pal, you might shut up, at least!"

"Don't you want to hear about the jolly old sights at Denderah, Mauly?" asked Nugent.

"Not at all—I mean, yaas!" amended Lord Mauleverer hastily. "Anythin' to keep Bunter from talkin'!"

"The celebrated Temple of Hathor is——" began Bob.

"Shut up!" roared Bunter. "Now, Mauly, I was saying——"

"Oh dear! Yaas!" murmured Lord Mauleverer. "Go it, old fat bean! Mind if I go to sleep?"

"Oh, really, Mauly, as I was saying, I'm not the fellow to brag or to make a song about what I've done—you know that! But did I, or did I not, get you away from those Arab beasts, Hamza and Yussef, when they bagged you the day we went to Karnak? Did I, or did I not, risk my life with a pluck that none of those fellows would have been capable of to rescue you?"

"No!"

"Ha, ha, ha!"

"Why, you ungrateful beast!" roared Bunter. "You jolly well know I did!"

"I know you were on the spot by accident, and in such a shivering funk that you jolly nearly left me to it!" said Mauly. "Is that what you mean?"

"No, it isn't!" roared Bunter. "And look at the night that Greek rotter, Kalizelos, got on the dahabiyeh after that silly scarab! Did I, or did I not, watch over your safety and save you?"

"No!" yawned Lord Mauleverer.

"Ha, ha, ha!"

"Of all the ungrateful rotters——" gasped Bunter.

"You got out in the night rooting after grub and butted into the Greek johnny, and were scared out of your wits!" yawned Mauleverer. "Is that what you mean, old top?"

"No wonder Shakespeare talks about the thankless tooth of a serpent's child!" said Bunter bitterly. "I'm accustomed to ingratitude! Look what I've done for these fellows! And are they grateful? No fear! But there's a limit, Mauly! You owe me your life! I'm not bragging of it; pluck happens to be my long suit! Kindest friend and noblest foe, and all that—that's me all over. Now, look here, Mauly, for some reason remittances haven't reached me since we've been on this holiday in Egypt——"

"I knew he was expecting a postal order!" murmured Bob Cherry.

"Ha, ha, ha!"

"Shut up!" roared Bunter. "I'm not going to sponge on you, Mauly. I'm not like some fellows I could name, I hope! But a loan till my remittance comes is quite a different matter. You've lent me a few piastres already——"

"A few thousand!" grinned Bob.

"Do shut up, Cherry! Now, look here, Mauly——"

Lord Mauleverer sat up.

"I see the point," he said thoughtfully. "The fact is, you men keep on telling me that nothing's safe in my pockets. You've made me hide that jolly old scarab of A-Menah, so that I shan't lose it. Those Arabs the other day at Karnak got a lot of money off me. On the whole, I think the best thing I can do is to hand over all the money I've got to Bunter."

"You silly ass!" bawled Johnny Bull.

"Good egg!" exclaimed Billy Bunter eagerly. "I'll take care of it for you, Mauly! Rely on me!"

Lord Mauleverer fumbled in his pocket. Billy Bunter watched him with his eyes almost bulging through his spectacles. Harry Wharton & Co. simply stared.

Lord Mauleverer was in the happy position of having more of that useful article, cash, than a fellow could possibly want. There was no doubt that he was careless with it. Backsheesh flowed from Mauleverer's pockets like a stream—or, rather, like a torrent. Hassan, the dragoman, was making a fortune out of him. Innumerable natives, all along the Nile, had lapped up the crumbs that fell from the rich man's table. Billy Bunter had used him like a bank in which he had an unlimited account. But this seemed to be rather the limit, even for Mauly. Placing his cash in the care of Billy Bunter was really an amazing proposition. There was little doubt that it would have been for Mauly's benefit to have a friend taking care of his cash for him. But dropping it into the Nile would have been about as useful as placing it in the fat hands of the Owl of the Remove.

Mauleverer seemed in serious earnest, however. He drew his Russia-leather purse from his pocket.

"Mauly, you ass!" exclaimed Wharton, almost aghast.

"You shut up, Wharton!" roared Bunter wrathfully. "Mauly knows a pal he can trust. Mauly isn't asking you to take care of his money for him, are you, Mauly?"

"No."

"He's asking me," said Bunter loftily. "He knows he can rely on a pal like me. You fellows can shut up."

"Well, fools and their money are soon parted!" remarked Johnny Bull.

"Thanks!" yawned Mauleverer.

"My esteemed idiotic Mauly——" murmured the Nabob of Bhanipur.

"Don't you men think it a good idea?" asked Mauleverer innocently. "You've told me often enough that I'm jolly careless. I own up—I'm careless. Well, this money will be safe with Bunter. I can leave it to his judgment to spend it how he thinks fit——"

"Oh crikey!"

"I leave it absolutely in his hands," said Mauleverer. "You don't mind, Bunter?"

"My dear chap—my dear old pal!" gasped Bunter. "That's all right! I'm your man! Hand it over!"

"It's a lot of responsibility off my hands, you see," Mauleverer explained to the staring five. "Bunter's willin' to take it on. That settles it. I'm goin' to hand over all my money to Bunter—every piastre I've got about me. Bunter can do as he likes with it. I leave it to him entirely."

"Dear old Mauly!" said Billy Bunter, his fat voice fairly thrilling with affection. "Rely on me!"

"Here you are, old chap!"

Lord Mauleverer opened his nobby purse. From the interior he extracted a nickel coin, which was called a "kirsch" in the native tongue, but more generally a piastre. Its value was twopence-halfpenny!

This he placed in the eager, outstretched palm of William George Bunter.

"There!" he said, and he replaced the purse in his pocket and sank back lazily in his chair.

Bunter blinked at the coin. He seemed hardly able to believe his little round eyes, or his big round spectacles.

"What—what—what's this?" gasped Bunter blankly.

"It's a piastre, old top."

"I know it's a piastre, you idiot! But what—what is it for?"

"It's all my money."

"Wha-a-at?"

"By the way," added Lord Mauleverer thoughtfully, as if he had just remembered something. "I shall have to drop into the bank before we leave Luxor and get some cash. I've entirely run out."

Bunter blinked at him. He blinked at the nickel coin in his fat palm. He blinked at Mauleverer again. He seemed bereft of speech. There was a sudden roar from the Famous Five.

"Ha, ha, ha!"

Bunter found his voice.

"Mauly! You silly idiot—you frabjous ass—you burbling chump——"

"Eh?" Lord Mauleverer looked surprised. "Are you calling me those fancy names because I'm trusting you with all my money, Bunter?"

"Ha, ha, ha!" yelled the Famous Five. They realised now that his lazy lordship had been gently pulling the fat Owl's podgy leg.

"Mean to say this is all the money you've got?" shrieked Bunter.

"Yaas!"

"Why, you—you—you idiot——"

"I feel that I can trust you with it, Bunter, old bean. Spend it how you like—use your own judgment——"

"Ha, ha, ha!" shrieked the juniors.

The expression on Billy Bunter's fat face might have made the statue of Rameses the Second smile.

"You—you—you——" gurgled Bunter. "You—you funny idiot! You slacking ass! You idiotic dummy!"

"Ha, ha, ha!"

"Anythin' the matter, old bean?" asked Lord Mauleverer, raising his eyebrows. "That isn't really the way to talk to a fellow who's trusting you with all his money."

"Ha, ha, ha!"

"Beast!" roared Bunter.

"My dear chap——"

"Yah!"

Billy Bunter hurled all Mauly's money—that single, solitary piastre—into the Nile. Then, with a sort of scorn, he rolled away, followed by a sleepy grin from Lord Mauleverer and a howl of laughter from the Famous Five.

After which Harry Wharton & Co. told Mauly all about the wonderful things they had seen that day at Denderah. Mauly did not mind. He went to sleep, and slumbered gently and peacefully while they told him.

THE SECOND CHAPTER.

Ructions on the River!

"CAMPING out?"

"That's it!"

"Rot!" said Bunter.

The song of the Nubian sailors, as they handled their long poles, sounded musically in the sunny morning. The great houseboat swung away from the Nile bank and floated out into the river. The Greyfriars tourists had "done" the eastern bank—Luxor, and Karnak, and the other wonderful things—and now the dahabiyeh was being poled across the Nile to the western bank, where many more marvels awaited them.

Hassan, the dragoman, was bursting with information respecting the Necropolis, the "City of the Dead," the Tombs of the Kings, the Tombs of the Queens—tombs, and tombs, and tombs!—that covered a vast space on the west bank of the Nile opposite Luxor. There were, as the dragoman told them gleefully, innumerable dead persons—more innumerable than in any part of Egypt hitherto explored by the Greyfriars party. Which, to Hassan's mind, at least, was an irresistible attraction.

The juniors had breakfasted on the balcony, under the awning, at the stern of the dahabiyeh. Billy Bunter was still breakfasting on the balcony when they went to the upper deck. The broad waters of the Nile glistened in the sunshine, and other dahabiyehs were to be seen, as well as a crowd of feluccas—some rowing with their great, heavy oars, others gliding under the big lateen sails. The Cleopatra was the largest, and handsomest dahabiyeh to be seen. Mr. Hilmi Maroudi, of Cairo, who had lent it to the Greyfriars party, was a millionaire, and his dahabiyeh was a palatial boat. The juniors watched the busy scene on the Nile with keen interest. Other tourists were going across to the western bank that morning, but most of them in the ferryboat or in hired feluccas.

Billy Bunter rolled up to the upper deck, after packing away several breakfasts, one after another, and he brought with him a big orange in either fat hand to wind up his meal. He found the Famous Five discussing what they were going to do on the western bank. And as soon as he learned that the idea was to leave the dahabiyeh tied up and camp out for a night or two ashore, Bunter stated his opinion—for what it was worth.

The chums of the Remove did not seem to consider that it was worth very much. They continued to discuss their camping arrangements, regardless.

"You'd like to go camping, Mauly—what?" asked Harry Wharton.

"Yaas."

"Look here, Mauly," said Billy Bunter. "What's the good of roughing it in a silly tent when you can come back and sleep comfortably on the dahabiyeh? You'd rather come back to the dahabiyeh, wouldn't you?"

"Yaas."

"You can't do both, fathead!" remarked Johnny Bull.

"Oh dear!" said Mauly.

Lord Mauleverer's system was to agree with every suggestion made—which was a little awkward when opinions differed.

Billy Bunter guzzled an orange, hurled the peel into the Nile, and swatted flies that had a fancy for the orange juice smeared on his fat face.

"Well, you can take this from me," he said. "I'm not going camping! If you camp out in a lot of putrid ruins you won't have my company!"

"I say, camping seems rather a jolly idea," remarked Lord Mauleverer thoughtfully. "Let's camp out, by all means!"

"Oh, really, Mauly!"

"Hassan can fix us up with all the things we need," said Bob.

The dragoman salaamed.

"On my head be it, sar!" he said. "Hassan is your dragoman. You trust Hassan. Everything shall be at the top of a hole, as you say in your noble English language."

"Everything shall be—what?" ejaculated Mauleverer.

"The esteemed Hassan means that the top-holefulness will be terrific," explained Hurree Jamset Ram Singh.

"Oh gad!" said Mauly, and the juniors chuckled.

A nasal voice, in emphatic tones, hailed the juniors on the dahabiyeh from a felucca on the Nile. In that felucca sat two tourists—one a tall, lean gentleman, with lantern jaws, the other a short, stout gentleman. Each of them wore a sun-helmet and smoked glasses, and carried a red-covered guidebook, and spat continually into the Nile. From which latter circumstance the juniors guessed that they were tourists from the great United States. It was the lean man who hailed the dahabiyeh.

"Say! You!" he called out. "You figure that you want to run down this doggoned felucca? I'll say you'd better tell your niggers to keep them pesky poles away."

The tall, bronze-complexioned reis, standing at the high helm of the dahabiyeh, glanced down at the felucca, but gave no sign. The singing Nubians poled on, unregarding. Billy Bunter sniffed. On board the most magnificent dahabiyeh on the Nile, Billy Bunter felt immensely superior to commonplace tourists in a hired boat. He sniffed to make that superiority clear to the commonplace persons. Harry Wharton & Co. looked down at the felucca. The small craft was cutting across the bows of the big craft, so they concluded that it was the felucca's own look-out if there was trouble, and left it at that. But Lord Mauleverer, with great politeness, raised his hat to the American gentlemen and answered in his most courteous tones.

"Sorry, sir! We'd much rather not run you down, as a matter of choice. But perhaps you wouldn't mind keepin' out of the way."

The lean gentleman gave him a glare.

"You bought the Nile?" he inquired.

"I think not," answered Lord Mauleverer thoughtfully. "I've been buyin' things ever since I've been in Egypt—the people here won't take no for an answer, you know! I can't remember everythin' I've bought! But I don't think the Nile was among my purchases."

The Famous Five grinned as his lordship made that reply with perfect gravity. The lean American stared at him.

"Say, bo, was you born funny?" he asked. "I'll say you don't want to shoot off your mouth too promiscus when you're talking to George Washington Jacks! George W. Jacks might step aboard that hooker and spank you, some!"

"My esteemed and ridiculous friend," said Hurree Jamset Ram Singh, "the spankfulness might be a boot on the other leg."

Mr. Jacks gave quite a jump. Hurree Jamset Ram Singh's English, learned from the wisest moonshee in Bhanipur, often had a surprising effect on strangers.

"Carry me home to die!" said Mr. Jacks. "Did you hear that, colonel?"

"Did I, colonel?" answered the fat man. "I'll say I did!"

Both the American gentlemen, apparently, were colonels, though they did not look like military gentlemen.

"Jevver hear anything like it, Colonel Skink?" asked G. W. Jacks.

"I'll say no, Colonel Jacks," answered Colonel Skink.

The dahabiyeh rolled heavily on. The little felucca, which was rowed by a couple of brown men, danced on the wash of the great houseboat. Some of the Nile washed aboard and wetted the feet of the two colonels, and angry remarks were made through the noses of Messrs. Jacks and Skink.

"Cheek!" said Billy Bunter.

He pushed his face into his second orange. Bunter liked oranges, and he enjoyed them—but it could not be said that his method of dealing with them was either cleanly or elegant.

Having gobbled the interior of that fat and juicy fruit, Bunter carelessly tossed the remains over the side of the dahabiyeh.

"Look out!" ejaculated Bob Cherry.

"Eh?"

"You fat ass!"

It was too late for Bunter to look out. The remnant of the orange had landed. Every bullet is said to have its billet, and the same rule seemed to apply to that juicy relic of Bunter's latest snack. It landed in the keen, sharp, penetrating eye of Colonel Jacks.

G. W. Jacks was standing up at the moment. The next moment he was sitting down. He sat down with a sudden concussion that made the light felucca rock. The roar that burst from G. W. Jacks might have been heard on both banks of the Nile.

"Oh gad!" ejaculated Lord Mauleverer. "You clumsy ass, Bunter——"

"Eh?" said Bunter. The short-sighted Owl of the Remove had not even seen where his missile had landed. "What's the row? I say, you fellows, what is that Yankee yelling about?"

Colonel Jacks was yelling wildly to his rowers. They stared at him dubiously, but obeyed. The felucca ran alongside the dahabiyeh, and the long-limbed American was aboard the Cleopatra almost in the twinkling of an eye. He was angry and excited—there was no doubt about his anger and excitement. There was orange-juice in his eye, which was uncomfortable and painful. And obviously he was convinced that the missile had been thrown intentionally—which was enough to annoy even a very good-tempered man. And the long gentleman from the U.S. did not seem at all good-tempered, anyhow.

"Hallo, hallo, hallo!" ejaculated Bob Cherry. "What——"

"Yarooooh!" roared Bunter.

Two bony hands were grasping Billy Bunter before that fat youth knew what was happening.

He was sprawled, face down, across a bony knee.

Spank!

"Whooooop."

Spank, spank!

"Yow! Wow!"

"Oh, my hat!" gasped Harry Wharton.

Spank!

"Yooop! Help! Rescue!" roared Bunter. "I say, you fellows——Whoooop!"

Spank, spank!

"I guess you can't get by with sauce to G. W. Jacks!" roared the lean colonel. "No, sir! I'll say nope, sir! I'll surely say nope! Not G. W. Jacks, sir! George W. Jacks doesn't stand for it, sir! Sure! Not in your lifetime, and some over! Nope!"

Spank, spank, spank!

Billy Bunter wriggled and raved. Harry Wharton & Co. gathered round and grasped G. W. Jacks on all sides. Bunter deserved to be spanked, perhaps, for landing the relic of a juicy orange in a stranger's eye from sheer carelessness. But the lean gentleman was overdoing it wholesale. The Famous Five grasped various parts of Colonel Jacks' bony person and yanked him away from the Owl of the Remove.

"Chuck it!" gasped Bob Cherry. "Keep your jolly old temper, old bean!"

"Yaroooh! Pitch him into the Nile!" yelled Bunter. "Whop him! Oh crikey! Rag him! Pull his nose! Yaroooh!"

"I'll say you'd better leggo!" roared G. W. Jacks, struggling in the grasp of the juniors. "Yep! I'll say so!"

But the juniors did not let go. The

excited transatlantic gentleman seemed rather too dangerous to be released. They led him to the side, and Wharton shouted to the dancing felucca.

"Catch!"

"Search me!" ejaculated the other colonel in the felucca, staring up in astonishment. "By the great horned toad, you can search me!"

The rowers held the felucca close alongside, and the Famous Five dropped the bony gentleman back where he belonged. The thin colonel went sprawling down, and the fat colonel, in an unfortunate moment for himself, stepped forward to catch him and help him land. His foot slipped in the rocking boat, and he missed G. W. Jacks. But G. W. Jacks did not miss him—G. W. Jacks landed on the back of his neck.

There was an agonised gurgle from the plump colonel as he was squashed in the bottom of the boat under the bony colonel.

"Ooooh! Great gophers! Yoooogh!"

"Thunder!" gasped Colonel Jacks.

"Ha, ha, ha!" came in a yell from the dahabiyeh.

The two colonels were wildly mixed up in the bottom of the felucca. The light craft rocked wildly, shipping water, which drenched over the two struggling and sprawling colonels. There was a cackle of laughter from the Nubian crew of the Cleopatra; even the grave reis condescended to grin.

The dahabiyeh rolled on, leaving the felucca behind. Two crimson and breathless citizens of the United States sorted themselves out at last, and sat and gasped for wind. The dahabiyeh rolled on, and they faded out of the picture, still gasping.

THE THIRD CHAPTER.

What is the Secret?

"WHAT about the jolly old prisoner?" said Bob Cherry.

The dahabiyeh was tied up once more on the western bank. Before the eyes of the Greyfriars tourists stretched the vast necropolis of ancient Thebes. Nearer at hand a crowd of donkey-boys already had their eyes on the tourists, and were already leading their animals towards the bank and shouting from the distance. Itinerant dealers in spurious antiquities were watching for them to come ashore.

Lord Mauleverer nodded thoughtfully as Bob referred to the prisoner of the dahabiyeh.

"Let's go down and see the jolly old bird in his cage," said Mauly, and the Famous Five followed him down to the cabins.

One cabin door was locked, and a Nubian was squatted outside on guard. He rose and salaamed and unlocked the door, and Lord Mauleverer stepped into the prison-cabin, with the Famous Five behind him. Kalizelos, the Greek, rose to his feet, his black eyes burning at the Greyfriars fellows. For a good many days now Kalizelos had been a prisoner on board the Cleopatra under lock and key. As Mauleverer stepped in the Greek looked as if he would spring on him like a tiger. Mauleverer smiled and waved him back.

"Keep your temper, old bean!" he said. "Hassan, knock him on the head if he cuts up rusty!"

"On my head be it, sar!" answered the dragoman, who had followed the juniors down, stick in hand.

Lord Mauleverer regarded the prisoner with thoughtful seriousness. Harry Wharton & Co. were smiling. Mauly's method of dealing with the Greek made them smile; but there was no doubt, at all events, that it was keeping their enemy out of mischief.

And there was no doubt that Kalizelos had asked for it. He had crept on board the dahabiyeh in the darkness of a night to steal the Golden Scarab—and Mauleverer had awakened with the Greek's knife at his throat! In Cairo the rascal had been handed over to the police, by Mr. Maroudi, the juniors' Egyptian friend; but he had escaped. Mauly was taking his own measures to see that the villain did not escape a second time. So far, those measures had been efficacious.

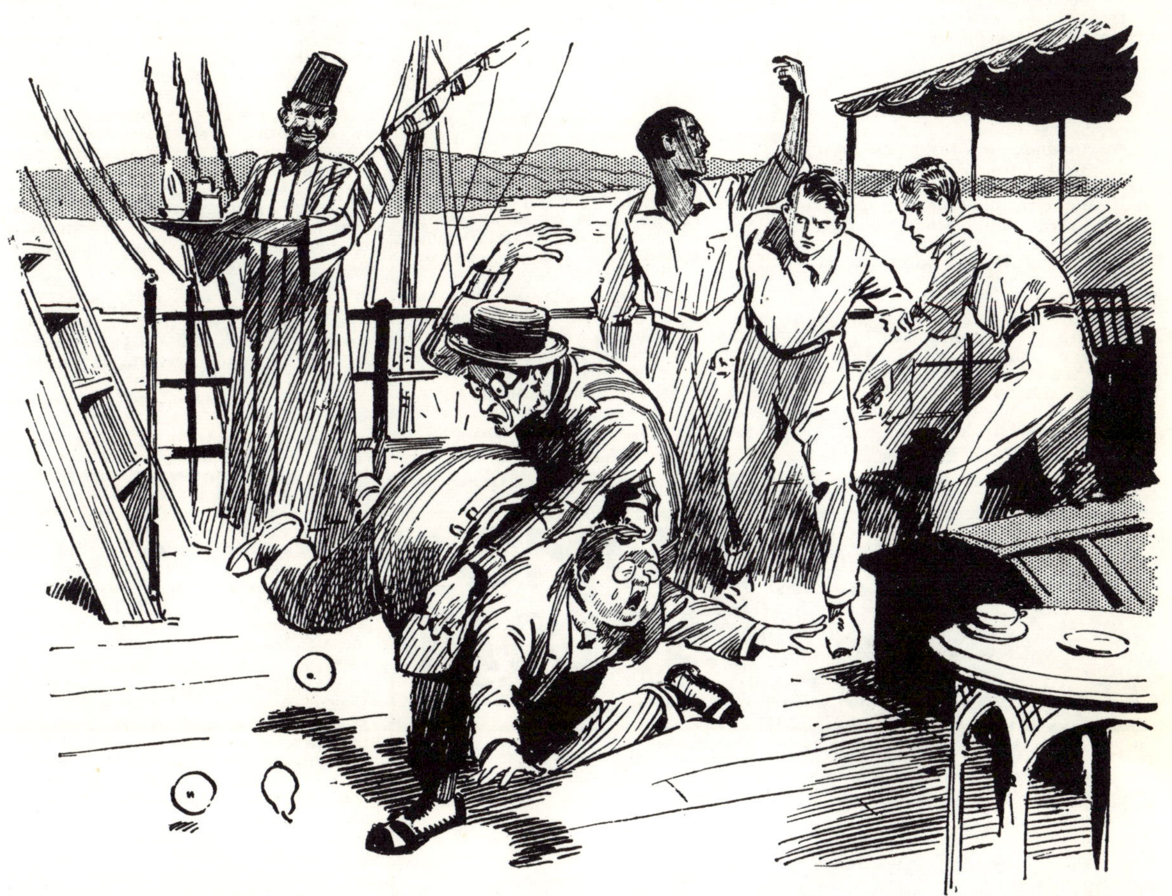

Two bony hands grasped Billy Bunter and he was sprawled, face down, across a bony knee. Colonel Jacks' hand rose and fell. Spank, spank, spank! "Yaroooh!" gasped Bunter. "I say, you fellows—whooop!" "I guess you can't get by with sauce to G. W. Jacks!" roared the lean American. "I'll surely say nope!"

"We're going away from the dahabiyeh for a day or two, Mr. Kalizelos," drawled Lord Mauleverer. "I'm givin' you another chance before we go. Are you comin' to terms?"

"Fool!" snarled the Greek.

"Look at it reasonably," urged Mauleverer placidly. "I've got the Golden Scarab that my father found in Egypt years and years ago. It's mine. It belonged to jolly old A-Menah three thousand years ago, in the reign of Ram—Ram—Ram—thingummy——"

"Rameses the Second!" grinned Bob.

"Yaas, I know it was Ram-somethin'. Jolly old A-Menah wore it as an amulet in those days, at the battle of What's-its-name, in Syria, and it seems to have brought him luck. He came back from the wars with a big diamond in his trousers pocket—if they wore trousers in the reign of Ram—Ram—Ram—thingummy! The story goes that the scarab will guide any Johnny who happens to hold it to that big diamond—the Eye of—of—of——"

"The Eye of Osiris!" prompted Bob.

"Yaas, that's it! Now, of course, I don't believe a word of it," said Lord Mauleverer cheerfully. "I can't quite swallow ancient Egyptian magic. But the trouble is that you do, Mr. Kalizelos. You keep on tryin' to get that scarab off me, and you've made things dashed unpleasant—shuttin' a fellow up in tombs, and so on. You can't expect a fellow to like it."

"Fool!"

"Your manners, old thing, are simply horrid," said Lord Mauleverer. "But never mind that. It seems that you got hold of an ancient papyrus, in your curio shop at Cairo, and learned the secret of the scarab. You're after that scarab like my friend Bunter after a jam-tart——"

"Oh, really, Mauly——"

"And a chap gets fed-up," said Mauleverer, shaking his head. "Now you've been obliging enough to drop into my hands, and I'm keepin' you where you can't do any more harm——"

"I demand to be handed over to the law!" said the Greek hoarsely.

Lord Mauleverer shook his head.

"You wouldn't—if you didn't fancy that you could wangle it to get away from the jolly old law," he answered. "I don't think a fearful lot of the law. It's rather a fishy bizney, even in my own country. In the East I've got an idea that it's largely a matter of backsheesh. You see, you got away in Cairo, old bean, and I can't help thinkin' you'd get away in Luxor. You're safer here."

"Fool!"

"Thanks! Now, there's two ways out of this difficult matter," said his lordship. "Either I can give you the scarab, or you can give me the secret. I'm not givin' you the scarab—it's mine. But I've got to draw your teeth! You see that?"

"Fool!"

"This sportsman doesn't seem to have a high opinion of my intellect, does he, you men? Never mind! Now, old top, if there's really a secret, cough it up. Once you've handed it over, you won't want the scarab, and I can get shut of you. I'd be thankful to see the last of you, believe me. You can see for yourself that it's the only way."

"Fool!"

Lord Mauleverer slipped his hand into his pocket and drew out the golden beetle, the cause of so many exciting adventures since the Greyfriars chums had started on their Egyptian holiday.

The Greek's eyes snapped at sight of it. Shaped like the sacred beetle of ancient Egypt, made apparently of solid gold, the amulet lay in Mauleverer's palm, glistening in the light. Often and often had the juniors handled it, wondering what was its strange secret—if any. They knew that the tiny picture-writing engraved on it told nothing but the name and title of A-Menah. That it had magic properties was hardly to be believed. How it could possibly guide its possessor to the Eye of Osiris was unimaginable. Yet the look on the Greek's face, the hungry greed that blazed in his eyes, the eager twitching of his features showed how strong was his belief.

It was obvious that Kalizelos could barely restrain himself from springing at the schoolboy earl and snatching at the scarab. Yet what secret could he have read in that ancient papyrus written by the scribe of A-Menah? What secret could there be in the golden beetle that no other eyes could read?

"There's the jolly old article," said Lord Mauleverer, holding it up. "It's mine, as I've mentioned. I'm not givin' it away—especially if it's a clue to a diamond worth a quarter of a million pounds. That's askin' rather too much of a fellow, what? Trot out the secret!"

"I will tell you nothing!" hissed the Greek.

"If you weren't so jolly savage about it, old thing, I shouldn't believe there was a giddy secret at all. But you're not the man to risk your life, and spend money like water, for the sake of a mere curiosity. I'm beginnin' to believe there really is a secret—though I can't begin to guess what it is. Won't you cough it up?"

"Never!"

"Most likely it's only gammon," said Mauleverer. "But if it turns out to be worth anythin', I'll do the fair thing. I'll stand you ten per cent of the loot, if I bag it. What?"

"That's a good offer!" grinned Bob Cherry.

"All or nothing!" muttered the Greek. "Fool! The scarab is valueless to you. You cannot read its secret. Only I can read it A thousand pounds—ten thousand pounds—sell me the scarab."

"Beats me hollow," said Lord Mauleverer. "This sportsman is in earnest, you men—he'd be glad to trot out ten thousand pounds for this scarab, which is worth about twenty-five for its metal. Do you get him?"

"It's pretty plain that there is a secret, and that Kalizelos knows it," said Harry Wharton. "But the scarab is yours, Mauly, and if it leads to a treasure, the treasure is yours."

"Quite! We can't let this man go," said Mauleverer. "Not unless he draws his own teeth by handin' over the secret. If I could trust him to let me alone, and let my scarab alone, I'd be glad to get shut of him. But——"

"It shall be mine!" snarled the Greek. "Your life, or a thousand lives, shall not stand in the way. I will gain my freedom—you cannot keep me on this dahabiyeh! Then for you, death; for me, the scarab!"

"Thanks for the tip," said Lord Mauleverer, slipping the sacred scarabæus of A-Menah into his pocket. "I'll see that you don't get loose—till you've coughed up that jolly old secret! Last time of askin'!"

"Fool!"

"I take that as an answer in the negative. Come on, you men!"

"Look out!" yelled Bob, as the Greek made a sudden, desperate spring.

Crack!

Hassan was looking out!

His stick whirled in the air, and came down with a loud crack on the head of Konstantinos Kalizelos.

The Greek gave a gasping cry, and rolled on the floor of the cabin.

Hassan chuckled.

"Hassan look out, noble sar!" he

said. "Hassan is your dragoman! You trust Hassan! Oh, yes!"

"Sorry, old thing," said Lord Mauleverer, politely, as the Greek sat up dizzily, clasping his head with both hands. "You asked for that—what? Ta-ta!"

The juniors left the cabin. The door was closed and locked on the Greek. His voice followed them in a string of fierce imprecations as they went.

Their faces were thoughtful as they returned to the deck. What was the strange secret of the scarab? It was an intriguing mystery. Looking at the golden beetle, they could not believe that it held a secret; but looking at the desperate Greek, they could hardly doubt it. Their minds seemed to sway to and fro on the subject.

"Better take it ashore with us, I think," yawned Lord Mauleverer. "That Greek sportsman is safe enough, but—— I don't fancy leavin' the scarab on the dahabiyeh with him while we're away for days."

"No fear," agreed Bob Cherry. "Mind you don't drop it in one of the jolly old tombs, though."

"I say, you fellows——"

"Hallo, hallo, hallo! Ready, Bunter?"

Billy Bunter fixed his eyes, and his spectacles, severely on the chums of the Remove.

"I'm ready, if we're going to have a car, and if we're coming back to the dahabiyeh for the night," he answered firmly. "If you're going to ride those beastly donkeys, and camp out among a lot of putrid old ruins, I'm not ready! I refuse to do anything of the sort!"

Bob Cherry chuckled.

"We're going to ride donkeys, and we're going to camp out for the night, old fat bean," he said.

"Yes, rather!"

"The ratherfulness is terrific, my esteemed fat Bunter."

Snort from Bunter.

"Then you can jolly well leave me out!" he snapped.

Bob Cherry took out his handkerchief.

"Excuse me while I cry for a few minutes, you men," he said. "Boo-hoo! We're going to l-lose B-B-Bunter! Boo-hoo!"

"You silly ass!" roared Bunter.

"Pardon these tears!" sobbed Bob Cherry. "Excuse my emotion! Boo-hoo!"

"Ha, ha, ha!"

"I mean it!" roared Bunter. "You can jolly well get on the best you can without me, see?"

"Boo-hoo!"

"Come on," said Harry Wharton, laughing.

And the Greyfriars party went ashore, Bob Cherry drying his tears; and Billy Bunter glared after them with a glare that almost cracked his spectacles.

THE FOURTH CHAPTER.

The City of the Dead!

"GREAT, enormous, and gigantic Ramesseum——" chanted Hassan.

Harry Wharton & Co., having "done" the Colossi of Memnon, arrived at the Ramesseum on donkey-back. Hassan's brown face fairly glowed with satisfaction. If there was anything the dragoman enjoyed more than cheating his lordly gentlemen it was pointing out to them the wonders of Egypt. And the Ramesseum, the gigantic temple built by Rameses the Second, was "some" sight.

The juniors dismounted from their steeds, which were left with the donkey-boys. Other tourists were on hand; and the ancient courts of the Ramesseum echoed to many languages—French and German, Arabic, English, and American.

It was a sunny day—and, of course, warm! It was going to be a real "beano," as Bob Cherry described it. The day was to be spent in donkey-riding among the ruins, seeing the sights; and instead of riding back to the Nile and the dahabiyeh, the party were going to camp out.

Within a short ride of the Tombs of the Kings was an estate belonging to Mr. Hilmi Maroudi, of Cairo, partly cultivated with orange-trees, partly desert. Mr. Maroudi, who had lent his magnificent dahabiyeh to his young friends, had told them of it, and that he had sent word to his manager to make them welcome if they gave the place a look-in. So while the juniors were sight-seeing with Hassan, the Nubians were conveying the necessary things to Mr. Maroudi's land for camping out.

When the day's ride was over, the juniors were to find the camp ready, the tent up, and the supper cooked—which was camping-out on very easy and agreeable terms. The friendship of Mr. Maroudi was helping to make their holiday in Egypt run on very pleasant lines.

Had Billy Bunter been able to see the party as they arrived at the Ramesseum, he would not have been able to observe any diminution of their cheery spirits on account of his absence. Indeed, from their looks, it might have been supposed that the chums of the Remove were rather bucked by Bunter's determination to stay on the dahabiyeh.

Clatter! Clatter! Clatter! came the beating of donkeys' hoofs, and the juniors glanced round at new arrivals. A nasal voice, which they had heard already that morning, came to their ears.

"Say, you! You black-faced bonehead! You want to take a cinch on this ornery cayuse, I'm telling you."

"Hallo, hallo, hallo, here come the jolly old colonels!" grinned Bob Cherry.

The two American gentlemen were in sight.

The tall, bony Colonel Jacks was struggling with a donkey that was trying to bolt. The donkey was so small, and the American gentleman was so long, that he could almost have touched the ground with his feet on either side of his mount by stretching out his lengthy legs. He had them doubled up, his bony knees jabbing at the donkey's ears. Perhaps that irritated the donkey. Anyhow, he was very restive, and G. W. Jacks was in difficulties, and yelling to his donkey-boy to control the steed.

The fat colonel, on the other hand, who was jogging on behind, was in no danger of his steed bolting. His unfortunate donkey looked on the point of collapse under his weight. Many Egyptian donkeys had suffered under Billy Bunter—but Colonel Skink was a heavier weight than Bunter, and he really looked as if he might turn his hapless moke into a pancake. The wretched donkey proceeded at a snail's pace, with an expression on his face that might have touched a heart of stone.

"Say, you bonehead!" roared Colonel G. W. Jacks, to his donkey-boy. "You hear me hoot? You hear me yaup? I'll say you want to take a cinch on this here cayuse!"

"Yes, sar!" gasped the donkey-boy. "Oh, yes, sar! Whack um, sar!" Probably the donkey-boy, whose English was limited, did not know any American at all, and had to guess what "taking a cinch" might possibly mean. Apparently, he concluded that the donkey was to be touched-up; and he touched him up, hard. The donkey jumped, and

FREE GIFTS FOR YOU!

A Special Announcement from Your Editor.

HALLO, CHUMS!—Here's some great news—not just ordinary great news, but something really extra special, and I want you to take most particular note of it.

In two weeks' time there will start in the MAGNET the BIGGEST COLLECTING BOOM that has ever been planned.

It is a tremendous scheme—record-breaking is a better description—and it will set all of you cheering lustily and congratulating yourselves that you are MAGNET readers. Now, read the following details carefully:

I have prepared a SPECIAL SERIES of SUPER STAMPS, and these reveal EVERY BOY'S WORLD in splendid coloured pictures. Six of these Super Stamps will be given away each week in every issue of the MAGNET for many weeks to come. These topping Super Stamps present the most fascinating pictures imaginable of railway engines, aeroplanes, ships, dogs, roughriders, and the art of self-defence—all beautifully coloured. The whole series of these Super Stamps comprises the mammoth total of 144 stamps, which are divided into six series of 24 stamps each! Got that?

Never has there been anything quite so good as this grand Free Gift Scheme. Our companion papers, MODERN BOY and RANGER will also give away each week six of these magnificent stamps.

This grand Free Gift Surprise to all MAGNET readers does not stop there. Every reader will have the chance of obtaining a tip-top Album specially designed to hold the whole collection of 144 stamps in its twenty pages. In next week's MAGNET I will explain how it is possible for every reader to secure this grand Album FREE, so make sure of your copy by ordering it NOW

Cheerio, chums!

YOUR EDITOR.

his rider's sharp, bony knees jabbed him behind the ears, and he jumped still more.

The donkey-boy whacked again, and whacked again. Colonel Jacks swayed to and fro on the donkey, yelling. That was not what he wanted at all. He wanted the restive donkey held back, not driven to greater speed. But the donkey-boy did not catch on, and he whacked with great vigour—unlimited whacking being in the nature of Egyptian donkey-boys.

"Oh, my hat!" exclaimed Harry Wharton, as the excited and exasperated animal broke into an infuriated gallop. "That sportsman is going to hit trouble!"

"Begad!" murmured Lord Mauleverer. "I fancy he's going to hit Egypt."

"Ha, ha, ha!"

Mauleverer was right.

Bony knees jabbing into him seemed to drive the donkey frantic. He galloped and plunged and roared, and suddenly put down his head and threw up his heels. G. W. Jacks shot over his head like a stone from a catapult and hit Egypt with a mighty smite.

"Oh crumbs!" gasped Frank Nugent.

"Him American gentleman him break him bones," remarked Hassan placidly.

"Well, he's got enough to spare!" murmured Bob.

Fortunately, the lean gentleman had not broken any bones. He sat up and stared after the donkey. That sagacious brute, relieved of his burden, was evidently desirous of keeping clear of it. He was going off at a gallop towards the Tombs of the Queens, with the perspiring donkey-boy raging in pursuit.

"Waal, I swow!" gasped Colonel Jacks. "I surely swow! Yep! I'll say I swow! By the great horned toad! You, Ephraim Skink, you ride after that doggoned burro and get him for me."

"I guess you want to tell me how to make this burro move, Colonel Jacks!" panted Colonel Skink, coming up at a snail's pace. "Yep, I'll say I want to know how to make this goldarned burro move!"

Colonel Jacks scrambled to his feet. He glared at the group of Greyfriars fellows, who were smiling. Then he started in pursuit of the runaway donkey, his long legs thrashing like flails. After him went the fat colonel, at a much slower pace. They disappeared from view beyond the Temple of Meremptah; and the grinning juniors turned back to the Ramesseum, the entertainment being over.

Harry Wharton & Co. found plenty to fill up the morning in the celebrated Ramesseum. After which, a luncheon-basket that had been brought on a donkey was unpacked, and they rested and lunched in the shade of a wide-spreading acacia.

In Egypt, it was an absolute necessity to rest in the midday heat. Not till well on in the afternoon did the tourists resume the exploration of the immense remains of the ancient Theban City of the Dead.

Then they rode up to Riban-el-Maluk to view the Tombs of the Kings. In that valley of the barren hills endless rock-tombs had been hewn by ancient hands. Most interesting to the juniors was that of Tutankhamen, of which Mauly's uncle, Sir Reginald Brooke, had told them. It was discovered in 1922 by Mr. Howard Carter and the Earl of Carnarvon. The mummy of the ancient king was still there, where it had been laid to rest so many centuries ago; but that the juniors did not want to see. But they explored the tomb; and then clambered back up the endless

steps to the valley, glad to get into the sunlight again.

By that time the sun was setting over the hills of the Libyan Desert, and the juniors had had enough of tombs; and though Hassan told them enticingly of "innumerable dead persons" that remained to be seen, they decided to start for camp.

Hassan led the way, by a rather rugged and tortuous path over the hills, to the estate of Mr. Maroudi. The gleam of the orange-trees against the dusty brown of the desert was a welcome sight.

"Hallo, hallo, hallo, there's the jolly old tent!" exclaimed Bob.

There was no road, only a donkey-track, which ran beside an irrigating canal. Beside the track, among a number of scattered acacias and tamarisk bushes, was a small tent.

The juniors drew rein and looked at it.

"That can't be our tent," said Harry Wharton. "It's not big enough for half of us."

"No, sar; that is not the tent of honourable lords," said Hassan, looking puzzled. "Great and luxurious tent for lordly gentleman is farther onward."

"Somebody else camping here?" said Johnny Bull.

"No person has leave to camp on land of great Maroudi," said Hassan. "Only my lordly gentlemen, who are friends of great Maroudi. This is tent of some common person who has butted in, as you say in English."

"Oh, my hat! It's the jolly old colonel's!" exclaimed Nugent.

A tall, lean man and a short, fat man came into view through the tamarisks. They stared at the Greyfriars fellows, who stared in return.

"Say, you bobbed up again!" said Colonel Jacks.

"The bobfulness is terrific, my esteemed transatlantic friend!" replied Hurree Jamset Ram Singh.

"You are camping here?" asked Harry.

"I'll say yep."

"But this is not of estimable permission!" exclaimed Hassan. "You have no affirmative leave from Mr. Maroudi."

Colonel Jacks looked at the dragoman.

"Who's Mr. Maroudi when he's at home?" he asked carelessly. Apparently, he had never heard of the Egyptian millionaire. "This here ground belong to him—hay? Perhaps he's the darky in the nightshirt who came along and blew off his mouth awhile back? Yep? Waal, I guess we're camping on this very identical spot, and I calculate that we ain't taking 'No' from a nigger! Nope!"

"I'll say nope!" chimed in Colonel Skink. "I'll surely say nope!"

Evidently the American gentlemen had made themselves at home on Mr. Maroudi's land without troubling about the formality of asking leave. The "darky in the nightshirt" to whom G. W. Jacks alluded was no doubt Mr. Maroudi's manager, who had come along to explain that it was private land —unheeded by the free-and-easy gentlemen from the United States.

Colonel Jacks turned a plug of tobacco in his mouth and spat. Colonel Skink followed his example.

"Say, since we've met up so handy," went on Colonel Jacks, "I've got suthin' to say to you guys for dropping me off your boat this morning! I've sure got a stick in my tent, if you'll hang on a minute till I get it!"

The long-legged colonel made a stride towards the tent. Harry Wharton & Co. laughed, and rode on without waiting for him to emerge. A grove of orange-trees hid the Yankee camp from their sight as they came in view of their own camping-ground.

A dark gentleman in a djubbah—probably the darky in the nightshirt who had interviewed the two colonels—came salaaming towards them. Black servants stood round and salaamed. A large tent stood by the orange-trees; and a camp-fire was lighted, which was needed, for after the heat of the day the night was cold. The dark gentleman spoke in Arabic, which was translated by Hassan, bidding them welcome in the name of Mr. Maroudi, and placing himself and all that was his at the disposal of the Faringhee lords.

"Jolly—what?" said Bob Cherry, as they sat down to supper round the jolly camp-fire.

"What-ho!"

There was no doubt that it was jolly. Mr. Maroudi's servants left them after supper, returning to their own quarters on a distant part of the estate, and the juniors sat and talked round the camp-fire, under the glittering stars of Egypt, Hassan hovering round them with a beaming, dusky face. And when the juniors turned in, in downy beds in the big tent, the dragoman stretched himself on a prayer-rug in the doorway—to sleep, as he told them, with one eye open to watch over the safety of his lordly gentlemen; a statement which the juniors took the liberty of doubting, for before they closed their own eyes the dragoman was snoring.

THE FIFTH CHAPTER.

Bunter on His Own!

"BEASTS!" growled Billy Bunter.

Billy Bunter was fed-up.

In one sense, he was more than fed-up; for he had spent a happy morning in taking a series of "snacks"—and every one of Bunter's little snacks would have made a square meal for any other fellow. That series of snacks had been followed by a Gargantuan lunch. Lunch had been followed by a nap, and nap by a substantial tea. Provender on board the houseboat was good and ample. Mr. Maroudi's own skilful Coptic cook was in charge of the commissariat, and he satisfied even Bunter. But even William George Bunter, at long last, grew fed-up with meals and intermediate snacks. He had a rather uncomfortable feeling in his circumference, and doubted whether he would enjoy his dinner that evening.

And he was fed-up with his own company. Bunter was gregarious. Camping out was rot; a comfortable cabin on the dahabiyeh was solid sense. But the other fellows had preferred their own "rot" to Bunter's solid sense, and Bunter had sniffed and left them to it. Now he wished he hadn't.

Even Bunter could not eat and sleep all day. When he was not eating or sleeping he wanted to talk. His fat voice was music to his own ears, if to no others. The Nubian sailors on the dahabiyeh did not understand English; the Nubian servants understood very little. The reis understood the language, but had no desire to use it as a means of conversation with Billy Bunter.

Indeed, the only living things on board the Cleopatra that had ever displayed any partiality for Bunter was the flies. One of Bunter's chief occupations was swatting the flies that loved him not wisely but too well.

Had the dahabiyeh still been tied up at Luxor, on the eastern bank, Bunter could have rolled ashore, and found

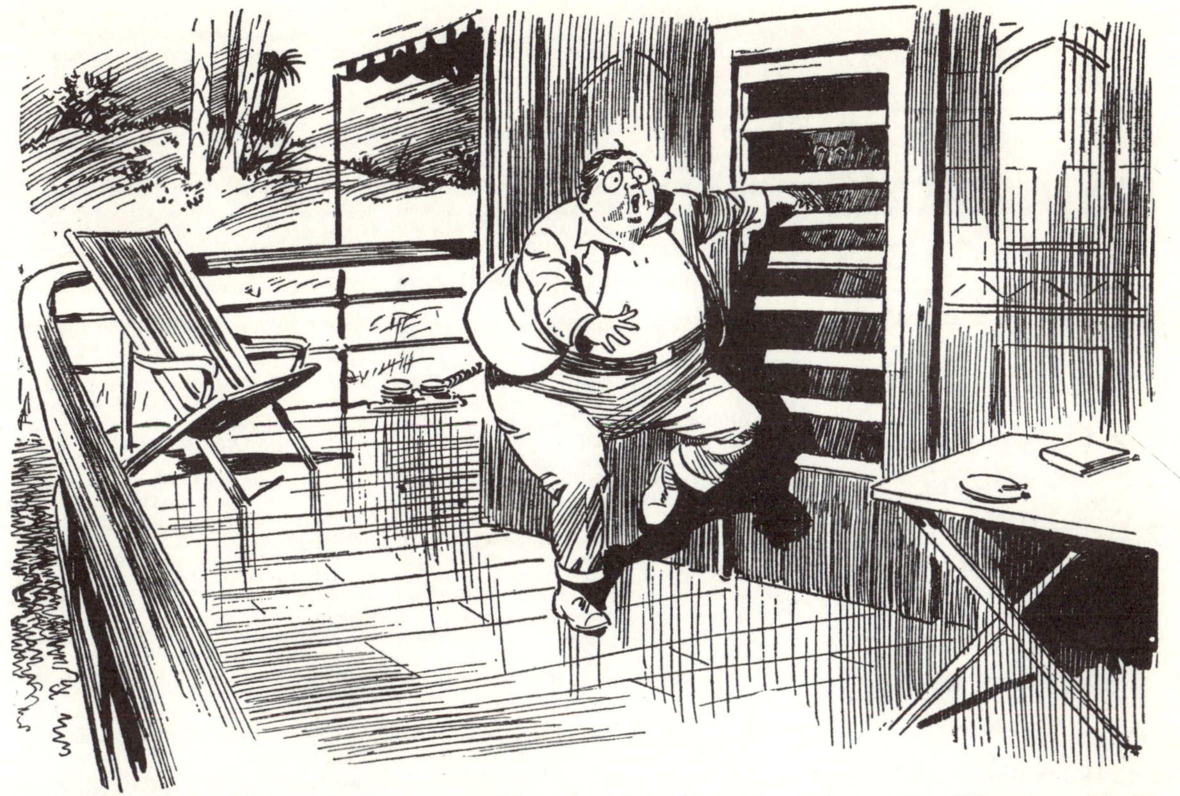

As Bunter put his hand through the slats a grasp of iron was laid on his wrist, and it was held as if in a vice. The fat junior gave a startled yelp. " Silence, pig ! " hissed Kalizelos. " One cry to the men on deck and I will twist your arm till the bones crack ! "

something to do in the town. But the Cleopatra was on the western bank now, and the broad Nile rolled between him and Luxor. Bunter blinked at the hills and valleys, at the towering Colossi, at obelisks and ruined temples and donkey-riders, and did not feel disposed to go exploring tombs on his lonely own.

It was just like those beasts, he reflected bitterly, to go off for the day and leave him on his own. It was true that he had refused to go with them; still, he might have consented if they had shown a proper yearning for his fascinating society. But they hadn't. If they had come back and begged him to think again, he might have consented to think again. But they hadn't.

"Leaving a fellow on his own!" grunted Bunter, blinking at the sunset over the Libyan Desert. "Beasts! After all I've done for 'em, too! It's always the same. A chap can't be open-hearted, generous, considerate, without meeting with beastly ingratitude on all sides!"

Bunter shook his head sadly over this. It was really a saddening reflection.

Leaning on the rail of the dahabiyeh, he blinked at the shore and debated whether he should go for a donkey-ride. He had had a lot of ill-luck with donkeys. Still, he was bored to the back teeth with hanging about the deck doing nothing. He was not hungry, and he was not sleepy, and a fellow had to do something. He had money in his pockets, too.

Lord Mauleverer had paid his visit to the bank before Luxor was left. When Mauly was in funds, Billy Bunter was in funds. He had borrowed a few thousand piastres from his lordship—the same to be "squared" out of some postal orders he was expecting next term at Greyfriars. He had almost made up his fat mind to go ashore and hire a donkey when he observed a figure in a dusty djubbah standing under a palm watching the dahabiyeh.

It was an Arab; he had been there some time, though Bunter had not specially noticed him before. Now that he did notice him, something familiar about the man struck Bunter. He fixed his spectacles on the dark face, but the distance was too great for recognition by the short-sighted Owl of the Remove. As he watched the man, another Arab came through the palms and joined him, and Bunter could make out the scar of an old knife-cut on the newcomer's cheek He gave a jump.

"Those villains!" he ejaculated.

He knew who they were now—Hamza, the man with the knife-cut; Yussef, the hawk-faced ruffian—the two Arab confederates of Kalizelos. For a moment Billy Bunter felt a spasm of terror. But he realised that he was safe on the dahabiyeh, with its numerous crew and crowd of servants—all, by the order of Hilmi Maroudi, devoted to the service of the Greyfriars party.

Reassured by that reflection, Bunter watched the two rascals curiously through his big spectacles. They were watching the houseboat, and there was little doubt that they had discovered or guessed at last what had become of their missing master, and knew that Konstantinos Kalizelos was kept a prisoner on board the Cleopatra.

The two Arabs came down to the bank at last, stepped on the gangway, and approached the side of the dahabiyeh. Moussa, the reis, waved them back. Bunter did not understand a word of what followed; Arabic volleyed to and fro between the two rascals and the tall, grave reis. The argument grew hot, and Hamza, the scarred man, suddenly drew a knife from under his djubbah and made as if to rush across the gangway.

The reis did not stir; but he called out, and a dozen of the Nubian sailors crowded to the spot, with staves in their hands. The scarred ruffian jumped back just in time to elude a blow that would have knocked him off the gang-plank into the mud of the Nile.

Moussa waved his hand and barked Arabic. Hamza and Yussef yelled back in the same tongue; and though Bunter did not understand, the words, looks and tones told him that they were hurling a storm of abuse at the reis. A faint flush showed under Moussa's dusky skin, and he rapped out an order to his sailors. Five or six of them ran across the gangway and began beating the Arabs with their staves.

Bunter grinned

"That's the stuff to give 'em!" he chuckled.

Yelling, the two Arabs beat a retreat and vanished beyond the palms. If they had entertained any idea of rescuing their master they had had to give it up now. The Nubian sailors came chuckling back to the dahabiyeh.

Hamza and Yussef were gone, but the sight of them caused Bunter to give up his idea of a donkey-ride ashore. Probably they would not have heeded the fat junior with whom they had no concern; but Bunter was not taking the risk. He loafed on the deck and yawned, and leaned on the side and blinked at the muddy bank of the Nile.

From a latticed window below, which was shuttered and fastened, he heard the sound of a voice and grinned. It was the voice of Kalizelos, the Greek; and though Bunter knew no Greek, ancient or modern, he did not need to be told that Kalizelos was uttering imprecations in the latter language. Doubtless, through the interstices of the shutter, he had seen his confederates and watched their retreat.

Bunter had forgotten the prisoner of the dahabiyeh, but he was reminded of him now. A thoughtful expression came over his fat face. Kalizelos knew the secret of the scarab, if it had a secret. It was a secret, if the Greek was well informed, worth a quarter of a million pounds! He had refused to reveal it to Lord Mauleverer as the price of his liberty; if there was, indeed, anything to reveal. Bunter was intensely curious on the subject, and he was idle and bored, and he resolved to have a talk with Kalizelos. It seemed possible to Bunter that a deep, wily, sagacious fellow like Bunter might be able to draw something out of the Greek.

Wild horses would hardly have dragged Bunter into the cabin within reach of the Greek's sinewy hands. But it was not necessary to go to the cabin. The window of the prison-room looked on the balcony that surrounded the stern of the dahabiyeh. That window was covered by a slatted shutter, which allowed the air to circulate freely, and through which it was easy to speak.

The fat Owl went below, walked through the passage and saloons to the balcony, and strolled round to Kalizelos' window.

He tapped.

There was a startled exclamation in the cabin. Bunter heard the Greek bound to the window. He grinned at the thought that perhaps Kalizelos supposed that it was one of his confederates coming to his aid.

There was a mosquito-net over the inside of the window. The Greek dragged it aside, and his olive face was pressed to the slats. Even with the shutter between, Billy Bunter felt a thrill of terror at the gleam of the jet black eyes.

The slats were about six inches apart, but they were strong, and the shutter was locked, the key taken away. Bunter was daunted only for a moment. Then he grinned.

The Greek glared at him like a caged wolf. Evidently he was surprised and not pleased to see Bunter's fat face outside.

"Hallo, old bean! Finding it warm in there?" asked Bunter genially.

"Fool!" snarled Kalizelos.

But his manner changed instantly. Perhaps the obvious fatuousness in Bunter's face gave him a gleam of hope.

"Boy! Listen!" He whispered through the slats. "A thousand pounds in English money to help me to freedom!"

"Oh crikey!" ejaculated Bunter.

He stared at the Greek, whose black eyes fairly burned at him through the slats.

"Are you watched? Can they see you?" breathed the Greek.

"Eh! No! They can't see me here from the deck," said Bunter.

"Help me! A thousand pounds——"

"Catch me!" said Bunter derisively.

The Greek eyed him evilly. He had set Bunter down as a hanger-on of the wealthy Mauleverer, and he had seen enough of the Greyfriars party to have learned a great deal about William George Bunter. He had hoped, at least, that Bunter could be bribed. But William George Bunter had his limit, though it was a wide one.

"You can wash that out, old bean," grinned Bunter. "Not that I believe you'd pony up; a knife in the back would be more in your line. He, he, he! But look here—about that jolly old scarab. Is there anything in the yarn, or are you gammoning?"

The Greek opened his lips for a savage retort. But again he changed his mind swiftly. The fierce scowl faded from his face and he smiled.

"My young friend, there is a secret, and it is worth a large fortune," he answered. "I have read it in the papyrus written by the scribe of A-Menah, which was to be given to his son Menarsis. This papyrus came into my hands, among many hundreds of papyri, in my shop in Cairo. But the secret is useless to me without the scarab and without my freedom. His lordship made me an offer this morning. You heard him. Now that I have had time to reflect I accept it. When will he return to dahabiyeh?"

"Not till to-morrow night, or the next day," answered Bunter. "But look here, you can tell me——"

His little round eyes gleamed with eagerness behind his big round spectacles.

"If I write it, can you carry the writing to his lordship and bring back the order for my release?" asked the Greek.

"Yes, rather!" said Bunter at once.

"I will write, then!"

The Greek fumbled in his pockets and produced a sheet of paper. He fumbled again, but his hand came out empty.

"I have no pencil. If you have a pencil——"

"Here you are!" said Bunter.

He fished out a stump of pencil from his pocket, and put his fat hand through the slats to hand it to the Greek. In a flash a grasp of iron was laid on his fat wrist and it was held as if in a vice. And as Bunter gave a startled yelp the Greek's voice came hissing:

"Silence, pig! One cry to the men on deck and I will twist your arm till the bones crack! Silence!"

THE SIXTH CHAPTER.
The Escape of Kalizelos!

BILLY BUNTER gasped.

The grip on his fat wrist was like steel. If it had been caught in a vice the fat junior would have had about as much chance of getting it loose again.

With a jerk the Greek had drawn the whole fat arm through the opening of the shutter-slats, so that Bunter's podgy chest was pulled against the outside of the shutter. Once his grip was on Bunter that was all he wanted.

"Oooooooh!" gasped Bunter.

"Silence, or——"

The Greek's voice was low and sibilant, and a twist of the fat arm in his grasp gave Bunter a hint of what to expect.

The fat Owl gurgled into silence.

His arm, stretched through the slats, gripped by the Greek, was at Kalizelos' mercy, and Bunter shuddered with fear and horror as he felt that warning twist. The Greek's powerful grasp could have broken his arm like a pipe-stem, and there was not the slightest doubt that he would do it if Bunter called for help, as readily as he would have broken the fat junior's neck to open a way of escape. It was a desperate man in the prison-room of the dahabiyeh; a man ready to take desperate chances, and as ruthless as a caged tiger.

Bunter, pulled against the shutter, gasped for breath, but gave no sound but a gasp. He dared not.

The Greek listened like a wild beast in the jungle. This was a chance for him, but a desperate chance. Outside his locked door a black Nubian squatted on guard, and if he learned what was going on the cabin would be entered at once and the prisoner overpowered. All depended on silence, and on the men on deck seeing nothing.

Bunter was silent; he dared make no sound. Too late, it dawned on his obtuse mind that the wily Greek had been tricking him. He had had no intention of revealing the secret. Bunter knew that now. He had tricked the obtuse Owl into placing an arm within his reach, and Bunter had fallen into the palpable trap blindly. The Greek had judged his character well; he would not even have thought of attempting such a trick on any other of the Greyfriars fellows. But he had counted on Bunter's stupidity, and not in vain.

Over the balcony was a sun-awning which screened it from the deck. The Nubian sailors could not see Bunter unless they looked down and pulled a corner of the awning aside; which, of course, they were not likely to do. Had the other juniors been aboard, some of them would have been on the balcony, but they were miles away. Only if some of the black servants came out on the balcony would Bunter's predicament be discovered. But that might happen any moment, as the Greek knew.

Bunter, his fat face white with terror, blinked through his big spectacles at the fierce eyes that glittered from within. Every instant he feared to feel his fat arm twisted and to hear the crack of breaking bones. His podgy heart almost died in his breast.

"Silence!" repeated the Greek, in a hissing whisper. "A single cry, and you know what to expect, fat fool!"

"I—I say——" Bunter whispered, even more faintly than the Greek. "I—I say, leggo! I—I say, you're hurting my arm! Ooogh!"

Kalizelos laughed savagely.

"I will break your arm to splinters if you do not give me the help I need!" he hissed.

"I—I—I—leggo! I say, I—I'll go round and unlock the door if—if you'll let go my arm!"

If Bunter expected the Greek to believe that mendacious promise, he was disappointed. A snarl answered him.

"I—I can't open the window, you know," breathed Bunter. "It's locked, and Hassan's got the key. It—it won't open. If—if you'll let go I—I'll go in and open the door——"

"Silence, fool!"

Bunter was silent. He was a helpless prisoner in the Greek's grasp, but what purpose the villain hoped to serve by his trick was a mystery to him. Certainly, Bunter could not have opened the locked shutter.

"You have a penknife—a pocket-knife. Give it to me with your other hand."

"I—I haven't——"

"I have seen you use it. Another lie, and I will break your arm like a reed!" snarled the Greek.

Billy Bunter fumbled in his pockets with his free hand. His pocket-knife was passed through the slats to the Greek within.

Even then, Bunter did not understand. The pocket-knife was useless as a weapon. But that was not what the Greek was thinking of.

He took the knife in his free hand and opened it with his teeth. Still holding Bunter's arm with his left, he used the pocket-knife with his right hand. Bunter heard a sound of clicking.

Then he understood. The Greek had used the knife to pick the lock of the window-shutter.

"Oh!" breathed Bunter.

The shutter opened outwards. Bunter hoped, for a second, that the Greek would have to let him go to open it. Once he was loose, one yell would warn every man on the dahabiyeh that the prisoner was escaping.

But Kalizelos was not likely to let him go.

He allowed Bunter's fat arm to slip out, still grasping his wrist, and keeping the fat hand within. That gave him room to open the unlocked shutter sufficiently to reach round with his other hand and grasp the fat junior by the collar.

CRACK A JOKE AND BAG A POCKET-KNIFE!

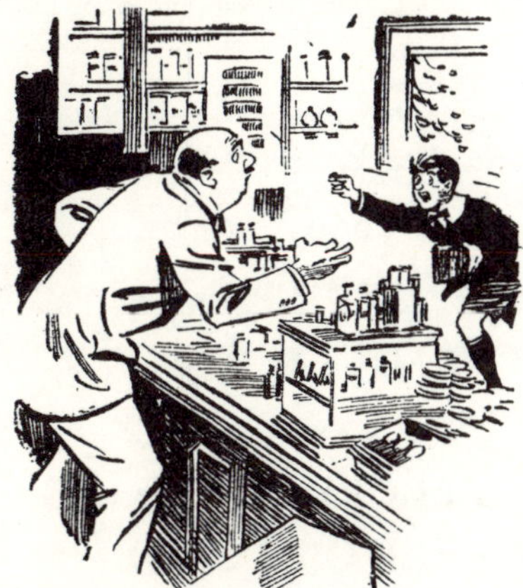

"I say," cried the little boy, as he dashed into the village store, "father is being chased by a bull!"

"Good gracious!" gasped the shopkeeper. "Er—er—what can I do?"

"Give me a roll of film for my camera, quick!" retorted the youngster.

The above winning effort was sent in by William Cain, of 14, Kennington Park Gardens, S.E.11, to whom one of these useful prizes has already been sent.

Then Bunter's fat paw was released and he jerked it away. The Greek's vice-like grip was on his collar now.

He pulled round the shutter, which swung wide open. Warning him, with a fierce glare, to be silent, Kalizelos pulled him in at the window. In a few moments Bunter was inside the cabin.

"One cry——" hissed the Greek.

Bunter did not utter a sound. Swiftly Kalizelos cut a sheet from the bed into strips and bound the fat junior hand and foot, gagged him, and laid him on the floor.

He drew a deep, deep breath as he turned to the window. The way of escape was open now.

Bunter watched him, with goggling eyes, as he climbed, actively as a cat, through the window, and dropped silently on the boat's balcony.

He vanished from Bunter's sight—and the fat Owl was thankful to see him go.

Kalizelos stepped softly across the balcony. The dahabiyeh was tied up close to the bank, and the gangway was run from the lower deck to the Nile shore. The distance was not too great for a spring by an agile man—and the Greek was agile as a tiger. Under the edge of the awning he paused for a moment. Some of the Nubian sailors on the forward deck were singing. The Greek was unseen, so far; but the moment he left the dahabiyeh he would be in full view of the whole crew.

With his teeth shut tight, the Greek stepped lightly on the rail of the balcony, balanced himself for a second, and sprang.

Thud!

The desperate spring reached the high bank, but he fell on his face there, clutching at the hard, dried mud, scrambling like a cat.

Instantly there was a shout from the deck.

The Greek heard the deep voice of Moussa, the reis, booming, and the patter of the Nubian sailors' running feet.

Desperately he scrambled up the bank and stood on his feet.

He gave one hurried glance back.

Moussa, standing on the upper deck, was waving his brown hands and shouting. Six or seven Nubians were rushing across the gang-plank to cut off the Greek's escape.

Kalizelos bounded away.

He had a start—not more than a dozen yards, but it was enough for the agile Greek. He ran like a deer, with the Nubians shouting behind. A few seconds, and he had disappeared behind a clump of palms.

The reis shouted frantically. The Nubians dashed in swift pursuit. Donkey-boys on the bank stared blankly. The Greek had vanished from sight, and he was not seen again. In a quarter of an hour the Nubians came back from the chase without even having set eyes on the escaping prisoner. Then Moussa came down to the prisoner's cabin to investigate, and his eyes almost bulged from his head at the sight of Billy Bunter, stretched on the floor, bound and gagged.

THE SEVENTH CHAPTER.

Stranded!

"OH crikey!"

That was Billy Bunter's first remark when he was released.

"Is he gone?"

"The son of a thousand pigs has escaped!" said the reis. "My lord's anger will be great. Upon your head be it!"

Bunter snorted.

"How could I help it, you silly idiot, when he grabbed me through the window? Don't be a silly ass!"

The reis gave Bunter a long, grave look and retired without saying anything more. He had bad news for Lord Mauleverer when he returned, but the fault was not his. There was nothing more to be done, and the reis therefore dismissed the matter from his mind and returned to his narghile.

Billy Bunter rolled, snorting, to the deck.

Bunter—so far as he could see, at least—was not to blame in the matter. The prisoner had escaped—which was unfortunate, but not Bunter's fault. He reflected bitterly that the other fellows, when they heard what had happened, would make out that he was to blame—as usual! Still, Bunter was used to injustice.

Certainly, he wished that he hadn't gone near the prisoner, as it had turned out. But it was too late to think of that, so Bunter did not think about it. What couldn't be helped, couldn't be helped. And that was that! If those inconsiderate beasts hadn't gone off for days, leaving Bunter on his own, it wouldn't have happened. Besides, Bunter had other matters to think about.

The really pressing matter to be considered was whether Billy Bunter was going to spend his time on the tied-up dahabiyeh, with no company but his own, or join the fellows in their camp on Mr. Maroudi's plantation. Bunter considered that pressing question as he blinked at the sunset over the Libyan desert.

It was easy enough to join the Greyfriars party, if he liked. The camp was only two or three miles from the Nile, and Bunter knew where it was. Mr. Maroudi's place was called Beni-Hasa, and any donkey-boy on the bank would be sure to know it. He had only to mount a donkey and say "Beni-Hasa," and the donkey and the donkey-boy would do the rest.

It was cooler now, and Bunter was utterly fed-up with the dahabiyeh and his own fascinating company. Also, he reflected, that if he butted in at the camp it might have an annoying effect on the other fellows—which was all to the good! It would show the beasts that he jolly well wasn't going to be left out of things.

Supper—an important matter—was pretty certain to be good. He knew what Mr. Maroudi's hospitality was like, and though the Egyptian gentleman was not there himself, he had sent orders to his people, and Bunter knew that Hassan had sent a messenger that morning to Beni-Hasa. Upon the whole, Bunter's fat comfort was not likely to suffer in camp—and, anyhow, if he didn't like it, he could ride back. All these important considerations having been duly considered, Billy Bunter made up his fat mind.

Having made it up, he rolled across the gangway to the bank.

"Donkey, sir!"

"Fine donkey, sir!"

"This magnificent donkey, sir——"

A dozen donkey-boys surrounded the fat junior at once. Billy Bunter carefully selected what seemed to him the quietest-looking donkey, and, with the help of the donkey-boy, scrambled into the red leather saddle.

"Where you go, sar? Ramesseum—Tombs of Kings—Tombs of Queens——"

"Beni-Hasa!" said Bunter. "You know Maroudi's plantation"

"Know Maroudi, sah! Know Beni-Hasa! Yes, sar!"

"Get on, then!"

The stick cracked on the donkey and they started. Billy Bunter cast a rather uneasy blink around him, remembering Hamza and Yussef. But it was an hour since he had seen the two Arab ruffians; they had long been gone. And there were plenty of people about. Bunter trotted away cheerfully, with the donkey-boy running behind, cracking his stick on the donkey.

The "City of the Dead" of the ancient Egyptian Thebes drew hardly a glance from Billy Bunter. He passed the "Tombs of the Kings" without even knowing that they were there. He gave attention to his surroundings when the donkey clattered up a rocky hill-path and he had to hold on with both hands to avoid slipping off.

Clatter, clatter, clatter!

"Oh lor'!" gasped Bunter.

He rocked and swayed in the saddle. The hills were low, but the path was not easy, even for a good rider. And Billy Bunter was the worst rider that ever was. And the small Egyptian donkey was feeling severely the terrific weight of the Owl of Greyfriars. Bunter had a strong suspicion that the donkey would throw him off if he could. He had, so to speak, been there before!

According to Billy Bunter, he was accustomed to backing magnificent hunters at Bunter Court. But he had had rotten luck in backing Egyptian donkeys. He held on for his fat life as he came out on the rocky slopes on the farther side of the hills. A patch of green showed against the brown of the desert in the sunset-lit west, and the donkey-boy pointed with his stick.

"Beni-Hasa, sar!"

The plantation was about a mile farther on, and a rough donkey-track led towards it down the hill. Clatter, clatter!

"Yarooooh!"

The donkey's hoofs slipped, and Bunter nearly took a header. He yelled to the donkey-boy.

"Here, you! Hold him! I'll get off!"

"Yes, sar!"

The donkey-boy held the animal, and Bunter dismounted. He decided to walk till the level was reached. Going down the hill was more risky than getting up, on donkey-back, and even Bunter could walk a half-mile downhill. He grunted and plodded on, and the black boy followed with the donkey.

Puffing and panting, the fat Owl reached the level at last, at the foot of the hill. The green plantation was only half a mile away now, gleaming against the brown desert in the last rays of the sun. The sudden twilight was at hand, but there was plenty of time to finish the ride before dark. But Bunter's donkey had his own ideas about that.

"Here, you! I'll get on now!" panted Bunter.

"Yes, sar!"

The donkey backed away.

"Bring that beast here, you dummy!" snapped Bunter irritably. "What's the matter with the silly brute?"

The donkey backed off farther. The donkey-boy shouted at the animal and brandished his stick, but that unfortunate donkey had had enough of his weighty rider. Perhaps he had supposed, when Bunter dismounted, that the fat junior was done with him. Anyhow, he was extremely unwilling to allow Bunter to mount again.

The donkey-boy grabbed at him, but the donkey jumped away and eluded the grab. With a clatter of hoofs, he dashed back the way he had come. Yelling, the donkey-boy dashed in pursuit.

"Oh crikey!" gasped Bunter.

He sat down on a rock to rest, while the donkey-boy caught the donkey. But the donkey-boy did not catch the donkey. Angry yells and a brandished stick behind his whisking tail, perhaps, did not encourage the animal to be caught. He clattered on, with his owner panting after him, and both of them disappeared from sight in a fold of the hills. Hoofbeats and yells died away in the distance.

Bunter sat and blinked in the direction in which they had disappeared. He was waiting for them to reappear.

Sunset deepened into dark. It was the brief twilight of the south, and night was at hand. It dawned on Bunter that the donkey-boy had not succeeded in catching the donkey, and that they were not going to reappear. That donkey was going all out for the Nile, and the donkey-boy was going all out behind him. And darkness dropped on the land of Egypt like a cloak, and the hills vanished from Bunter's sight.

"Oh crikey!" gasped Bunter.

For the second time that day Billy Bunter was left on his own. But his last state was worse than his first! This time he was left on his own on a barren hillside, three miles at least from the dahabiyeh, and without the remotest possibility of finding his way back to it—even if his fat legs had been equal to the tramp across rough hills. Billy Bunter sat and blinked in utter dismay.

There was no going back! That was certain! He had to go on—on foot! And if he missed the track——

"Beasts!" groaned Bunter.

Mr. Maroudi's plantation was a cultivated patch on the edge of the desert. If Bunter missed the track, he was likely to go wandering into the Libyan Desert. He groaned.

The bright stars of Egypt were coming out in the sky. Eastward of Bunter, towards the Nile, the hills lay a black mass. There was no sign or sound of the donkey-boy, or of any other living being. Westward, in the gleaming of the stars, he was comforted to make out a dark mass which could only be the orange plantation. And he found, too, that the donkey-track that led to Beni-Hasa was very clearly marked—so clearly marked that even Bunter could hardly miss it in the bright starlight.

There was no danger, after all, of wandering into the remote recesses of the Libyan Desert. He had only to follow the donkey-track till he reached the Greyfriars camp, and if he missed the camp he would arrive at the plantation and its buildings. That was a comfort—but he had to walk half a mile at least, and he groaned as he started, after a long, long rest!

He tramped on with bitter feelings in his podgy breast. This was the sort of thing a fellow had to stand, after all he had done for a set of ungrateful rotters! Likely as not, they had turned in already—fat lot they cared about Bunter! With deep wrath and indignation, and at the pace of a very old and very tired snail, Billy Bunter plodded along the rough donkey-track, stopping every now and then for a rest on a boulder.

The track wound among acacias and clumps of tamarisk bushes. Suddenly in the opening of some acacias, Billy

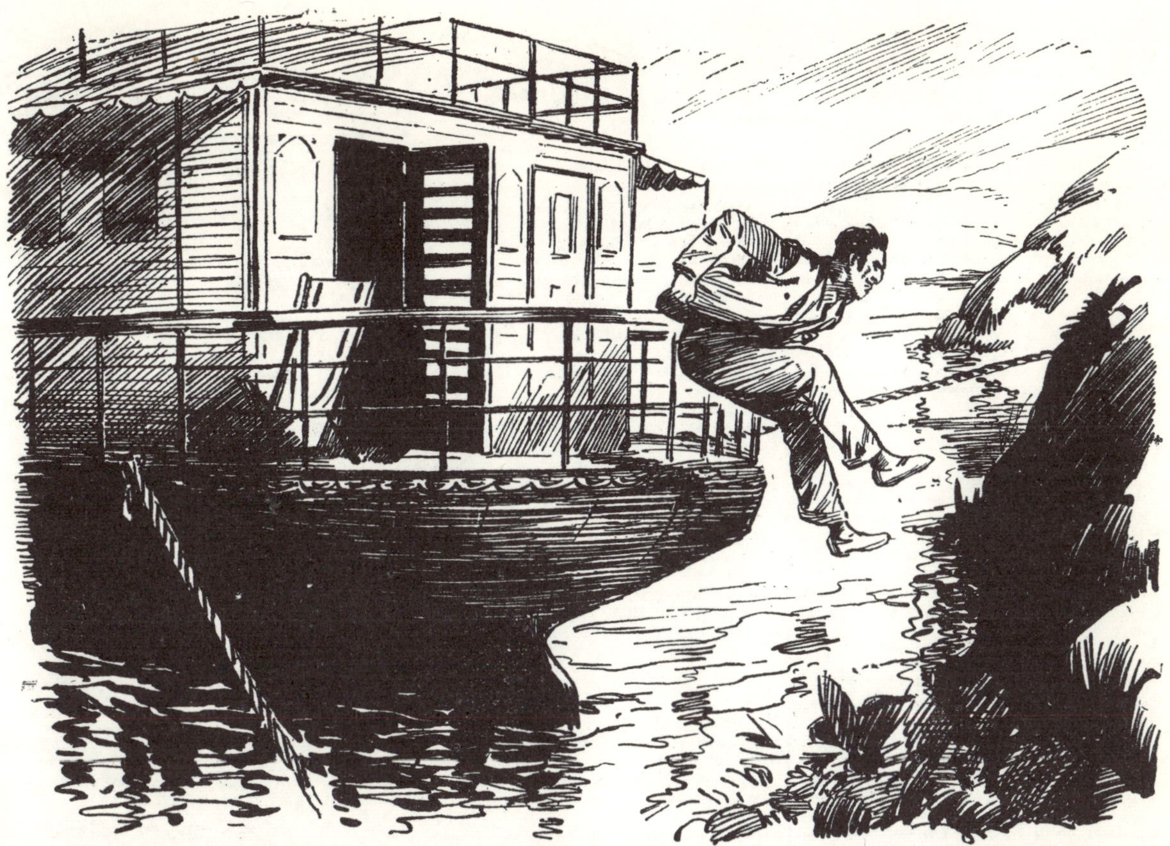

As silently as a cat, Kalizelos crept along under the edge of the awning. With his teeth shut tight, he stepped lightly on to the rail of the balcony, balanced himself for a second, and then made a desperate spring for the high bank!

Bunter spotted the starlight glimmering on a tent. He halted, gasping for breath, and ejaculated:

"Beasts!"

THE EIGHTH CHAPTER.

Bunter All Over!

BILLY BUNTER stood in the starlight, blinking at the tent.

It was dark and silent; the occupants, evidently, had turned in for the night.

They had not waited supper for Bunter. True, they had not known that he was coming along. But Bunter was hungry by this time and he reflected bitterly that the beasts did not care whether he had any supper or not.

In the starlight and the shadow of the thick acacias the tent was dim to the view. But Bunter noticed that it was not a large tent; certainly not so large as he would have expected, considering the number of the party. It looked as if he was not going to be so comfortable, after all, as he had taken for granted. Packed in a poky little tent—Bunter sniffed.

There was a gleam in Bunter's eyes behind his spectacles He had had many trials that day, and his temper had suffered. Here he was, tired and hungry—and there were those beasts, sleeping as if he did not matter! It would serve them jolly well right to loosen the tent-pegs and bring the tent down on their nappers!

It was easy enough—for evidently the occupants of the tent were fast asleep. Bunter grinned a sour grin. The only drawback to that justifiable little scheme of vengeance was that the fellows might kick him afterwards. Still, they would suppose that the tent had come down by accident—and Bunter was prepared to deny having been anywhere near it when it fell.

Bunter was tired, but not too tired to give these unfeeling beasts what they deserved. He crept cautiously towards the tent, over the rough ground.

The tent-flap was closed and fastened. As he listened near it he heard a sound of sleepers breathing within.

Fast asleep, the beasts—but they were going to wake up jolly suddenly! The fat junior crept stealthily round the tent, jerking out peg after peg.

There was a sudden collapse.

"He, he, he!" chuckled Bunter.

The canvas billowed on the ground. In two places it was shoved up from underneath, evidently where two heads butted up at it. There was a muffled roar from the interior.

Billy Bunter backed away. His idea was to retreat to a distance, and come on the scene when the juniors struggled out of the fallen tent—as if he had just arrived! Then even those suspicious beasts could hardly suspect that he had had a hand in the collapse of the tent!

That programme was not carried out, however. At the second step, Bunter caught his foot in a trailing tent-rope, and went sprawling

"Ooooogh!" he gasped.

He rolled down a rough slope, and brought up against the trunk of an acacia-tree, with a bump. There he lay gasping, quite winded.

From the wallowing canvas, extraordinary noises were proceeding. Obviously, the occupants of the tent had been awakened very suddenly, and were very startled, and still more exasperated. Two voices rang out into the night—only two, and neither of them was a Greyfriars voice. Bunter, as he sprawled gasping for breath under the shadowy acacia, heard those two voices—in amazement and dismay.

"Say, what's got this doggoned tent?"

"I'll say you never fastened them pegs safe, Colonel Jacks."

"Forget it, you pie-faced bonehead! I fastened them pegs as safe as any ornery pegs ever was fastened, Ephraim Skink!"

"I guess it looks like it, you gink! Hyer's this thundering tent down on our cabezas——"

"I'm telling you I fastened them pegs safe——"

"And I'm telling you you're the biggest bonehead from Boneheadville! Yep! You want to l'arn to fasten a tent-peg! Yep! You surely do!"

"You pie-faced geck——"

"You ornery gink——"

Two frantic figures were struggling under the wallowing canvas, as the two colonels slanged one another. There was a sudden yell.

"Great gophers! Keep your hoof out of my doggoned eye!"

"Keep your pesky eye away from my foot!"

"I guess I'll——"

"Aw! Can it, Colonel Skink! You surely do blow off your mouth a lot too much, and I'm telling you so."

"You pesky bonehead, if you'd fastened them pegs——"

"I'll say I fastened them pegs, sir, and I'll say that some guy has come along and hooked them out! Yep! And I'll say that I'm going to cinch that guy and give him ginger!"

A long, lean figure struggled, at last, out of the wallowing canvas. It was followed by a gasping fat figure.

Billy Bunter sprawled in the dark shadow of the acacia, almost frozen with

(*Continued on page* 16.)

The SCHOOLBOY PRO

By Dicky Nugent

I.

"HALF a sardeen and one stale biskit!" eggsclaimed Jack Jolly of the Fourth Form at St. Sam's, gazing reflectively at the study table. "Is this all we've got for tea to-day, you chaps?"

"'Fraid it can't be helped, Jack," said Merry, with a shrugg. "We've all run out of munny—and there's not much chance of getting any more for another week, worse luck!"

"Fammine is staring us in the fizz!" remarked Bright sadly.

"Well, something will have to be done—or somebody!" sighed Jack Jolly. "I wish I knew an easy way of earning a fiver!"

No sooner had the words left his lips than Tubby Barrell poked his boolit head round the study door.

"Letter for you, Jolly!" he annowneed. "I brought it up from the letter-rack to save you the trubble. If it contains a remittance I trussed you'll show your grattitude by lending me five bob till the weather breaks!"

Jack Jolly took the letter and opened it. As he read it, he uttered a gasp of sheer serprize.

"Well, if this isn't the giddy limmit! Just read it for yourselves!"

Merry and Bright and Tubby Barrell peered over his sholders to read the letter. This is what they read:

"Dear Master Jolly,—I am riting on behalf of the Muggleton Rovers Footbawl Club to ask whether you can play senter-forward for us against Slushford United in the Leag match on Saturday. Our usual senter-forward, Dixie Bean, has unforchunitly broken his nee, dislocated his sholder, ricked his ankle and sprained his rist, in addition to developing mumps, measles and hooping-coff, so he can't turn out for us. You are the only man we can think of to get us out of our difficulty. We are willing to pay Five Pounds for your services, but you will have to fill up the enclosed Professional Form and return it to us before the match. Awaiting your decision,

Yours trooly,

GEORGE PLAYFAIR
(Sekretary)."

"Oh, good!" eggsclaimed Merry and Bright together as they reached the end of the missive.

"Saved in the nick of time, by Jove!" said Jack Jolly. "To-morrow's Saturday, and there's no special junior match on. I can turn out for the Rovers, and we shall be in a land flowing with milk and hunny again!"

"Yes, rather!"

"I'll fill in this form immejately," went on Jack. "Lend me your fountain-pen, Bright!"

Jack Jolly & Co. forgot their pangs of hunger now. It was a grate honner and privilege for a meer junior like Jack Jolly to play for a famus Leag team like Muggleton Rovers, and the Co. felt awfully eggsited about it.

"Better not let the Head know about it," said Merry, as Jack Jolly sined the all-important form on the dotted line. "Rather a pity you let this fat idiot Barrell into the secret, for it's ten to one he'll give you away!"

"Beests!" snorted Tubby Barrell, as he rolled away.

The Co. speedily forgot the fat junior's eggsistence. They went downstairs, posted the completed form, and then walked back to the House arm-in-arm in grate spirrits. Afterwards they went to the Junior Common-room.

They hadn't been in that sellybrated apartment more than a brace of shakes before there was a hevvy tramp of hob-nailed boots outside, and Dr. Alfred Birchemall, the revered and respected headmaster of St. Sam's, strolled in.

Then came the bomb-shell!

"Boys," said the Head, addressing the crowded Common-room, "I have an annowncement to make to you! I have notissed lately that some of you make a praktiss of attending the professional footbawl matches in Muggleton. I do not approve of such praktiss. From now on anyone caught going there will be birched black and blew. You savvy?"

"We savvy, sir!"

"All serene, then; mind you don't forget it!" said Dr. Birchemall, retiring from the Common-room with a breef nod.

The door closed behind him, and Jack Jolly & Co. were left looking at each other like follows in a dreem.

Outside, the Head pawsed to chuckle into his beard.

"Ha, ha, ha!" he gurgled. "Little do they guess that I am only doing this so that nobody shall see me go to watch the match myself! Having drawn Slushford United in the Masters' Sweepsteak, I am anxious to watch them make mince-meat of Muggleton; but it wouldn't do for the juniors to know that! Ha, ha, ha!"

And the Head returned to his study, fairly rocking with merriment.

———

II.

"BEND over!"

The cry rang across Dr. Birchemall's study like a pistol-shot.

It was just after dinner the following day, and the Head had summoned Tubby Barrell into his illustrious prezzence. Immejately Tubby arrived Dr. Birchemall had seezed a birch and barked out that stern command.

"But, sir," gasped the fat junior in dismay, "I haven't done anything!"

"I am quite aware of that, Barrell!" was the Head's retort. "I am meerly going to birch you becawse I have just had a rather hevvy dinner, and I feel like a little exercise before I go out! Bend over and don't argew the toss!"

Tubby Barrell groaned and was just about to bend over when a sudden thought struck him.

"I say, sir," he gasped. "Suppose I told you about some Fourth Form chaps who're going to break bounds this afternoon, do you think you mite let me off then?"

Dr. Birchemall lowered his upraised birchrod.

"I trussed you're not thinking of pulling my leg, Barrell. Becawse if you are——"

"Nunno, sir!" said Tubby hastily. "The fact is, sir, Jack Jolly and his friends are going to Muggleton to watch the footbawl match to-day—or, at least, two of them are. Jolly himself is playing senter-forward for Muggleton Rovers!"

The Head recoiled as from a blow.

WOULD YOU BELIEVE IT?

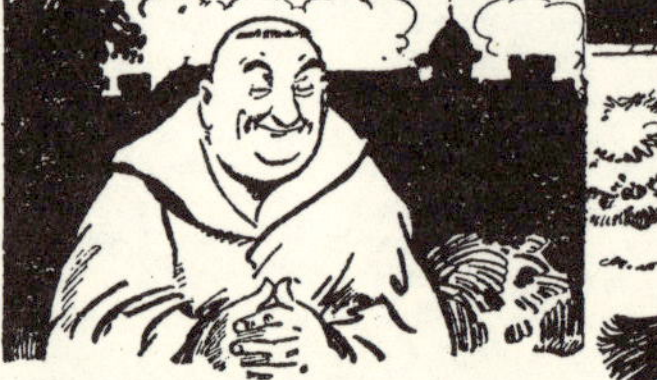

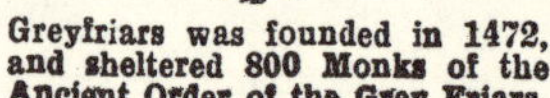

Greyfriars was founded in 1472, and sheltered 800 Monks of the Ancient Order of the Grey Friars.

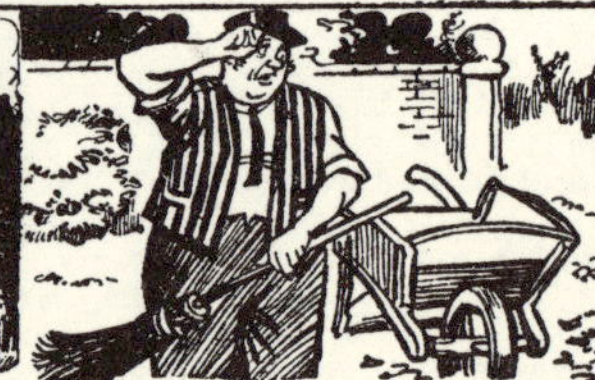

Gosling, the school porter, has completed twenty years' service, and hopes to double this!

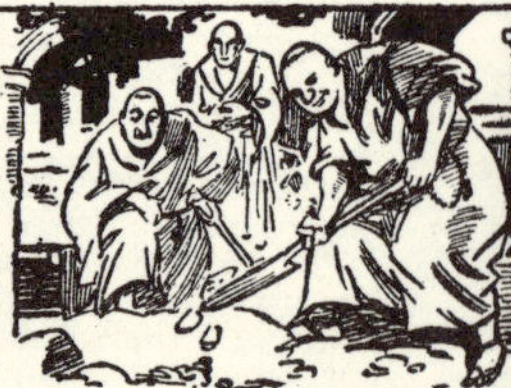

The old Grey Friars suffere[d] death rather than reveal whe[re] their treasure was hidden.

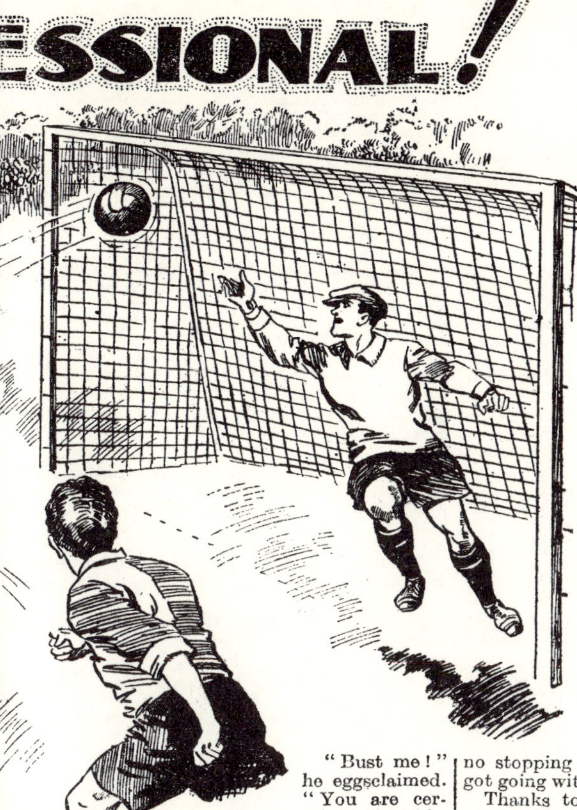

"Bust me!" he eggsclaimed. "You are certain of this, Barrell?"

"Absolutely positive, sir!"

The Head flung his birchrod into a corner of the room.

"Very well, Barrell," he said. "It is not my praktiss to encurridge sneaking, but under the circs I'll let you off with a cawtion. You may go!"

"Thank you, sir!" mermered Tubby, and he rolled out of the Head's study at express speed.

"Playing senter-forward, is he?" mermered Dr. Birchemall when he was left alone. "Well, he'd better not score any goals against my sweepsteak team or there'll be the dickens to pay! Perhaps I'd better disguise myself before I set out!"

After a moment's thought he divided his beard into two sections, then wound them round his neck and tied them in a not. By the time he had finished his sellybrated face fungus looked just like a silk muffler!

Thus disguised, the Head set out for Muggleton. Half an hour's sharp walking brought him to the Rovers' ground. He paid his shilling entrance fee and entered the ground just as the Rovers were turning out.

"Play up, the Rovers!" roared the home supporters.

A few moments later the Slushford United team appeared, and Dr. Birchemall gave a deffening cheer.

"Good old United!" he roared. "Nock spots off 'em! Make rings round 'em! Run the nitwits off their giddy feet!"

"My hat! It's the Head!" eggsclaimed Merry, who was standing only a few yards away. "Now we know why the old buffer put the ground out of bounds—he wanted to be able to let off steam without being spotted by anyone belonging to the skool!"

"That's it, right enuff!" nodded Bright. "I wonder if he'll reckernise Jack Jolly?"

That question was soon answered, for as soon as the Rovers began attacking and Jack Jolly took the ball into the United's territory the Head started rattling out a steady fire of orders, which showed that he was well aware of the skoolboy pro's eyedentity.

"Kick it out, Jolly! Let the United have it! Don't be greedy! If you shoot, I'll simply pulverise you when we get back to St. Sam's!"

But Jack Jolly was not to be intimmidated by the Head's prezzence, uneggspected as it was. Once he got going at footbawl there was no stopping him, and he seemed to have got going with a vengenz on this occasion.

Thanks to his efforts, the score stood at 5—nil in the Rovers' favour at half-time.

III.

About half-way through the interval, Dr. Birchemall sneaked down to the players' dressing-rooms underneeth the stands.

"Mite a bloke speak to the new senter-forward Jolly?" he asked the door-keeper, slipping a small copper coin into the man's hand as he spoke.

"Yes, sir; I'll fetch 'im out at once," said the man.

He was as good as his word. Jack Jolly was standing before the visitor in a brace of shakes.

The first thing the skoolboy professional did was to burst into larfter.

"Oh crums, sir!" he gasped, wiping the tears of merriment from his eyes. "Eggscuse my larfter, but you really do look a commical site with your wiskers tied round your neck!"

Dr. Birchemall's skollerly fizz blushed almost skarlet.

"I don't pretend to understand how you have pennytrated my clever disguise, Jolly!" he snorted. "But since you have, I will admit it: I am your headmaster. I will also admit that I came down here to offer you a bribe to lose the game. But under the circs, I will withdraw the bribe and threaten you instead. Understand, then, that unless Slushford United win to-day I intend to birch you black and blew. You get me?"

"Ratts, and many of 'em!" said Jack Jolly cheerfully.

Before the Head had recovered from his astonishment Jack Jolly had vanished.

The second half commenced, and Jack Jolly, the skoolboy professional, fairly let the fur fly. Goals piled up merrily, and the cheering was simply deffening.

Unable to stand it any longer, the Head made his way down the terracing, jumped over the barrier on to the field itself, made a dash for Jack Jolly and seezed him by the ear.

"Jolly!" he cride. "I forbid the banns—I mean, I forbid you to play a minnit longer! Return with me immejately to St. Sam's to receeve the punishment you so richly deserve!"

"Leggo my ear!" howled Jack Jolly. "Can't you see the game's in progress?"

The Head larfed harshly.

"What care I for the fact of the game being in progress—yoooooop!" he conclooded, sitting down suddenly as the ball smote him in the chest.

During the next few seconds the Head lerned to care quite a lot about the game being in progress. The game seemed to eddy around him, and he was jumped on and trampled on and kicked and biffed till he felt sorry indeed that he had ever herd the mention of a game of footbawl.

"Ha, ha, ha!" roared the spectators.

Evenchally, Dr. Birchemall mannidged to crawl off the field of play. He spent the remainder of the match being revived by the Second-Aid Detachment!

Pheep!

The game ended at last. The Rovers had won by 14 goals to nil, Jack Jolly having scored all 14! With gleaming eyes, the Head descended on the incoming players and grabbed Jack Jolly.

"Follow me!" he hist feercely.

He rushed the brethless junior off the ground to the street outside, hailed a passing taxi, rained instructions to the driver, and stormed at Jack Jolly all the way back to St. Sam's.

Mr. Lickham, the master of the Fourth, was waiting at the school gates to greet Dr. Birchemall.

"Congratulations, sir, on winning the Masters' Footbawl Sweepsteak!" he cride.

The Head of St. Sam's jumped.

"Wha-a-at?" he yelled.

"Didn't you know, sir?" asked Mr. Lickham in serprize. "I thought I'd told you that you had drawn Muggleton Rovers this week!"

Dr. Birchemall gasped.

"But—but I thought you said something about Slushford United?"

"Yes, sir, I mentioned that the Rovers were playing them. So they were; and they have licked them by a record score. So you win the hansum prize of five-and-sixpence!"

"M-m-my giddy aunt!" stuttered the Head.

That was all he could say for a time. At last, however, he turned to Jack Jolly, fairly beaming all over his fizz.

"Jolly, my dear boy," he said, "you can consider that birching off. I wouldn't dreem of birching such a fine footbawler and true sportsman as yourself. Thanks awfully, instead!"

"Don't mensh, sir!" grinned Jack Jolly. "May I go now?"

"Certainly—and thanks once again, my dear boy!"

Jack Jolly & Co. were in high spirits at the thought of collecting Five Pounds from the Muggleton Rovers' Footbawl Club!

THE END.

(If you want another long laugh be sure and read "'SAMSON' STRONG OF ST. SAM'S," next week's corking yarn by our youthful laughter-merchant, Dicky Nugent.)

GREYFRIARS FACTS WHILE YOU WAIT.

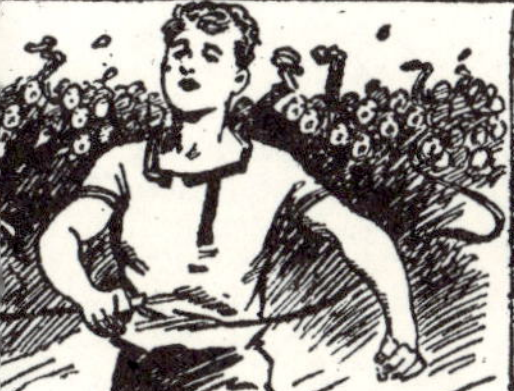

Cherry is the Mile Champion of the Remove. His time is 4 minutes 59 seconds.

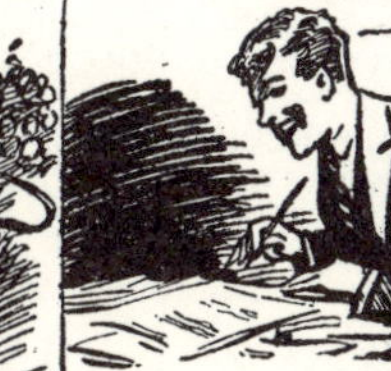

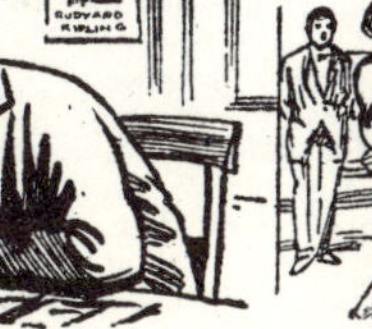

Dick Penfold writes poetry all day and every day. He hopes to become Poet Laureate.

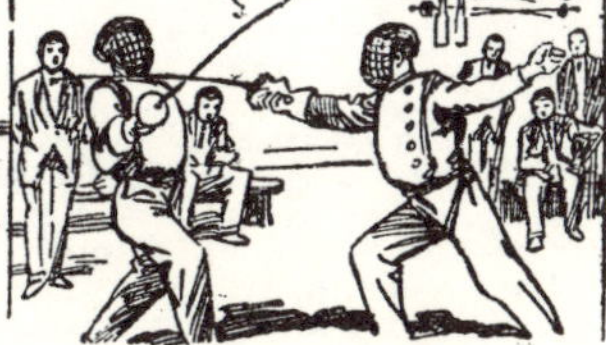

Wharton and Vernon-Smith recently fought a draw in the Foils' Championship of the Remove.

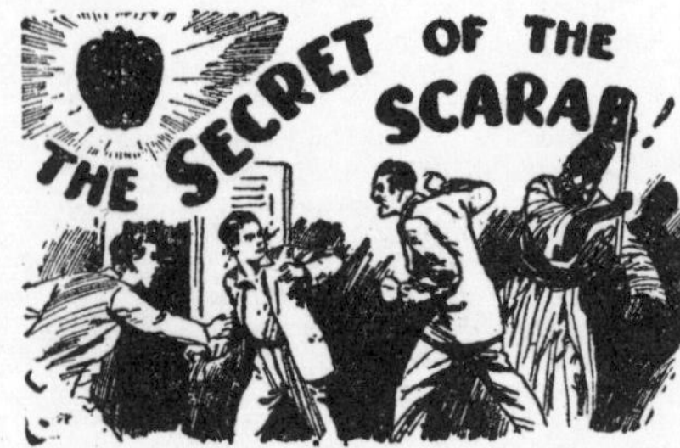

(*Continued from page* 13.)

terror. He realised now that he had made a little mistake. This tent, only too obviously, was not the Greyfriars tent. Its occupants were not the Greyfriars juniors; but the two Yankee gentlemen of the felucca—and the lengthy gentleman, who was raving with wrath, was the very gentleman who had spanked Bunter on the dahabiyeh that morning! Bunter had not forgotten that hefty spanking! He hugged the shadow of the acacia, not daring to run for it into the open starlight.

"Say, you!" roared Colonel Jacks, glaring round him. "Say, where are you? I want to see the pie-faced gink that let down this tent!"

"Aw, don't I keep on telling you that you never fastened them pegs——" gasped Colonel Skink.

"You ornery pie-can, don't I keep on shouting that I fastened them pegs safe!" roared Colonel Jacks. "Don't I keep on yauping that some guy has moseyed along and let that goldarned tent down on us!"

"Waal, who'd do it, you gink?"

"One of them pesky sons of John Bull, what we had a rookus with on the Nile, Ephraim Skink! They're camping near by. I'll say——"

"Oh, guff!" said Colonel Skink. "You never fastened them pegs——"

"If you want to be gouged, Ephraim Skink, you'll keep on yauping that I never fastened them pegs!" bawled Colonel Jacks. "I'll tell you that it was a pesky trick, jest to get our goat—yep! I'll tell a man, sir! And I guess I'm after that guy, sir, and if I don't spread him out over Egypt in small pieces, sir, you can call me a boob, sir."

The long-legged colonel, as he glared round in search of the suspected practical joker, did not see the fat figure crouching in the shadow of the acacia. But he caught a glimmer of Bunter's spectacles from the shadows, and gave a roar.

"Say, you! I guess you're my mutton."

The long legs whisked like lightning. Billy Bunter leaped up with a howl of terror.

Before the long-limbed American gentleman could reach the acacia, the fat Owl bolted back to the donkey-track, and raced away.

Tramp! tramp! tramp! came the colonel's pursuing footsteps after him. Both the colonels had a clear view of Bunter in the starlight, and recognised him.

"I swow!" ejaculated Colonel Skink. "I guess you touched the spot, Colonel Jacks—it was one of them pesky sons of John Bull——"

"I guess I got him!"

But G. W. Jacks had not quite got Bunter.

Bunter was going strong along the donkey-track. G. W. Jacks raced after him! Bunter had simply no chance in the race. He heard the footsteps thundering behind; he felt an outstretched bony hand graze his shoulder. In sheer terror, the fat junior stumbled over and fell.

The next instant, Colonel Jacks was sprawling over him. His bony head hit the donkey-track, with a loud concussion.

There was a fearful howl from G. W. Jacks.

Bunter scrambled up.

Colonel Jacks, sprawling, was clasping his bony head with both hands, and howling with anguish. Bunter did not stay to listen. He circled round the damaged colonel, and raced on, and vanished.

G. W. Jacks hardly saw him go. His head, evidently, was damaged. His head was hard, but Egypt was harder. For several minutes the hapless colonel sat clasping his head, and emitting howls of anguish and wrath.

When he staggered to his feet, at last, the night had swallowed Bunter. Colonel Jacks limped back to his tent and his companion.

"You get that guy?" asked Colonel Skink.

"I'll say nope!" gasped Colonel Jacks. "But I'm going to get him! Them guys are camped up the road somewheres. You get hold of a stick, Colonel Skink, and mosey along with me! I guess we're going to knock spots outer the whole doggoned outfit! Yep! I'll say so, a few."

"I should smile!" agreed Colonel Skink.

And there was a stick grasped in a bony hand, and another stick grasped in a fat hand, as the two exasperated colonels started up the donkey-track to search for the camp of the Greyfriars party.

THE NINTH CHAPTER.

The Enemy!

HARRY WHARTON stirred, and opened his eyes.

He raised his head, and looked round him in the darkness of the big tent.

Some sound or movement had awakened him.

He could hear the steady breathing of his friends, still fast asleep. But the deep snore of Hassan, the son of Suleiman, sleeping on the prayer-rug outside the door-flap, was no longer to be heard.

Wharton smiled sleepily. Hassan slept on the rug outside, under the stars, to watch over the safety of his lordly gentleman—but Wharton had heard him snoring before he dropped off to sleep himself. As the snore was not now audible, he concluded that the dragoman had awakened, and made some movement that had disturbed his slumber. He laid his head on the downy pillow again, and closed his eyes.

If he dreamed, he little dreamed of what was happening within a few yards of him, outside the tent-flap. Danger was not in the thoughts of the Greyfriars juniors.

Kalizelos, the Greek, had been in a Cairo prison, when Sir Reginald Brooke had trusted the juniors up the Nile in Mr. Maroudi's dahabiyeh. He had escaped and tracked them up the river of Egypt; but he was a safe prisoner, locked in a cabin on the Cleopatra; and so there was nothing to be feared from him. Had Wharton been aware that the Greek had escaped from the dahabiyeh, certainly he would not have felt so secure. But he had no suspicion of that.

He closed his eyes and dozed again; and if a faint sound came from without, he did not notice it.

But in the glimmer of the stars, there was a strange scene outside the tent; hidden from the juniors by the canvas flap, Hassan, the dragoman, would have done well to sleep with one eye open, as he had stated that he would do. Both his eyes were shut fast, when groping hands seized him in the gloom, and a dhurra sack was slid over his head, and pressed over his mouth by sinewy hands, blinding and silencing him.

That was why Hassan's snore had ceased; if the captain of the Greyfriars Remove had only known it!

Hassan was awake—wide awake—and struggling, silently, but savagely. He was a powerful man; and though he was a rogue to the finger-tips, he was no coward, and under his smiling, beaming politeness, he had all the fierceness of his Arab race. But he ceased to struggle, as the keen edge of a knife was pressed to his ribs.

A cord was run round the sack, gripping it over his mouth to gag him. Then he was lifted to his feet, with the point of the knife touching his ribs. Not a word was spoken, not a whisper; but Hassan knew that if he gave the alarm, the keen blade would be driven home, and he would be a dead dragoman. He submitted to his fate with oriental passiveness, though watchful as a cat for a chance at his assailants.

With a grip on either arm, and the knife still pressing him, he was walked away silently.

The dragoman was alarmed; but more astonished than alarmed. He did not think of the Greek, whom he believed to be still a prisoner on the dahabiyeh. He could only suppose that bedouin thieves from the desert had chanced on the camp, and that was surprising enough, for such outrages, though not unknown, were extremely rare so near to the Nile and Luxor. And not three hundred yards distant was the house of Mr. Maroudi's plantation manager, and the mud huts of two or three score of fellahin who worked for him.

Hardly a mile distant was the rest-house belonging to Thomas Cook & Co., the tourist firm. If his assailants were bedouin thieves from the desert, they were thieves with a more than usual amount of nerve.

He walked on quietly between his unseen conductors. They stopped at a distance of about a hundred yards from the tent, and the sack was taken from Hassan's head.

He blinked round him, with startled eyes.

He was standing under an acacia, shadowed from the bright starlight. But he could make out the two Arabs who gripped his arms—Hamza and Yussef. And he could make out a third man who stood by the tree waiting—and he caught his breath as he recognised Konstantinos Kalizelos. He understood it all now.

The Greek's black eyes glittered at his startled face. Kalizelos spoke in Arabic.

"Dog of a dragoman! Speak low—your life is in my hands."

"That is known to me, O effendi!" said Hassan, in the same tongue. "But remember that I am under the protection of the great Maroudi, who will demand life for life."

"Maroudi is in Cairo," sneered the Greek. "Can Maroudi, powerful as he is, save your life, jackal of the streets of Cairo?"

"Maroudi's arm is long," said the dragoman composedly. "His greatness has promised me reward and protection, for serving the Faringhees faithfully. If my life is taken, he who takes it will die under the kourbash."

Yussef and Hamza stood silent. The hawk-faced Arab was still holding the knife to the dragoman's side. But Hassan had no doubt that it was fear of the vengeance of Hilmi Maroudi, that held back the thrust. If the Greek did not fear the powerful Egyptian, his followers did.

"Enough!" snarled Kalizelos. "What is your jackal's life to me? It is the young English lord that I seek. Speak the truth to me, or the protection of Maroudi will not save you from having your lying tongue cut out, dog of a dragoman. The young lord is in the tent?"

Hassan made a sign of assent.

"His friends are with him?"

"All but the small fat lord, who remained on the dahabiyeh."

The Greek grinned sourly. He had good reason for knowing that the "small fat lord" had remained on the dahabiyeh.

"And the scarab?" asked Kalizelos, his black eyes glittering. "Is that in the keeping of the English lord?"

"I know not, effendi."

"You would have me believe that anything passes without your knowledge, you lying jackal! Take care!"

"By the beard of the Prophet, I know nothing of the scarab, effendi," answered Hassan. "Do I even know why you seek it? It is a trifle in my eyes—I have seen many such. As for the fable that it will guide its possessor to the Eye of Osiris, what is that but an old woman's tale? I am a civilised Arab, effendi, I believe nothing."

The Greek gave a curt laugh.

"If you believed the tale, Hassan, you would have stolen the scarab long since, in spite of your fear of Maroudi," he said.

"It is true!" assented the dragoman. "For so large a sum as a king's ransom, I would dare Maroudi's vengeance, and even slay the young lord with my own hands." Hassan made that statement with perfect calmness. "Is it not written that the slaying of an unbeliever is pleasing in the eyes of the Prophet? But there is no truth in the tale, and if you believe it, effendi, your senses must be touched with madness."

"Enough!" snarled the Greek. "If the boy has the Golden Scarab, it will fall into my hands when I seize him. If it is hidden on the dahabiyeh, it shall be given to ransom his life, and the lives of his friends. The old man Brooke will give it freely to save him, when my message reaches him from the heart of the Libyan desert."

He snarled an order to the two Arabs, and they placed Hassan against the acacia, and proceeded to bind him to the trunk.

The dragoman's eyes burned. But he did not resist. The Greek had taken the knife from Yussef's hand, and he was ready to strike if the dragoman raised his voice. A shout might have reached the tent, but a shout would never have been uttered.

"Effendi!" said the dragoman quietly. "I am in your hands—and the young lords are at your mercy. But remember that Maroudi is powerful. The King of Egypt is not so powerful as he. In this land there is no corner that will hide you from his vengeance, if you harm the foreigners whom he has taken under his noble protection."

"Silence!" snarled the Greek.

At a sign, the dragoman was gagged.

The three rascals stood near him, in low - voiced consultation. Hassan watched them, with burning eyes. He had failed in his trust, and he feared Maroudi. To the Greyfriars juniors Hassan was a dragoman who was paid for his services; and they trusted him because they had found him faithful. They knew that he was a rogue, as a matter of course; but supposed that he was a rogue who knew on which side his bread was buttered. They never dreamed how much they owed to Hilmi Maroudi, and that it was fear of the Egyptian millionaire that kept Hassan true to his trust.

That fear was shared by Yussef and Hamza, and to a lesser extent by the Greek. It was fear of the Egyptian that had led Kalizelos to attack him in Cairo, when Wharton and Bob Cherry had saved Maroudi's life. Hassan, as he watched the three shadowy figures, and listened to their low muttering, was thinking with dread of being called to account by Maroudi for having failed to protect the schoolboys in his charge.

The muttering ceased at last. The three dim figures crept away in the gloom, in the direction of the schoolboys' tent. Hassan watched them go, with a heavy heart. His "lordly gentlemen" were at the mercy of their enemy now, and he could not help them or warn them. For his "lordly gentlemen," except from the point of view of backsheesh, the faithful Hassan cared nothing—but he cared very much for his own dusky person, and his face was troubled as the three shadowy figures flitted away in the starlight.

(*Continued on next page.*)

THE TENTH CHAPTER.
Captured!

KALIZELOS drew aside the tent-flap, and stared into the dark interior of the tent.

Behind him crept the two savage-faced Arabs, with long bedouin knives in their dusky hands. In the Greek's olive hand was an automatic. From the tent came a sound of steady breathing, and the Greek grinned with triumph. Before him lay the Greyfriars party, buried in slumber, without a suspicion of danger.

As the starlight streammed in at the opening, he could make out the sleepers, dimly and faintly—six of them, though he could not recognise them individually in the gloom. Harry Wharton & Co. were at his mercy—if they attempted to resist, the six unarmed schoolboys had no chance against three armed ruffians. Kalizelos' look was gloating. The dragoman, bound to a tree at a distance, could not help; there was no help for the Greyfriars juniors.

Bob Cherry stirred, and raised his head from the pillow. A draught of the night wind, through the opening, had disturbed him. He opened his eyes, and blinked at the starlight—and at the dark figure that blotted it.

"What——" ejaculated Bob.

For a second he supposed that it was Hassan, looking into the tent. But the next moment he knew that it was not Hassan.

He bounded to his feet.

"Hallo, hallo, hallo! Wake up, you men!" shouted Bob.

"Eh—what?"

"What the thump——"

"What's the row?" came Lord Mauleverer's sleepy drawl. "Let a fellow sleep, old bean! It isn't mornin' yet."

"Kalizelos!" gasped Harry Wharton, his startled eyes turning on the olive face in the starlight. "My hat! The Greek!"

"Kalizelos—here!" stuttered Nugent.

"Oh gad!" gasped Lord Mauleverer.

The juniors scrambled to their feet, wide enough awake now. They stared in amazement and dismay at the Greek, in the opening of the tent, and the two dark figures behind him, knife in hand.

"Yes—it is Kalizelos!" said the Greek. "Stand quiet—and do not think of resistance—I will riddle you with bullets if you lift a hand."

The bluish barrel of the automatic glimmered as he raised it.

"Oh, my hat!" breathed Johnny Bull.

Harry Wharton clenched his hand.

"You scoundrel! So you have escaped from the dahabiyeh!" he said between his teeth.

"As you see!" grinned the Greek. "I warn you not to resist. I am not here to shed blood, but if you give trouble I will shoot you down like a jackal in the desert."

The juniors stared at him. The apparition of the Greek took them utterly by surprise. Not for a moment had they dreamed that the desperado could escape from the locked cabin on the dahabiyeh. They had not counted on the fat fatuousness of Billy Bunter.

"Your lives are in my hands," said the Greek quietly. "Take care!"

"Hassan!" shouted Bob Cherry.

Kalizelos laughed.

"Hassan is already taken care of," he said. "Your dragoman is a prisoner, my young friend. Hassan was taken first of all. Step out from the tent."

"You scoundrel!" breathed Wharton.

The juniors exchanged glances, but they did not stir.

Kalizelos muttered in Arabic, and

Yussef and Hamza entered the tent. They drove the schoolboys out at the point of the knife.

It was impossible to resist. The Greek was not keen to shed blood, whether from reluctance to commit so terrible a crime, or from a lurking fear of the vengeance of Hilmi Maroudi or of the law. Probably from a mingling of motives. But he was in deadly earnest, and prepared for bloodshed if it was necessary to gain his ends.

Had the juniors flung themselves at him, as they longed to do, the automatic would have spat death on the instant. They could read as much in the glittering black eyes. With deep rage in their hearts the Famous Five filed out of the tent, driven by the bare knives in the hands of the Arabs. Lord Mauleverer followed them, yawning. His lazy lordship did not seem at all excited. He only rubbed his sleepy eyes as he came out, and yawned portentously.

Between the tent and the donkey track the six juniors were lined up. A grunt in Arabic from Kalizelos and their hands were bound behind their backs by Hamza.

Then Kalizelos slipped the automatic back into his pocket, and at a sign from him the Arabs' knives disappeared.

He fixed his eyes on Lord Mauleverer.

"My turn now, my lord," he said, with a grim smile.

"Yaas," assented Mauleverer. "Every dog has his day, you know. But I wish you'd left your call till the mornin'. I'm frightfully sleepy!"

"The scarab, my lord!" said the Greek.

"Dear man," said Lord Mauleverer negligently, "do you know, I fancied you were goin' to mention that. Sort of obsession of yours, isn't it? Well, you can search me, as the gentleman from the United States would say."

Harry Wharton & Co. stood glumly silent. It had seemed only judicious to bring the Golden Scarab with them rather than to leave it on the dahabiyeh during an absence of days. But if the scarab was, as the Greek believed, worth a fortune of a quarter of a million pounds, that fortune was in the hands of the Cairo plotter now. He had only to search.

Kalizelos looked at Mauleverer, long and hard. Then, with a muttered word to the Arabs to guard the prisoners, he went into the tent.

The juniors waited with grim faces. Only Lord Mauleverer did not seem to lose his cheery equanimity. To Wharton's astonishment, he even caught a wink from his lordship.

Kalizelos was a long time in the tent. It was evident that he was making a thorough search of the juniors' belongings.

But he emerged at last, with dark disappointment in his face. He strode straight towards Lord Mauleverer. Obviously he had not found the Golden Scarab in the tent, and he suspected that Mauleverer might have placed it in the pocket of his pyjamas—as the juniors also supposed must be the case.

The Greek did not speak, but he searched the schoolboy earl thoroughly. To the surprise of the Famous Five, the scarab did not come to light. They would have supposed that Mauly had forgotten, after all, to put it in his pocket when he left the dahabiyeh. That would have been rather like Mauly. But they had seen him put it in his pocket. Yet the Greek's meticulous search had failed to reveal it, and they could only wonder whether Mauleverer had dropped it somewhere during the day's ride. In the circumstances they hoped that he had.

"Where is the scarab, my lord?" asked Kalizelos at last in a low, bitter voice.

"Find out, old bean," answered Lord Mauleverer coolly.

The Greek's hand slid into his pocket, where he had placed the automatic. Lord Mauleverer laughed.

"No, my lord," said Kalizelos, his voice trembling with rage. "No, I shall not blow your foolish brains out."

"I rather fancied not," agreed Lord Mauleverer cheerfully. "You'd have to ladle out a fearful lot of backsheesh to save your neck if you did—what?"

"That is not my reason, my lord. The scarab will ransom your life and your liberty. It is hidden on the dahabiyeh. Be it so! There, I cannot reach it. But it will be given to me for your ransom, my lord, unless the old man Brooke chooses to leave you to die a jackal's death in the desert!"

He rapped out an order in Arabic, and Hamza hurried away through the acacias. Kalizelos turned to the juniors again, with a bitter look.

"I have sent for donkeys," he said. "I have had time to lay my plans since I left your dahabiyeh. In ten minutes Hamza will return with donkeys, and you will ride with me into the desert."

He waved his hand to the dusky west.

"Maroudi's plantation, where you have camped, is the last cultivated land in this direction," he said. "Beyond lies the Libyan Desert. In an hour we shall be far from all known tracks. The sands of the desert will hide you from all knowledge. We are not near Cairo now. We are far up the Nile. Here, we are on the border of the wilderness. Do you dream that the police, even the soldiers, will track you in the recesses of the desert?"

"Oh, my hat!" murmured Bob Cherry.

The juniors gazed at the bitter, savage face of the Greek. There was no doubt that he meant every word he uttered.

And there was no doubt that he could carry out his intention. Hardly a mile away the Nile rolled, with dahabiyehs and feluccas on its tide. Across the Nile was the city of Luxor. Yet where they stood was on the very edge of the great African desert—wastes of trackless sand, where no man wandered save the roaming bedouin, drifting from oasis to oasis.

The land of Egypt consists only of the cultivated banks of the Nile, and all along the great valley a traveller may stand with one foot in cultivated land, the other in the desert. Civilisation jostles primitive barbarism at every step. It seemed like some nightmare to the juniors. But it was no dream; it was terribly real. It was in the power of the Greek to carry them off into the untrodden heart of the desert, and that was his intention.

In silence they waited for Hamza to return with the donkeys. Lord Mauleverer broke the silence.

"Look here, you men, I'm not seein' you landed in this! Say the word and——"

The Greek's eyes glittered.

"Give up the scarab and I am done with you," he said. "I will leave you here, unharmed. You are nothing to me. It is the scarab and the Eye of Osiris that I seek. Give up the scarab——"

"Never!" said Harry Wharton curtly.

"But——" said Mauleverer slowly. He was not thinking of himself.

"Chuck it, Mauly! You're not giving in to that scoundrel!" grunted Johnny Bull.

"You all say the same?"

"Yes, ass!" said Bob.

"The samefulness is terrific!"

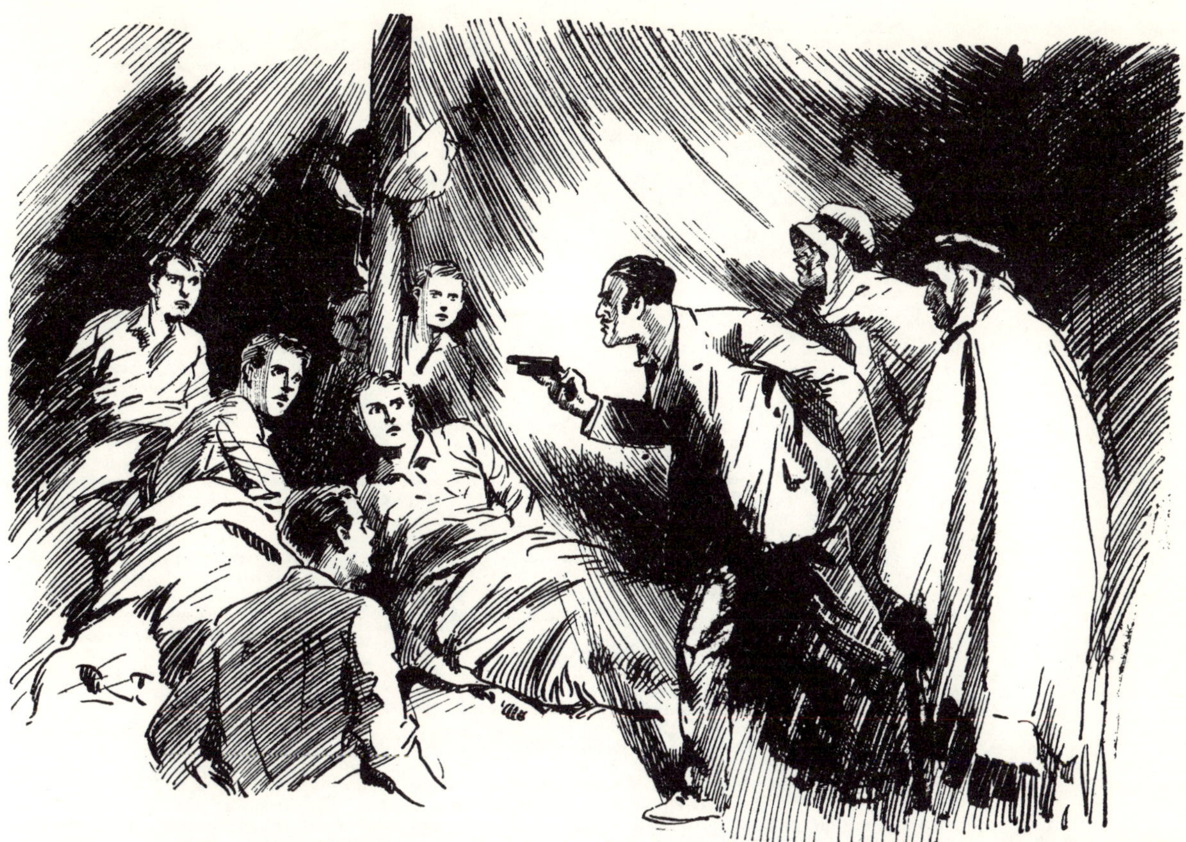

" Hallo, hallo, hallo ! " shouted Bob Cherry. " Wake up, you men ! " The Greyfriars juniors rose from their beds and stared in amazement and dismay at Kalizelos, automatic in hand, and the two dark figures behind him. " Remain still," said the Greek, " or I will riddle you with bullets ! "

"Good men!" said Lord Mauleverer. And he said no more, and, in silence again, the Greyfriars juniors waited for the return of Hamza.

THE ELEVENTH CHAPTER.
A Surprise for Bunter!

BILLY BUNTER halted.

He had to halt.

He puffed, he panted, and he blew.

Had the bony paw of the long-legged colonel been fairly on his fat shoulder, Bunter would have had to halt.

Flesh and blood could do no more.

Bunter was always short of wind. What wind he had had been utterly expended in that wild race along the donkey track of Beni-Hasa.

He halted by a fringe of tamarisks along the track and panted for breath, and gasped and gurgled.

For a minute or two no sound reached his ears, save his own gasping and gurgling. He mopped perspiration from his fat face in streams. He wiped his spectacles and jammed them again on his fat little nose. He gasped and gasped and gasped.

Then he listened. But there was, so far, no sound of pursuit. He was glad to remember that the bony colonel had damaged his head when he smote the donkey track with it. He hoped that Colonel Jacks was too damaged to resume the pursuit. He hoped vengefully that he was severely damaged—awfully damaged. He almost hoped that he was quite brained!

If the beast was still after him, he was not at hand yet. Perhaps the two beasts were coming together. In that case the long-legged colonel would probably accommodate his pace to that of the short-legged colonel and Bunter would have breathing space.

Anyhow, he had to rest! If a lion of the Libyan desert had been behind him Bunter could hardly have put on a spurt.

Satisfied that there was no immediate danger in the rear, Billy Bunter breathed more freely. He was fatigued and winded, warm and damp, feeling altogether extremely uncomfortable and frightfully exasperated. Having recovered his wind a little, he blinked about in the starlight for a sign of the Greyfriars camp, wondering dismally whether he might have passed it in his frantic flight from G. W. Jacks. Once he got into camp all would be well; even those beasts, ungrateful as they were to a fellow who had done so much for them, could hardly fail to protect him from the angry Yankees. But where was the camp?

A glimmer of white canvas, the flutter of a coloured flag from a tent-pole in the starlight, caught his eyes. Ahead of him, off the donkey-track and among the acacias, stood a great tent—any fellow but Bunter would have spotted it long ago. It was not fifty yards away, and clearly visible in the bright light of the stars of Egypt.

"Oh, good!" gasped Bunter.

This must be the Greyfriars camp. Bunter blinked inimically at the tent. He listened again, but still there was no sound from the rear. He stirred at last and crept along the donkey-track towards the big tent. The beasts were fast asleep, of course, and Bunter was going to wake them up, as he woke up the two Americans. But he did not want to make another mistake and get a fresh party of strange excursionists on his track. He was going to make sure this time that it was the Greyfriars tent before he pulled up the tent-pegs.

He crept with great caution among the tamarisks and acacias along the donkey-track, blinking at the tent as he advanced. A sound of voices reached his ears in the quiet night, and he paused and listened. The beasts were not asleep, after all! He spotted moving figures before the tent and blinked at them in astonishment. There was no light in the tent or in the camp, save that of the stars. But it was clear that the Greyfriars fellows were not in bed. And a voice that came through the silence made Bunter jump and thrill with sudden terror. He did not catch the words, but he knew the musical voice of the Greek, Konstantinos Kalizelos.

Bunter stood rooted among the tamarisks.

So many troubles had fallen on Billy Bunter since he had left the dahabiyeh that he had forgotten all about the Greek. He remembered him now.

"Oh lor'!" breathed Bunter, palpitating.

It dawned on his fat mind that the Greek had lost no time in making use of his freedom. No doubt Hamza and Yussef had joined him; most likely they had spied on the Greyfriars party, and knew where the camp was. Anyhow, the Greek was there—that was certain. And Bunter realised what had been the result of his fatuous folly. Kalizelos and his confederates were there—which meant that the juniors were at the mercy of their enemies.

For a long minute Bunter stood

rooted with terror; then he moved to an opening of the bushes and peered at the camp, now not ten yards from him. He could see the juniors standing in a row, with their hands tied behind them —Lord Mauleverer and the Famous Five, evidently prisoners. He could see Kalizelos, the Greek, and Yussef, the Arab. Hamza was not there, neither could he see anything of the dragoman.

"Oh crikey!" groaned Bunter.

He was thankful that he had not run on as far as the tent. That would have landed him in the soup along with the others. As matters stood, no one in the Greyfriars camp knew, or suspected, that he was at hand. Kalizelos, if he thought of him at all, thought that he was still on the dahabiyeh. That was a comfort.

Had Billy Bunter been of the stuff of which heroes are made, no doubt he would have considered at once the possibility of helping the juniors out of their scrape. That did not occur to Bunter. It was obvious—to Bunter—that he could not help them, and he was thankful that his own fat person was safe so long as he kept in cover. He hugged his cover in the tamarisks and watched the strange scene through his big spectacles.

What it meant he could not make out. They appeared to be waiting for something. Bunter knew that Lord Mauleverer had taken the Golden Scarab with him that day, but he could guess that the Greek had not found it, or he would have vanished at once with his prize. Except to get possession of the mysterious scarab, he had no concern with the Greyfriars party, and did not care two straws about them. But what were they waiting for? The sound of voices had died away, and they were waiting in silence. For what?

A clumping of donkeys' hoofs from the distance beyond the acacias answered the question.

Hamza, the scarred Arab, came into view in the starlight leading a string of donkeys. He led the animals up to the group standing before the tent. Bunter blinked on in amazement. The voice of the Greek came to his fat ears.

"For the last time, my lord! If you would save yourself and your friends from the desert, place the Scarab of A-Menah in my hands! A message to the dahabiyeh——"

"Nothin' doin', old bean!" came the quiet drawl of Lord Mauleverer.

"My lord, if you will ransom yourself and your friends with the Golden Scarab, I will trust to your word of honour and release you to fetch it and place it in my hands."

"Bow-wow!"

"What—what did you say?" exclaimed the Greek.

"Bow-wow!"

"Fool!" snarled Kalizelos.

He turned to the Arabs and snarled an order in Arabic. The two ruffians led the juniors towards the donkeys.

Billy Bunter understood now. They had been waiting for Hamza to bring the donkeys, and they were to be taken away, prisoners, into the wastes of the Libyan desert.

"Oh crikey!" breathed Bunter.

He could not help them! He did not even think of trying to help them. But he was utterly dismayed and horrified. His fat heart almost died within him as he realised the fate that hung over the Greyfriars juniors. For once, William George Bunter was not thinking wholly of himself. If there was a chance of getting help——

Somewhere on Beni-Hasa was the house of Mr. Maroudi's manager. But Bunter did not know where, or at what distance. A mile away was Cook's rest-house; less than that the custodians of the Tombs of the Kings. But they were too far away for help. Then into Bunter's fat brain flashed the recollection of the two Americans. Their camp was not distant—and in all likelihood they were following him along the donkey-track. Colonel Jacks and Colonel Skink, of course, were beasts; they were looking for Bunter to whop him. But they were white men, and surely——

Billy Bunter did not stop to think it out. It was the only chance of helping the Greek's prisoners—the only chance of saving them from vanishing into the wastes of the desert. He backed out of the tamarisks, crept to the donkey-track, and, after an anxious blink behind to make sure that the bushes screened him from the Greyfriars camp, he started back the way he had come, running as if his fat life depended on his speed.

THE TWELFTH CHAPTER.

U.S.A. to the Rescue!

"CARRY me home to die!" ejaculated Colonel Jacks.

"Search me!" exclaimed Colonel Skink, equally astonished at what they saw.

The long colonel and the short colonel were tramping up the donkey-track, stick in hand, looking for the Greyfriars camp. Neither of them had the slightest doubt that the collapse of their tent was a "lark" of the English schoolboys. They were wrathy, and they meant to find the schoolboys' camp, and wade in with the sticks and impress upon the minds of those sons of John Bull that they could not lark with impunity with citizens of the great United States.

They halted in sheer amazement at the sight of a fat figure racing towards them, with a pair of big spectacles flashing back the light of the stars.

"I guess it's that fat guy I took a tumble over!" gasped Colonel Jacks. "I'll say he's coming back to ask for it."

"I kinder calculate he's going to get it, too, where it will hurt!" said Colonel Skink.

"You've said it!" agreed Colonel Jacks.

And the two transatlantic gentlemen, grinning, waited for Bunter to come up. Why he was running back, fairly into their vengeful hands, was a mystery to them, but there was no doubt that they were glad to see him.

Bunter sighted them, but he did not stop, and did not dodge away into the bushes as he saw them, as they fully expected. He came puffing and panting on. And as he drew nearer, Messrs. Jacks and Skink discerned the terror in his face and stared at him curiously.

"Say, there surely can't be a lion around loose," murmured G. W. Jacks. "I'll say that fat guy has got the wind-up."

"If he ain't scared stiff I've never seen a scared guy!" said Colonel Skink. "I'm sure glad I packed my gun for this trip."

"They let on that you don't want a gun in Egypt these days," said Colonel Jacks, slipping his hand into his hip-pocket. "But that fat guy surely does look as if suthin's the matter with Hanner, Ephraim Skink, and I'm powerful glad that I packed my hardware."

Bunter came panting up. He gurgled as he came:

"Help!"

He staggered from sheer exhaustion as he reached the two Americans. G. W. Jacks put a hand to his fat shoulder to steady him. He was not thinking now of giving the fat schoolboy what he deserved. It was plain that the matter was serious.

"Say, bo', I guess you're safe hyer," said G. W. Jacks quite kindly. "Take a cinch on yourself, sonny! What's the rookus?"

"Spill it, son!" said Colonel Skink encouragingly.

"Help!" groaned Bunter. "They've got them——"

"Who've got who?"

"My friends, the Greyfriars fellows—they're prisoners—they're going to take them into the desert!" gurgled Bunter. "A Greek villain and two Arabs—oh dear!"

Breath failed Bunter, but he grabbed

the lean colonel's arm with one hand and pointed with the other, gasping spasmodically:

"Help—help them! Oh crikey!"

The two Americans stared at him blankly for a second. Then they exchanged a glance, and a bony hand and a podgy hand grasped a revolver from a hip pocket.

"I guess we chip in hyer, Ephraim Skink!" said Colonel Jacks briefly.

"You said it!" assented Colonel Skink.

Leaving Bunter spluttering helplessly, the two Americans ran up the donkey-track in the direction from which Bunter had come.

Colonel Jacks' long legs whisked like lightning; Colonel Skink's short fat legs went like machinery behind him.

The long-legged colonel was the first to sight the Greyfriars tent, glimmering in the stars. He came through the tamarisks like a charging giraffe. But the fat colonel was not far behind.

Kalizelos and Hamza were holding the donkeys. Yussef was forcing the juniors to mount them, heaving them roughly into the saddles as their hands were bound.

Colonel Jacks burst on the scene like a thunderbolt. If he had had any doubt of Bunter's startling statement he had proof of it now; a single glance told that the Greyfriars fellows were prisoners in lawless hands, and were about to be carried away on the donkeys. The starlight glimmered on Colonel Jacks' revolver as he charged up.

"Say, you!" he roared, his powerful voice breaking on the silence like a thunderclap. "Say, I guess you want to let up on this stunt, and I'll say you want to let up sudden! Get me?"

The juniors, amazed, stared round. The two Arabs started, and flashed out their knives. Kalizelos, gritting his teeth, spun round, his automatic leaping to his hand.

"Drop it!" roared Colonel Jacks.

The Greek's weapon gleamed up.

Bang!

Undoubtedly it was fortunate, for the Greyfriars fellows and for G. W. Jacks himself, that the long-legged colonel had 'packed his gun' for his trip to Egypt. It was Colonel Jacks who fired, before the desperate Greek could pull trigger, and Kalizelos gave a fearful cry and staggered back, his pistol-hand sagging down. At that desperate moment there was no doubt that the Greek would have shot down the stranger who had butted in. But the long-legged colonel had got in first.

"Oh gad!" gasped Lord Mauleverer.

The donkeys, startled by the shot, reared and plunged. Kalizelos staggered against an acacia, his olive face white as chalk, his left hand pressed to his right shoulder, where the American's bullet had struck. Hamza and Yussef, knife in hand, leaped towards the long-legged American.

Bang, bang, bang!

Both the Americans were shooting now. Harry Wharton & Co. hardly knew what was happening. With their hands bound they could not control the excited, plunging donkeys, and they pitched helplessly off the animals, and sprawled on the ground. As they rolled over, some of them had a glimpse of Hamza and Yussef running for their lives. Bang, bang, bang! roared the six-shooters, and bullets knocked up the dust at the heels of the two Arabs as they fled.

"Oh, my hat!" gasped Bob Cherry. He sat up dizzily. The frightened donkeys were racing away, and Bob caught a glimpse of the Greek, wounded as he was, clutching at one of the fleeing animals with his sound arm. He saw Kalizelos drag himself desperately across the donkey's back, and the animal galloped away with him.

"Good gad!" stuttered Lord Mauleverer. "What—who——"

"It's the jolly old Yankees!" gasped Bob.

Bang, bang, bang!

"Say, you!" roared Colonel Jacks, as he loosed off shot after shot. "Say, you want to hump it, you! You want to light out! You want to beat it! You want to beat it spry and sudden! Yep!"

Bang, bang!

The Greek and the two Arabs were "beating it" as "sudden" as they could. They had already vanished into the night. But the two excited colonels seemed to be enjoying the fireworks, and they emptied their "guns" after the vanished fugitives. Not till the last cartridge was expended did they cease to throw lead into space.

Then Colonel Jacks calmed down and chuckled.

"I'll say this was some circus, Ephraim Skink!" he remarked.

"I'll surely say so!" agreed Colonel Skink.

"I opine that them guys lit out like they was sent for!" chuckled Colonel Jacks. "And I'm sure glad I packed my hardware for this trip!"

"Search me!" agreed Colonel Skink.

The long-legged colonel strode towards the Greyfriars juniors. The fat colonel pumped in breath after his run.

G. W. Jacks looked at the juniors with a cheery grin on his bony, lantern-jawed visage.

"Say, I guess them guys had you'uns by the short hairs," he remarked.

"You guess right, old bean," answered Bob Cherry.

"The guessfulness is terrifically correct, my esteemed and ridiculous Yankeeful friend," said Hurree Jamset Ram Singh.

Colonel Jacks chortled, apparently entertained by that reply from the Nabob of Bhanipur. He drew out an enormous clasp-knife, opened it with his prominent teeth, and cut the schoolboys' bonds. With deep thankfulness, Harry Wharton & Co. found themselves free once more.

THE THIRTEENTH CHAPTER.

Where the Scarab Was!

"I SAY, you fellows!"

Six juniors jumped.

A fat figure rolled up in the starlight, gasping. Harry Wharton & Co. gazed in amazement at the Owl of the Remove.

"Bunter!" ejaculated Frank Nugent.

"The esteemed and idiotic Bunter!" exclaimed Hurree Jamset Ram Singh.

Bunter mopped his perspiring brow, gasping and panting. Billy Bunter had followed the two colonels to the spot—but at a safe distance. Not till he was sure that the enemy had been put to flight did the fat Owl venture on the scene. The juniors were amazed to see him; they had supposed Bunter to be sound asleep on the dahabiyeh. They little guessed, so far, how much they owed to the intervention of the Owl of the Remove.

"How on earth did that fat frog hop here?" asked Johnny Bull.

"Oh, really, Bull——"

"I guess that's the fat gink that put us wise!" said Colonel Jacks. "I surely opine I owe him a lambasting!"

"Here, you keep off!" exclaimed Bunter. "I say, you fellows, it's pretty lucky that I came after you—what? Where would you be now if I hadn't come?"

"What the thump——"

"I decided to come after you," explained Bunter. "I knew you'd land in some trouble without me——"

"You fat owl!"

"Looks as if I was right!" grinned Bunter. "Those beasts had you all right, and if I hadn't spotted them and fetched these Yankee chaps where would you be I'd like to know."

"My hat!" Harry Wharton stared blankly at the grinning Owl. "Did Bunter bring you here, Colonel Jacks?"

"I guess he put us wise," said G. W. Jacks. "We was arter him for pulling down our tent, and he came cavorting back, scared stiff, and told us about them guys. And we sure did raise the dust getting here, didn't we, Ephraim Skink?"

"We surely did, Colonel Jacks," answered Ephraim Skink.

"We don't know how to thank you, sir," said Harry. "You've saved us, and you'll believe that we're grateful."

"The gratitude is terrific and preposterous, esteemed colonel."

Colonel Jacks waved a bony hand.

"That's O.K., sonny," he said. "I guess we wasn't letting the niggers get away with this, was we, Ephraim Skink?"

"We surely was not, Colonel Jacks," answered Ephraim Skink.

"And seeing what's happened we're letting you off the lambasting we was going to put across," added Colonel Jacks generously.

Harry Wharton & Co. looked at him. They were genuinely grateful to the two Americans, and anxious to show that they were thankful for the immense service the colonels from the U.S.A. had rendered them. But if Messrs. Jacks and Skink had started in to "lambaste" the party, they would probably have met with a surprise.

"Yep!" assented Colonel Skink. "Nary lambasting."

"But what—what have we done?" asked Harry. "You don't mean to say you were still bothering about that little accident on the Nile——"

"Aw, can it!" said Colonel Jacks. "Didn't you and that fat guy bring our tent walloping down on our cabezas——"

"Oh, my hat! Certainly not!"

"They wasn't in it, Colonel Jacks," said Ephraim Skink. "I guess it was that fat guy on his lonesome. We didn't see the other guys."

"Oh, sure!" assented G. W. Jacks. "I guess you've said it!"

"Bunter, you fat villain, have you been playing tricks on these gentlemen?" exclaimed Lord Mauleverer.

"Oh, no! I never pulled out the tent-pegs," said Bunter hastily, with an

(*Continued on next page.*)

uneasy blink at the two colonels. "Besides, I thought it was your tent."

"Why, you pernicious porpoise!" exclaimed Bob. "You were going to pull down our tent——"

"Well, leaving a fellow on his own—serve you jolly well right!" said Bunter indignantly. "I've had a fearful time following you—my donkey ran away, and I had to walk, and——"

"Ha, ha, ha!"

"Blessed if I see anything to cackle at! Of course, I thought it was your tent," said Bunter, "and I was jolly well going to bring it down on your nappers, blow you! How was I to know anybody else was camping here? Not that I did it, you know," added Bunter, blinking at Colonel Jacks. "The fact is I was nowhere near the place—I never even saw your tent——"

"Carry me home to die!" ejaculated Colonel Jacks, staring at Bunter. "I'll say that guy is some liar!"

"Oh, really, you know——"

"Where's Hassan?" asked Nugent suddenly.

"I say, you fellows, I'm fearfully hungry——"

"By gum! Where's Hassan?" exclaimed Bob. "He was gone when those rotters fetched us out of the tent? If they've harmed him——"

"We'd better look for him at once," said Harry. "That brute Kalizelos has done something with him——"

"I guess you better stay right here," said Colonel Jacks. "Them guys might be hanging round looking for another chance at you. I guess I'll mosey round and find your dragoman."

"You said it," said Colonel Skink.

The two colonels started to search for Hassan. Harry Wharton & Co. went into the tent and dressed themselves. They were not thinking of sleep again that night. While they dressed Billy Bunter searched for provender, and, having found it, settled down to dispose of it internally.

"Jolly lucky that fat idiot turned up," remarked Bob Cherry. "If he hadn't roused out the Yankees——"

"The luckfulness was terrific," remarked Hurree Jamset Ram Singh.

"But what became of the scarab, after all?" asked Nugent. "You had it in your pocket, Mauly, when we left the dahabiyeh?"

"Yaas!" Lord Mauleverer grinned. "But it wasn't in my pocket, old bean, when that Greek Johnny looked for it. I put it in my pyjama pocket for safety when I turned in."

"But he searched you——"

"Yaas; but you see I've got a lot of presence of mind," explained Lord Mauleverer cheerfully. "As soon as the sportsman woke us up I reached for that jolly old scarab at once, and, bein' in the dark, he didn't spot me. Did you hear me scratchin' while the Greek was talkin'?"

"Scratching! No!"

"Lucky you didn't, or he might have, too," said Mauleverer placidly. "You see, I slipped my little paw under that jolly old rug that's spread on the ground and scratched a little hole in the sand and left the scarab in it. An' it's there now."

"Carry me home to die, as Colonel Jacks would say!" ejaculated Bob Cherry.

"Ha, ha, ha!"

"The presence of Mauly's preposterous mind was truly terrific," declared Hurree Jamset Ram Singh.

Lord Mauleverer turned back the Turkish prayer-rug that covered the floor. Under it was the sandy soil.

Mauly blinked at the sand.

"Blessed if I can see the place now," he remarked. "You see, I poked it under the sand and covered it, and now——"

"We'll jolly soon find it," said Bob.

The juniors chuckled. They realised that when Kalizelos had been speaking to them in the doorway of the tent Mauly, in the darkness, had been concealing the scarab of which the Greek was in quest. They had never suspected his lordship of possessing such prompt presence of mind.

Bob turned on an electric torch, and the juniors scraped up the sand till the scarab was revealed. There was a glitter of gold in the light.

"Yaas, there it is, safe and sound," yawned Lord Mauleverer; and he picked up the scarab of A-Menah and transferred it to his pocket. "Dear old Kalizelos never guessed that it was under his feet when he was searchin' our clobber in the tent."

"I say, you fellows——"

"Hallo, hallo, hallo! Bursting?" asked Bob Cherry.

"I say, is there any more grub?"

"He's scoffed the lot!" said Bob, in wonder. "Where on earth has he put it?"

"Oh, really, Cherry——"

"Poor old Bunter! He's only had enough for about seven or eight fellows," said Bob sympathetically. "He will have to endure the pangs of hunger till Maroudi's people bring along brekker in the morning!"

"Well, I've had a snack," said Bunter. "I can sleep now! I think I'll turn in. I suppose you fellows are going to keep watch."

"Naturally," answered Bob. "Could we find anything better to do than to sit round keeping watch while you snore?"

"All right, then!" said Bunter. "Mind you don't go to sleep—those beasts might come back, you know. You'd better get those Yankees to stay, too—it will be safer! They're beasts, but they'll keep the other beasts off—see? Keep watch till morning, old chaps, and wake me when they bring breakfast—not before."

"On my head be it!" said Bob Cherry solemnly.

"Ha, ha, ha!"

And Billy Bunter, having stacked away all the available provisions, rolled into the tent, rolled into the nearest bed, and in about ten seconds his deep snore was awakening the echoes of the land of Egypt.

Harry Wharton & Co. joined the two Americans in searching for the dragoman. In spite of Billy Bunter's injunctions he was left to snore unwatched. It was some time before Hassan was discovered, bound to the acacia in the deep shadow of the branches, and it was Bob Cherry who finally spotted him.

"Hallo, hallo, hallo! Here he is!" roared Bob.

There was a faint mumble from the gagged dragoman. The juniors gathered round him and released him.

"My lordly gentlemen!" exclaimed Hassan, in great relief. "It is enormously enjoyful to behold you as safe as a house, as you say in the English language! Wahyat-en-nabi! O noble sars, I fell into the hands of those sons of dogs and pigs, and I was without power to aid my magnificent lords, for which reason my heart was very heavy! To see you in enjoyment of safety and freedom what is called in English a sight for sore eyes!"

Hassan returned to the camp with the juniors. He left them there and hurried on to the plantation buildings to call a number of the fellahin a keep guard for the remainder of the night. The two Americans remained in the camp till Hassan returned with two or three dozen natives, armed with stout staves.

"I guess you-uns will be O.K. now," said Colonel Jacks. "But if there's any more trouble you put G. W. Jacks wise, and I guess we'll see you through. Ain't that so, Colonel Skink?"

"You said it!" agreed Colonel Skink.

"We're awfully obliged to you," said Harry Wharton. "If you hadn't chipped in we should be prisoners now, miles away in the desert. We really don't know how to thank you."

"That's all right, sonny," said Colonel Jacks affably. "I allow it's up to the U.S.A. to see John Bull through—yep! Didn't we win the War for you? I'll say yep! Good-night!"

"Didn't you which?" gasped Bob Cherry. "Oh—ah—yes—quite—just so—my hat! Thanks no end! Good-night!"

And the long colonel and the short colonel faded out, leaving the Greyfriars fellows grinning.

THE FOURTEENTH CHAPTER.

Bold Bunter!

"READY, Bunter?"

"No!" hooted Billy Bunter.

"Come on, fathead!"

"Shan't!"

Billy Bunter did not "come on." William George Bunter was comfortable and lazy, and did not want to move.

Donkeys and donkey-boys had arrived at the camp in the morning, and the Greyfriars party had ridden to the Tombs of the Queens, and other "sights" of the Theban Necropolis. Whether their enemies were lingering in the vicinity they could not tell, but they knew that the Greek, at least, had been wounded, and it was likely that he was hors de combat for the time, at least. And in the day-time, with plenty of tourists, guides, and donkey-boys about, there was no danger to be looked for.

They returned to the camp of Beni-Hasa for lunch and rest, and in the afternoon prepared to start to the dahabiyeh on the Nile. Now that Kalizelos was free again, and once more on the track of the Golden Scarab, the juniors agreed that the camping-out had better be given up.

Hassan was urgent that they should return to the safety of the dahabiyeh. And it was in the care of the dragoman that Sir Reginald Brooke had trusted them up the Nile "on their own." In the camp, on the edge of the desert, Hassan pointed out that the enemy might swoop down on them in the night, perhaps in strong force.

A scrap with some gang of armed and savage bedouins, in the pay of the Greek, could only have ended one way, as the juniors admitted, so it was decided to go back to the houseboat.

Marvellous to relate, Billy Bunter was prepared to brave the dangers which the other fellows thought it only prudent to obviate.

Bunter was tired. He was fat. He was lazy. He had eaten enough lunch for three or four. He had napped only a couple of hours since lunch. And the danger was not near at hand. So Bunter was not prepared to shift. No doubt, when it grew dark, funk would have supervened. But in broad daylight, with no enemy in sight, Bunter was as bold as a lion.

"It's sickening," said Bunter, glaring at the Famous Five through his big spectacles as he sat up on a rug under a shady tree. The beasts had disturbed

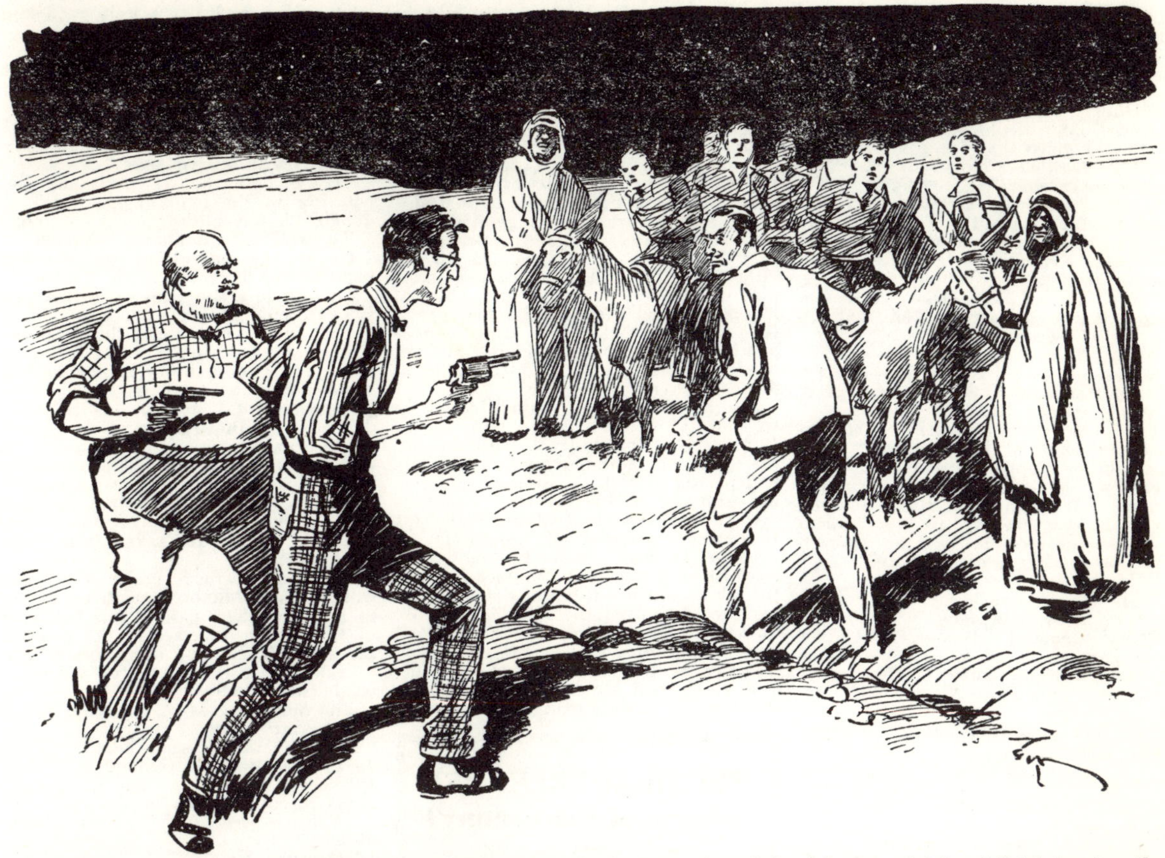

Harry Wharton and Co. were about to be carried away on the donkeys when Colonel Jacks and Colonel Skink burst on the scene like a thunderbolt. "Say you!" roared the former, levelling his automatic at Kalizelos. "I guess you want to let up on this stunt, and let up sudden! Get me?"

him in a prolonged nap, so Bunter was naturally bitter. "I was against this idea of camping out—you know that. Now we're here, let's stick it out! What are you afraid of? I'm with you!"

"Get up, idiot!" said Bob Cherry.

"Shan't! Hassan can fetch Maroudi's niggers to keep guard to-night. And there's those Yankees, too," said Bunter. "And I've no doubt that Greek beast has cleared off—likely as not pegged out by this time, in fact. Anyhow, I'm here to protect you, same as I did last night. Keep a stiff upper-lip, and don't be frightened."

The Famous Five looked at him. Lord Mauleverer grinned. Billy Bunter sat and blinked with scorn.

"It's the limit," he said. "Never saw such a set of funks! Frightened at a shadow! I'm jolly well not going to be frightened away—I can tell you!"

"You piffling porpoise!" said Bob Cherry, with a deep breath. "You were scared out of your silly wits last night."

"Yah!"

"And if Kalizelos showed up to-night with some gang of Arabs from the desert, you'd have a fit."

"Yah!" repeated Bunter.

"Besides, we've invited those Americans to come on the dahabiyeh."

"Blow 'em!"

"They're going to ride back with us."

"Rot!"

Probably Billy Bunter would have been jerked off his rug, and bumped on the hard, unsympathetic surface of Egypt at that stage, but for the fact that the two Americans came up the donkey-track just then. Bunter had his back to the donkey-track, and did not see them coming. His spectacles were fastened on the Greyfriars fellows with ineffable scorn.

"I say, you fellows, pluck up a little courage!" he admonished. "Be men, you know—like me!"

"My lordly gentlemen, the donkeys are ready!" said Hassan.

"You can shut up!" said Bunter. "We're not going! If you're frightened, you can clear off—see? If you fellows are frightened, run away as soon as you like! Leave me to face danger alone! I'm the man for it!"

"Ye gods!" murmured Bob Cherry.

"I must say I'm ashamed of you fellows," said Bunter. "Dash it all, have a little pluck! If there's any danger to-night, wake me up! I'll see you through! And now I'm going to sleep. You can't expect me to sit up in this heat, listening to you babbling about your funk. For goodness' sake, take example by me, and have a little pluck! Do I care for danger?"

Colonel Jacks and Colonel Skink had arrived under the tree. They stood looking down at Billy Bunter's portly back, listening to him, and grinning. After their experience of him the previous night, they seemed to find the fat Owl's valorous words entertaining.

"Why," went on Bunter, still blinking with devastating scorn at the exasperated juniors—"why, if those beasts showed up again this minute, do you think I should care twopence? Not me! I'd jolly well like them to, in fact! I'd show you fellows how to buck up!"

Colonel Jacks closed one eye at the juniors over Billy Bunter's unconscious head. Then, stooping behind Bunter, he suddenly grasped him by the back of the neck. His large, bony hand closed like a vice on that fat neck, and there was a startled yell from Bunter.

"Ooooop!"

"Dog of a Faringhee, die, by the beard of the Prophet!" roared Colonel Jacks, in Bunter's startled ear.

"Ow! Oooh! Help!" yelled Bunter, wriggling frantically. "I say, you fellows, help! Keep him off! He's got me! Yarooooh!"

Billy Bunter had not the slightest doubt that he was in the grasp of a savage Arab. G. W. Jacks, evidently, had a playful sense of humour.

"Bismillah!" he roared. "Inshallah!"

"Yaroop! Keep him off!" shrieked Bunter. "Help! Help! I say, you fellows, rescue! Help!"

"Ha, ha, ha!" yelled the juniors. The sudden evaporation of Billy Bunter's courage was too much for them. They shrieked.

"Help!" roared Bunter. "Leggo! Help! Yarooooh!"

With that iron grip on the back of his neck Bunter could not turn his head, and see who was behind him. His terrified mind pictured a ferocious Arab, and he palpitated with horror. It might have occurred, even to Bunter, that if a ferocious Arab had seized him from behind, Harry Wharton & Co. would hardly have stood roaring with laughter. But William George Bunter was too scared to think of that, or anything else, save the iron grip on the back of his fat neck.

"Help! Rescue!" shrieked Bunter. "Oh crikey! Mercy! Spare my life! It wasn't me! Yarooooh! Mercy!"

"Ha, ha, ha!" shrieked the juniors.

"Buck up, Bunter!" chortled Lord

Mauleverer. "You're not afraid of a jolly old Arab, you know!"

"Set us an example, old fat bean!" chuckled Bob Cherry.

"Ha, ha, ha!"

"Help! Whoop! Yooop! Mercy!" roared Bunter.

"Say, I guess that fat guy will have a fit!" drawled Colonel Skink. "He sure is some boob!"

G. W. Jacks, with a chuckle, released Bunter's fat neck. The fat Owl made a bound to his feet, and, without a backward glance, jumped away. He dodged behind the juniors, yelling.

"Keep him off! Oh crikey! Hassan, help! Harry, old chap! Bob, old fellow, help! Keep him off!"

"Ha, ha, ha!"

"You silly owl!" roared Bob Cherry. "It's not an Arab! Shut up, you ass!"

"Oh!" gasped Bunter.

From behind the Famous Five he ventured to blink at his assailant. His eyes almost popped through his spectacles as he saw the two grinning colonels. It dawned on Billy Bunter's fat brain that his leg had been pulled.

"You—you—you beast!" he gasped. "W-w-w-was it you collared me?"

"Ha, ha, ha!"

"I'll say it was," chortled Colonel Jacks. "Haw, haw haw!"

"Oh!" gasped Bunter. "I—I—I knew it was you, of course. I—I knew it was you all the time. I—I—I bet I made you think I was frightened! He, he, he!"

"I'll bet you did!" agreed Colonel Jacks.

"I'll say so," chuckled Colonel Skink.

"Well, are you ready to start now, Bunter?" asked Harry Wharton, laughing.

"No; I'm jolly well not!" Billy Bunter had recovered now. "And if you fellows are funky——"

"Bump him!" said Bob Cherry.

"I say, you fellows, leggo! Oh crikey!" howled Bunter, as the Famous Five grasped him, and he smote the sandy soil with a mighty smite. "Yaroooh! I say, you fellows, I'm ready! I'm waiting! Whoop!"

Bump!

"Yow-ow-ow!"

"Now get on your donkey, and shut up!" said Bob. "If you say another word, you fat, funky frump, I'll jolly well kick you!"

"Beast!" roared Bunter.

Thud!

"Ow!"

"Have another?" asked Bob. "Another word, and——"

Billy Bunter did not say another word. He clambered on his donkey, and the Greyfriars party started for the Nile.

THE FIFTEENTH CHAPTER.

Very Hot Coffee!

MOUSSA, the reis, greeted the Greyfriars juniors with grave salaams as they came on board the dahabiyeh.

From Moussa they learned how Kalizelos had made his escape; details which Billy Bunter had not thought it worth while to mention. It was probably only the presence of the visitors on board that saved the fatuous Owl from being kicked from one end of the Cleopatra to the other. But in the presence of the two transatlantic gentlemen, Bunter could not be dealt with as he deserved.

Bunter, unaware of his narrow escape, was by no means pleased by the presence of those two citizens of the United States. G. W. Jacks' little jest at his

expense had roused his wrath, and he bestowed a good many inimical blinks on the long-legged colonel; which G. W. Jacks did not even notice. Indeed, he did not seem to observe Bunter at all; which added to the irritation of the most important member of the party.

Messrs. Jacks and Skink were very pleased to pay that visit, for two good reasons—they had discovered that Mauleverer was a "real live lord," which was naturally very gratifying to true republicans; and they were going to get a lift on the Cleopatra up the Nile as far as Armant, their next stopping-place, which saved the cost of hiring a boat. And the juniors, grateful for the help the two Yankee gentlemen had rendered in the hour of need, were only too glad to make as much of them as possible.

Bunter did not share that feeling in the least. G. W. Jacks had chased Bunter up a donkey-track with the full intention of "lambasting" him. He had played a trick on Bunter, frightening him out of his fat wits. And he disregarded the fat Owl as if the fat Owl was a person of absolutely no account at all. Billy Bunter would have liked to punch G. W. Jacks' nose—though he did not think of doing so. He had not forgotten the spanking G. W. Jacks had given him, and he did not want any more. But as the dahabiyeh was cast off from the bank of the Nile, and while Lord Mauleverer was politely showing the visitors over Mr. Maroudi's

magnificent houseboat, Bunter stated his views to the other fellows.

"I say, you fellows, I don't want those Yankees here," he said. "I can't make out what you've brought them on board for."

"Forgotten already what they did for us last night?" asked Nugent.

"Oh, rot!" said Bunter. "Nothing to make a song about! Besides, I did it all, really—I fetched the beasts and saved you from danger—I'd like to know what would have happened without me——"

"Without you, you fat idiot, Kalizelos would still be locked up in his cabin," growled Johnny Bull. "Shut up!"

"Well, I'm fed-up with those Yankees," said Bunter firmly, "and I can tell you, I don't want them here—especially that cheeky rotter Jacks. I've a jolly good mind to tell them so."

"Get ready to be dropped in the Nile if you do!" said Harry Wharton.

"The dropfulness will be terrific, my esteemed idiotic Bunter," assured Hurree Jamset Ram Singh.

Bunter's fat lip curled.

"So you're putting those Yankees before me, after all I've done for you," he said. "Talk about a serpent's child being more ungrateful than a thankless tooth——"

"Ha, ha, ha!"

"Well, let 'em look out, that's all," said Bunter darkly. "That cheeky beast smacked me—and played a rotten trick on me, and I've a jolly good mind to punch his nose——"

"You'd want a ladder to get to it, old fat man," grinned Bob. "And he might spank you again. And we won't stop him next time."

"I'm not going to have a row with the fellow," said Bunter loftily. "But I can jolly well tell you——"

"Hallo, hallo, hallo!" exclaimed Bob, pointing to the bank, from which the dahabiyeh was gliding away. "Look!"

"Kalizelos!" exclaimed Wharton.

Under the palm-trees on the high bank of the Nile, stood the Greek, his right arm in a sling, his olive face pale. He had suddenly appeared through the palms, and was watching the dahabiyeh as it glided up the Nile. As he caught the eyes of the juniors turned on him, his clenched fist at them, his pale face his clenched fist at the, his pale face distorted with rage. Bob Cherry politely raised his hat in response, with a cheery grin. The Greek's brow grew blacker, and his jetty eyes burned.

"We're not done with that merchant yet," remarked Johnny Bull. "All Bunter's fault! Let's kick him."

"Beast!"

The Greek stood under the palms watching the dahabiyeh with bitter rage in his face. The palms, and the figure of the Greek, faded into the distance. He was still standing there, his burning eyes fixed on the group of schoolboys when the dahabiyeh glided round one of the many curves of the Nile, and he was lost to sight.

"I'll say this is some boat!" Colonel Jacks' nasal voice resounded. "Yep, I'll surely say this is some boat, and I guess it cost a heap of dollars."

"You've said it!" agreed Colonel Skink.

"Gentlemanly lords," said Hassan, "coffee is prepare on a balcony."

"Tea's ready," said Harry. "This way!"

They descended to the stern balcony, where Colonel Jacks stretched his long limbs in a long cane chair; and another chair creaked and groaned under the weight of Colonel Skink. The two American gentlemen were in high good-humour, and so were the Famous Five, and Lord Mauleverer beamed. Only Billy Bunter's fat face wore a frown. But nobody seemed to observe that William George Bunter was dissatisfied. So far as the two colonels were concerned, Bunter might have not been there at all; which was naturally annoying to a fellow who knew his own importance, if nobody else did.

"I'll say this is good coffee," said Colonel Jacks, having drained his seventh cup. "Yep! I'll certainly say so!"

A Nubian servant took the bony colonel's cup to refill it. Billy Bunter dropped into a chair beside Colonel Jacks. There was a gleam in Billy Bunter's eyes, behind his big spectacles. Also Billy Bunter had something in his fat hand. Hurree Jamset Ram Singh, who was on Bunter's other side, gave a slight sniff, and glanced at the fat Owl's closed hand. He scented pepper.

"My esteemed Bunter——" murmured the nabob.

Bunter blinked at him.

"It's all right, Inky! I haven't got anything in my hand," he whispered. "If you think I went down to get a packet of pepper from the cook, you're jolly well mistaken. What should I want pepper for?"

"My only esteemed hat!" murmured the nabob.

"Nothing of the sort," said Bunter airily. "You needn't blink at me in that suspicious way, Inky! Mind your own bizney, see!"

Hurree Singh grinned.

He looked away from Bunter; but the corner of his eye was on the fat junior. Bunter's manner was so excessively sly, that it would have aroused the least suspicious person's suspicions had anyone observed him. Only the nabob, as it happened, was observing him; but the Nabob of Bhanipur was observing him very keenly indeed—out of the corner of his eye.

Colonel Jacks' cup was set before him again. It was undoubtedly good coffee, made by Hassan's own hands; but it was Billy Bunter's idea that the bony colonel was not going to enjoy that cup, at all events.

"I say, you fellows!" exclaimed Bunter suddenly. "What's that on the bank? Is it an elephant?"

He pointed with his empty hand towards a fringe of date-trees on the bank of the Nile, near which some fellahin were working a shaduf. The tea-party looked round in the indicated direction, certainly not expecting to see an elephant wandering along the Nile.

All eyes being off him—except the corner of one very keen eye—Billy Bunter reached out his other hand over the colonel's coffee-cup. The contents of the paper packet in his fat paw shot into the colonel's coffee.

Really, it was very slyly done; Billy Bunter was displaying uncommon wiliness. Hurree Jamset Ram Singh winked into space.

"Blessed if I can see any elephant!" said Bob Cherry. "There's a shaduf—is that what you took for an elephant, you owl?"

"The seefulness of an esteemed elephant is not terrific," remarked Hurree Jamset Ram Singh.

"I guess you're dreaming, son," said Colonel Jacks. "I surely don't spot any pesky elephant."

The tall colonel stood up, to stare at the slowly gliding bank. Billy Bunter grinned, and took a sip of his own cup of coffee. The pepper was in Colonel Jacks' coffee now, and when he had finished looking for a non-existent elephant on the bank of the Nile, there was a surprise in store for him.

Hurree Jamset Ram Singh touched the fat Owl gently on the arm.

"My esteemed Bunter," he murmured, "did you drop that hundred-piastre piece on the deck?"

"Eh? Yes!" said Bunter, promptly. "I had one in my pocket—in fact, I heard it drop! Where is it, old chap? It's mine!"

Bunter bent down, blinking eagerly for the Egyptian pound on the deck. Hurree Jamset Ram Singh reached out and changed Bunter's coffee-cup for that belonging to Colonel Jacks.

Both the colonels had stood up to stare at the bank, and did not observe his action. But Wharton and Bob Cherry observed it.

"What the thump——" began Bob.

Hurree Jamset Ram Singh closed one eye, and Bob, puzzled, broke off. He realised that the nabob had had some reason for changing the coffee-cups, though he could not begin to guess what it was.

"I say, Inky, where's that quid?" exclaimed Bunter, still blinking anxiously at the deck. "I say, where did you see it?"

"The seefulness was not preposterous, my esteemed Bunter!"

"You silly ass!" roared Bunter. "Mean to say you were pulling my leg?"

"The pullfulness of your fat leg is terrific."

"Yah!"

Colonel Jacks sat down again, and lifted his coffee-cup. Billy Bunter watched him, with fascinated eyes, behind his big spectacles. The bony colonel gulped down the coffee, and Bunter watched for the explosion. But it did not come!

"I'll say that's pesky good coffee!" said G. W. Jacks.

"Oh crikey!" gasped Bunter.

Unless the bony colonel had an inside lined with zinc, Bunter simply could not understand it. He knew that he had dosed the colonel's coffee with hot red pepper, and he had expected something like an earthquake when G. W. Jacks swallowed it. Instead of which, the colonel smacked his lips over the coffee and pronounced that it was good!

Bunter was unaware, so far, that the peppered coffee-cup was now standing in the place of his own! That was a discovery he had yet to make!

"My absurd Bunter," murmured the nabob, "your excellent and idiotic coffee will be getting cold——"

Bunter snorted. His trick had failed—how, he could not imagine. Colonel Jacks evidently was none the worse for it. The fat Owl picked up his own cup, and gulped down the coffee.

The next moment there was a fearful roar.

"Yurrrrrrrgggh!"

"My esteemed Bunter——"

"Urrrrrrrggghh!"

Billy Bunter bounded to his feet. He spluttered and sputtered, gasped and gurgled, coughed and sneezed! Water streamed from his eyes, and he clasped both fat hands to his burning mouth. It was quite a large dose of pepper that Bunter had so slyly slipped into the coffee. It was hot pepper—frightfully hot pepper! He had meant it to give the coffee-drinker a shock—and it did!

"Yaroogh! I'm burned!" yelled Bunter. "Oh crikey! Ooooogh! Pip-pip-pip-pepper—— Yarooooooch!"

"Pepper in the coffee!" exclaimed Bob Cherry. Then he understood and roared: "Ha, ha, ha!"

"Say, bo', what's biting you?" exclaimed Colonel Jacks. "I'll say this is some rookus you're kicking up. Yep!"

"Sure!" said Colonel Skink.

"Ooooough! Wooough! Ooooch! Atchooh-shoo-oooh! Ow! Gug-gug-gig!" gurgled Bunter wildly.

"What the dickens——" exclaimed Nugent.

"Urrrrrrrrggggh!"

Billy Bunter staggered away, spluttering, gasping, coughing, sneezing, and clasping his scorching mouth. How he had come to swallow the peppered coffee himself, Bunter did not know. But he knew that he had! Only too well he knew that! He staggered away, emitting sounds of woe and anguish, leaving some of the tea-party staring, and some of them grinning. And he stayed away—and was not even missed!

THE END.

(The final story of this rollicking fine holiday series is entitled: "THE EYE OF OSIRIS!" You'll find it in next week's MAGNET. *Also, look out for full particulars of our AMAZING FREE GIFT SCHEME in this issue.)*

OUR THRILL-PACKED HIGHWAYMAN STORY.

THE RED FALCON!

By ARTHUR STEFFENS.

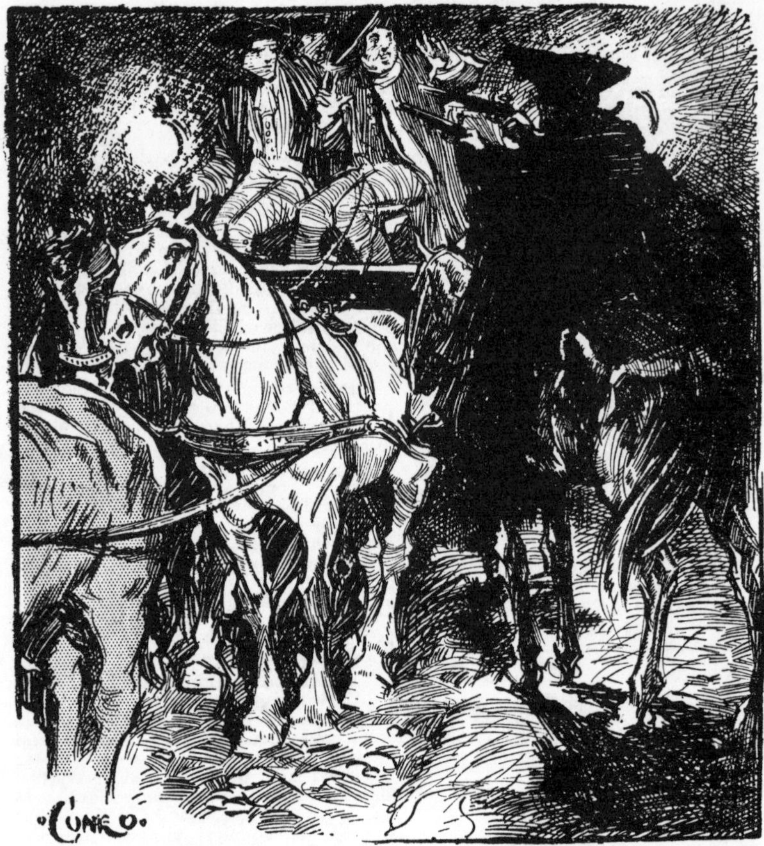

READ THIS FIRST.

Convicted of robbing the Earl of Huntford of a diamond star, Hal Lovett and Jerry McLean are conveyed to the convict hulk Ethalion, anchored at Woolwich—Hal to serve a sentence of seven years and McLean to await deportation. As the result of a prearranged plan, the convicts fire the ship, and Hal and Jerry escape in the blackness of the night, eventually reaching Blackheath, where they seek sanctuary in an inn named The Swan With Two Necks.

The Spy!

JERRY McLEAN leant back in his seat and sipped contentedly the hot grog which Peter Davey had prepared for him.

The change from Newgate Prison and the convict hulks at Woolwich to this cosy pew in the coffee-room of the Swan With Two Necks was unbelievable.

"So you are going to stand by my friend, eh, Peter?" he asked, as he drummed his fingers upon the tablecloth.

"Of course," answered Peter Davey, sipping at his steaming glass and smiling back at McLean. "I've never forgotten the day you first drove up to the inn, sir, with four of your friends in a barouche and ordered the best dinner I ever served. It marked the turn in my fortunes, sir. Nor am I likely to forget how often you come and spent money to help me along, and how you gave me five hundred guineas, refusing to take security, when I told you I had the bailiffs in the house. I always reckon you saved my life as well as my fortune, sir, and you can count me as your best friend."

"Even though I am an escaped convict, Peter? If they take me and my pal here now it may mean Tyburn Tree instead of transportation for me, and perhaps hanging for Hal. If in the event of our capture it were known that you tried to help us, why——"

"I'm going to help you," vowed Peter Davey, "and so——"

"Then don't 'sir' me; call me Jerry," said McLean, rising from his place and stretching his arms lazily. "And let's to bed. I'll be better able to tell you how you can help me and my pal when my brain has been cleared by a much needed sleep."

Jerry slipped past Hal Lovett on to the sawdust-covered floor of the coffee-room, and was about to speak again when a creaking on the stairs made him rush out into the hall. He was just in time to see a thick ankle, clad in grey hose and a heavy-soled shoe, turn the angle of the staircase leading to the bed-rooms of the inn. The ankle seemed familiar.

"Peter," said Jerry, when he returned, "are you sure you can trust your potman—Tom Kinch?"

"Ay!" replied Peter Davey. "Tom's been wi' me since a lad, and though he grumbles sometimes I put that down to the rheumatiz."

"Grumblers are people I don't trust," remarked Jerry McLean, with a frown, as he took his candle and lighted it.

He proceeded up the stairs, followed by Hal, who still kept the rug Jerry had stolen from the traveller on Blackheath wound tightly around him so as to conceal his convict's suit of rough brown cloth, the landlord bringing up the rear.

The passage on the first floor was empty. Peter himself showed Hal into a bed-room, the diamond-paned windows of which stood open on the latch, and then accompanied McLean to a room farther along the corridor.

After bidding the two "Good-night!" he pursued his way to his own bed-room.

McLean entered his room, turned the key in the lock, and shot the bolts home with much ado. Immediately afterwards he silently drew the bolts and slowly turned the key again. His sharp ears had caught stealthy footsteps in the passage. He heard a heavily built body go slowly by. Breathlessly he waited, listening, until, hearing no further sound, he whipped the door open and sprang out into the passage.

He sprang so quickly that Tom Kinch had no time to rise. Jerry caught him crouching with knees bent and eye set to the keyhole of Hal's bed-room door.

Hal, Jerry learned afterwards, had taken the key out of the lock before entering his room, had shot the bolts home, but had not placed the key back in the lock, so that Tom Kinch was able to command a full view of the room.

Tom Kinch had seen enough—a boy in the act of removing a water-soaked convict's suit of brown cloth.

Jerry took in the evil smile on the potman's face, and bridled as he saw him screwing his hands together in satisfaction as he watched.

Jerry McLean was so startled that for a moment he could not act. Then, as the full significance of the potman's treachery sank home, he ran two paces and drove his right boot with its heavy sole against the softest part of Tom Kinch's anatomy, hurling him from his crouching position flat on to his face on the floor.

Kinch bumped the door of Hal's room as he went down, and Hal, alarmed by the sound, unbolted the door and came out into the passage.

He was just in time to see Tom Kinch rise and hurl himself at Jerry.

Jerry was much the smaller man, but he was as hard as nails.

Turning the potman's futile blows aside without an effort, he hit him back with smashing blows to the head of the staircase, where Kinch for a moment rallied desperately.

Stooping, Kinch tore a heavy brass rod from the top step and drove it down at Jerry's bobbing head. But the rod clattered from his hand to the floor as Jerry again struck home with left and right, till at last Kinch toppled backwards, hitting almost every one of the stairs as he bumped and rolled to the bottom.

Printed and published every Saturday by the Proprietors, The Amalgamated Press, Ltd., The Fleetway House, Farringdon Street, London, E.C.4. Advertisement offices: The Fleetway House, Farringdon Street, London, E.C.4. Registered for transmission by Canadian Magazine Post. Subscription rates: Inland and Abroad, 11s. per annum; 5s. 6d. for six months. Sole Agents for Australia and New Zealand: Messrs. Gordon & Gotch, Ltd., and for South Africa: Central News Agency, Ltd.—Saturday, September 17th, 1932.

"You say one word to a living soul about what you've seen to-night," cried Jerry, as he leaned over the baluster rail, "and I'll carve every ounce of flesh from your bones with my sword, you sneaking hound!"

"What did he see, Jerry?" asked Hal Lovett wonderingly.

"You in your convict's brown, boy," answered Jerry grimly. "Why, lad, you've the trousers on now. But I've a notion he won't split, so go you to bed and get some sleep."

McLean Buys a Horse!

HAL LOVETT took the precaution to lock as well as bolt his bedroom door after the adventure with the potman, and no sooner had he set his head upon the soft pillow than he drifted off into a deep and health-restoring sleep.

In the morning Jerry McLean entered his room, after knocking, accompanied by the landlord of the Swan With Two Necks.

Peter Davey bore some clothes draped over his arm, which he tumbled on to the bed.

"I borrowed them from a young nevvy of mine who lives down in the village, laddie," he said, smiling a greeting. "You're about his height and size, and they should fit. Slip 'em on and come down to breakfast in the bar parlour along o' me and the missus."

Eagerly Hal donned the borrowed clothes, finding them only a trifle on the large size. It was the best suit he had ever worn, in spite of it's having been much used.

Rags and a convict's garb, saving only the cheap clothes Jerry McLean had procured for him whilst they were languishing in Newgate Gaol, were the things he had been accustomed to wearing. Hal Lovett eyed himself proudly in the glass before he went down to breakfast.

After a hearty meal Peter Davey led Hal and Jerry to the shade of a spreading walnut-tree at the end of a lovely garden.

"And now what's to do, Jerry McLean?" he asked. "There's a scare in Blackheath village over the robbery last night. A rider came in from Woolwich just after sunrise, and he said that the hulk Ethalion was burnt right down to the water's edge. They say four guards are missing, and more than twenty convicts either escaped or were drowned. Among the convicts reported missing are Jerry McLean and Hal Lovett."

Peter spoke in a low, tense whisper, his eyes roaming about the garden the while.

"It won't be safe for Hal and me to stay here in our present guise, Peter," answered Jerry, his face set hard. "But I want you to help me."

"I promised to help. Tell me what you have in mind?"

"I want a horse," answered McLean. "No ordinary hack, but a blood horse, all fire and speed and stamina. My life may depend upon the speed of my horse, Peter."

"Do you mean you'll turn highwayman?" Peter Davey's voice was still hushed.

"I have no choice," rejoined Jerry McLean. "If they take me now they'll hang me. If I tramp the country with Hal, we would both be taken in a few hours. And, don't forget, the boy and I were innocent, in spite of our conviction, Peter."

"You shall have a horse," the landlord promised.

"And I shall need some money. I require a complete new outfit, Peter, and some arms. So does the lad."

"I'll lend you a hundred golden guineas, Jerry."

McLean clasped the landlord's hand.

"Let me have the money, friend, and secure me the horse, and you'll not have to do more for me."

"I'll drive you along to Squire Chelvey's," said Peter Davey. "He bought a hunter in the spring, but the mettled beast proved too much for him, and he wants to sell. There, Jerry, you'll find as fine a horse as ever jumped a five-barred gate."

Peter Davey's words proved correct, for after he had had his cob harnessed up to a gig and driven them to Deep End Manor, Squire Chelvey's house, Jerry was shown the finest horse he had ever seen.

Peter had introduced Jerry to the squire as a prospective purchaser, and though Chelvey looked suspiciously at Jerry's rough clothes, he ordered a groom to lead Galloper out into the stable yard.

It proved to be a great, upstanding, deep-toned bay, with magnificent shoulders, and it pawed the stones impatiently, as if aching for a gallop.

POCKET WALLETS FOR BUDDING POETS!

Compile a Greyfriars limerick as good as the one here, chum, and win one of these handsome prizes!

When Wharton asked Bunter to tea,
Fat William was chuckling with glee.
He ne'er dreamt at all
They were tea-ing in Hall,
He thought they were out for a spree!

The above winning effort was sent in by Norman Smethurst, of 36, Ladysmith Street, Shaw Heath, Stockport.

As Squire Chelvey approached it, pointing out its outstanding qualities with his cane, the horse showed the whites of its eyes, and its ears flattened. The vicious snap it made at him caused the squire to leap out of distance hastily, and lowered the price of the hunter perhaps five-and-twenty guineas.

"If your friend has a mind to buy, Peter," said the squire, "I'll take five-and-thirty guineas for him. He cost me two hundred only a month or two ago."

The bay was saddled and harnessed. Borrowing a riding-whip from the groom, Jerry set his hands upon the horse's high shoulders, and leapt up into the saddle.

As the horse swerved and tried to unseat him, he steadied it and turned it towards the open gate. The next moment Jerry McLean was galloping away along the chestnut drive, with Squire Chelvey, the groom, and Peter and Hal staring after him in blank amazement.

Jerry returned about a quarter of an hour later, pulling up the steaming and foaming horse and slithering lightly to the ground.

"He's a grand horse," he said. "If Squire Chelvey still wants to sell, I'll have him, Peter."

During Jerry's absence, however, Squire Chelvey had changed his mind. Until he had seen McLean treat the horse as if it were an ordinary hired hackney he had doubted whether anybody could ride the brute. But since it had been proved otherwise, why should not he keep the horse himself? There was not another in the neighbourhood to equal it.

Squire Chelvey roared to his groom to hold the horse steady. Then, taking the whip, he hauled himself up into the saddle.

"Why, Peter," he shouted, "if your friend finds him so easy to ride, I'll not sell. I'll keep him for myself. I'll——"

He broke off suddenly, for at that moment the bay began to pace sideways along the cobbled yard. At the end, it turned and swung its heels up high, bringing them down again with a crash that struck sparks from steel shoes and stones. Then up on its hind legs it reared until the squire came near to sliding out of the saddle. The next moment the forelegs crashed to the stones, and off went the horse. Instead of making for the drive, however, it galloped through a narrow gate which opened on to a path that led in turn to a vegetable garden. There, without the slightest hesitation, Galloper deposited the squire bodily in the midst of a patch of cabbages, after which it came ambling back to allow the groom to take it and lead it to its box.

"Curse the cross-grained brute!" roared the squire as he came back, his face crimson with indignation. "Your friend can have him. And if he don't lead the beast away from my stables at once, by gad, I'll get my gun and shoot it!"

Jerry McLean paid over thirty-five golden guineas out of the hundred Peter Davey had lent him and returned to the Swan With Two Necks Inn on horseback, riding beside the gig.

When he dismounted in the stable yard of the inn, and a groom came to take the reins, Jerry saw Tom Kinch standing in the open doorway. Jerry had already told Peter Davey what had happened the previous night. As he eyed the evil-looking rascal, whose left eye was almost completely closed, he said to Peter once again:

"Peter, is it safe to trust that rascal Kinch?"

"You needn't go worrying yourself about him, Jerry," answered the landlord. "I've read Tom the Riot Act. He'll stay mum. And, what's more, I've told him that he's not to leave the inn. Tom Kinch is all right. I've had more than one highwayman sleep overnight at the Swan With Two Necks, and Tom's known of it, but he hasn't said a word. Tom knows which side his bread is buttered You can trust Tom."

Outfits for Two!

HAVING bought the horse he so badly needed, Jerry McLean set himself to his next task, which was to secure a complete change of clothes for himself and a fresh and more presentable rig-out for Hal Lovett. As these clothes could not be procured out of London Town, Jerry booked seats for himself and Hal on the London coach.

They drove away from the inn at half-past nine the following morning, and rattled their way through pretty villages and past turnpikes to the sound of the posthorn.

Jerry and Hal were just two ordinary passengers who attracted little notice as they sat on the front seats, with their hats drawn down over their faces and their arms folded, pretending to be half asleep.

With a rattle and a clatter the coach rolled over the stone-paved streets of the borough and on to Westminster, where it crossed the bridge without check at the toll-gates and drew up outside the Golden Cross at Charing, where Jerry and Hal climbed down.

"I'm taking you to Sloman's, Hal," said Jerry. "He's a good sort, though he did pay me the price of rags for the fine wardrobe I sold him. We'll buy all we need there, with the exception of the horse you want. And we'll go back by the coach which starts from the Cross at eight o'clock. It will be better for us to return to Peter Davey's inn under cover of darkness.

Hal had no option but to place himself in Jerry's hands. And, besides, he was conscious of an ever-growing affection for his dare-devil friend.

Together they shouldered their way amongst the crowd, without arousing the slightest suspicion, until they were in the neighbourhood of Seven Dials.

Here the flaring drinking-shops were full, and drunken men were quarrelling or fighting in the streets.

Jerry pushed open the door of an ill-lit shop, and drew Hal in, to the ring of a shrill-toned doorbell.

In the darkness a tall, bent figure rose to meet them. It was Sloman, who rubbed his hands together as he studied the two through piercing eyes.

Sloman seemed to recognise Jerry, for he let out a low chuckle, and then reached for a tinder-box.

Two flickering candles soon allowed him to see more clearly, and after a quick glance from Jerry to Hal he hastened to the street door, locking and bolting it.

"I read you were missing from the burnt-out hulk, Mr. McLean," croaked Sloman, "and I thought you might have been drowned. But I'm glad to see you're alive. What can I do for you and your friend?"

"This is Hal Lovett, Sloman," said Jerry, introducing the boy. "I want clothes for him and for me—second-hand, but good—riding kit down to boots and spurs, and some more ordinary garb. You can add two brace of pistols, with their cases, and powder and ball. Add some hats in the mode, and two well-balanced hangers. Then we shall need underclothing and cravats, and two wood chests to pack the things in."

"Quite a wholesale order!" said Isaac Sloman, showing his teeth in a spreading grin.

"And I pay cash, Isaac," said Jerry, as he banged a bag purse down on the counter, striking out of it a ring of gold. "Jerry McLean never let a friend down yet. Let's have the best you've got, and name your own price. I know I can trust you."

Sloman bowed low, then led the way, candle in hand, up a creaking, winding, darkened stairway to the floor above. Here Hal and Jerry found a good supply of second-hand clothes, and soon furnished themselves with all they needed.

Within a couple of hours the two sallied forth clad in semi-fashionable clothes of goodly cut. Each wore a new and modish three-cornered hat upon his head and carried gloves and a cane.

At their heels staggered two porters, each carrying a wooden chest to the doors of the Golden Cross Hotel. Tied to each chest was a formidable-looking hanger, or cutlass, in its scabbard.

Isaac Sloman had arranged to send down two second-hand saddles—with holsters complete, and furnished with horse-pistols—to the Swan With Two Necks by a later coach.

From the door of his shop he gave them his blessing as they parted.

"You always treated me like a gentleman, Mr. McLean," he said, "and if I have been able to help you in any way I am delighted. May good fortune continue to shine on you and your friend! And if ever you have need of me, I am yours to command."

"That's what I call a friend," said Jerry, as they paced along in front of the porters. "He has given us more than our money's worth, and, though I am nearly at the end of Peter Davey's hundred guineas, we are fully equipped for action—barring your horse, Hal."

Jerry and Hal were approaching the Golden Cross, when they espied a Bow Street Runner striding towards them, his hat on one side of his head, his red waistcoat showing a bright splash of colour.

Instinctively they hesitated, but in a moment moved on.

Hal felt his heart beating quickly; but there was no cause for alarm, for the Bow Street officer scarcely gave them a glance as he swaggered by.

At the Golden Cross, McLean gave the porters a handsome tip and directed them to take the chests to the yard to await the starting of the coach; then he led Hal away to a chophouse, where they ate in a quiet corner, drawing only an occasional stare from the aproned waiter.

The coach rolled up to the Golden Cross punctual to time, and, their boxes having been stowed away, Hal and Jerry clambered up beside the driver.

To the blare of the post horn and the clatter and clink of harness and the beat of thudding hoofs, the coach rattled off.

Onward they went through New Cross until they were out in the open country, where the night was scarcely pierced by the lights from the coach lamps.

Only when a tollhouse and its shut gate loomed up ahead, or if they passed a country house, did a glimmer of light shine anywhere, and the signposts loomed up like ghosts as they rattled on.

Even the villages were in darkness, and the only break was when they stopped to change their steaming team, and the passengers alighted for refreshments.

Jerry and Hal had maintained a silence which amounted almost to churlishness in the mind of their driver, who attempted to joke with them. But joking was dangerous for two escaped convicts who were being hunted high and low.

At a smashing pace the horses tore along through the leafy lanes. Soon they would be at the Swan With Two Necks—and home.

In a whisper Jerry told Hal that they must reach the heath soon. The driver was laughingly telling the passengers on his left about the farmer who, two nights ago, had been robbed of his clothes and his horse by one of the convicts who had escaped from the hulks, and how he had run six miles home to his wife in his shirt. They were laughing at the story, when all of a sudden a horseman rode out of the shadows into the road in front of them. A seam of fire seared the blackness of the night, and as a ball whistled close to the driver's ear a deep, stern voice called upon him to "Halt!"

(It looks as if Hal and Jerry have bumped up against another bit of bad luck, doesn't it? You'll be thrilled more than ever, chums when you read next week's gripping instalment.)

FREE—FIRST 6 SUPER PICTURE-STAMPS NEXT WEEK

The MAGNET 2d

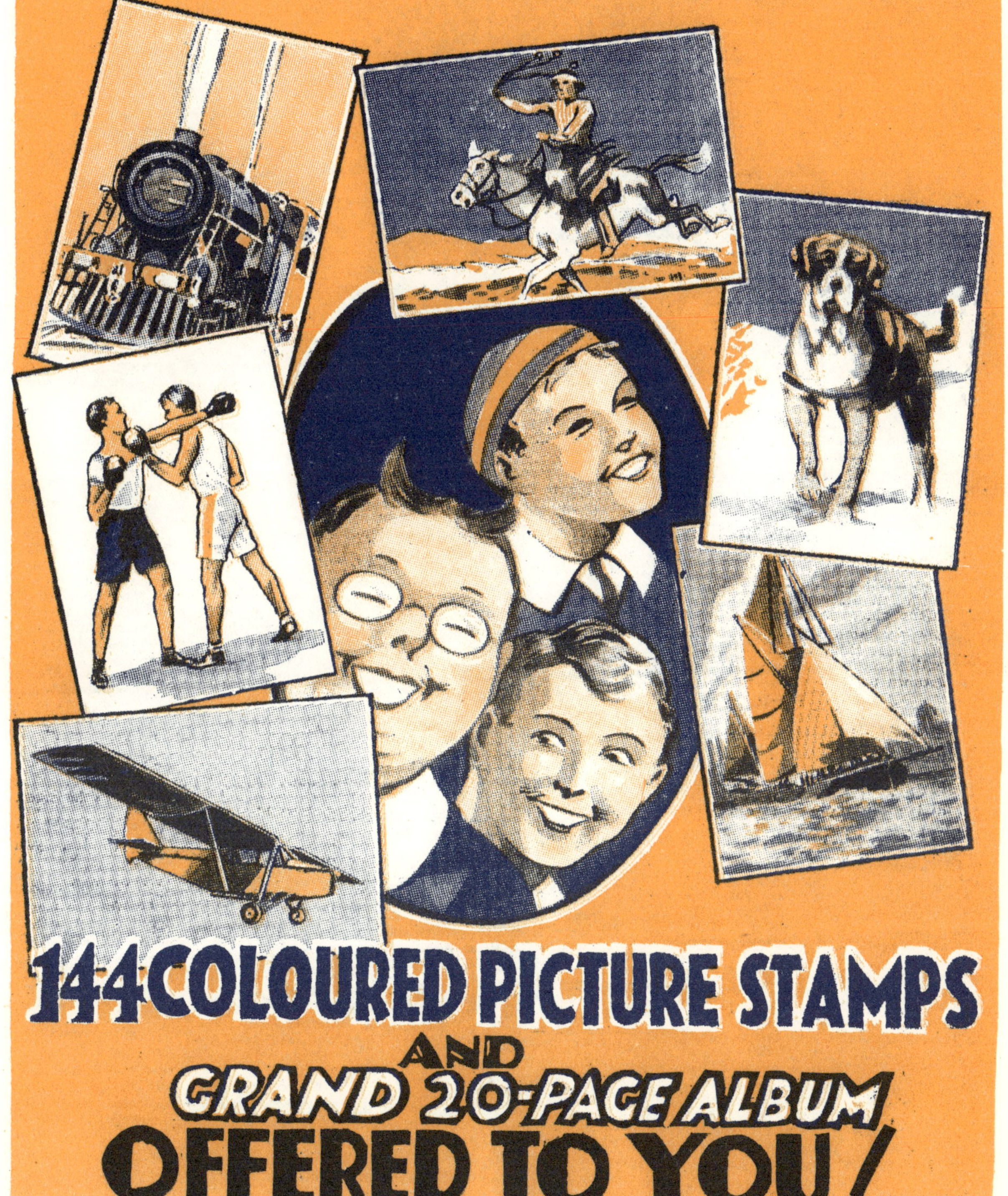

No. 1,284. Vol. XLII. EVERY SATURDAY. Week Ending September 24th, 1932

A MAGNIFICENT LONG COMPLETE TALE OF TREASURE-SEEKING IN EGYPT—

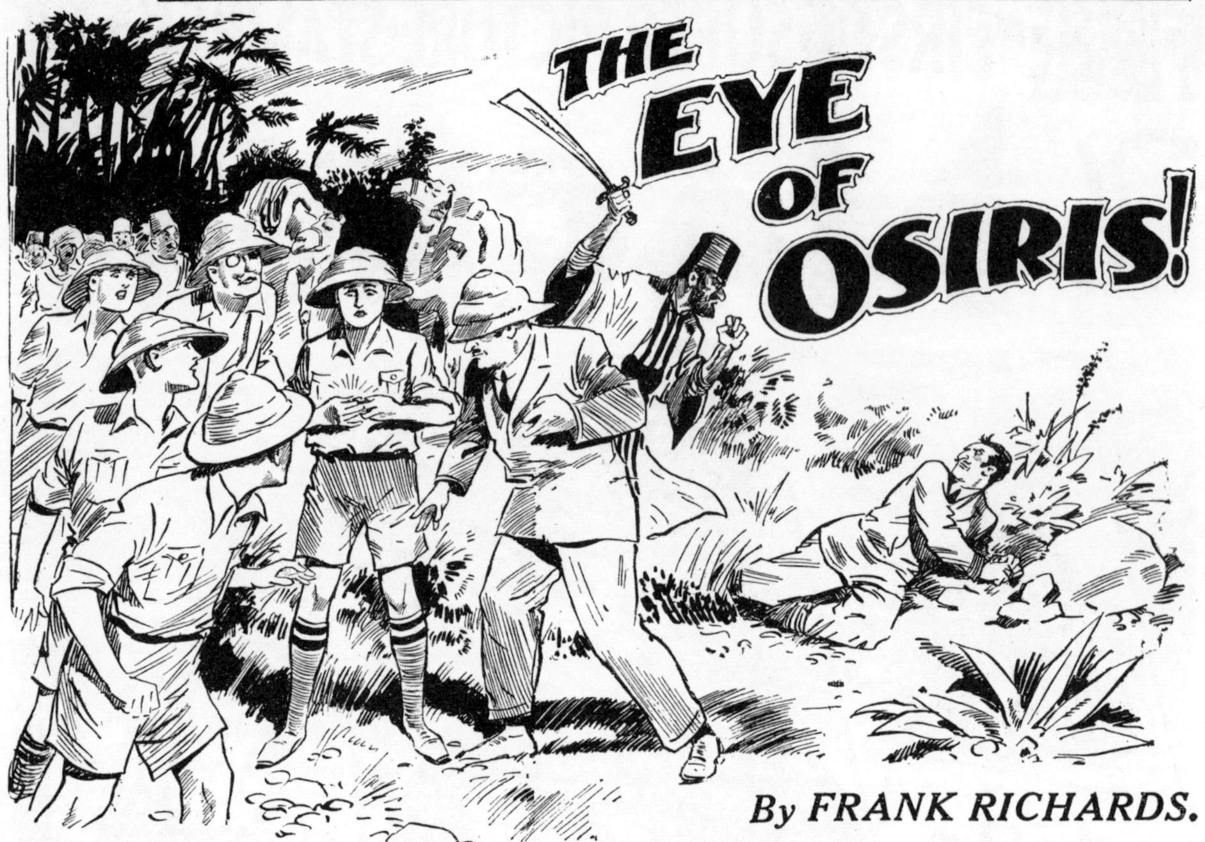

THE EYE OF OSIRIS!

By FRANK RICHARDS.

THE FIRST CHAPTER.
Halt!

BILLY BUNTER sat down.

It was hot in the land of Egypt.

Bunter was tired.

Having walked nearly half a mile, Billy Bunter felt that his fat little legs had done enough.

A shady sycamore grew beside the sandy track that led towards the Nile. Billy Bunter turned from the track, plumped down under the shade of the wide-spreading branches, and leaned back against the trunk. He took off Lord Mauleverer's best Panama hat and fanned his heated fat face.

Harry Wharton & Co. halted. They stared at Bunter. Only another half-mile ahead of the juniors the Nile rolled and gleamed in the sun, and they could see their dahabiyeh tied up to the bank and the figures of the Nubian sailors on deck.

The Greyfriars tourists, on their way up the Nile in the houseboat, had taken a walk ashore that morning. Under the guidance of Hassan, the dragoman, they had "done" some ancient rock tombs. Bunter hadn't "done" the tombs. Bunter had sat under a date-palm and disposed of a large bag of sticky Turkish sweetmeats he had thoughtfully brought with him. The Famous Five and Lord Mauleverer had walked miles. Bunter hadn't! So anyone who did not know Billy Bunter might have supposed that he was good for the walk back to the Nile. It was only a mile. But half a mile was enough for Bunter—in fact, too much.

So he sat down. Harry Wharton & Co. were rather anxious to get back to the dahabiyeh for lunch. Bunter, for once, wasn't! With several pounds of sticky sweets in his capacious inside, Bunter for once didn't mind being late for lunch—in fact, he wasn't ready for lunch. What he wanted was a rest. What the other fellows wanted was a trifling consideration to which Billy Bunter naturally gave no thought.

"Well," said Bob Cherry at last, "how long are you going to squat there, Bunter?"

"I'm tired!" said Bunter, with calm dignity.

"The tirefulness must be terrific after the walkfulness of an esteemed half-mile!" remarked Hurree Jamset Ram Singh.

"It's hot!" said Bunter.

"Hotter for you than for us?" asked Johnny Bull.

Snort from Bunter! He disdained to reply to that frivolous question.

"We've got to get on, fatty," said Frank Nugent—"we want our lunch, you know!"

Bunter's fat lip curled.

"I can't make out why some fellows are always thinking of grub," he said. "It's a bit sickening."

"Oh, my hat!"

"You fat cormorant!" roared Bob Cherry. "You've been guzzling all the morning and we've had nothing since brekker!"

"I may have had a snack," said Bunter. "It's not much I eat, as you know. You fellows seem to think of nothing else. For goodness' sake stop worrying about your blessed insides and sit down and rest for an hour or so."

Lord Mauleverer grinned. The Famous Five looked at William George Bunter as if they could have eaten him. They were not blessed with appetites like Bunter's, but they had healthy appetites of their own. They were already rather late for lunch on the dahabiyeh, which the Coptic cook was certain to have all ready for them. They had been thinking of putting on speed for the last half-mile. Bunter, evidently, was thinking otherwise.

The fat junior blinked at them severely through his big spectacles.

"I say, you fellows, don't be pigs!" he admonished. "For goodness' sake think of something else beside meals—think of me! I don't mind being late for lunch. And I'm tired. If one of you fellows would fan the flies off I could get a nap! Don't be so jolly selfish, you know. If there's one thing I never could stand it's selfishness."

"Oh, great pip!"

"You fat chump!" exclaimed Harry Wharton. "Get up and come on!"

"Shan't!"

"Oh, come on, you men!" grunted Johnny Bull. "I'm hungry! That fat ass can stay here as long as he likes, and be blowed to him!"

"We can't leave the howling idiot here," said Harry. "Bunter, you duffer——"

Snore!

Bunter's eyes closed behind his spectacles. No doubt the Owl of the Greyfriars Remove considered it best to put an end to the argument by going to sleep.

"Bunter!" roared Bob Cherry.

Snore!

"You fat piffler——" bawled Bob.

"Oh, really, Cherry! I wish you wouldn't roar like a mad bull when a fellow's fast asleep!" said Bunter peevishly.

"Lug him along by the ears!" said Bob. "We can't leave him here! Take hold of his ears—plenty of room for the lot of us!"

"You cheeky beast!" roared Bunter. "Look here, you fellows, I'll come if I don't have to walk! What about Hassan carrying me?"

"Oh, my lordly gentlemen!" exclaimed Hassan, in dismay at the idea. "Oh, sar, I am as strong as King Rameses, but not strong enough for that, sar."

"Don't you be cheeky," said Bunter. "I say, you fellows, Hassan can take me on his back—you fellows can help. After all, it's not far—the river's in sight. Don't be slackers!"

Hassan, the dragoman, looked quite uneasily at the juniors. He was eager to oblige his "lordly gentlemen"—unwilling to reply in the negative to any request. But the prospect of having Billy Bunter's avoirdupois landed on his back evidently dismayed him. Neither did the idea of rallying round Hassan and helping to support Billy Bunter's uncommon weight seem to appeal to the chums of the Greyfriars Remove.

"Perhaps I find a donkey, sars!" suggested Hassan. "I go and run with a prompt dispatch and find one donkey to carry noble fat lord, sars."

"Well, that's all right," said Bunter. "I'm considerate, I hope—I'll wait here till Hassan fetches a donkey from somewhere, you fellows. If it's a quiet donkey—not like those beasts at Luxor—I'll ride it! Mind there's a comfortable saddle, Hassan!"

"There's no donkeys near at hand, anyhow," said Harry. "For goodness' sake, Bunter, don't be such a fat slacker! Get up and get on!"

"Yah!"

"What about kickin' him?" asked Lord Mauleverer, as if struck by a sudden bright idea. "I can't very well kick Bunter, as he's my jolly old guest, but I'll walk on while you fellows kick him—what!"

"Ha, ha, ha!"

"Beast!" roared Bunter.

"Look here, Bunter——" said Nugent.

"I wish you'd stop talking when a fellow wants to go to sleep. If you're not going to fan the flies off I don't want you here! I'll wait till Hassan brings the donkey, and you fellows can get off to your guzzling!" added Bunter scornfully.

Lord Mauleverer made a sign to the dragoman, and Hassan departed in quest of a donkey. All along the Nile donkeys and donkey-boys were to be found in their myriads—the difficulty, as a rule, was not to hire a donkey if a fellow set foot on shore. But, as so often happens in this troublesome universe, a thing that could be had in abundance when it wasn't wanted was not to be found when it was wanted. No donkeys or donkey-boys were to be seen, and the dragoman had to walk back to the native village near the rock tombs to fetch one.

The Famous Five glared at Bunter. Bunter shut his eyes once more—he snored.

"I'm going!" growled Johnny Bull.

"Hold on!" said Harry. "We can't leave him here, old chap. That villain Kalizelos has been watching us ever since we left Luxor, and those two Arab rascals, Hamza and Yussef might be about. Mauly's uncle has told us that when we go ashore we've got to keep together. Look here, Bunter, if we leave you here something may happen to you!"

Snore!

"Suppose that Greek villain, Kalizelos, dropped on you?"

Snore!

"Suppose those Arabs got after you——"

Snore!

"Will you come on, you fat frump?" bawled Johnny Bull.

Billy Bunter's eyes opened with an exasperated blink.

"No, I won't!" he hooted. "There isn't any danger—besides, if there was I shouldn't be funky, like you fellows! Get out, and let a fellow sleep!"

"You fat idiot——"

Snore!

Harry Wharton & Co. exchanged a glance. Bunter could not be left on his own. He had to get a move on. Kicking him seemed the only resource, and the Famous Five were prepared to take that measure. But Lord Mauleverer interposed.

"Go easy, old beans!" murmured his lordship. "Kickin' Bunter as far as the Nile will take as long as waitin' for Hassan to come back with the donkey. And I've got rather a wheeze."

Stepping back out of hearing of the fat Owl, Lord Mauleverer whispered. There was a chuckle from the Famous Five. Mauly's wheeze, whatever it was, seemed to catch on, and to console the chums of the Remove for the postponement of their belated lunch.

"Good-bye, Bunter!" roared Bob Cherry.

The juniors tramped away. Bunter opened his eyes, and blinked after them, and saw the six fellows disappear beyond the tamarisk bushes along the sandy path. With a grunt of satisfaction he closed his eyes again, and sank into balmy slumber, and his deep snore echoed along the bank of the Nile.

———

THE SECOND CHAPTER.

The Kidnapping of Billy Bunter!

BILLY BUNTER woke suddenly. He woke with a startled gasp. He had been dreaming—a happy dream of a spread in a Remove study at Greyfriars.

Bunter, on the whole, had enjoyed his holiday in Egypt. The grub had been good. And if the grub was all right, everything was all right, from the point of view of William George Bunter. Still, he was not sorry at the prospect of returning to Greyfriars for the new term. He was not anxious to see the Head or his Form master, Mr. Quelch, or to grind at lessons in the Remove Form-room. But he looked forward to dropping into the school tuckshop.

He had not forgotten Mrs. Mimble's doughnuts. And whilst he admitted that the grub on the dahabiyeh was good—distinctly good—he pined for the jam tarts of his native land. And as he slept and snored under the shady sycamore, he was dreaming of a spread in Smithy's study in the Remove passage at Greyfriars, and of an unlimited supply of juicy, flaky jam tarts that went down like oysters. It was a happy dream, and he smiled in his sleep.

He ceased to smile and ceased to sleep as a dusty dhurra-sack was suddenly whipped over his head, and drawn down over his fat shoulders.

"Ooooooh!" gasped Bunter.

He blinked dizzily.

He could see nothing!

Hands were on him on all sides, and they drew the rough sack down round about him, and a rope was run round it and tied.

Then he was jerked to his feet.

He stood gasping, blindfolded by the sack, and sneezing as some of the dust got into his fat little nose. He could not possibly see his assailants, but he knew that there were at least four or five pairs of hands on him. He could hear the movements of a donkey close at hand.

"Ow! Help!" roared Bunter. "I say, leggo! Yooop!"

"Bismillah!" came a deep voice through the sack. "Mashallah! Woshy-bosh bash-bash wushy-tush!"

"Oh crikey! Those beastly Arabs have got me!" gasped Bunter. "I say, leggo! I'm not Mauleverer! Mauly's got that beastly scarab! He's on the dahabiyeh! I'll show you the way, if you like! Oh crikey!"

"Inshallah! Wooosh-kooosh!" said the deep voice. "Coshy-boshy-wosh-bump!"

Bunter did not know much Arabic. He had learned the word "backsheesh," like all travellers in the East, his first day there. Such ejaculations as "Bismillah," and "Inshallah" he had heard among the natives along the Nile. But the rest of the talk was unintelligible to him, though he had no doubt that it was Arabic. If it was, it was a kind of Arabic that would have puzzled and perplexed any Arab.

"Kooosh!" said another deep voice. "Wooosh! Hacky-cracky-backy-bang!"

"Bunky-bunky-bump!" said another voice.

Evidently there was a gang of them, all speaking in that strange tongue, which was Arabic to Bunter's terrified ears.

He felt himself lifted from the ground. From the panting among the unseen gang, it was clear that the kidnappers had to exert themselves to get him up. But they got him up, and he was planted in the saddle of a donkey.

"Yoo-hoooh—woosh!" said a savage voice. "Kosh! Bosh! Pong!"

The donkey started.

Bunter heard the tramping feet of the kidnappers round him. He swayed and lurched in the saddle, spluttering with terror.

He had no doubt in whose hands he was.

Kalizelos, the Greek, had tracked the Greyfriars party up the Nile, and they had had more than one narrow escape from him and from Yussef and Hamza, his Arab confederates. Kalizelos was in quest of the Golden Scarab, which he believed to hold the secret of the lost treasure of the reign of Rameses the Second. Why the ruffians should have seized Bunter was not clear, for the scarab belonged to Lord Mauleverer, and they could not suppose that he had entrusted it into Billy Bunter's keeping. But they had seized him—for here he was, blindfolded in a dusty sack, stuck on a donkey, riding away in the midst of the ruffians to parts unknown.

At Luxor the juniors had had a narrow escape of being taken away into the desert by the Greek. Now Bunter realised that he was for it. He could not see in what direction he was being taken, but he had no doubt that the villains were heading for the sandy wastes of the Libyan desert.

"Help!" yelled Bunter suddenly.

A hand jabbed at the sack that enveloped him, and a deep voice growled in threatening accents:

"Boosh! Whup-whup-kooosh! Bashy-pashy-wang-bang—skooop!"

Bunter shuddered.

He did not, of course, understand the words; but the tone in which they were uttered was blood-curdling!

He did not yell again.

The donkey tramped on. On and on and on, till suddenly there was a halt. Muttering voices came through the sack.

"Booosh! Wishy-washy-whoop!"

"Cous-cous mashallah pong!"

"Hicky-chicky-wicky-wumps!"

"Osh-kosh! Yo-ho ping-pong pump!"

Bunter was lifted from the donkey after that muttered consultation. His feet landed on the earth, with strong hands grasping him on both sides. He shuddered at the touch, in his mind's eye picturing the fierce, dark faces of the savage desert Arabs by whom he was surrounded. Kalizelos could not have been among them. The Greek would have spoken to him in English. Some fierce gang of bedouins, most likely.

Forced forward by the grasp on his fat arms through the sack, Bunter tottered on his way. To his astonishment his feet no longer trod sandy earth, but hard wood. He might have fancied that he was crossing the gang-plank from the bank of the Nile to the deck of the dahabiyeh. But that, of course, was impossible if he had been taken away into the heart of the desert by a gang of kidnapping Arabs.

"Oooshywoooshy-wops!" said a deep, growling voice.

Bunter was still walking on wood, which felt exactly the same as the deck of the dahabiyeh under his feet. He was taken down three shallow steps. A door opened.

"Kooosh!" came the savage growl.

He was led into a room.

Bump!

He roared as he landed on the floor in a sitting position.

Slam! A door closed!

Billy Bunter was left alone.

He sat in the sack, gasping. Evidently this unseen room was to be his prison, and the beasts had left him tied in the sack. For several minutes he dared not move, lest the villains should return.

But there was no sound of returning footsteps. The silence reassured him at last. He began to struggle with the sack.

To his intense relief he found that the rope tied round him was very loosely tied. The kidnappers seemed to have been careless with their prisoner. The rope fell away as Bunter struggled. He worked the sack upward, and got it clear of his fat shoulders, his fat face, and his head. He gasped with relief when it was off at last.

"Oh lor'!" gurgled Bunter.

He picked himself up, set his spectacles straight on his fat little nose, and blinked round him.

He was in a room with a latticed window, and through the lattice he could see the glimmer of sunshine on water. Apparently his prison was near the Nile. There was one door, and Bunter rolled to it, and stood listening with a palpitating heart. From a little distance a sound came to his ears. It was a sound of laughter. Apparently the kidnappers were laughing over their success in seizing the most important member of the Greyfriars party.

"Beasts!" groaned Bunter.

Within sound of the villains Bunter dared not open the door. He perceived, with an astonished blink, that it was fastened only by the latch, and it would have opened to his fat hand. Undoubtedly those kidnappers were very careless with their valuable prisoner. But the fat Owl dared not venture out in sight of the desperate villains. He rolled across the room and blinked through the slats of the latticed window.

It was the Nile that rolled before him. He could see across the wide river the roofs of Assuan glistening among date-palms, and two or three dahabiyehs were in sight, as well as a dozen or more native feluccas. And now it dawned on Bunter, to his further astonishment, that the room in which he was imprisoned was a cabin on some vessel on the Nile. He could hear the wash of the water past the hull below.

The kidnappers had not, after all, taken him away into the desert on donkey-back—they had brought him to the river, and on board some vessel—perhaps a houseboat belonging to Kalizelos! That seemed probable to Bunter.

With a trembling fat hand he felt over the slatted shutter at the window. It opened to his touch. Even the window was not fastened by those careless kidnappers. Bunter blinked down at the rolling Nile, and shook his head. Swimming did not appeal to him—he did not like the idea of crocodiles.

A native felucca, gliding by at a little distance, slowed down, two brown faces turning towards the fat face that blinked out of the cabin window. One of the boatmen held up bunches of dates, evidently having those succulent articles for sale. Bunter's eyes gleamed behind his spectacles. He signed to the natives to approach with the boat.

They pulled in.

Billy Bunter put his head out of the cabin window, and blinked to and fro, and up and down. From the deck above he could hear a sound of moving feet and of native voices, but no one was looking over the side. The felucca's mast was down, fortunately; the boatmen were rowing, not sailing. Bunter hoped that the boat might approach without being observed by the men on the upper deck.

The felucca glided under Bunter's window. One man held on, the other held the bunches of dates, in the belief that that was what the foreign tourist wanted. But Bunter, for once, did not want something to eat. To the utter amazement of the boatmen, he clambered through the window, hung on by his fat hands, and dropped into the felucca.

They fairly goggled at him. Why a white man should leave a dahabiyeh in this extraordinary way was a mystery to the Nile boatmen.

Bunter bumped.

"Oooooh!" he gasped.

But there was not a second to lose! Any instant, eyes might stare down from the deck and his escape be cut off! Bunter gasped, gurgled, and pointed to the eastern shore, where the roofs of Assuan glistened in the sun. With the other hand he showed a handful of piastres, which he had fortunately borrowed from Lord Mauleverer that morning.

"Assuan—quick!" he breathed.

"Yes, sar!" stuttered one of the astounded boatmen.

And they shoved off, and pulled for the shore.

THE THIRD CHAPTER.

The Flight and the Pursuit!

"HA, ha, ha!"

That merry sound of laughter was ringing in the dining-saloon of the Cleopatra, the magnificent dahabiyeh which Mr. Maroudi, of Cairo, had lent to the Greyfriars party, and in which Harry Wharton & Co. were "doing" the Nile up to the First Cataract.

The chums of the Remove had arrived late for lunch. They were enjoying it all the more for that reason. Still more were they enjoying their little jest on the fat and fatuous Owl of the Remove.

Billy Bunter had discovered that he was a prisoner on board a dahabiyeh. But he had not discovered that the dahabiyeh was the Cleopatra. He had heard the sound of laughter—but he had not realised that it proceeded, not from a gang of Arab kidnappers, but from the chums of Greyfriars. Not for a moment had it dawned on Bunter's fat brain that his kidnappers were the Famous Five of Greyfriars, and that he was a "prisoner" in a cabin only a few yards from the saloon where they sat at lunch.

The juniors were wondering how long it would be before those interesting facts dawned on William George Bunter.

They really expected that Bunter would discover how matters stood as soon as he got the sack off his head.

But lunch was nearly over now, and the fat Owl had not emerged from the cabin where he had been placed.

From the dining-saloon the juniors could see along the passage that divided the cabins, and Bunter would have been in view had he emerged.

But he did not emerge.

Apparently he was still under the impression that he was a kidnapped prisoner in lawless hands, and that state of affairs made the juniors yell.

"Is that silly ass still sitting there with the sack on his silly head, I wonder?" remarked Bob Cherry.

"Ha, ha, ha!"

"He needed a lesson," said Harry Wharton, laughing. "Well, he's getting it! I dare say he will sit there, too funky to move, till we go and root him out."

"Ha, ha, ha!"

"We will give him a look in after lunch," chuckled Frank Nugent. "Or shall we leave him there till we get to Assuan?"

"Ha, ha, ha!"

Nubian servants glided to and fro, waiting on the juniors. Their black faces wore cheery grins. Everybody on board the dahabiyeh had seen Billy Bunter brought on board, enveloped in a sack, and taken to an unoccupied cabin. What such an extraordinary proceeding meant the natives did not know; but no doubt they realised that it was a jest at the expense of the fat Owl. Even Moussa, the grave reis, had grinned at the sight of him in the sack. How long he was going to stay in that cabin, under the impression that he was a kidnapped prisoner, was quite an interesting question.

The juniors intended to leave him till after lunch, anyhow, if he did not come out of his own accord before. That afternoon the dahabiyeh was going on to Assuan, which was in sight, where the party were to meet Mauly's uncle, Sir Reginald Brooke, and his friend, Mr. Maroudi, the Egyptian millionaire, who had lent them the dahabiyeh. The holiday was drawing to a close, and only a few more days remained on the Nile, which were to be spent on a trip above the cataract, to see the great Assuan Dam, and the Nubian Nile above.

Harry Wharton & Co. would have been quite pleased to follow the great river up to Khartoum and the Sudan, and even to the Great Lakes where it had its source; but Greyfriars and the new term claimed them. Also, Sir Reginald Brooke had completed the business in the Fayyum which had brought him out to Egypt.

There was a hurried footstep in the cabin passage, and Hassan, the dragoman, came into the dining-saloon.

The dragoman was grinning.

"Lordly gentlemen!" he exclaimed.

"Hallo, hallo, hallo!"

"Oh, sars!" exclaimed Hassan. "The little fat lord——"

"Bunter?" exclaimed Harry Wharton. "What about Bunter?"

"Magnificent, sar, he has escaped!" gasped Hassan.

"What?" roared the juniors.

"Good gad!" ejaculated Lord Mauleverer, in amazement. "What the dooce——"

"He call a boat from a window of a cabin, sars!" gasped Hassan. He make boat peoples in a boat row him away, sars!"

"Great pip!"

"Oh, my hat!"

The juniors jumped to their feet. They stared at Hassan, and at one another, and then burst into a roar of laughter.

"Ha, ha, ha!"

"Escaped!" yelled Bob Cherry. "Oh, my only summer hat! Bunter escaped from the jolly old kidnappers——"

"Ha, ha, ha!"

"He go very fast, sars!" said Hassan, his brown face wreathed in grins. "He hold up handful of piastres to boatmen—he point to eastern bank—he say 'Quick, quick, quick!'"

"Ha, ha, ha!" shrieked the juniors.

They had wondered how long Bunter would remain a prisoner in a cabin a few yards away. But they had never dreamed that he would escape by the window, in a boat on the Nile. They had not suspected the fat Owl of such resource. Evidently Bunter was desperate!

"Oh crikey!" gasped Bob, wiping away his tears. "This is too jolly rich!"

"The richfulness is truly terrific!" chortled Hurree Jamset Ram Singh.

"We'd better get after him!" gurgled Nugent. "Goodness knows where he will get to!"

"Ha, ha, ha!"

Forgetful of their unfinished lunch, the Greyfriars fellows rushed on deck. Moussa, the reis, and the Nubian sailors, were staring after a felucca that was pulling hard up to Assuan, on the other bank. Two brown men were pulling for all they were worth. In the stern sat a well-known fat figure. A fat face was turned, to stare back at the dahabiyeh, and the sunshine flashed on a pair of large spectacles.

Billy Bunter was blinking back with terrified eyes behind his spectacles. Partly owing to his short sight, and partly to his state of palpitating funk, he did not recognise the dahabiyeh, or the black sailors who stared at him from the deck.

But he knew that his escape had been seen, for he could see that the sailors were staring after him, and he was in momentary fear of pursuit. He blinked back from moment to moment in dire terror, and from moment to moment urged his rowers to greater efforts. The two Nile boatmen were doing their best, but the felucca was slow and heavy, and progress was not swift.

Harry Wharton & Co. stared after the fugitive, hardly believing their eyes. Bunter was in desperate flight. Evidently he had not the faintest suspicion that it was the Cleopatra and the Greyfriars party from which he had escaped.

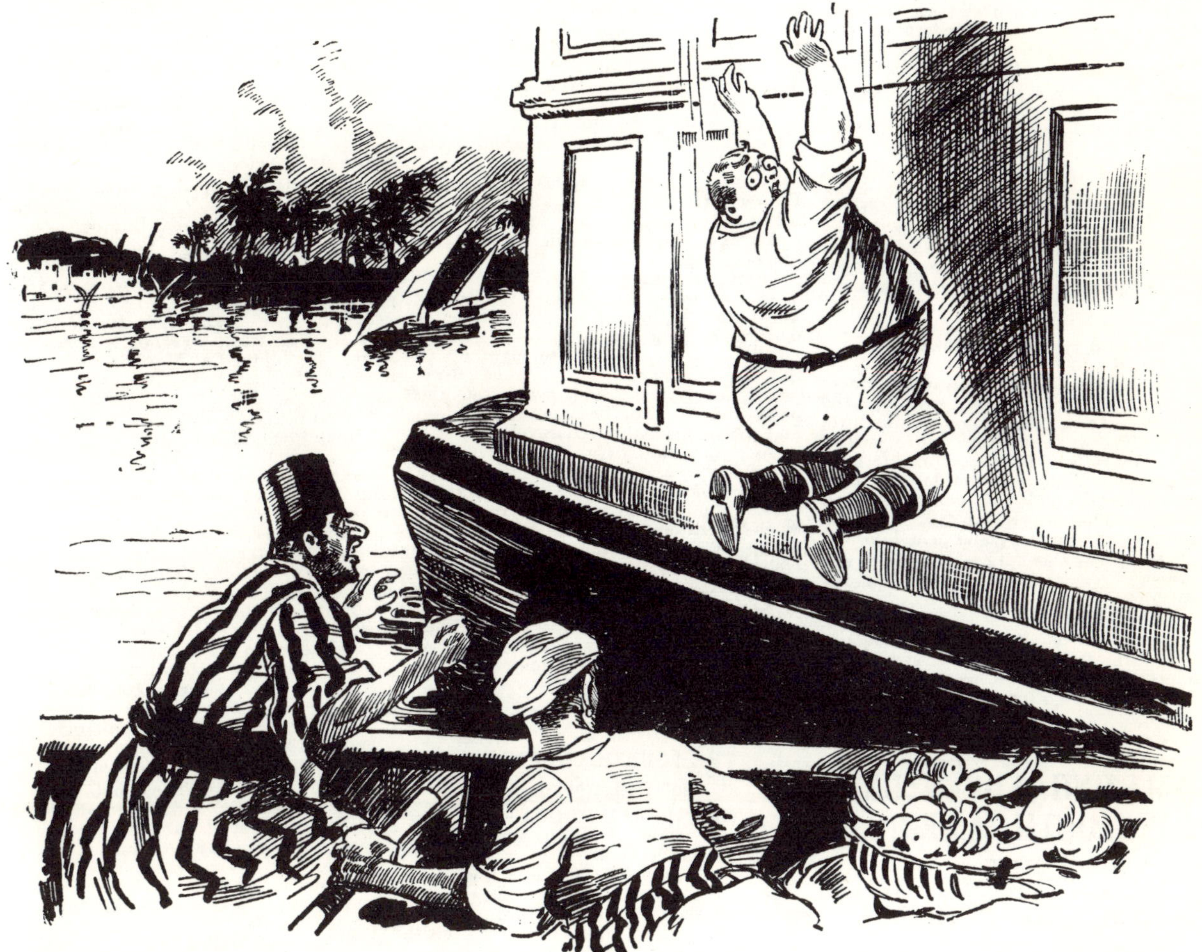

Bunter signed to the natives to approach, and the felucca glided up to the side of the dahabiyeh. Then, to the utter amazement of the boatmen, the fat junior clambered through the window, hung on by his fat hands, and dropped into the felucca!

"Ain't he the jolly old limit!" gasped Bob.

"Ha, ha, ha!"

"Small fat lord enormously frightened, sars," grinned Hassan. "He has the cold foot, as you say in English."

"Get after him," said Harry Wharton. "We're going on to Assuan, anyhow, so we may as well get under way. Tell the reis to get going for Assuan, Hassan."

"Yes, sar!"

Moussa called orders to the Nubian sailors. The gangway was taken in, and the dahabiyeh poled off from the bank. The current was against the houseboat; but the wind, as usual, blew from the north, and the lateen sail was hoisted. The huge boat rolled into motion and glided on the track of the felucca.

The juniors saw Bunter turn his head again and give a jump at the sight of the dahabiyeh under sail.

The fat owl knew that he was pursued now.

At the distance, no doubt, he did not make out the white faces on the dahabiyeh, or perhaps his terrors transformed them into fierce Arab faces. The juniors saw that he was waving and shouting to his boatmen, though he was too far away for his voice to be heard.

"They're hoisting the sail!" yelled Bob.

"It's going to be a jolly old race!"

"Ha, ha, ha!"

The Nile boatmen pulled in their oars and hoisted the lateen sail of the felucca. As the wind caught it the little craft danced away much more swiftly on the Nile. Bunter blinked back anxiously. Time had been lost in hoisting the sail and the dahabiyeh had gained. Bunter yelled to the boatmen, and now the juniors could hear him.

"Buck up, you beasts! Row, you rotters! Oh crikey! Quick—quick—quick!"

"Ha, ha, ha!"

The boatmen put out the oars again, and, with sail and oars going strong, the felucca gained on the heavy dahabiyeh. Bunter increased his distance again, and he gasped with relief as he blinked back once more.

"Bunter will beat us to Assuan at this rate!" chuckled Bob Cherry.

"Ha, ha, ha!"

"Row, brothers, row!" chortled Nugent.

"Ha, ha, ha!"

In the felucca Billy Bunter mopped his streaming brow and gasped. He was gaining ground slowly but surely. Barring accidents the felucca would beat the dahabiyeh in the race to the landing-place at Assuan. Little dreaming that it was the Greyfriars party in pursuit, Bunter urged on his rowers to greater efforts. Even Bunter realised that it was rather extraordinary for a gang of kidnappers to venture to pursue him on the Nile in this way, in full sight of the city of Assuan and of a hundred pleasure-boats and trading feluccas. Still, they were doing it; there was no doubt that they were doing it, for there was the dahabiyeh from which he had escaped rolling on his track, its huge lateen sail bellying in the wind from the north.

"Quick, quick, quick!" gasped Bunter. He held up a large handful of Lord Mauleverer's piastres to encourage his boatmen. "Quicker, quicker, quicker!"

The felucca surged on.

At Assuan—if he reached it—Bunter knew that he would be safe. Even a desperate gang of kidnappers would hardly dare to pursue him right up to the landing-place. Yet, as he drew nearer to Assuan, and people on the bank and in other boats stared at him and his felucca, the dahabiyeh was still rolling on behind. Close to the landing-place the boatmen took in the big sail and tooled the felucca in with their oars. Bunter had won the race; the enemy were beaten. Yet, as he blinked back, he saw the big dahabiyeh still rolling on, coming right into Assuan after him!

"Quick!" he gasped.

And the felucca shot on to the landing-place; the Greyfriars fellows, in the dahabiyeh behind, shrieking with laughter as they watched.

THE FOURTH CHAPTER.

Not Dangerous!

SIR REGINALD BROOKE removed his eyeglass from his eye, rubbed it, and jammed it back into his eye again and stared. The old baronet could hardly believe his eye or his eyeglass. Mr. Hilmi Maroudi, the Egyptian, who was walking with Mauly's uncle down the Shari-el-Manshiya at Assuan, stared also, almost startled for once out of his impassive, Oriental calm. The lean, tall English baronet, and the plump Egyptian gentleman were equally astonished at what they saw on the Nile.

"Good gad!" said Sir Reginald blankly. "What does this mean, I wonder?"

"It is perhaps some schoolboy jest," suggested Mr. Maroudi.

Walking down the Shari-el-Manshiya towards the river, the two gentlemen had sighted the Cleopatra in the distance on the Nile. They came down to the landing-place to meet the Greyfriars fellows when they arrived. Then they spotted the fleeing felucca.

Plenty of other people had spotted it and were staring at it. Billy Bunter's frantic gesticulations to his boatmen were rather calculated to draw attention. With his terrified eyes almost popping through his spectacles, his fat hands waving, Bunter was urging on his boatmen to unheard-of efforts. Why he was in such a fearful hurry, the Nile boatmen did not know, but they were doing their best at the urgent behests of the fat Faringhee.

"It is the boy Bunter!" said Sir Reginald. "A foolish boy—— But what——"

"He appears to be frightened!" remarked Mr. Maroudi.

"But why?"

Mr. Maroudi shook his head.

Why Bunter should be fleeing in terror on the sunlit Nile, with the houseboat following him, the other fellows laughing on deck, was a mystery which the Egyptian gentleman could not solve.

They walked down to the landing-place to meet the felucca as it came in. It was well ahead of the slower dahabiyeh.

The boat bumped, and Bunter made a jump ashore. He slipped and stumbled and sprawled fairly at the feet of Mauly's uncle.

Sir Reginald stooped, grasped him by a fat shoulder, and lifted him. There was a howl of terror from Bunter.

"Ow! Leggo! Help! Police! Fire!"

"You absurd boy, cease these antics!" thundered Sir Reginald. "What do you mean by this, Bunter?"

"Oh!" gasped Bunter. He realised that this, at least, was not a ferocious Arab. He blinked at Mauly's uncle and recognised him. "Oh, it's you! Save me!"

"What?"

"Keep them off!" panted Bunter.

"Keep who and what off?" almost shrieked Sir Reginald. He was beginning to wonder whether this was sunstroke.

"Those beasts—those Arab villains!" gurgled Bunter, blinking round in terror at the Nile. "They're after me! That dahabiyeh——"

"That dahabiyeh!" articulated Sir Reginald.

"Yes; they're the kidnappers——"

"The—the—the kidnappers?"

"Ow! Yes! They got me! I escaped——"

"You escaped from that dahabiyeh!" exclaimed Mr. Maroudi, quite forgetting his Oriental calm in his amazement.

"Oh dear! Yes! They put a sack over my head and kidnapped me, and took me on that dahabiyeh!" groaned Bunter. "I got out of a window into that felucca and—and escaped——"

"Goodness gracious me!" ejaculated Sir Reginald, staring blankly at the fatuous Owl.

Mr. Maroudi smiled.

"It is a schoolboy jest," he remarked. "The high spirits of exuberant youth, my good friend."

"'Tain't!" roared Bunter indignantly. "I tell you I was kidnapped, and they're still after me! They're coming here! Let's get out of this!"

Another moment and Billy Bunter would have been tearing up the Shari-el-Manshiya at top speed. Fortunately Sir Reginald grasped him again in time.

"Stop!" gasped the old baronet.

"Leggo! I'm not going to be kidnapped again!" shrieked Bunter. "Leggo, you old donkey——"

"What? What?"

"Beast! Leggo! They're after me!" roared Bunter. "Help!"

"My dear boy, you are in no danger," said Mr. Maroudi gently.

"Beast! They're after me! Leggo!"

Sir Reginald compressed his grip on the scared Owl's collar. Billy Bunter had drawn enough public attention

(*Continued on page 8.*)

OUR GREAT PICTURE STAMP COLLECTING SCHEME

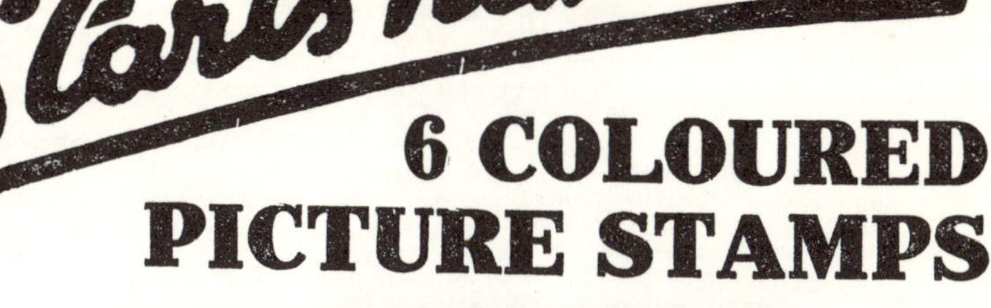

6 COLOURED PICTURE STAMPS

FREE

each week in The MAGNET

The most fascinating collecting scheme ever devised is about to commence. You will get your first six picture stamps in the MAGNET next Saturday. In the complete collection there will be 144 DIFFERENT PICTURE STAMPS, each measuring $2\frac{1}{4}$ x $1\frac{1}{2}$ inches, showing EVERY BOY'S WORLD IN PICTURES. They are divided into six sets illustrating such thrilling subjects as ROUGH RIDERS, AEROPLANES, SHIPS, RAILWAY ENGINES, DOGS, and the art of SELF-DEFENCE. Think of the fun you'll get swapping with your pals—two boys working together will each be able to get a complete collection. More details will be given next week when you get your first six stamps.

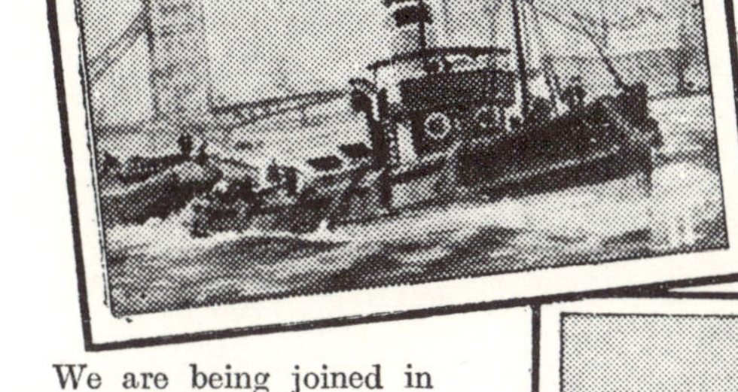

We are being joined in this great scheme by our two companion papers—

MODERN BOY

and

The RANGER

Both these papers will give picture stamps every week, and by taking them as well as The MAGNET you will make sure of the complete collection, and have some extra stamps for swapping.

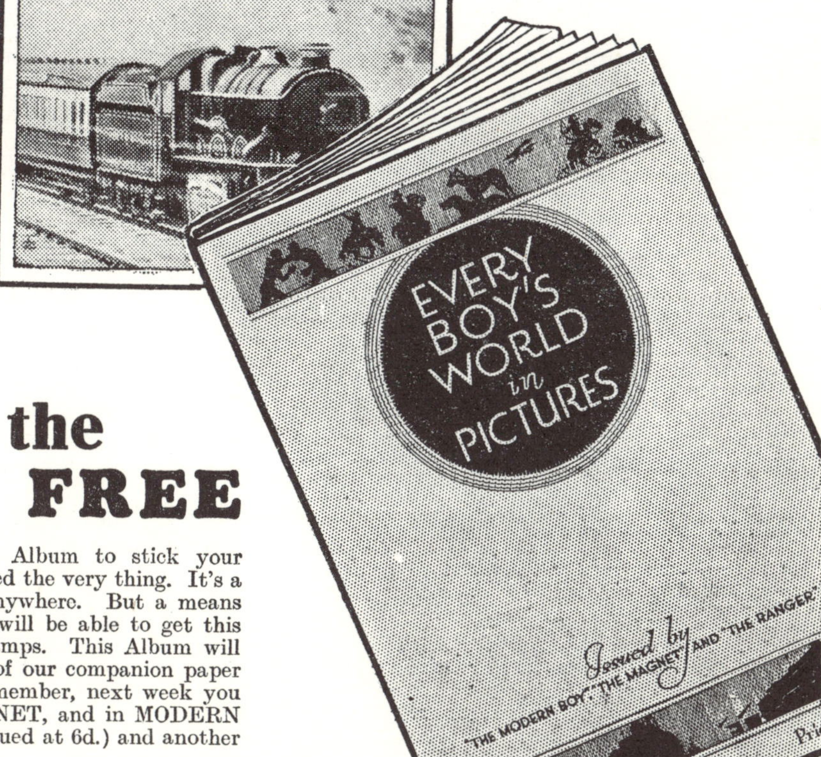

How to Get the ALBUM FREE

Of course you will want an Album to stick your stamps in, and so we have designed the very thing. It's a real topping album worth 6d. anywhere. But a means has been devised by which you will be able to get this Album FREE as well as the stamps. This Album will be given away with every copy of our companion paper MODERN BOY next week. Remember, next week you will get six stamps in The MAGNET, and in MODERN BOY you will get the Album (valued at 6d.) and another six stamps.

THE EYE OF OSIRIS!

(*Continued from page 6.*)

already. Sir Reginald did not intend to let him go charging up the Shari-el-Manshiya to the astonishment of all Assuan.

"You utterly absurd boy!" snorted the old baronet. "Calm yourself——"

"Leggo!"

"You are in no danger——"

"Help!"

"That dahabiyeh is the Cleopatra."

"Police!"

"It is Mr. Maroudi's dahabiyeh——"

"Eh?"

"My nephew and his friends are on board——"

"Wha-a-at?"

"It is some absurd practical joke!" snorted Sir Reginald. "Have you not sense enough to see that you are in no danger, you stupid boy?"

Billy Bunter blinked round at the dahabiyeh. The Nubian sailors had lowered the sail, and were poling in to the landing-place. The Cleopatra was so near now that even the short-sighted Owl of the Remove could make out the grinning faces of the Greyfriars juniors on the deck.

His eyes bulged through his spectacles.

"Hallo, hallo, hallo!" roared Bob Cherry. "You've beaten us, Bunter! Some race, old fat bean!"

"Ha, ha, ha!"

"The racefulness was terrific!" chortled Hurree Jamset Ram Singh.

"I—I—I say, it—it's those beasts!" gurgled Bunter. "I—I—I thought it was a gang of Arabs. Oh lor'! B-b-but I was—was kidnapped. I—I was shoved in a sack. Oh, the rotters!" gasped the fat Owl as he realised, at last, how his podgy leg had been pulled.

"Absurd!" snapped Sir Reginald. Mauly's uncle had reached a sedate and serious age, and had no use for practical jokes.

"A little jest!" smiled Mr. Maroudi. "Boys will be boys, my dear friend."

The dahabiyeh ranged up to the landing-place, and the gangway was run out. Lord Mauleverer and his friends came ashore, and greeted the baronet and the Egyptian gentleman.

Billy Bunter looked on, his fat face crimson with wrath.

He had been made a fool of. There was no doubt about that. Those rascally, desperate kidnappers who had shoved the sack over him and talked such extraordinary Arabic, were the Greyfriars juniors; and it was from a cabin on board the Cleopatra that he had made his desperate escape. Even William George Bunter's self-satisfaction and conceit failed him now, and he looked, and felt, a complete ass—as indeed he was!

"Oh, the beasts!" he mumbled.

"Herbert, this is really—really——" rumbled Sir Reginald.

"Only a joke on the jolly old Owl, nunky," said Lord Mauleverer. "My idea entirely. Bunter bein' my guest, I couldn't very well kick him. I'm sure you would not approve of my kickin' a guest, uncle——"

"Upon my word!" gasped Sir Reginald.

"So we pulled his jolly old leg instead," said Mauleverer. "But we never guessed he would escape from the dahabiyeh. Ha, ha, ha!"

"Ha, ha, ha!"

The juniors roared. They could not help it. Bunter's dramatic escape from the dahabiyeh and his wild race for freedom were really too rich. Mr. Hilmi Maroudi was grinning, and even Sir Reginald's severe old face broke into a smile.

"Well, well, it was only a jest," said Sir Reginald. "The foolish boy has attracted a great deal of attention. Bunter, you should be more sensible, and you should not be so easily frightened. Now, my boys, we will go for a walk round Assuan, and then to tea at the Ghezireh Palace Hotel, with our good friend, Mr. Maroudi."

"Come on, Bunter!" chuckled Bob. "That is, if you feel sure that we're not jolly old kidnappers, after all."

"Ha, ha, ha!"

"Yah!" snorted Bunter. "Go and eat coke! Yah!"

And the fat Owl rolled down the gangway to go on board the dahabiyeh. Apparently, he was fed-up, for the present, with the Greyfriars fellows, though he was no longer in a state of terror. As he rolled across the gangway his two boatmen yelled and gesticulated excitedly. Bunter had forgotten them; but they had not forgotten Bunter. With a grunt the fat Owl handed over the promised piastres and rolled on board. For once the fat and fatuous Owl of Greyfriars was anxious to get out of sight.

Harry Wharton & Co. enjoyed a walk round the interesting city of Assuan and tea at the Ghezireh Palace Hotel with Mr. Maroudi, minus the company of William George Bunter. Bunter was sulking on the dahabiyeh, like Achilles in his tent. But the loss of his fascinating society did not seem to have any depressing effect on the merry juniors. Indeed, they seemed to enjoy it.

THE FIFTH CHAPTER.
Bunter Hits Back!

BILLY BUNTER was wrathy.

He was indignant.

He was vengeful.

He longed to make those beasts who had pulled his podgy leg to such an absurd extent sit up!

From the dahabiyeh he watched them strolling away in a cheery crowd, with the tall Sir Reginald and the plump Mr. Maroudi, and Hassan, the dragoman, fluttering round them like a gorgeous tropical butterfly.

They disappeared from his sight along the busy Shari-el-Manshiya, and Bunter snorted with wrath and scorn.

"Beasts!"

People on the shore, people in dahabiyehs and feluccas, were still glancing at Bunter. His wild flight had attracted a lot of attention, and people naturally wondered what was up. Many staring eyes followed him to the dahabiyeh. On board that craft the Nubian sailors were grinning; and Bunter did not need to ask what they were grinning at. He did not need to inquire what caused the smile on the grave bronze countenance of Moussa the reis.

He rolled below, red and wrathful. He was ready for lunch now—more than ready. In fact, much more than ready. He lunched amply, but he detected lurking grins on the faces of the Nubian servants. He was really glad to get out of the sight of derisive eyes and roll into his cabin for a nap. He napped, and rose again for an early tea and sat on the boat's balcony eating Turkish Delight until he could dispose of no more and Turkish Delight ceased to be delightful.

Sticky and sulky, Bunter brooded over his wrongs. Bunter, as a rule, was not a fellow to bear malice. Seldom did the sun go down on his wrath. Now he was deeply incensed, and yearning to make those beasts sit up. They had shoved a sack over him, making him think he was kidnapped; talked a lot of rot which he had fancied was Arabic, uttered by ferocious Arabs; and, worst of all, he had set the dahabiyeh chortling from end to end by his dramatic escape and his frantic flight. Bunter realised that he looked a fool —and he did not realise that he seldom looked anything else. So his wrath was deep!

And Mauly was at the bottom of it! Mauly, whose devoted pal Bunter had been, had actually propounded that wheeze! The ingratitude of it stung Bunter—after all he had done for Mauly!

In Shakespeare, that rather unreasonable old gentleman, King Lear, remarks: "How sharper than a serpent's tooth it is to have a thankless child!" In the same way, and with really more reason, Bunter reflected how bitter it was to have a thankless pal! He had done a lot for Mauly—accompanied him on his holiday to Egypt, borrowed his best Panama hat, worn his clothes, spent his piastres—in fact, he had been a devoted pal, sticking closer than a brother, or even a leech!

And this was his reward!

It would serve Mauly jolly well right to chuck him, and turn down the whole party. Bunter was tempted to do it. Crushing the ungrateful Mauly with gleaming eyes of scorn, he would turn his back on him and shake the dust of the dahabiyeh from his feet! Leaving the party to get on the best they could without him, Bunter would depart, on his dignified own! The difficulty was that he would have to borrow the fare home from Mauly—and borrowing the fare from him, while crushing him with scorn, might spoil the effect.

On reflection, Bunter decided on less drastic measures. Mauly deserved punishment, but not, after all, such a knock-out blow as the loss of Bunter's society.

Billy Bunter rolled into Mauleverer's cabin. An idea was working in his fat brain. In Mauly's cabin was the Golden Scarab.

The ancient scarabeus of A-Menah, once worn as an amulet by that old warrior of Rameses the Second, had been the cause of many adventures since the Greyfriars fellows had landed in Egypt. Kalizelos, the Greek, was in desperate quest of it, and, according to his own statement, he knew the mysterious secret of the scarab, and in his hands it would have guided him to the treasure of Osiris. From a prosperous merchant in Cairo the Greek had become a hunted futigive, through his fierce and lawless attempts to possess himself of the scarab. And the Greyfriars fellows had come to believe, at last, that that ancient Egyptian relic really was a clue to treasure, though in what way they could not imagine.

Often and often they examined it, wondering what could be the secret that the Greek had read in an old papyrus, written by a scribe three thousand years ago at the order of A-Menah. They even had a lingering idea that they might guess the secret and lift the treasure during their holiday on the Nile. And, if the tale was true, the treasure was worth lifting, for it was the famous diamond called the Eye of Osiris, which had never been seen since

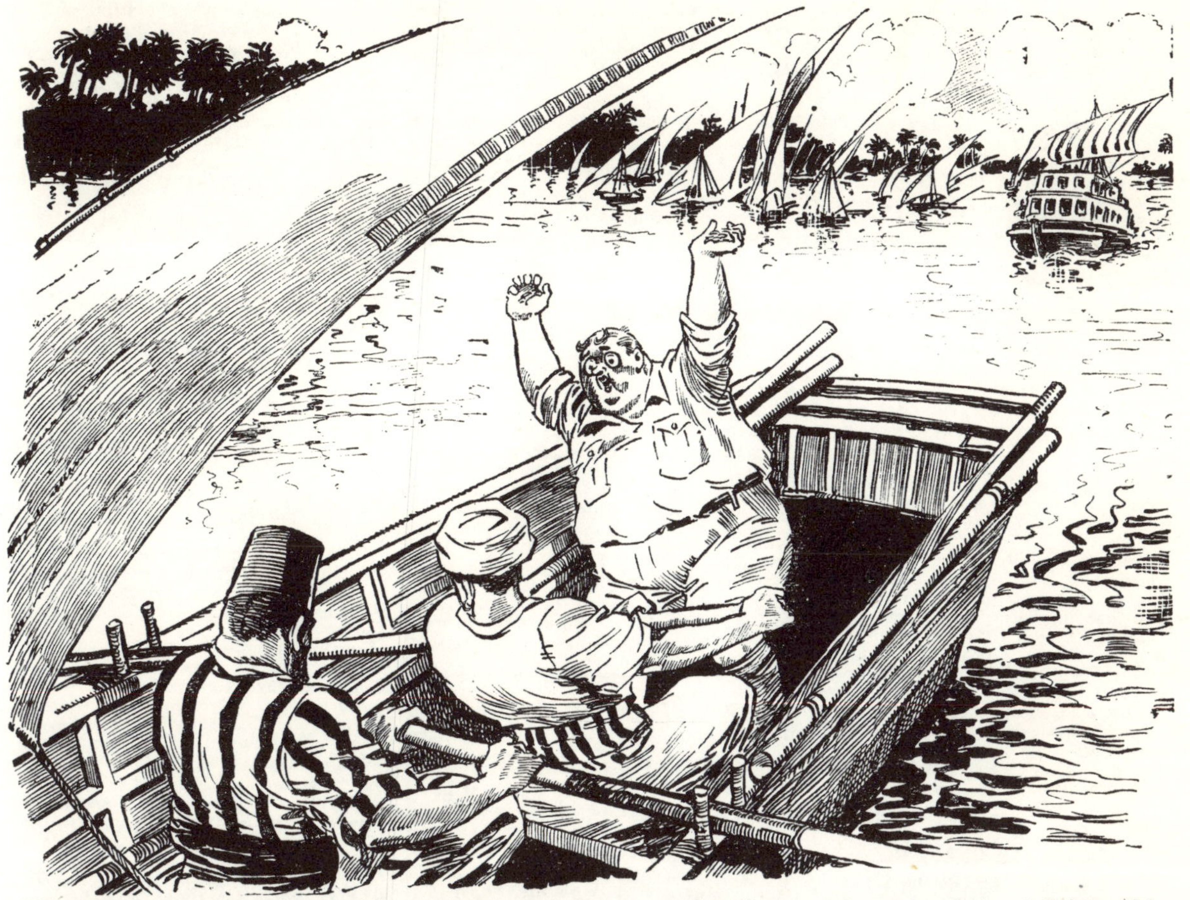

Little dreaming that it was the Greyfriars party in pursuit, Bunter urged on the rowers to greater efforts. "Quick, quick, quick!" he gasped, holding up handfuls of piastres to encourage his boatmen. "Quicker, quicker, quicker!"

the reign of Rameses the Second. Described in ancient papyri as worth many a king's ransom, it was supposed to be worth a quarter of a million pounds in modern money.

Billy Bunter shut the cabin door and blinked round the room, with a fat grin on his face.

Lord Mauleverer, certainly, was keen to keep possession of the mysterious scarab, but his lordship was careless, and the old relic had had many narrow escapes. For which reason, Mauly's friends had made him secrete it in a hiding-place in his cabin, where it was safe from thievish hands.

Bunter was not supposed to know anything about that. But Billy Bunter often knew things that he was not supposed to know. The Peeping Tom of Greyfriars had a way of finding things out, and he was, as a matter of fact, perfectly well aware of the scarab's hiding-place. It was from sheer inquisitiveness that Bunter had pried into that matter, for he was not in the least interested in the scarab, and did not dream of believing for a moment that it was a clue to a treasure. But he was going to put his knowledge to account now.

The fat Owl, of course, had no intention of "pinching" the scarab! He was going to abstract it from its hiding-place and hide it somewhere else—to punish Mauly for his ingratitude.

That would make Mauly sit up!

Bunter rolled across to Lord Mauleverer's dressing-table. On that table stood an ivory box containing an ointment that was used for sunburn.

Billy Bunter poked his fat fingers into the ointment and scooped up the Golden Beetle, which was hidden under it, wrapped in paper.

He gave a fat chuckle.

He unwrapped the greasy paper from the scarab, and tossed it out of the window into the Nile.

The Golden Scarab lay in his fat palm. Bunter blinked at it.

It was nothing but a beetle, made of gold, with the name and title of A-Menah inscribed on it in the picture-writing of ancient Egypt.

It looked as if it was made of solid gold, and, if that was so, it was worth perhaps twenty or thirty pounds for the metal.

"Silly ass!" murmured Bunter, thinking of Kalizelos. Whatever it was that the Greek had read in the old papyrus, written by the scribe of A-Menah, it seemed scarcely possible that this golden beetle could be a clue to a vast treasure.

According to ancient tradition, it would guide its possessor to the "Eye of Osiris," a tradition founded, no doubt, upon some inaccurate knowledge of what was written in the old papyrus that had fallen into the Greek's hands.

Unless it had some magical properties of some sort, the thing seemed impossible. And it was scarcely possible to believe in magic.

Moreover, the scarab had been for years in possession of Lord Mauleverer's father, and of Mauleverer himself, and certainly it had guided neither of them to the Eye of Osiris.

Bunter's opinion was that it was all "rot," an opinion that Harry Wharton & Co. would have shared, but for the desperate attempts of Kalizelos to lay hands on the scarab.

Anyhow, whether it was valuable or valueless, Bunter had it now! He slipped it into his pocket and rolled out of Mauly's cabin and went to his own.

His next proceeding was to find another hiding-place for the scarab, where the beasts would never find it. Later on, Bunter would let Mauly have it back—after duly punishing him for his ingratitude to a faithful and devoted pal! For the present it was going to remain safely hidden, in Billy Bunter's keeping.

Billy Bunter considered that matter deeply. He was still considering it deeply, when there was a tramp of feet on the gangway and a sound of cheery voices on the deck. Harry Wharton & Co. were returning to the dahabiyeh.

"Oh lor!" ejaculated Bunter.

Swiftly he stuffed the Golden Scarab into a matchbox, and slipped the matchbox into his trousers pocket. It was out of sight there, and later he could find a safer hiding-place for it. He rolled out of his cabin with a fat grin on his face.

"Hallo, hallo, hallo!" roared Bob Cherry. "Here we are again! Look out for kidnapping, Bunter!"

"Ha, ha, ha!"

Billy Bunter snorted.

"Perhaps you fellows had better look out!" he said, with a fat sneer.

"Mind your eye, you men!" gasped Bob. "Bunter's going to whop us all round."

"Spare us, old fat man!" yawned Lord Mauleverer.

"You've treated me rottenly!" said Bunter, with a disdainful blink at the cheery juniors through his big spectacles. "After all I've done for you, you've treated me rottenly! Perhaps you'll be sorry for it! Perhaps you'll be sorry you left me on my own this afternoon! Wait and see!"

"My esteemed, idiotic Bunter——" said Hurree Jamset Ram Singh.

"I'm not going to tell you anything!" said Bunter mysteriously. "I may or may not have paid you out for playing rotten tricks on a fellow! That's telling!"

"What have you been up to, you fat frog?" asked Harry Wharton.

"Find out!"

"I know what he's done!" said Bob.

Bunter jumped.

"You beast, what——"

"He's scoffed all the grub on the boat and left nothing for supper!" said Bob. "Is that it, Bunter?"

"Ha, ha, ha!"

"You silly ass!" roared Bunter.

"Well, what have you been up to, if you've been up to anything?" asked Nugent.

"That's telling!"

"Fathead!" said the juniors together.

Bunter intended to keep it a dead secret that he had played tricks with the Golden Scarab. But Bunter had his own inimitable way of keeping a secret. Certainly his mysterious hints might have roused suspicion if the juniors had given them attention. But they didn't! Dark and mysterious hints from Billy Bunter did not even rouse their curiosity. They only concluded that Bunter was talking rot, as usual, and let it go at that.

THE SIXTH CHAPTER.

A Ducking for Bunter!

"ENORMOUS dam, triumphant exhibition of wonderful skill of British engineers, at which it is proper to gaze with considerable wonder——"

Hassan, the dragoman, was at it as the dahabiyeh rolled up the Nile above Assuan. But the Greyfriars fellows did not need the dragoman's descriptions to interest them in the mighty Assuan Dam.

It was one of the wonders of Egypt, as wonderful as the Pyramids, and a great deal more useful.

The juniors, as they looked at it, could not help feeling proud of the work of British engineers.

Above Assuan is the First Cataract of the Nile, and there the great dam, designed by Sir William Willcocks, was built by the British firm of Aird.

More than 500,000 million gallons of water are stored in the vast reservoir barred by the dam, which turns the Nile above the Cataract into an immense lake, storing the water that comes down from Central Africa.

Water is precious in Egypt, which has scarcely any rain. But for the Nile, the country could never have existed.

In the huge dam are no fewer than 180 sluice-gates for regulating the flow of the precious water, which, when the Nile is low, is let out with great care to fill the irrigation canals of Lower Egypt.

Millions and millions of gallons of precious water, which once ran to waste into the Mediterranean, are stored up till needed. Indeed, when the engineers have finished their work on the Nile, probably not a drop of water from that great river will reach the sea at all—every drop being needed by the industrious fellahin for their crops.

By the Navigation Canal on the west side of the mighty dam, through a series of locks, the dahabiyeh floated slowly onward, to the upper waters of the Nile.

"Some job!" said Bob Cherry, as he gazed at the great dam. "Beats the jolly old Pyramids hollow, what? If you ask me, old Cheops would have shown a lot more sense if he had built this dam instead of the Great Pyramid!"

"The morefulness of the sense would have been terrific!" agreed Hurree Jamset Ram Singh. "But the ancient Egyptians had not the wonderful common sense of the esteemed and ridiculous English."

Even Billy Bunter condescended to bestow a blink or two on the Assuan Dam. In that triumph of British engineering skill lay the cause of much of the wonderful fertility the juniors had seen in Lower Egypt.

"This great work shall go to commence in the year 1898!" chanted Hassan. "Historic foundation-stone is laid by noble highness Duke of Connaught. Enormous and gigantic triumph of estimable British engineering persons! Yes! Island of Philae, once extremely bootiful spot, now generally submergeful in waters of dam, to ruin of vegetation, also great damage to wonderful temples which are usually washed over by Nile waters. When waters go low, temples emerge, and may be seen by interested eye of tourist, but receding waters leave slime on temple walls, covering the same with what you call muck in the bootiful English language."

The great barrage was left behind, and the dahabiyeh rolled on to Philae, the island in the Nile that was once a beauty spot, but which has been sadly marred by the building of the dam.

When the reservoir is full the island is flooded; but in the autumn the sluice-gates are opened to allow the stored water to flow down into the canals of Egypt; and then the level of the Upper Nile sinks, leaving slimy walls and rotting vegetation to greet the eyes of the tourist; and so the Greyfriars fellows were able to go ashore and explore the temples of Philae.

"Think you'd better come, Bunter?" asked Bob Cherry doubtfully.

"Eh! Why not?" asked Bunter. "You're taking a lunch-basket, I suppose?"

"Ha, ha! Yes. But——"

"But what?" grunted Bunter.

"That gang of kidnappers will be there!" said Bob. "The same gang that got you last time, you know."

"Beast!"

It was only a little joke of Bob's; but Billy Bunter drew from it the inference that his company was not wanted. For which reason, Billy Bunter determined to go; though, as a matter of fact, he would rather have loafed on the dahabiyeh.

"Here we see great Temple of Isis!" Hassan was full of information, as usual. "This temple built by Ptolemy Philadephus, lordly gentlemen! Completion of great work by Energetes the First——"

"Oh, chuck that!" said Bunter peevishly.

"My noble sar!" ejaculated Hassan.

"Dry up!" said Bunter. "You talk too much!"

Billy Bunter was peevish! It was, as usual, a hot day; and, also as usual, the innumerable flies of the Nile haunted Bunter. The traces of his last meal on his fat face attracted them. When Bunter was peeved he was not polite.

As a matter of fact, the other fellows would have enjoyed the wonderful sights of Egypt more, if the dragoman had not talked so much. But Hassan felt it his duty to impart information—and he did his duty manfully.

"Shut up, Bunter!" growled Johnny Bull.

"Yah!" replied Bunter elegantly.

"My esteemed and idiotic Bunter——"

"Yah! I say, you fellows, let's chuck this and have lunch," said Bunter. "I'm fed-up with temples and tombs and Hassan jawing."

As it was only an hour since breakfast, the suggestion of lunch did not catch on. Really, the party had not landed on Philae to sit under a tree and watch Bunter eat.

They rambled on; listening more or less to Hassan. They had to listen also to a series of discontented grunts from Bunter. Bunter rolled after the other fellows, wishing he hadn't come! Instead of tooting about mucky old temples and things, he might have been stretching his fat limbs in a deckchair on the Cleopatra, under a shady awning, and eating! So might the other fellows, if they had had as much sense as Bunter!

"Here we take care, lordly gentlemen," said Hassan, as the party came to a wide ditch that was full of water and mud, left from the last high water of the Nile, and which was crossed by a plank.

"I say, you fellows, what about lunch——"

"Oh, come on, fatty!"

"Look here, what about going back to the dahabiyeh——"

"Buck up!"

"I'm tired!"

"Well, sit down and rest, and we'll pick you up coming back," said Harry Wharton. "We'll leave the lunch-basket with you, if you'll agree not to scoff more than nine-tenths of the grub."

"Just like you, to want to leave a fellow on his own after bringing him all this way!" snorted Bunter. "Just like you, I must say!"

"Oh, kick him!" said Johnny Bull.

"Beast! Lot of rot, I call it, mooching about a beastly island and listening to that silly nigger jabbering," said Bunter.

"Hassan!" said Lord Mauleverer.

"Oh, yes, my noble sar!"

"You can kick Bunter if you like."

"Oh, noble sar!" said Hassan.

"Oh, really, Mauly——"

"Let's get on," said Bob, and he marched across the plank, followed by the rest in single-file.

Bunter remained on the edge, blinking across uneasily. The Famous Five looked back at him.

"Are you coming, Bunter?" bawled Bob Cherry.

"That plank's not safe!" hooted Bunter.

A SPLENDID PRIZE GOES TO

E. Raymond, of 128, Albany Street, Regent's Park, N.W., who sent in this winning Greyfriars limerick:

Vernon-Smith, of Greyfriars School,
Is often an arrogant fool.
But as Redwing's his chum,
Some sense he can drum
Into Smithy, who's just like a mule!

Readers are invited to send in original Greyfriars limericks. Handsome POCKET WALLETS are awarded for all efforts published.

"We've crossed it, you fat duffer!" answered Nugent.

"I'm not going to be ducked in mud to please you!" roared Bunter. "I know it's exactly what you would like; but I'm jolly well not going to do it, see?"

"Stay where you are, and be blowed!" snorted Johnny Bull.

"Beast! You fellows hold the plank," said Bunter. "You'll only have to stand in up to your knees to hold it."

"Oh crikey!" gasped Bob. "Is that all?"

"That's all! Get to it," said Bunter. "Don't stand around slacking!"

Somehow, the prospect of standing up to their knees in slimy mud, holding a muddy plank for Bunter to cross, did not seem to appeal to the Famous Five. Bunter blinked across at them impatiently.

"I'm waiting!" he hooted.

"The waitfulness will probably be terrific!" chuckled Hurree Jamset Ram Singh. "There is too much mudfulness for my absurd self, my worthy Bunter."

"Well, let that nigger step in and hold it," said Bunter, with a glare at the dragoman. "What's he here for, except to make himself useful? Are we going to pay him for nothing?"

Hassan's eyes gleamed for a moment. Effusively polite and amiable as the dragoman was, his politeness sometimes wore a little thin under the stress of Billy Bunter. Perhaps Bunter did not care. There was no doubt that when Bunter was tired and peevish his manners were not those of the very best circles.

"Oh gad!" said Lord Mauleverer. "Can you help him across, Hassan? Take hold of his ears and lift him."

"On my head be it, noble lordly sar!" answered Hassan.

He went back across the plank to assist Bunter.

"All safe as a house, sar, as you say in English," said Hassan encouragingly. "Hassan is your dragoman, sar—you trust Hassan! I take one hold on your noble arm, sar, and help your majestic feet on a plank."

"Well, take care," grunted Bunter. "All you niggars are such clumsy fools."

"Oh, sar!" murmured Hassan. "I take an enormous care of so noble a lordly gentleman, sar! On my head be it!"

"Don't jaw!" said Bunter.

"Ain't he a dear?" murmured Bob Cherry. "Doesn't he encourage a man to give him a helping hand? Asks for it, doesn't he?"

The juniors watched Bunter's progress across the plank. As a matter of fact, it was quite safe without Hassan holding him. As another matter of fact, it was quite unsafe with Hassan holding him.

In the middle of the plank, Hassan suddenly slipped.

"Look out!" gasped Bob.

Hassan did not fall from the plank into the ditch. He stumbled, and regained his footing quite actively. But in doing so, he released Bunter's arm, and at the same time, jerked him violently to one side.

Bunter staggered on the plank.

"Oooogh!" he gurgled.

Splash!

Bunter sat in the ditch.

Luckily, it was not deep. As he sat in it, the soft, liquid mud came up only to his chin.

"Oh crumbs!" gasped Bob Cherry.

"Groooooogh!" came from Bunter. "Oooooch! Woooooooh!"

"Oh, sar, what a terrible accident!" gasped Hassan. "This lordly gentleman has fallen from a plank! Wahyat-en-nabi!"

ALL ABOUT NEXT WEEK'S FREE GIFTS!

CHEERIO, CHUMS!—I expect you are beginning to get excited over our Magnificent Free Gift Collecting Scheme. Well, when you open next Saturday's bumper number of the MAGNET, you will find inside the first Six Grand Super Stamps, starting you on the greatest Collecting Scheme ever devised for boys. These Super Stamps are beautifully finished in three colours, and you will feel instantly that you must collect them. The whole series, showing "Every Boy's World in pictures," consists of 144 Stamps in six sets of 24 Stamps, each set illustrating a different subject, such as dogs, railway engines, aeroplanes, roughriders, ships, etc.

Six Super Stamps will be presented free to MAGNET readers each week for many weeks to come, while our companion papers, RANGER and MODERN BOY, will also contain six Free Stamps. In addition, a magnificent 20-Page Album, priced at sixpence, has been produced to hold the whole series of 144 Stamps—and this you can get FOR NOTHING! You simply buy next week's issue of the MODERN BOY and—hey presto!—you have the Album FREE. Don't miss this wonderful chance of getting the special Album, which will hold the six sets of Stamps! Then week by week you can stick in the Stamps by means of the gummed backs, and by judicious "swapping" of your spare Stamps, you will be able to make up the six complete sets. The collecting of the Stamps is a fascinating pastime that will give additional interest to the scheme.

Remember, chums, SIX SUPER STAMPS will be given away Free in next week's MAGNET, in next week's RANGER, and in next week's MODERN BOY, while the latter paper will also contain a splendid ALBUM FREE! Why not start off your collection with all three publications?

THE EDITOR.

"Grooogh! Woooh! Help!" shrieked Bunter. "I'm sinking! I'm drowning! I'm just going to be suffocated! Yaroooh!"

"Pull him out, Hassan!" shouted Harry Wharton.

"Yes, sar! I pull out this noble lord with a prompt despatch!" answered Hassan obediently.

He knelt on the plank, reached at Bunter and grasped him firmly by the back of the collar. With a squeezing, squelching sound, the fat junior was drawn up from the clinging mud. He glared furiously at the dragoman as he dragged.

"You clumsy fool!" he hooted.

Squelch! Perhaps by accident—or perhaps not by accident—Hassan let the fat Owl slip again, and Bunter sank into mud once more. Reaching after him, Hassan somehow pushed the top of his head, and Bunter's face went under the mud this time. It came up smothered, with the fat junior snorting like a grampus.

"Grooogh! You silly, clumsy fool of a nigger!" spluttered Bunter.

"Oh, sar!" gasped Hassan.

"Ooooooch! Groooogh! Gug-gug-ug! Oh crikey! I'm smothered! I'm suffocated! I'm chook-chook-chook-choked! Urrrrgggh!"

"This was one sad and lamentable accident, sar——"

"Beast! Gimme out!" howled Bunter. "You clumsy dummy, gimme out! You silly chump of a nigger—— Oooough!"

Once more Hassan was clumsy, and Bunter ducked into mud again. He was a hill of mud when he was pulled up.

Perhaps it dawned upon Bunter that these lamentable accidents were likely to continue so long as he called Hassan fancy names. Or perhaps the mud made utterance difficult. Anyhow, this time Bunter held his peace till the dragoman had dragged him on the plank.

Once there, Bunter scrambled back to the side he had started from. In his present state Bunter was not inclined for further exploration of the island of Philae. Bunter was not a whale on washing, but even Bunter realised that he needed a wash now, and needed it badly. He squelched ashore, gurgling.

"Lordly gentleman, you desire that I help you across a plank one more time?" asked Hassan politely.

"Beast!" gasped Bunter.

"Oh, sar!"

"Blow you!" roared Bunter.

And he started back to the dahabiyeh, squelching mud at every step. Hassan crossed the plank once more, and rejoined his lordly gentlemen—who were grinning. They had a strong suspicion that Bunter's mud-bath had not been entirely accidental. Still, there was no doubt that Bunter had asked for it. So they went cheerfully on their way, and explored Philae—what time Billy Bunter, on the dahabiyeh, was cleaning off mud.

THE SEVENTH CHAPTER.

The Desert Sheikh!

"THE real, genuine, jolly old desert!" said Bob Cherry.

It was a few days later, and night lay on the Nile.

High over the great river of Egypt soared the moon, shedding silver light on the rolling river, on the high brown banks, and on the desert that lay on either side.

The dahabiyeh was tied up to the bank for the night, many a long mile from Assuan, and well on the way to the Second Cataract. Still a great distance ahead of them was Wady Halfa, which marked the limit of Upper Egypt, beyond which lay Nubia and the Sudan.

The spot where the houseboat was tied up was a lonely one.

Here the belt of cultivation on either side of the Nile narrowed, and Upper Egypt was hardly a mile in width, including the river. Beyond, east and west, lay the desert.

It was to the west that Bob Cherry was looking, over vast wastes, marked by lines of low, sandy, and rocky hills, where the Libyan Desert stretched away to the great Sahara.

No glimmer of light was to be seen on either bank.

The chums of the Remove seemed to have Africa to themselves.

After supper they had come up to the upper deck, to look at the desert in the moonlight, and chat before turning in.

The silence and solitude of the desert impressed the minds of the Greyfriars juniors, as they sat in the deckchairs and looked away to the west. Even Billy Bunter felt a little of the influence of the calm, still night and the illimitable desert. But Bunter did not give such trifling matters much thought. Neither was he, for once, sleepy.

Bunter had done uncommonly well at supper. Mr. Maroudi's Coptic cook had produced a wonderful ragout, which all the juniors had pronounced ripping—and of which Billy Bunter had had so many helpings that he was feeling a little uneasy. Billy Bunter's idea was that a fellow could not have too much of a good thing—but just now he was feeling as if a fellow, after all, could!

"Only a few days more!" said Frank Nugent. "We shall get a look at Wady Halfa, and then we turn back. Anybody willing to miss the new term at Greyfriars and go on to the Great Lakes?"

The juniors chuckled. There were plenty of attractions at the old school, especially with the football coming on; but they would have been more than willing to give the new term a miss and keep on to the very end of the river of wonders.

But that was not to be! After reaching Halfa, the dahabiyeh was to turn back for Assuan, where Sir Reginald Brooke and Mr. Maroudi were staying. Mr. Maroudi's househoat was to be handed back to its owner, and the old baronet and his flock were to take the train back to Cairo, for the return to England. Only a few days more—but the cheery chums of Greyfriars were going to make the most of them—little dreaming, at that moment, how those days were destined to be spent.

"Well, we've had a ripping time," said Bob Cherry. "That bounder Kalizelos has made it rather exciting at times——"

"We seem to have seen the last of that sportsman," remarked Lord Mauleverer. "He seems to have chucked up his stunt of gettin' hold of my jolly old scarab."

"Still got it safe, Mauly?" grinned Bob.

"Oh, yaas!"

As it was hidden in what was supposed to be a perfectly safe place, it had not occurred to Lord Mauleverer to look at it, and so he had not yet missed it! Mauly and the other fellows supposed that it was still safe in the ivory box of ointment in Mauly's cabin. Bunter could have told them differently, had he liked. But he did not like! The beasts were going to have the shock of their lives when they missed it.

"I suppose Kalizelos has chucked it?" remarked Harry Wharton thoughtfully. "He was wounded, you know, when those American johnnies chipped in to help us when he got hold of us near Luxor. Well, if he's chucked it, all the better—though I'd have liked to know what was the secret of the scarab."

"Same here!" assented Bob.

"The samefulness is terrific!" remarked the Nabob of Bhanipur. "It is a terrific and preposterous mystery!"

"Grooooough!" came from Bunter.

The juniors looked round at him again. Bunter rose from his chair. He had doubted whether he had overdone it at supper. Now he no longer had any doubts; he knew that he had.

"Feeling the strain, old fat bean?" grinned Bob. "I told you to let that seventeenth helping alone."

"It was only the eleventh, you beast," answered Bunter, "or the twelfth, at the the most! I haven't had too much supper, and I don't feel at all upset. I'm not a fellow for stuffing, I hope—like some fellows I could name. I—I think a walk would do me good!"

"Roll round the deck," said Bob. "You can't go ashore."

"I can jolly well do exactly as I like, I suppose?" retorted Bunter.

"Look here, you ass——"

"You fellows afraid to step off the boat?" sneered Bunter. "Do you think that Greek blighter is hiding behind one of those rocks? It's a lovely night for a stroll."

"That's so," agreed Bob, with a glance at the Nile shore. "But——" He glanced at the captain of the Remove.

Harry Wharton shook his head.

"Nothing doing," he said. "Mauly's uncle told us not to go ashore except at the show places, where there's crowds, and it's safe. We're bound to play up."

"The boundfulness is terrific!"

"I say, you fellows, don't be such rotten funks," said Bunter. "Be men, you know. Like me."

"Cheese it, fathead!"

"Yah!"

Billy Bunter rolled down the steps to the lower deck. The gangplank was in position, from the lower deck to the bank. There was nothing to prevent Bunter from walking ashore, if he liked. He blinked very cautiously at the bank. Bathed in bright moonlight, it was almost as light as by day. Bunter stepped on the gangway.

Harry Wharton called down from the upper deck.

"Come back, you ass!"

"Rats!" retorted Bunter independently. And he rolled across the gangway to the bank.

"Who's going to lug him back by his ears?" yawned Bob Cherry. "Bunter, you howling ass, come back, you frabjous fathead!"

"Yah!"

Billy Bunter strolled along the high bank. He was only a few yards from the juniors on the dahabiyeh, with a strip of mud and water between. They frowned at him, and Bunter grinned back derisively. He put a fat thumb to his fat little nose and extended his fingers.

"You silly owl!" roared Johny Bull.

Bunter added his other hand, with the fingers extended. That disrespectful gesture was intended to show his contempt for the Greyfriars fellows. The effect was rather spoiled, however, by an orange which Bob Cherry suddenly whizzed ashore at the fat and derisive Owl.

Bang!

The orange landed on Bunter's fat chin. He sat down quite suddenly on the bank of the Nile.

Bump!

"Good shot!"

"Ha, ha, ha!"

"Ow! Beast!" roared Bunter. He scrambled up and, instead of putting his fat fingers to his podgy nose again, he shook a plump fist at the grinning juniors on the houseboat.

Then he walked on, and a fringe of tamarisk bushes hid him from their sight.

Behind the tamarisks, Billy Bunter sat down on a rock and grinned. His idea was to give the juniors the impression that he had walked on, and was, like Felix, still walking. From his cover, he could hear the voices on the dahabiyeh in the still quiet of the night.

"Where has that fat idiot got to?" he heard Bob Cherry ask.

Bunter chuckled silently.

"Oh, let him rip!" growled Johnny Bull. "If he loses himself it won't be much loss."

"Beast!" murmured Bunter.

"We shall have to go after the fat chump if he doesn't show up soon," said Harry Wharton. "We'll jolly well kick him all the way back!"

"Hear, hear!"

Thud, thud, thud! There was a sudden sound of horse's hoofs on the silent shore. From an opening in the rocks at a distance from the bank, an Arab horseman appeared suddenly in sight. In white burnous and turban, with his dark aquiline face and black eyes glinting in the moonlight, he was a rather startling figure. The juniors gazed at him.

"A jolly old Arab from the desert!" said Bob Cherry. "Nice of him to show up and let us have a squint at him."

"Bismillah!" breathed Hassan, the dragoman.

The dragoman's startled tone drew the glances of the juniors upon him. Hassan stood with his eyes fixed on the horseman, who was riding down to the Nile-bank, and there was something like fear in his brown face.

"You've seen that Johnny before, Hassan?" asked Bob.

"It is Abdurrahman, the sheikh!" said Hassan, in a low voice. "How dares he ride so near the Nile. The soldiers at Wady Halfa would be seeking him if they knew—yet he dares to show himself! Inshallah!"

The juniors exchanged rather startled glances.

"Who—what is he then?" asked Harry.

"He is a robber of the desert, sar," answered Hassan. "He is a sheikh of the Baggara, and as a boy of ten he fought in the Khalifa's army at Omdurman, against the great Lord Kitchener!"

"Oh, my hat!"

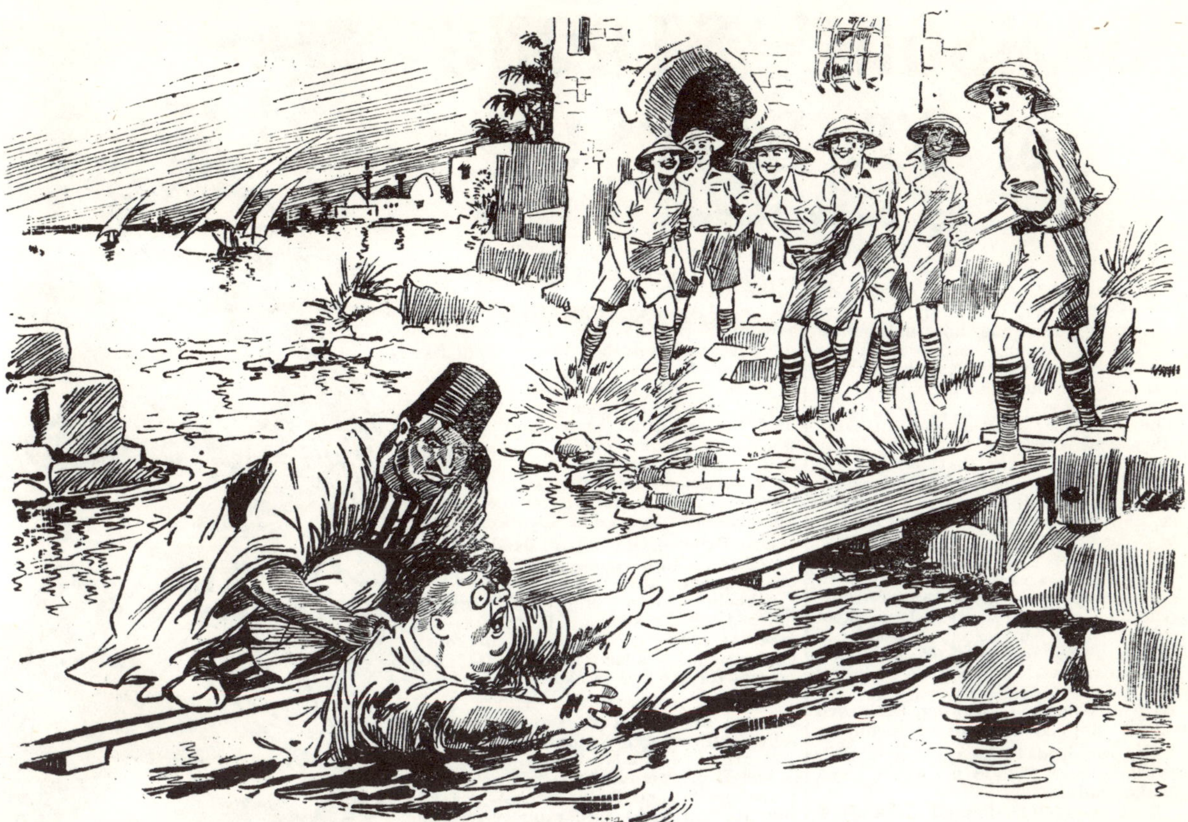

"Yes, sar!" said Hassan obediently. "I pull out this noble lord with a prompt despatch!" He bent down, and grasped Bunter firmly by the back of his collar. With a squeezing, squelching sound, the fat junior was drawn up from the clinging mud.

With deeper interest, the juniors bank. Wild and fierce and savage he looked, as was natural in one of the fierce Dervishes who had fought under the Khalifa, and who, since the re-conquest of the Sudan, had preferred the life of a robber in the desert to submission to the Anglo-Egyptian rule. It was amazing to see such a man riding on the banks of the Nile. His life was forfeit a dozen times over, and it was only in the trackless, sandy wastes of the desert that he could find liberty and safety.

"What on earth is he doing here, then?" asked Nugent.

"That is only known to Allah!" said the dragoman, but his face was troubled and uneasy.

The horseman clattered down to the bank. He rode a magnificent black Barbary horse, which he handled to perfection. He came down to the water's edge with such a rush that the juniors wondered whether he would pitch headlong into the Nile. Within two or three feet of the shore gangway he pulled in his horse so suddenly that it reared and pawed the air. There he halted and sat his horse motionless as a statue, in startling contrast to his swift activity of a moment before.

"What on earth does he want here?" muttered Wharton.

Hassan breathed hard and deep.

"Gentlemanly lords, I will draw in the gangway," he said. "It will be wise to push off and cross to the eastern bank of the Nile!".

"Oh, my hat!" ejaculated Bob Cherry. "You don't think——"

"Where the Sheikh Abdurrahman rides, his followers ride," said the dragoman. "It has never been known for the robbers of the desert to ride to the Nile—but Abdurrahman is here! What this may mean I do not know, my noble sars, but I have great fear that we are in what you call, in English, a queer street."

"Phew!"

The juniors were startled now. It seemed incredible that wild Arabs from the Libyan Desert could have any design of attacking a holiday houseboat on the Nile. Yet what else could the wild sheikh's presence portend—for, unless for some very special reason, the desert robber would never have ventured to ride within fifty miles of the Nile. Sir Reginald Brooke had impressed on the juniors never to leave the dahabiyeh except at well-known stopping-places. But he had never dreamed of danger to them on the houseboat itself—and such a thought had never crossed the minds of the juniors. But they had to think of it now—as they watched the dark-faced ruffian from the desert, sitting his horse on the bank.

"The sooner we get to the other bank the better, I think!" muttered Nugent. "If that fellow's got a gang with him like himself——"

"That fool Bunter!" breathed Wharton. "We can't leave him behind—oh, the silly fathead!"

"Look!" breathed Bob.

Hassan had gone down to the lower deck. But as he approached the gang-plank, the horseman drew a long-barrelled, silver-mounted pistol from his girdle, and lifted it. Over the levelled weapon, he shouted to the dragoman in Arabic.

"Wahyat-en-nabi!" gasped Hassan, and his brown face was almost grey with fear.

He returned to the upper deck without touching the gangway and without calling the crew to pole off. The juniors looked at him.

"What did the man say?" asked Harry quietly.

"Oh, my noble sar!" said Hassan, "he say we stay here in this place, or he shoot! No one can dare to disobey the Sheikh Abdurrahman—he has taken many lives! Alas, noble sars, we are in one queer street!"

Wharton set his lips.

"That means that that scoundrel has ridden ahead to keep us here while his men come up, you fellows!" he said.

"Looks like it!"

"We'd chance his pistol and sheer off—only—that fool, Bunter——"

The juniors stared along the bank for Bunter. They had seen nothing of him since he had disappeared behind the tamarisks. Whether he was near at hand, or far away, they did not know. And they were not likely to see anything of him now.

The sight of the wild Arab horseman had caused Billy Bunter's eyes almost to pop through his spectacles, and his fat heart to quake with terror. He could not get back to the dahabiyeh without passing the savage horseman, who was halted close to the gang-plank. Wild horses would hardly have dragged Bunter into view while the savage Arab was there.

He squatted in the thickness of the clump of tamarisks, palpitating with terror, only anxious to keep out of sight. And from the shadowy rocks farther back from the river there came a sound of many hoofs, a glancing of turbans and burnouses in the moonlight, a squealing of camels. A bunch of dark-faced riders came in sight on the bank,

(*Continued on page 16.*)

"SAMSON" STRONG of ST. SAM'S!

By Dicky Nugent.

I.

JACK JOLLY & CO., of the Fourth at St. Sam's, were standing at the skool gates one fine half-holler-day, wondering how to spend the afternoon without spending any munny, when a weerd newcomer rolled up on the seen.

The newcomer was dressed in skool clothes and a cap. But the funny thing about him was that he stood at least 6 feet 3 inches in his sox. He had a grate, bull-like neck, a beefy face, collyflower ears, and leg-of-mutton fists.

"Grate pip!" eggsclaimed Jack Jolly, rubbing his eyes in astonishment. "This chap's a giant—a veritable Carnera! Yet he's dressed in skool clobber! Who can he be, I wonder?"

"He's going to speak to us," said Frank Fearless. "Perhaps we shall find out!"

As Frank finished speaking, the weerd stranger stopped in front of them.

"Hi, you brats!" he said, in a ruff, savvidge voice. "Show me where I can find the 'cadmaster!"

"Brat yourself!" flashed back Jack Jolly, undawnted by the newcomer's tremenjous size. "Who are you, anyway?"

The big fellow seemed quite taken aback by Jack Jolly's fearless retort, and he clenched his fists, while grate nottid veins stood out on his forrid, as though he was tempted to give the kaptin of the Fourth a savvidge, brutal punch on the dial. But he evidently changed his mind again, for he unclenched his fists and allowed the nottid veins to sit down again.

"My name's Meakin Mild!" he growled. "I'm a new boy at this 'ere college, and I want to see the 'cadmaster!"

"My hat!"

"Where does 'e 'ang out?" asked Meakin Mild, with renewed feerceness.

"Over there, old bean!" replied Frank Fearless, pointing to the Head's house.

Jack Jolly & Co. watched the eggstraordinary stranger out of site with feelings that were too deep for words.

"I fansy we're not going to like this new chap," mermered Jack Jolly, when Meakin Mild had disappeared into the Head's house. "There's something pekuliar a b o u t h i m—something sinnister!"

While the juniors were diskussing the new boy, Meakin Mild was being ushered into the prezzence of the Head. His behaviour in front of the majestick Dr. Birchemall, however, was in vivid contrast with his behaviour in front of Jack Jolly & Co. He farely cringed and grovelled as the Head swept his eagle eye over him.

"Please, sir," he said, "I should very much like to join your skool as a junior skoller."

"Bust me!" mermered Dr. Birchemall, eyeing the newcomer in grate astonishment. "How old are you, my man—I mean, my boy?"

"Please, sir, I'm fifteen next birthday!"

"Well, I'm jiggered! I should have taken you for fifty, at least!" said the Head. "Anyway, I'm afraid it's impossibul; you have to apply years in advance to get into a famus skool like St. Sam's."

Meakin Mild frowned for a moment. Then his face brightened up a bit again, and he dived a large hand into his pocket and drew out a thick wad of crisp, russling notes.

"I forgot to menshun, sir," he said, "I have plenty of cash on me, and I am prepared to pay in advance."

Dr. Birchemall's eyes fixed rather greedily on those notes, and his manner changed notissably.

"Ahem! Why didn't you say so before?" he asked. "If that is the case, of corse, I can perhaps make an eggseption for once. Shall we say five pounds for the first week?"

"That'll suit me all right, sir!" grinned Meakin Mild, counting out the notes with a grimy fourfinger. "'Ere you are—five pun!"

The Head snatched the five notes and transferred them to his pocket, regarding Meakin Mild rather queerly as he did so.

"Thanks!" he said. "I must say, judging by what I have herd of you, so far, that the fiver will be earned. Your grammar is really shocking. Fansy saying 'five pun'! Why, any idiot knows the correct eggspression is 'five quid'—I know it myself!"

"Sorry, sir!" grinned Meakin Mild.

"Well, well, we shall soon lick you into shape, I suppose!" sighed the Head. "You will be placed in the Fourth Form to begin with!"

Five minnits later Meakin Mild was walking out of the Head's study a registered skoller of St. Sam's. He didn't look a bit like a fellow who would soon be licked into shape. On the contrary, he looked the kind of fellow who would soon want to lick St. Sam's into shape himself!

II.

"MEAKIN MILD!"

"'Allo!"

Mr. Lickham, the master of the Fourth, jumped. It was in class on the following morning, and Mr. Lickham had decided to test the new boy's nollidge. But that "'Allo!" was uneggspected, and, instead of going straight on to the test, Mr. Lickham could only stare at the new skoller.

"Meakin Mild!" he gasped.

"You've said that once already, old cockerlorum!" growled Meakin. "Wodger want?"

"Few!" wissled the Fourth.

Mr. Lickham seemed to be on the verge of paralissis.

"Meakin Mild!" he roared. "I was warned by the 'eadmaster that you were a somewhat pekuliar boy, who has had no education or tooition in good manners. But for that sercumstance, I should cane you very seveerly——"

"Ha, ha, ha!" roared Meakin. "You'd walk into trubble if you did!"

"What?"

Mr. Lickham flew into a towering rage, picked up his cane, and approached Meakin.

"Bend over, boy!" he thundered.

To the utter amazement of the master of the Fourth, Meakin Mild wrenched the cane from his hand.

An instant later the serprizing new boy went one step further.

WOULD YOU BELIEVE IT?

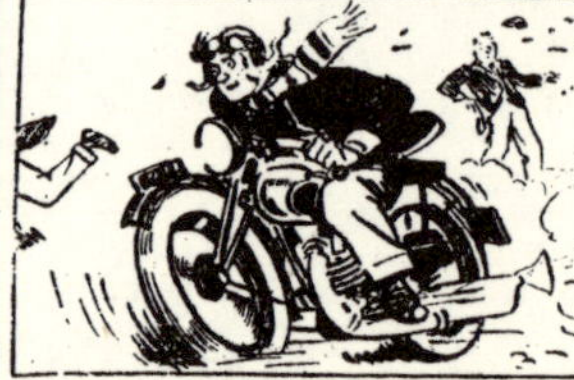

Horace Coker owns the most powerful motor-bike in or around Greyfriars, and yearns to become a track-rider!

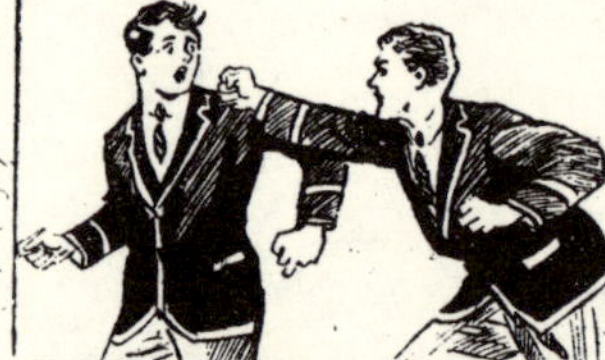

Although Frank Nugent takes girls' parts in Remove theatricals, he carries a hefty punch for those who call him a "milk-sop."

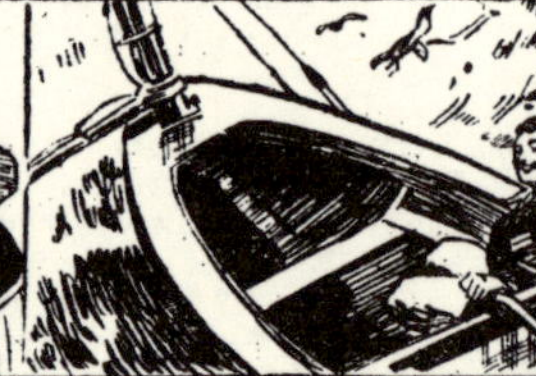

Tom Redwing has the sea in hi blood, and is never happier tha when sailing in Pegg Bay

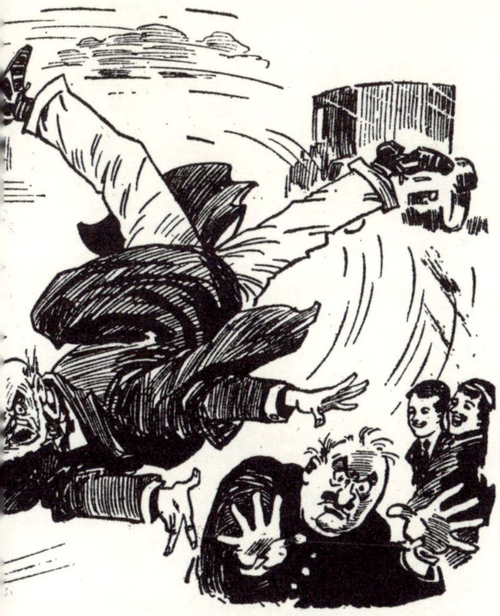

Seezing Mr. Lickham by the skruff of the neck, he lifted him clean off his feet, and started belabouring him for all he was worth! A verritable rain of blows dessended on the unforchunit Form master's anatomy, and Mr. Lickham emitted a series of wild howls.

"Yarooo! Whoooop! Ow-wow-ow!"

Jack Jolly started to his feet.

"I say, you chaps, we can't allow this!" he cride. "Reskew, St. Sam's!"

"What-ho!"

The Fourth didn't intend to sit idly by and watch manslawter committed before their eyes. They leaped over the desks to the front of the class, and farely flung themselves at Meakin Mild.

How the kontest would have gone can only be conjectured, for before it had really started Dr. Birchemall rushed into the Form-room.

"Bless my sole! What ever's the meaning of this here?" he asked, in shocked, though cultured, axxents. "Back to your desks at once, the lot of you! Mr. Lickham! Kindly eggsplain the meaning of this riot!"

"It's this—this hooligan!" gasped Mr. Lickham, pointing a trembling fourfinger at the gigantic new boy. "He started walloping me with my own cane!"

Dr. Birchemall frowned.

"You are using strong langwidge, Lickham! Let me tell you that I have a very high opinion of Mild; if he set about you, I'm pretty sure he had good cawse!"

"Quite right, sir!" said Meakin Mild. "That old gent wanted to cane me—me, you know!"

"Preposterous!" eggsclaimed Dr. Birchemall. "I wonder you're not ashamed of yourself, Lickham, using such brutal methods on a meer lad! Kindly leave him alone for the future!" Then he turned to Meakin Mild and wispered: "By the way, Mild, what about settling up for your second week in advance?"

"Plezzure, I'm sure!" grinned Meakin Mild, passing over a crisp, russling fiver. "That right?"

"Right as rain, thanks!" smiled the Head. "Now return to your desk, Mild, and if Mr. Lickham or anybody else tries to booly you, just come and see me!"

With that, the Head russled out, leaving Mr. Lickham and the Fourth almost overcome.

It was clear to everyone now how matters stood. Meakin Mild was an ally of the Head, and was evvidently being given a free hand to do just as he liked. The outlook for the Fourth was black indeed!

III.

AFTER the insident in the Form-room, Meakin Mild farely ran amok at St. Sam's. He walked round the old skool, doing just as he pleased, and boolying to his hart's content. Not sattisfied with tweaking fags' noses and twisting their ears, he nocked Fourth-Formers' heads together, tripped up stately prefects, and even jumped on Mr. Justiss' toes!

Natcherally, there were protests. Masters and prefects swarmed round the Head's study like bees round a jam-pot, and a score of voices clammered for Mild's immejate eggspulsion. But the Head turned a deff ear to all appeals.

But Nemmysis was rappidly overtaking the Carnera of St. Sam's, and his rain as the booly of the skool was destined to end very shortly in a most untimely manner.

It was Jack Jolly who brought it all about.

The leader of the Fourth was sitting in his study in the evening, talking things over with his pals as he glarnsed through the daily newspaper. The problem of Meakin Mild was worrying Jack considerably. As he talked his brow was corrugated, his jaw like iron, and his eyes like steel. Jack Jolly felt that he was on his metal.

All of a sudden he jumped to his feet.

"Grate pip!" he eggsclaimed. "Just look at this, you chaps!"

Fearless and Merry and Bright crowded round him and peered over his sholder at the newspaper.

Staring them in the fizz was the ugly, but unmistakable fotograph of the man of the moment—Meakin Mild!

"Meakin Mild—by all that's wonderful!" breethed Frank Fearless.

Jack Jolly smiled grimly.

"I'm not so sure about the 'Meakin Mild,' he said. "Judging by what they say here, that's not his name at all! Read this!"

The amazed Fourth-Formers read the paragraph underneeth the foto. This is what they saw:

"Above is a fotograph of 'Samson' Strong, a notorious crimminal, who varies the monotony of 'all-in' wrestling by indulging in frekwent highway robberies with violence. The perlice are anxious to get in touch with Strong, who was last seen near Muggleton, after raiding a costumier's, where he pinched an outsize in skool suits."

"Grate pip! Then that's the mystery about him!" gasped Merry. "He's not a skoolboy at all, but a fugitive from justiss!"

"Few!"

"I'm going to wring up the perlice!" declared Jack Jolly.

The young kaptin was as good as his word. He got on to Inspector Smart, of the Muggleton Perlice, and in a very short space of time a perlice-van was roaring up the carriage-drive to the Skool House.

"Quick! There's your man!" said Jack Jolly, who was waiting for them at the top of the steps. Before Samson Strong could say 'Nife!' the peelers were upon him!

Dr. Birchemall's face, when he was told that his faverite pupil was an old lag, was a site for gods, men, and little fishes.

"Villan! Skoundrel! Double-dyed deceever!" he cride, shaking a bony fist at the Carnera of St. Sam's. "How dare you besmirch the fare name of this grate skool with your evil prezzence? Avaunt! Take him away, inspector, and throw him into your deepest and darkest dunjon!"

The green eyes of Samson Strong gleemed as he herd that stern speech. He was thinking of the fivers the Head had been very pleased to take from him only a few hours since.

"Mite I 'ave a word with you afore I go, sir?" he asked humbly.

Dr. Birchemall eyed him rather craftily, wondering whether he was going to hand over the swag into his keeping.

"Very well; release him for a minnit, inspector."

Inspector Smart nodded, and released Samson Strong, who then went close up to the Head.

Instead of whispering and handing over the munny, as the Head had hoped would happen, the criminal seezed Dr. Birchemall by the beard, yanked him off his feet, and started swinging him round and round in a circle.

When he did let go, evenchally, the Head's speed was so tremendous that he flew through the air above the heads of the spectators, to land with a terrifick crash in the branches of one of the trees!

"Yaroooo!" shreeked Dr. Birchemall from that dizzy hite.

"There! Perhaps that'll lern you not to turn agin a man arter you've bin taking 'is munny!" said "Meakin Mild." "Now, inspector, I am ready to take my grool!"

And the Carnera of St. Sam's stepped into the perlice-van to be taken away to his richly-deserved punishment.

It is hardly necessary to add—but we will add it, all the same—that St. Sam's breethed a grate sigh of releef to see the back of him!

THE END.

GREYFRIARS FACTS WHILE YOU WAIT!

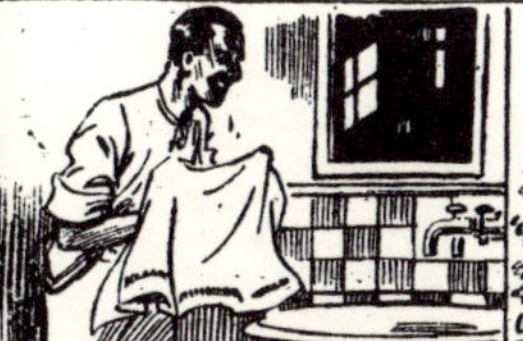

ar-off Bhanipur, "Inky" had with his morning ablutions. he Remove dorm., "Inky" ies himself—and prefers it!

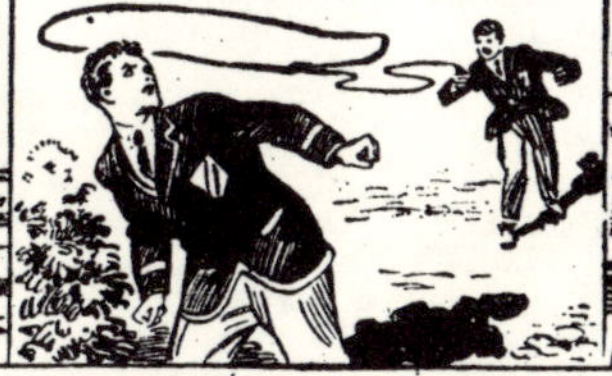

Tom Brown, the New Zealand junior, is an adept with the lariat, and has "roped up" more than one astonished victim.

Dr. Locke reads the works of Plato, Euripedes, and Aeschylus—for relaxation!

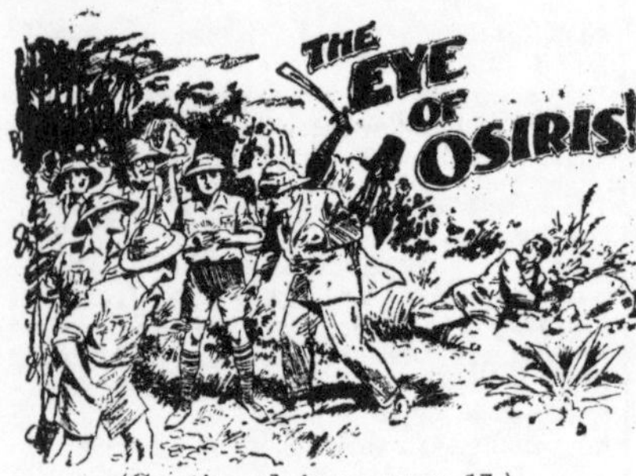

(*Continued from page* 13.)

and among them was a man with an olive-skinned face—a face that the Greyfriars juniors knew only too well.

It was Konstantinos Kalizelos!

THE EIGHTH CHAPTER.
In the Hands of the Enemy!

"KALIZELOS!"

Harry Wharton breathed the name.

The juniors understood now.

It was their enemy, the relentless seeker of the Golden Scarab, who was riding down to the Nile with the desert robbers.

"My hat!" murmured Bob Cherry.

The reis and the Nubian crew were up now. They stood in a startled crowd, staring at the men on the bank.

Motionless as a statue the Sheikh Abdurrahman sat his black Barbary horse, the long-barrelled pistol in his hand. But when Moussa made a movement towards the gang-plank the pistol was raised, and the reis stepped back again.

It was long since they had seen anything of Kalizelos, and they had begun to think that the Greek had given up the quest of the Golden Scarab. But it was clear now that he had been only biding his time.

Evidently the dahabiyeh had been watched on its way up the river, and the Greek had picked time and place for an attack. Fugitive as he was, he had plenty of money, and "backsheesh" had hired Abdurrahman and his gang of desert robbers.

Even the desperate dervish would hardly have ventured on a raid on the Nile shore, so far from his den in the recesses of the desert, at the risk of being cut off by the Egyptian soldiers at Wady Halfa. Many eyes must have seen the savage troop, and news of their coming would spread swiftly. The days of dervish raids were long over. In a few hours at the most the Camel Corps from Wady Halfa, mounted men from a dozen posts on the Nile, would be riding to intercept the desert troop. It was not a raid on Nile villages and plantations. The savage troop had one object, and one object only. The Greyfriars schoolboys understood that quite well. The Greek had planned a swift ride from the desert, the seizing of the dahabiyeh, and a swift ride back into the remote wilderness. Only swiftness could spell success, and even minutes might make the difference between success and failure.

Abdurrahman had dashed ahead on his swift horse to make sure that the dahabiyeh did not push off from the bank before the tourists could take the alarm at the sight of the desert troop. Sitting his black horse, pistol in hand, he kept guard while the rest of the gang came up.

There was a scared murmur from the Nubian sailors on the lower deck. They watched the Arabs with terrified eyes. Bared scimitars gleamed in the hands of the dusky ruffians riding down to join their chief. It was scarcely possible to think of resistance, and the crew of the Cleopatra were not thinking of it. With a clatter and a jingle and a squealing of camels the Arabs came on, and the juniors on the upper deck caught the triumphant grin on the olive-skinned face of Konstantinos Kalizelos. The Greek had won at last!

Harry Wharton set his lips.

"We've got to chance it," he said in a low voice. "We can pick Bunter up later. He will have sense enough to keep out of sight when he sees that gang. We've got to get the dahabiyeh away before that gang can get on board."

"And there's no time to lose," said Bob. "Come on."

"Oh, lordly gentlemen," gasped Hassan, "your noble lives will be taken! The sheikh will shoot with a pistol——"

"Tell the men to push off, Hassan, at once!"

"Oh, sar, under the eyes of Abdurrahman they will not dare——"

"Come on!" snapped Wharton.

He ran down to the lower deck, followed by his comrades. He caught Moussa, the reis, by the arm.

"Push off from the bank at once!" he exclaimed.

Moussa made a gesture towards the savage sheikh.

"Effendi, it is death!" he said.

"Get hold of the poles, you men," said Harry.

He ran to the side, one of the sailors' poles in his hands.

The man on the black horse raised his pistol, his eyes scintillating over it in the moonlight. He aimed it at Wharton.

"Unbelieving Faringhee," he said in a deep voice. "Stand back!"

Unheeding the Arab, Wharton drove the pole at the steep bank. There was a flash in the Arab's eyes, and he pulled the trigger. Bob Cherry grasped Wharton by the shoulder and dragged him back. It was only in time; the bullet crashed in the deck a foot from the captain of the Greyfriars Remove, and the report of the pistol roared and echoed along the Nile.

"Chuck it, old man!" muttered Bob. "Nothing doing!"

The sheikh had drawn a second pistol from his girdle. He raised it, aiming at the group of Greyfriars juniors.

Wharton dropped the pole.

His face was pale with anger, and his teeth set. But he realised that, as Bob said, there was nothing doing. The juniors were unarmed, and at the mercy of a ruthless ruffian with firearms in his hands. Almost incredible as it might have seemed, there was no doubt that the dervish would have shot them down like rabbits if they had attempted to push off.

"Lordly sars," groaned Hassan, who had followed the juniors down, "do not anger that terrible man—it is death!"

"If a fellow had a chance——" muttered Johnny Bull, between his teeth.

"The chancefulness is not great," said Hurree Jamset Ram Singh, shaking his head. "We must bear it grinfully."

"Can't be helped," said Lord Mauleverer. "It's the scarab that rotter is after; that's all they want! Kalizelos has got us this time! But who the dooce would have thought it?"

With a trampling of hoofs the Arab gang reached the bank. There were more than a score of the desert riders, and some of them were leading spare camels. Kalizelos dropped from his camel and came on the gang-plank. Behind him followed Hamza and Yussef. Abdurrahman and his men remained on the bank.

Kalizelos stepped on the deck of the dahabiyeh.

He gave the juniors a mocking salute.

"We meet again, my lord!" he said.

"Yaas," assented Lord Mauleverer placidly. "You've got a rotten way of turnin' up like a bad penny, Mr. Kalizelos. Can't say I'm pleased to see you."

"Do not think of resistance," said the Greek quietly. "I have hired Abdurrahman and his men at a great price to give their aid, and resistance is useless. They will remain on the bank unless I call them here; but I warn you that if those savage robbers are once let loose on the dahabiyeh, and blood is shed, they are not likely to leave a man alive."

Looking at the dark, savage faces on the bank the juniors could quite believe it.

"Give me the scarab!" continued Kalizelos. "Give me what I seek, and I will ride away with my men and you will see us no more. You may go peaceably to your beds as safe as any other tourists on the Nile. But lose no time; I have not even seconds to waste."

The Famous Five stood silent.

It was useless to attempt a futile resistance, which would only have been the signal for a massacre.

"You hear me, Lord Mauleverer?"

"Yaas."

"Give me the scarab!"

"Rats!"

"Is it on board the dahabiyeh?"

"Find out!"

The Greek's black eyes glittered.

He spoke in Arabic to Yussef and Hamza, and the two Arabs approached Lord Mauleverer. Swiftly they searched the schoolboy earl; Mauleverer submitting to the search with cheerful equanimity, as there was no help for it. Then each of the juniors was searched in his turn.

The Greek stood biting his lips with impatience. With equal impatience the Arabs on the bank waited and watched.

Every man in the gang was anxious to get finished and ride; every moment on the banks of the Nile was fraught with peril for them. Probably a hundred startled fellahin had seen the wild riders as they came, and were already carrying the news of their coming to the military posts along the river. The raiders could not get through too swiftly.

The Greyfriars fellows were well aware of that. Every moment there was a chance of help appearing in sight, and every moment that their enemy lost was a gain to them.

Kalizelos muttered in Arabic again and hurried below, followed by Yussef and Hamza. The juniors heard them searching in Mauleverer's cabin.

They waited.

The hiding-place of the Golden Scarab in the box of ointment was a safe one, and the juniors believed that it was still there. If the Greek found it he was not likely to find it in a hurry.

Kalizelos came back to the deck, leaving his confederates still searching in the cabin. His olive face was pale with rage.

"The scarab is hidden?" he said in a low, hissing voice.

"Yaas," assented Lord Mauleverer.

"Will you tell me where it is hidden?"

"No!"

"You would like to delay me till the soldiers arrive from Wady Halfa!" said the Greek bitterly. "But you will not succeed, my lord. I have no time to search the dahabiyeh for a secret hiding-place. Neither would Abdurrahman and his men consent to wait so long; they are already impatient to be gone. We shall ride—and you will ride with us! The old man Brooke will give the scarab for your lives and your liberty. Let him refuse, and the crows of the Libyan Desert will pick your bones."

He snarled out the words.

"Here, at any moment, rescue may come," he said. "But do you dream that rescue will follow when we have ridden at great speed into the heart of the desert? Do you fancy that the soldiers will track down Abdurrahman, who has defied the Egyptian Government for thirty years? Do you think that the sands of the desert will leave a track to be followed? Fool, while there is yet time, give me the scarab!"

Lord Mauleverer yawned.

"Answer me, fool!" snarled the Greek.

"I've answered you, old bean," drawled Lord Mauleverer. "If you want that jolly old scarab, look for it and find it."

"Bind them!" snarled the Greek, in Arabic.

Hamza and Yussef proceeded to bind the hands of the Greyfriars fellows behind their backs. Hassan's hands were bound, also.

Moussa and the Nubian sailors looked on in silence. They could not help. It needed only a call from the Greek to bring the wild crew of desert robbers on the dahabiyeh, scimitar in hand. With their hands bound, the six schoolboys and the dragoman were hustled to the side. There was a thoughtful expression on Lord Mauleverer's face, but he uttered no word till the two Arabs began to drive the prisoners across the gangway to the bank. Then the schoolboy earl broke his silence at last.

"Hold on a tick, Mr. Kalizelos!" he drawled.

The Greek signed to the Arabs to stop and turned eager eyes on Mauleverer.

"Speak!" he snapped.

Lord Mauleverer looked up and down the bank of the Nile in the bright, clear moonlight. But if help was coming it was not in sight. Harry Wharton & Co. understood what was in Mauly's mind. He had delayed matters as long as he could in the hope of help coming. He had hoped that a long search on the dahabiyeh would delay the enemy still more, and give time for rescue to arrive. But the Greek was too cunning for that, and there was nothing more to be done.

"Look here, Mr. Kalizelos," said Lord Mauleverer quietly. "This is between you and me. May I ask you to leave my friends out of it?"

"Fool!"

"Shut up, Mauly!" growled Johnny Bull. "You're not going to let them have the scarab. We can stand it if you can."

"Not a word, Mauly!" said Harry.

Lord Mauleverer shook his head.

"The game's up, old beans," he said quietly. "If that brute had got us away that time near Luxor there was a chance of rescue. But there's no chance here! A day's ride from here will take us into the Sahara! I'd stand it on my own, but I can't see you men landed in it!"

"Fathead!" growled Bob Cherry.

"My esteemed idiotic Mauly——"

"'Nuff said!" interrupted Lord Mauleverer. "The old bean's got us by the short hairs. I brought you fellows out to Egypt for a holiday, not to get you kidnapped in the desert. Kalizelos, old thing, tell your thieves to fetch up an ivory box from my dressing-table."

The Greek's black eyes snapped.

He ran below, and came back almost in a moment, with the ivory box of ointment in his dusky hand.

"This?" he explained.

Lord Mauleverer nodded.

"Yaas."

"It is here?"

"Yaas."

With a blaze in his eyes, his olive-skinned face irradiated with triumph, the Greek scooped the ointment out of the box. Harry Wharton & Co. watched him in grim silence, Hassan, the dragoman, in great relief. For his own sake, Lord Mauleverer would not have yielded; to save his comrades he was giving up the Golden Scarab, at last, into the greedy hands of the Greek. But there was a surprise in store for the Greek, and for the Greyfriars juniors.

The ointment that had hidden the

(*Continued on next page.*)

scarab in the ivory box was scooped out. But there was no glitter of gold in the moonlight. The box was empty! The scarab was gone!

THE NINTH CHAPTER.

The Ride in the Desert!

"GONE!"

Lord Mauleverer uttered the word, in tones of blank astonishment.

The Famous Five stared.

Hassan gave a groan of disappointment.

The olive face of Kalizelos worked with rage. He hurled the ivory box on the deck with a crash that broke it into a score of pieces. He turned to Lord Mauleverer, convulsed with fury.

"Fool, you would trick me, to waste time!" he hissed. "Do you think that the soldiers from Wady Halfa are already on their way, liar and fool?"

Mauleverer compressed his lips.

"The scarab was there!" he said.

"It is false!"

"I suppose a rascal like you wouldn't understand that a fellow would not tell lies," remarked Lord Mauleverer reflectively.

"Where is the scarab?" hissed the Greek.

"Ask me another!"

"What the thump can have become of it?" exclaimed Bob Cherry in wonder. "It was in that box, packed under the ointment!"

"Looks as if somebody spotted it and pinched it," said Mauleverer. "I'm sorry for this, you chaps! I'd have let them have it, like a shot, to save you from his clutches. Now there's nothin' doin', unless that cheery old bean will take my word for it that I don't know what has become of the scarab."

"Am I a child, to be deceived by a trick?" said the Greek hoarsely. "For the last time, Lord Mauleverer, will you give up the scarab?"

"Can't!"

"Where is it?" hissed Kalizelos.

"Haven't the foggiest."

"Enough!"

The Greek snarled an order in Arabic, and Yussef and Hamza drove the juniors across the gangway to the bank. As they stumbled on the shore Hassan turned his eyes imploringly on Lord Mauleverer.

"Oh, noble sar!" he groaned. "I beg you in the name of the Prophet, to give up the scarab to this Greek. What is the value of such a trifle, lordly sar, to your noble lordship? These men are fierce as the lions, and all our lives are worth nothing in the desert of Libya."

Mauleverer glanced at him.

"Didn't you hear me tell the old bean that I haven't the foggiest idea where the jolly old scarab is, Hassan?"

"Oh, sar! Think yet once more, noble sar, before you anger these terrible men. I, Hassan, the son of Suleiman, have told many lies, sar, but I would not dare to lie to these men."

"Oh gad!" said Mauleverer.

"You silly dummy," growled Bob Cherry. "The scarab's been taken. Nobody here knows where it is."

"Lordly sar, I swear that the telling of lies to these men is useless," urged Hassan. "There is yet time to speak the truth my noble lord, and save us all from knock into a cock hat, as you say in the English language."

Evidently Hassan, no more than the Greek, believed that the scarab was lost. Lying was the dragoman's usual resource in a difficulty, and it did not ever occur to his Oriental mind that the Faringhees might be more particular in such matters. Lord Mauleverer shrugged his shoulders and walked up the bank, and the unhappy son of Suleiman groaned in despair.

No time was lost now. The Greek and every lawless ruffian in his gang was in a state of trepidation, casting uneasy glances up and down and across the river in the bright moonlight. Already the delay had endangered the retreat of the gang of desert robbers.

The schoolboys and the dragoman were hoisted on the spare camels and the whole party turned from the Nile. Bound on the camels, the prisoners rode away from the river, in the midst of the Arabs, Abdurrahman leading the way on his black Barbary horse.

From the dahabiyeh the reis and the Nubian sailors stared after them. And from the clump of tamarisks on the bank, where he lay hidden, in mortal terror, Billy Bunter watched them through his big spectacles, and gasped with relief when the shadows of the desert swallowed them from sight. Billy Bunter, no doubt, was concerned for his schoolfellows, but there was still less doubt that he was more deeply concerned for himself!

With a rapid beat of hoofs, the party rode away from the river. The sheikh galloped in advance, and after him thundered the camels, driven to speed by blows and cries from their riders.

Every man was glancing to right and left as he rode. Abdurrahman and his men well knew that such a raid was a desperate one, and the delay on the dahabiyeh had added to their danger. They feared every moment to see armed riders start into view in the moonlight.

Eagerly the Greyfriars juniors looked back as they rocked and bumped along on the tall, swaying camels. What the desert robbers feared, was what the prisoners hoped.

There was a sudden shout from one of the robbers. It was echoed by others, as he pointed to the south. In the glimmering moonlight a camel-rider appeared in sight, and there was a gleam of a carbine-barrel in the light of the moon.

"That's a gipsy soldier!" breathed Bob Cherry.

The Sheikh Abdurrahman shouted to his followers. The ride, or rather the flight, had been swift before; now it was doubly swift. With fierce and savage blows and hoarse yells, the desert robbers drove the swaying camels onward, and it seemed to the juniors that they were rushing through the night at almost the speed of an express train. The way lay through a defile in a range of low sandy hills; and looking back now, they could see the Nile no longer, and the camel-rider they had glimpsed for a moment had vanished.

"They're after us, anyhow!" said Johnny Bull.

Thud, thud, thud, thundered the galloping hoofs.

Beyond the low, sandy hills lay a plain of sand, across which the riders tore at their fastest speed. Then they rode through a defile in rocky hills again, still keeping up the desperate pace. Again and again, they passed through ranges of low hills, clattering among dark limestone boulders—again and again, vast stretches of sand flashed under the thudding hoofs. Hour after hour passed, and still the wild ride went on without a pause.

And the hopes of the Greyfriars fellows died away. They had no doubt that the news of the raid had spread; that mounted men would be seeking the Arab raiders up and down the Nile and across the western desert. But the sand and rocks left no trace of the fleeing robbers; and once in the illimitable spaces of the desert, pursuit was a practical impossibility.

For hundreds of miles the desert stretched, sandy, barren, uninhabited; with only the eyes of the birds of prey to watch the wild riders as they passed. Search for the prisoners, when they had vanished into the desert, was like a search for a needle in a haystack—a very small needle in a very large haystack. The Greek had won at last. There had been a chance that rescue might come, while the raiders were still in the valley of the Nile; but that chance had failed. There was no hope now.

No hope—and the juniors realised it. Long, long miles lay between them and the Nile now. The bright moonlight showed them only barren stretches of sand, and ranges of rocky hills. And still the camels thundered on, while the night grew older and the moonlight gave place to dawn.

Weary, aching from the jolting and bumping of the camels, with tired eyes, the Greyfriars juniors watched the sun rise on the desert. The rays of the rising sun glimmered over immense solitudes. The pace was slower now; even the hardy Baggara camels were growing fatigued; and the juniors could see, too, that the raiders had now little or no fear of pursuit. But the ride still went on, farther and farther into the trackless wastes.

It was like some terrible nightmare to the Greyfriars juniors. Only a few hours ago they had been chatting in the deckchairs in the dahabiyeh, in fancied security, discussing the new term at Greyfriars. From civilisation they had fallen, at one fell swoop, into primitive barbarism. Houseboats and the Nile, guides and donkey-boys, temples and tombs of past ages, had given place to the desert—the raw and savage desert, where life was held cheap, where savage men roamed as fierce and untamed as in the earliest ages of the world.

Through a long and weary morning the ride went on, more slowly, but without a halt until the heat of noonday approached. Then even the hardy robbers of the Libyan Desert were weary. They halted at last, in the midst of a stone-strewn, sandy plain, at a spot where a group of scrubby acacias grew, the only vegetation within reach of the eye. Evidently there was a spring at the spot, and water was to be found, known to the desert riders. The camels laid down to rest, and the prisoners were unbound from the humps on which they had swayed and jolted so long and so wearily. Their hands were released also; and they were given dry dhurra bread and brackish water. They ate and drank mechanically, almost too fatigued to stir. The Greek came over to them with his black eyes smouldering.

"Do you dream that we may be followed and that you may be found by your friends?" he asked.

"Doesn't look a healthy chance!" said Lord Mauleverer.

"The Golden Scarab will be your ransom! I will give you pen and paper and you shall write to the old man Brooke, at Assuan. The dragoman will carry your message!"

Lord Mauleverer made no answer.

"I know you, my lord!" said the Greek bitterly. "You would perish here in the desert before you would yield! I know you! That is why I

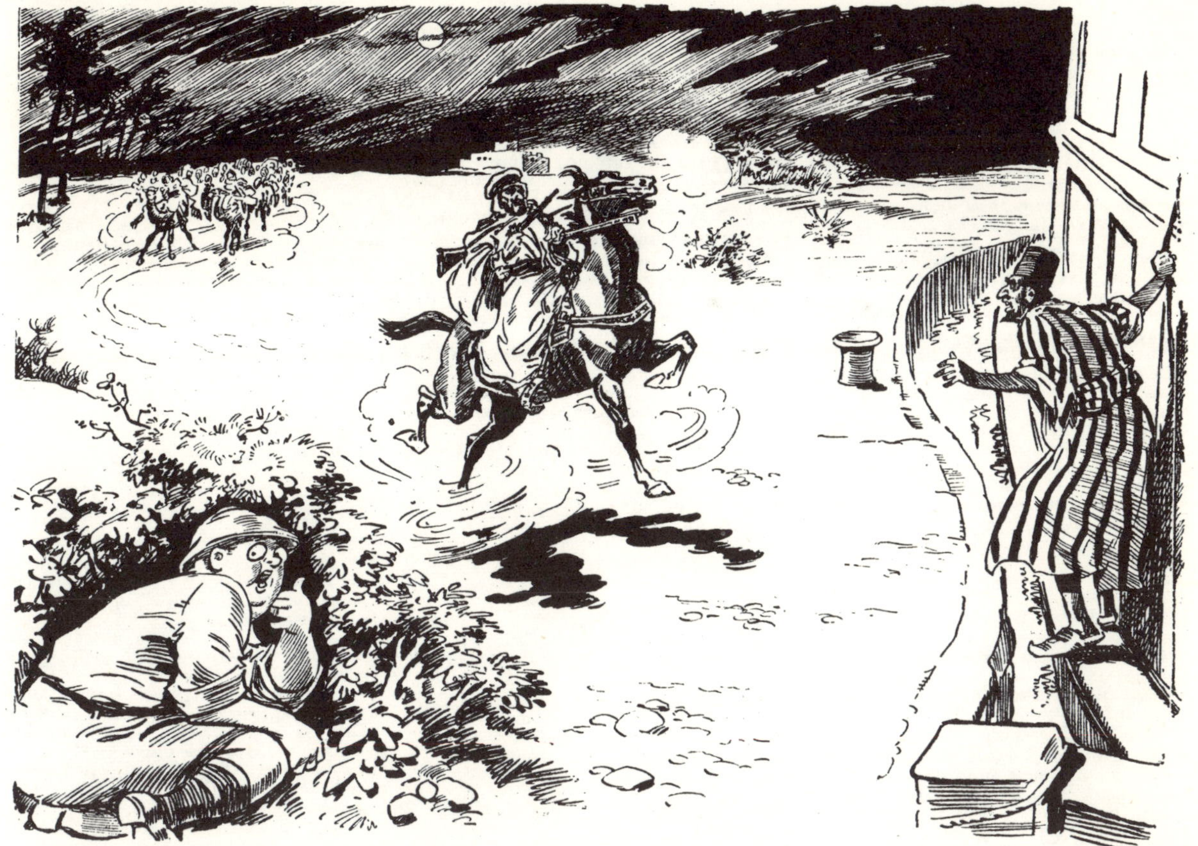

Quaking with terror at the sight of the wild Arab horseman, Bunter squatted in the thickness of the clump of tamarisks, anxious to keep out of sight. From the shadowy desert farther back, a bunch of dark-faced riders came in sight, riding fast for the dahabiyeh !

have brought your friends to die with you if you do not yield! Do you dream that I will show them mercy?"

"You don't look it," said Mauleverer.

"To save them, if not to save yourself, will you write to the old man Brooke? Only the scarab will ransom you."

"I've told you," said Mauleverer calmly, "that I know nothin' of the scarab. It was hidden in the ivory box; and someone must have taken it, as it was not found there. If you want the scarab, you must find who has taken it."

"Fool!" hissed the Greek. "Will you lie to me, when your life and the lives of your friends hang upon a thread?"

Mauleverer shrugged his shoulders.

"As you will, my lord!" snarled the Greek. "I can afford to wait! You will not escape from my hands! I leave you unbound—attempt to escape if you choose!" He waved his hand at the vast desert. "Leave this camp, and do you think you could find your path back to the Nile? Do you not know that you would perish of thirst in the sands? Yet I will warn you that if you take a step beyond the camp the Arabs will ride you down and spear you. Take thought, my lord—I can afford to wait! Either the Golden Scarab shall be placed in my hands, or you and your friends die in the desert! Dream of escape and rescue if you choose—you will soon come to your senses!"

The Greek swung away.

The Greyfriars fellows exchanged glances.

"Looks as if we're booked!" said Bob dismally.

"I'm sorry for this, you fellows!" said Mauleverer in a low voice.

"Not your fault, fathead!"

"I'd give the scarab like a shot to see you fellows clear! You know that, don't you?"

"But what the dickens has become of it?" said Bob.

"Goodness knows! Somebody on the dahabiyeh must have spotted where it was hidden and pinched it. Can't expect Kalizelos to believe that, though—he's not a trustful sort of johnny."

"Well, we're for it," said Harry Wharton quietly. "We've got to keep a stiff upper lip and see it through! Never say die! I'm glad Bunter's out of it."

"Oh, sar!" mumbled Hassan. "If you will write a writing to the noble lord Brooke, I, Hassan, the son of Suleiman, will carry it to Assuan—and surely you will not lose so many lives for a scarab?"

The juniors made no reply to that. They stretched themselves on the hard ground under the acacias and slept the sleep of utter weariness.

THE TENTH CHAPTER.

All Right for Bunter!

"OH lor'!" groaned Billy Bunter. He mopped the perspiration from his streaming brow.

Bunter's little fat legs were almost dropping off with fatigue. But he plugged desperately on in the blazing sunshine.

Bunter had watched the desert raiders ride away with the prisoners; thankful to see them go, thankful that he had not been on board the dahabiyeh when they came. Not till the wild riders had vanished did the fat junior venture to crawl out of the clump of tamarisks.

Then he did not return to the dahabiyeh. There was no safety on the houseboat of Mr. Maroudi. Bunter did not know whether the raiders might return—he did not even know whether any of them might have remained on board. He turned his face to the north, following the course of the Nile, and tramped away as fast as his fat legs could move, only anxious to get out of the danger-zone.

Mile after mile the fat Owl tramped on, guided by the river till the night was gone and the new day came. He might have obtained help at more than one village along the Nile; but at the sight of a turban or a tarboosh, the fat junior dodged, palpitating, out of sight, dreading an enemy. He was a little comforted when daylight came; but his fat legs were aching, and he groaned and grunted as he plugged on. How many miles he had covered he did not know; but he knew that he was now at a great distance from the dahabiyeh, and there had been no pursuit. Apparently, the Greek, whom he had seen among the raiders, had not given him a thought, and had forgotten his fat existence; and for once, Billy Bunter was glad to be forgotten.

The sun rose higher, and Bunter's fat brow streamed, and his fat legs ached as he tramped down the rolling Nile. Flesh and blood could stand no more, and Billy Bunter came to a halt at last.

His first thought had been simply to escape and get out of danger of sharing the fate of the Greyfriars party.

But as his terrors diminished, the fat Owl ceased to think wholly of himself, and gave a thought or two to the fellows who had been carried off into the Libyan Desert.

He had to get help somehow. Sir Reginald Brooke was at Assuan, waiting for the return of the dahabiyeh there, and Mauly's uncle was the man to take the matter in hand. Bunter did not know how far he was from Assuan, but he knew that it was many miles.

His fat little legs could carry him no farther, and he stopped under the shade of a date-palm, and grunted and groaned.

Every dark face on the Nile-shore was, to Bunter's terrified mind, an enemy or a possible enemy. A dozen times, at least, he had dodged out of the sight of a harmless fellahin.

But the sight of a fruit-boat on the Nile was reassuring. A felucca, with a cargo of fruit aboard, rowed by six brawny brown men, was coming down the river, and appeared in Bunter's sight as he stood panting under the palm. Even Bunter could not fear that the natives on the boat had any connection with the Sheikh Abdurrahman's gang of desert robbers.

He waved a fat hand and shouted to the boatmen.

Brown faces turned towards him inquiringly.

"Hi!" roared Bunter. "Stop! Give me a lift to Assuan! Hi!"

The rowers slowed down, still staring, and talking to one another in rather excited tones. The boat pulled in to the bank at last.

Two or three of the natives spoke to Bunter, but it was in a language of which he did not understand a word. But with gestures they invited him on board the felucca, and he plumped down into a seat with a gasp of relief.

"Assuan!" he gasped, pointing down the river.

The answer was in Arabic, but the brown men bent to their oars again and rowed on.

The felucca was slow, but it was ten times as fast as Bunter's tired, fat legs could have carried him on. Six long, heavy oars pulled steadily, and the heavy craft rolled on its way. The rowers gave the fat junior many curious looks as he sat and mopped his perspiring face, gasping for breath, and dabbed at flies. Obviously, they were interested in him.

It occurred to Bunter at last that they knew what had happened on the dahabiyeh, and guessed that he was one of the party of Faringhees that had been attacked by the riders from the desert.

He realised that the reis, and the Nubian crew, would have spread the news of the outrage long before this, and that it must have run like wildfire up and down the Nile.

Such news was certain to cause a sensation, and to spread far and wide, and Bunter realised, too, that most likely it had already reached Assuan. It was more than probable that Sir Reginald Brooke had already heard it.

Slowly, but steadily, the felucca pulled on down the Nile, under the blaze of the Egyptian sun.

Chug-chug-chug-chug!

It was an hour later that Bunter heard, without heeding, the chugging of a motor-boat on the river.

The motor-boat was coming up from the direction of Assuan and the Nile Dam. Bunter gave it a blink through his big spectacles, without interest. He had a glimpse of a white man's face looking towards him, and caught the gleam of an eyeglass in the sunlight.

There was a shout, and the felucca's crew ceased to row, and the motor-boat ran down on them. Bunter gave a yelp.

"Get on! Get on, I tell you! Get on to Assuan, you dummies! I jolly well won't pay you anything if you don't hurry!"

"Bunter!"

The fat junior gave a jump. It was the voice of Sir Reginald Brooke, calling to him from the motor-boat.

Bunter blinked round in amazement.

Beside the tall baronet stood the plump figure of Mr. Hilmi Maroudi of Cairo. Both were staring at Bunter, evidently astonished to see him in the felucca coming down the Nile.

"Oh!" gasped Bunter.

Mr. Maroudi spoke to the felucca's crew in Arabic, and the fruit-boat ranged alongside the motor-craft. Sir Reginald stretched out a hand to the fat junior and helped him on board. A handful of piastres were tossed to the brown men in the felucca, and they rowed on down the river.

The motor-boat immediately resumed its way up the Nile. Billy Bunter stood and gasped and mopped his brow, and blinked at Mauly's uncle through his big spectacles.

He could see the lines of deep anxiety in Sir Reginald's face, and guessed that the old baronet had already heard the news; indeed, he could guess, further, that it was the news of the raid that had brought Sir Reginald and his Egyptian friend up the Nile from Assuan that morning.

"Take courage, my dear friend," said Mr. Maroudi, in his low, pleasant voice. "This is one of the boys who has escaped—perhaps the others——"

"Bunter! Where is my nephew?" asked Sir Reginald, speaking quietly, but with a shake in his voice.

"They've got him!" gasped Bunter.

"Who?" snapped Sir Reginald.

"That beast Kalizelos——"

"You are sure it was the Greek?"

"I saw him!" groaned Bunter. "That Greek villain, and a swarm of awful Arabs—horrible-looking, savage beasts they——"

"News has reached Assuan of the attack on the dahabiyeh," said Sir Reginald, in the same quiet tone. "We have heard, so far, that a number of desert robbers attacked the houseboat and took away the schoolboys. We supposed that all had been taken—yet you are here——"

"I was ashore," explained Bunter. "I'd gone for a walk on the bank, and I jolly well kept out of sight when I saw them."

"That was fortunate, my young friend!" said Mr. Maroudi.

"Yes—just luck!" gasped Bunter. "But for that, I should be with them now—jolly lucky I was on shore! It couldn't have happened better, really! I might have been in the hands of those awful villains, along with the other chaps!"

Mr. Maroudi gave him a rather curious look, and Sir Reginald Brooke emitted a snort. Perhaps both the gentlemen considered that Billy Bunter might have evinced some desire to share the fate of the party, to sink or swim together. Such an idea as that was certainly not likely to occur to the fat mind of William George Bunter. He was sorry for the other fellows—but deeply thankful that he was not in their company. Matters were bad enough—but they might have been worse!

"Then my nephew and his friends are all prisoners?" asked the old baronet.

"All but me!" said Bunter.

Another snort from Sir Reginald, which might have implied that he did not count the fat Owl among his nephew's friends. Bunter wondered what the old donkey was snorting for.

"You saw them taken away?" asked Mr. Maroudi.

"Yes—tied on camels," said Bunter. "Kalizelos was there, and those two Arab beasts Yussef and Hamza, and a crowd of savage brutes——"

"I cannot understand it," said Sir Reginald. "The attack can only have been caused by that scoundrel Kalizelos' desire to possess the Golden Scarab. My nephew would never have submitted on his own account, but I should have expected him to give the scoundrel whatever he asked, to save his friends from savage enemies——"

Bunter gave a start.

"Oh crikey!" he ejaculated.

Sir Reginald stared at him, with a frown.

"They cannot have seized the scarab," went on the old baronet. "That is all that the Greek desired. I am convinced that he would have been willing to leave the party alone, had he gained what he wanted. No doubt it was safely concealed, and my nephew refused to reveal it. Yet, to save his friends, I should have expected——"

"Oh crikey! I—I say, I—I've got the scarab!" gasped Bunter.

"What?"

"I'd forgotten about it!" gasped the fat Owl. "I've got it in my pocket now! Mauly couldn't have handed it over, if he wanted to! Oh lor'!"

Sir Reginald stared at him.

"You have the scarab? How did it come into your hands, pray?"

"Oh! I—I—Mauly handed it to me to keep safely, you know!" stammered Bunter. "Being his best pal——"

"Nonsense!"

"Oh, really, sir——"

"If you have the scarab, let me see it!" snapped Sir Reginald. "I am quite assured that my nephew would never place it in your hands!"

"Well, here it is," grunted Bunter sulkily, and he fished out the matchbox from his pocket and opened it. "I've got it safe all right! Mauly trusted it to me, you know—he's got more faith in me than in the other fellows, of course. I never found where he had hidden it, you know."

"What?"

"I'm not the fellow to spy anything out, I hope," said Bunter, with dignity. "As for taking the rotten thing to hide it, to make Mauly sit up for being such a beast, I never even thought of such a thing."

Snort from Sir Reginald.

"Give it to me!" he grunted.

He took the Golden Scarab from the fat Owl. He scanned it carefully, and Mr. Maroudi's dark eyes dwelt on it curiously.

"This is the Scarab of A-Menah," said Sir Reginald, with a grunt. "But for this foolish boy's crass trickery my nephew might have ransomed himself and his friends by giving it up to the Greek."

"Perhaps it is fortunate," said Mr. Maroudi softly, "for your nephew and his friends will be rescued, my good friend; and the scarab is safe."

"It is of little value. I fail entirely to understand the Greek's desire to possess it, at the cost of danger and crime." Sir Reginald slipped the golden beetle into his pocket. "The legend attached to it can be nothing but a fable. I would gladly give it, and a thousand such, to see my nephew safe once more."

"That is the Greek's design," said Mr. Maroudi quietly. "But I have some power in this land, my good friend, and I am here. According to the report received at Assuan, it was the Sheikh Abdurrahman, once a follower of the Khalifa, who attacked the dahabiyeh with his men. If that is ascertained beyond doubt——"

"This boy may know!"

"You saw the leader of the desert riders, my young friend," said Mr. Maroudi. "You can tell us something of him."

"A fierce-looking beast with a hooked nose," said Bunter. "I heard Hassan tell the fellows on the dahabiyeh that he was the Sheikh Abdurrahman. Never heard of him before. Hassan said that the beast had fought as a boy against Kitchener at Omdurman."

Mr. Maroudi's face lightened.

"Then there is no doubt!" he said. "It is Abdurrahman, the robber of the Libyan Desert, who has aided the Greek in this raid!"

"Is that good news?" asked Sir Reginald, staring at the Egyptian. "I have heard of the man—a desperate and savage outcast, stained with the blood of many murders——"

"But a man who is known to me, and with whom I have eaten salt!" said the Egyptian tranquilly. "And now that I am assured, my good friend, that it is the Sheikh Abdurrahman into whose hands our little friends have fallen, I shall answer to you that I can save them. Upon my head be it!"

Billy Bunter blinked at the Egyptian, and then blinked round the motor-boat. He was wondering if there were any provisions on board. Fortunately there were, and Bunter sat down to a meal and forgot his troubles—and still more easily the troubles of the other fellows—as he packed away the foodstuffs, and the motor-boat chugged on swiftly up the Nile.

THE ELEVENTH CHAPTER.

The Messenger!

NIGHT in the desert!

Tall, feathery palms waved their fronds in the light of the moon.

Far and wide, on all sides of the little oasis, stretched the Libyan Desert, glimmering in the moonlight, trackless, arid, illimitable.

Only a line of low, rocky hills, in the distance, broke the level of the desert.

Save in that one spot, where the oasis was fed by a spring, all was sandy, arid, barren. From the shadows of the barren plain came a distant sound, which the Greyfriars fellows thrilled to realise was the roar of a roaming lion.

After the noonday halt the desert raiders had pushed on again, ever and ever westward, deeper and deeper into the desert. Through the long, sunny afternoon they had ridden, and under the burning sunset, and till the moon rose in the velvety sky. Then they reached the oasis—evidently a place well known to them—and camped for the night.

The juniors wondered whether this was the final halt. They heard the talk among the Arabs without understanding it. But Hassan told them that the next morning the ride was to go on, farther and farther. Desperate ruffian as the Sheikh Abdurrahman was, he feared vengeance for so daring an outrage as a raid on a dahabiyeh on the Nile, and he intended to put a vast distance between himself and possible pursuit by the Egyptian troops. The halt at the oasis was only for a rest till dawn, as Hassan learned from the talk of the Arabs.

There was something like despair in the hearts of the schoolboys. The desert had swallowed them, far from help and hope. It was not even possible to pay the ransom demanded by the Greek, for the Golden Scarab had vanished, and Lord Mauleverer knew no more than the Greek where to lay hands on it. Unless there was pursuit and rescue they were doomed to leave their bones in the desert, and how could rescue reach them in the trackless wilderness of sand and rock?

Yussef and Hamza had put up a tent for the Greek, the hardy desert robbers wrapping themselves in their cloaks to sleep on the earth by the sides of their camels. Of the juniors, Abdurrahman and his men took little or no notice. They were not concerned with them. At a word from the Greek who had hired them they would have cut off the schoolboys' heads, without a moment's hesitation or remorse; but so long as Kalizelos desired to keep them prisoners, the Arabs left them to themselves.

Escape was impossible; the juniors hardly thought of it. They were left unbound; but the swift camels could have run them down at once if they had wandered from the camp. And escape into the arid desert meant nothing but death by hunger and thirst. Once, when Johnny Bull moved out beyond the sleeping camels to look across the plain, a blow from the butt of a spear drove him back again, and the look of the Arab who drove him in showed that he would willingly use the point if the junior resisted.

A supper of dhurra bread and dates and water was given to the prisoners. Hopeless as their position seemed, the juniors were keeping up their courage. It was Hassan who was plunged into the depths of woe. He was wanted only as a messenger to take word from Mauleverer to his uncle; and when he was no longer wanted, if it was certain that no message would be sent, Hassan expected to be knocked on the head as a useless encumbrance.

Hassan, torn and soiled and dusty, looked little like the gorgeous, smiling dragoman who had guided the juniors at Cairo and Luxor, and sailed with them on Mr. Maroudi's dahabiyeh. If Hassan retained any hope, it was not in the Egyptian authorities, or in Sir Reginald Brooke, but in the power of the Egyptian millionaire, Hilmi Maroudi, the protector of his "lordly gentlemen." But the dismal, dolorous expression on Hassan's brown face showed that he doubted whether even Hilmi Maroudi's arm could stretch across the Libyan Desert to save them.

After they had eaten their supper the juniors sat under the tall palms of the oasis, and wached the moonlit plain. The camels and the Arabs were sleeping, and Kalizelos, in his tent, was perhaps sleeping, too; perhaps dreaming of the "Eye of Osiris," which he now believed to be almost in his grasp. Two or three of the savage outcasts were keeping watch, and a faint mutter of Arabic reached the juniors as the ruffians talked together.

The moon that sailed high above the desert was the moon that had shone down so peaceably the previous night on the juniors on the dahabiyeh; the same soft and silvery light fell in a flood on the desert, yet it seemed to them that they were in a different world. So, indeed, they were, for they had dropped back from the twentieth century into the ages of barbarism.

"We're for it, and no mistake!" said Bob Cherry, breaking a long silence. "I'm glad Bunter's out of it!"

"Yes, that's so much to the good," said Nugent. "Lucky the fat idiot took that stroll ashore last night, after all."

"Well, it would make matters worse if we had him grumbling and grousing here!" grunted Johnny Bull. "Thank goodness we haven't!"

"The thankfulness is terrific!" murmured the Nabob of Bhanipur.

There was silence again.

Through the silence there came a sound from the distant desert. The juniors saw the Arab sentinels start up, and stare away across the plain in the brightness of the moon.

"That's a horse or a camel!" said Bob. "I—I wonder—— Hassan, old bean, do you think there's a chance they've got after us?"

Hassan shook a dismal head.

"No, sar. We are in one queer street," he answered lugubriously. "The soldiers will seek, but they will not find. That is a deadly cert, as you say in your language."

Thud! Thud! Thud!

The beat of swift hoofs was clearer now. A horseman was riding towards the camp at the oasis at a furious speed.

The juniors rose to their feet and looked across the sand. Far away in the moonlight they sighted the figure of an Arab rider on a powerful horse.

"One of the gang, I suppose," said Nugent, with a sigh. "Nobody can know where to look for these villains except their friends."

Hassan fixed his eyes on the approaching horseman. It was evident that the dragoman had no hope that the rider's coming meant rescue. But a strange expression came over his face as the galloping horseman drew nearer and clearer in the light of the moon.

"Bismillah!" muttered Hassan. "It is Selim, the son of Mustapha, who comes—Selim of Shellal, who has served the great Maroudi."

"You know the man?" asked Harry.

"Hassan knows all peoples in valley of the Nile, sar," said the dragoman, with a touch of his old manner. "Yes, sar, Hassan know everything! Selim, the son of Mustapha of Shellal, rides with the caravans that do business for the great Maroudi. Many times I have seen him. By the beard of the Prophet, it may yet be possible that the great Maroudi may help us, even here in the Libyan Desert. His power is great."

All the Arabs were on their feet now, watching the horseman as he came. The dark, fierce eyes of the Sheikh Abdurrahman were fixed on him. But there was no hostility in their looks. It was plain that Selim, the son of Mustapha, was known to them, and known on friendly terms. The juniors did not understand.

"You say that that man is in the service of Mr. Maroudi?" asked Harry Wharton.

"Yes, sar."

"Then how can he be friendly with these robbers and thieves—they look as if he was a friend."

Hassan grinned.

"Oh, sar, in the desert it is different!" he said. "On the banks of the Nile Selim would not call the Sheikh Abdurrahman his friend. But in the desert I think he pay backsheesh to the sheikh, to permit the caravans to pass in safety. Abhurrahman is one terrible man, my lordly sar; he is feared in the desert. And if Selim pay him backsheesh, no robber of Libya dare to lay one finger on the great Maroudi's caravans."

"Oh!" said Harry. He understood now how an agent of Mr. Maroudi might have dealings with a robber chief of the desert. It was plain, at all events, that Selim was known to the horde; some of them made him welcoming gestures as he galloped up.

The Arab pulled in his horse, foaming and dust-covered, showing very plain signs of having been driven hard. He leaped lightly to the ground, approached Abdurrahman, and salaamed before the sheikh. They proceeded to talk in Arabic; but they stood too far away for Hassan and the juniors to hear what they said. The Greyfriars fellows watched curiously.

It was clear that Selim had ridden desperately hard from the Nile, to reach the camp at the oasis. His brown face was caked with dried sweat and the dust of the desert, and his horse, powerful beast as it was, was almost exhausted. He was speaking breathlessly, but urgently, to the sheikh, and from time to time Abdurrahman nodded his head as he replied in curt tones.

Many times, as they stood speaking, both of them glanced towards the tent of the Greek, Kalizelos, as the juniors did not fail to notice. Once they caught a cruel, sardonic grin on the sheikh's hard, brown face, as he looked towards the tent of the sleeping Greek.

"I wonder——" muttered Bob.

"I, Hassan, do not understand!" muttered the dragoman. "They do not talk of the safe passage of a caravan, my lordly sars; they speak of the Greek, for they look towards the tent of that son of ten thousand dogs and pigs! Wahyaten-nabi! May it be that the power of Maroudi may reach us here!"

The juniors looked at one another, with beating hearts. They would have given much to hear, and to understand, the talk between the desert sheikh and the man who had ridden in such desperate haste from the distant Nile. Twice or thrice they saw the black eyes of Selim rest on them, and they knew that he was speaking of them.

Hassan made an attempt to edge nearer to the speakers, but a threatening gesture from an Arab drove him back. There was little, perhaps, on which to build hope, and yet all the prisoners in the camp in the oasis felt that the coming of Selim from the Nile spelled hope for them.

THE TWELFTH CHAPTER.
Hope!

KALIZELOS, the Greek, stepped out of his tent under the palm-trees, in the sunrise of the Libyan Desert. He glanced towards the Greyfriars juniors with a grim smile on his olive face.

Harry Wharton & Co. were already up, and eating a breakfast of maize bread and dates—their eyes turning incessantly to the east—the direction of the distant and unseen Nile. From that direction, if rescue came at all, it would come, and though it seemed like hoping against hope, the chums of the Remove hoped.

Selim, the man from Shellal, on the Nile, was still in the camp; they had seen him among the robbers. He had not approached them, but his presence seemed to give hope. He was at least some sort of a connection between them and their Egyptian friend, Hilmi Maroudi.

The hope that was in the hearts of the schoolboys was reflected in their faces, and the Greek read it there, and it brought a grim smile to his olive visage. So far as Konstantinos Kalizelos could see, at all events, there was no hope for his prisoners. Surrounded by savage Arab robbers, and the boundless desert, they were in his hands like birds in a cage.

The Greek, after glancing at the juniors, stood looking about him before the tent. The juniors heard him call to one of the Arabs, who shook his head in reply. Hassan, the dragoman, started a little, and his keen eyes flashed towards the Greek.

"Inshallah!" murmured Hassan.

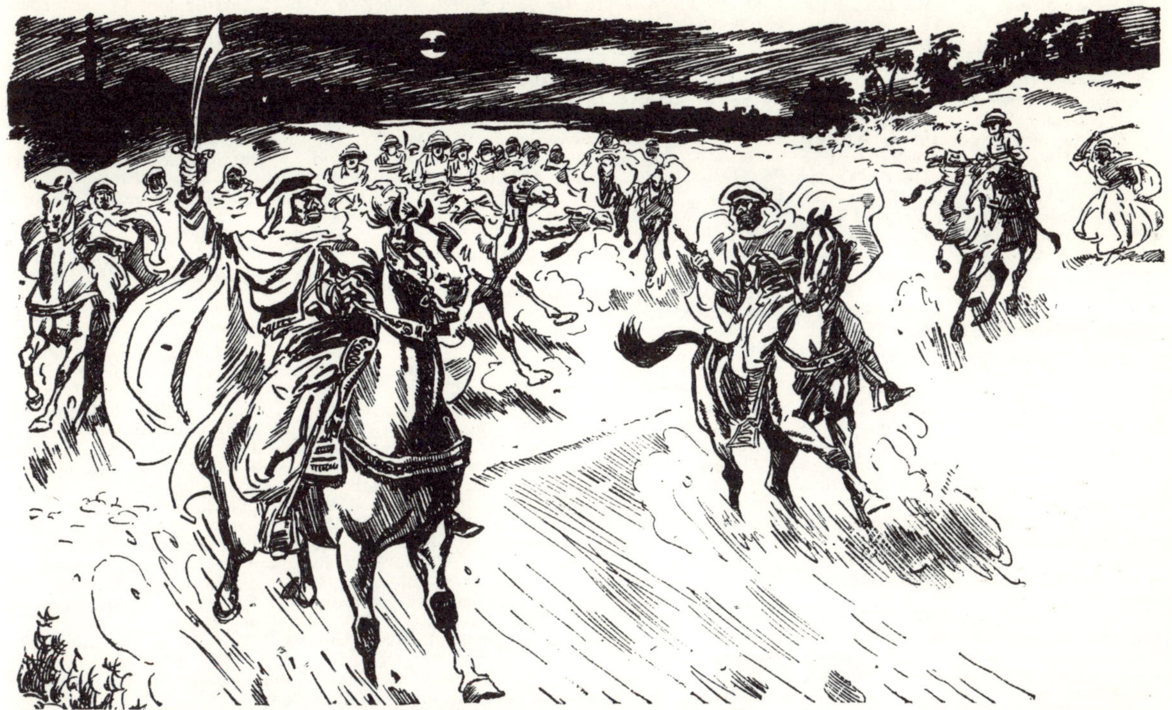

Harry Wharton & Co. were bound and hoisted on the spare camels and, with a rapid beat of hoofs, the party rode away. The sheikh galloped on in front, and after him thundered the camels, driven to speed by blows and cries from their riders!

"What's up, Hassan?" asked Harry Wharton. He could see that the dragoman had been struck by what was said in Arabic between the Greek and the robber.

"This is one strange thing," said Hassan. "Kalizelos, he ask where are his Arabs—Yussef and Hamza. The man he ask do not know."

"They're in the camp somewhere, I suppose," said Harry.

"I do not see them, noble sar," answered Hassan, "and I remember that I hear in the night a sound of camels that go fast. This is strange."

The juniors watched the Greek rather curiously.

It was easy to see, from where they sat under the palms, over the whole of the little oasis, which was merely a small bunch of palms in the midst of the desert. Now that they gave the matter attention, they could see that Yussef, the hawk-faced Arab, and Hamza, the man with the scar, were not present. The look of the Greek was perplexed and angry. It seemed that the Greek's two native confederates had left the camp during the night, evidently without the knowledge of their master, and had not returned.

They saw Kalizelos approach the Sheikh Abdurrahman, who was standing in the sand watching the east, like the juniors.

A murmur of voices reached their ears, but they understood nothing of the Arabic. But Hassan, who caught the words between the man from Cairo and the Arab sheikh, breathed hard.

"This is very strange!" he repeated.

"Construe!" grinned Bob. "Tell us what they're saying, Hassan."

"Somethin's going on, you men," murmured Lord Mauleverer. "I can't make it out, but I sort of fancy things ain't so rosy for Kalizelos as he fancied they were."

The juniors could see that Kalizelos was puzzled and irritated, while the sheikh, on the other hand, was cold and curt.

"Kalizelos, he want to know where are his servants, Yussef and Hamza," said Hassan. "Abdurrahman say that in the night they take camels and ride. The Greek he very angry. He do not understand why is this. He is what you call in English, riddled."

"Puzzled!" grinned Bob.

"Yes, sar, he is puzzled and riddled to a great and considerable extent," said Hassan. "This is a very strange happening!"

The Greek at last went back to his tent.

Abdurrahman stared after him for a moment, and the juniors read in his hard face the cold, ironical, sardonic smile they had seen on it before. If the Greek was puzzled, the Greyfriars fellows were equally so. It looked as if there was some rift in the lute, as if matters were not going as smoothly as before, between the Greek and the desert thieves he had hired for his work. How and why, the prisoners could not guess.

"Oh, sars!" breathed Hassan. "You see that look of the sheikh? He is a terrible man! Kalizelos has paid him much backsheesh for this work. But what faith is there in a thief of the desert? Oh, sars, I think I see in this the hand of the great Maroudi!"

"Maroudi!" repeated Bob.

"Maroudi is a great and powerful man," said Hassan. "He is as rich and powerful as a caliph! Is he not the friend of my lordly gentlemen, who saved him the life when Kalizelos attacked him in his palace at Cairo? Oh, sars, I think it may be the will of Allah, and of Mahomet, his Prophet, that Maroudi may save us yet!"

"He will have to get a move on, if we're going on into the desert," said Nugent, with a faint smile. "You heard the scoundrels saying that we ride again at dawn, Hassan."

"It is true," said the dragoman. "But there is a change. The camels still lie in the sand; there is no sign that we ride. And now it is long past dawn, my noble sar."

"There's Selim!" muttered Johnny Bull.

The man from Shellal passed in sight of the group of juniors. He gave them a glance as he passed, with a smile and a flash of white teeth. But he did not approach the group, passing on and joining Abdurrahman, and standing by his side watching the desert to the east.

The prisoners in the oasis felt their hearts beating more quickly.

Something—something strange and mysterious, behind the scenes—was going on in the Arab camp, that was clear. What ever it was, did it mean hope to the prisoners? They could not help thinking that it did.

At all events, there was no sign of the robbers breaking camp. The camels lay undisturbed, the Arabs loafed and lounged idly among the palms. Abdurrahman stood like a statue gazing across the desert to the east.

It could scarcely be for pursuers, for enemies, that he was watching. At a hint of danger the desert thieves would have been in the saddle, fleeing for their worthless lives. For whom, for what, was the sheikh watching?

Then from the sunlit level of the sandy plain to the east two moving dots came in sight. They were evidently horsemen approaching the camp at a gallop, though at present mere moving specks in the great distance. Harry Wharton & Co. watched them with their hearts in their eyes. It was for these riders, it was clear, that the sheikh was waiting and watching. Who were they? What did their coming portend?

The thudding of hoofs was heard at last. Closer and clearer came the two galloping riders. One of them wore the Egyptian tarboosh, the other a white man's pith helmet. There was something familiar about both of them, more and more so as they drew nearer. But the schoolboys hardly dared to believe what their eyes told them.

"One of them's Maroudi!" said Bob in a low voice, breaking the tense silence.

"And the other——"

"Nunky!" said Lord Mauleverer quietly.

"And that means——" said Bob, with a deep breath.

"It must mean that we're saved!"

"The savefulness is terrific," chuckled Hurree Jamset Ram Singh.

"Great and powerful is Maroudi!" grinned Hassan. "Oh, my lordly gentlemen, the day you gain the friendship of that great man is a day worthy to be marked with a white stone. It is Maroudi! There is no God but one God, and Mahomet is his Prophet!"

With a thudding of hoofs, a jingle of spurs and bridles, the two horsemen dashed up to the oasis and dismounted.

THE THIRTEENTH CHAPTER.

The Golden Scarab Gives Up Its Secret!

THE Sheikh Abdurrahman salaamed low before Hilmi Maroudi. The Egyptian gave the juniors a glance and a smile, and then plunged into talk with the desert sheikh in Arabic. Sir Reginald Brooke came over to the juniors.

"Jolly glad to see you again, nunky!" said Lord Mauleverer.

"The gladfulness is terrific, esteemed and venerable sir!" declared Hurree Jamset Ram Singh.

"What-ho!" chuckled Bob.

Hassan, the dragoman, was salaaming to the old baronet as if he had a spring in his back. The dragoman almost capered with joy.

"Thank Heaven I find you safe, my boys," said Sir Reginald, "and thank Heaven again for such a friend as Mr. Maroudi!"

"Then it's all right?" asked Harry.

Sir Reginald smiled.

"I believe so, or I should not be here without help. Where we are, I have no idea, but Mr. Maroudi knows the desert as well as he knows the streets of Cairo. I gather that he has some influence over these wretches. I trust to him entirely. He is a wonderful man."

"And Bunter?" asked Bob. "Seen anything of Bunter?"

"Bunter is safe," said Sir Reginald. "We came on him on the Nile and took him back to the dahabiyeh with us. He is there now. The troops are out from Wady Halfa searching for these villains, but they have, of course, no knowledge where to look for them. But for Mr. Maroudi——"

The schoolboys glanced towards the Egyptian. He was in deep talk with the sheikh. Evidently it was an amicable interview. Even the fierce, proud sheikh of the desert was treating the Egyptian with marked respect. No doubt "backsheesh" figured in the talk.

Abdurrahman, who had hired himself and his gang to the Greek for a great price, was no doubt prepared to betray the Greek for a greater price. Treachery came as easily to him as breathing. Fear of Maroudi's power counted for much; backsheesh, it was probable, counted for more. Obviously Maroudi had counted on success when he rode out with only a single companion to meet the robbers at the solitary oasis in the Libyan Desert. The schoolboys did not know, or care to know, the details of that talk, but they knew that Hilmi Maroudi had saved them.

"I was surprised, astounded, when Mr. Maroudi proposed to me to ride into the desert, and without armed forces," went on Sir Reginald. "But he pointed out that even if guided, the troops would have had no chance of running down such elusive scoundrels in their native desert; moreover, the desert Arabs are much more likely to kill their prisoners than to allow them to be rescued. It seems that Mr. Maroudi dispatched a swift rider to reach these Arabs and detain them till he could arrive. All has gone as he told me, though I hardly dared to believe that it would be so. He is a wonderful man and a faithful friend. My dear, dear boys, you are saved!"

"Hallo, hallo, hallo!" ejaculated Bob Cherry. "Look!"

There was the sound of a struggle, and a yelling voice, hoarse with rage. Kalizelos, the Greek, had seen the arrival of the baronet and Mr. Maroudi from his tent, staring at them with amazed and unbelieving eyes. For several minutes the Greek stood like a man in a trance.

Then he rushed towards the sheikh. Three or four of the robbers, closing round, grasped his arms.

The Greek, mad with rage, struggled furiously.

Abdurrahman gave him one cold, careless glance over his shoulder and turned his head away again and resumed his conversation with Maroudi. The Egyptian did not deign to look at him at all.

Struggling, shrieking, foaming at the mouth with rage, realising at last that his treacherous allies had turned on him, the Greek tore and wrenched in the grasp of the Arabs.

He was borne to the ground, and a camel-rope was knotted round him, securing his arms and legs.

He lay a helpless prisoner under the palms, spitting like a cat with fury. His screaming voice rang through the oasis and echoed far on the desert. Abdurrahman turned his head again and snapped a word in Arabic. One of the robbers approached the Greek and struck him with the flat of a scimitar. It was a hint to be silent, and Kalizelos, grinding his teeth, was silent.

"Looks as if the jolly old Greek has lost this game, after all," remarked Lord Mauleverer.

"Just a few!" grinned Bob Cherry.

The conference between Maroudi and the sheikh ended at last. Abdurrahman salaamed low, evidently satisfied with the outcome. He called an order to his men and they ran to their camels. The long-legged beasts lurched up from the sand.

"They're going!" breathed Bob.

Abdurrahman mounted his black Barbary horse and placed himself at the head of the troop. Once more he saluted Mr. Maroudi, and then, with a clatter and a jingle, rode away into the desert, to the west, followed by his crew. With a thudding of hoofs, a squealing of camels the whole gang of robbers disappeared into the waste of sand.

Glad enough were the Greyfriars fellows to see them go.

Mr. Maroudi came up to the schoolboys with a smile on his dark, plump face.

"We meet again, in happy circumstances, my little friends," he said. "Now we have but to ride back to the Nile, and I have prevailed on that very great scoundrel, Abdurrahman, to leave you camels to ride. This is a happy day."

"You've saved us, sir," said Harry Wharton. "It's not easy to tell you how grateful we are!"

"Did you not save me, in my house at Cairo?" smiled Mr. Maroudi.

"It is a tit for a tat, as you say in the noble English language," chuckled Hassan.

"The gratitude of our ridiculous selves is both terrific and preposterous, absurd sir!" said Hurree Jamset Ram Singh.

Mr. Maroudi grinned.

Then his face became grave as he glanced at the writhing Greek. A gleam shot into his dark eyes.

"We have to deal with Kalizelos!" he said. "The crimes of this man have filled the cup to overflowing, and it is fitting that he should not live to do more evil."

"Oh gad!" exclaimed Lord Mauleverer. "Hold on, sir! That johnny won't do any more harm. The scarab's lost."

Kalizelos writhed over and fixed his black eyes on the schoolboy earl. Mauleverer gave him a cheery nod.

"You may believe me now, old bean, though you're not a trustin' sort of johnny," he said. "I told you the scarab had been pinched on the dahabiyeh. Even a doubtin' Thomas like you will believe me now you hear me tell my uncle so—what?"

The Greek made no reply.

"My dear boy," said Sir Reginald Brooke with a smile. "The scarab was lost, but it has been found. It was that stupid boy, Bunter, who removed it from the hiding-place on the dahabiyeh."

"Bunter!" exclaimed the juniors.

"Oh gad! If I don't kick that fat villain from one end of the dahabiyeh to the other——"

"He handed it over to me, and I have it here," said Sir Reginald, and he drew the Golden Scarab from his pocket.

"Great gad!"

In the old baronet's hand the Golden Scarab glistened in the sun. The Greek's eyes snapped as he saw it.

"That's the jolly old article!" said Lord Mauleverer. "Perhaps it's just as well, as things turned out, that that fat idiot played silly tricks with it. Kalizelos would have had it." He gave the Greek a grin. "Feel inclined to cough up the giddy old secret now, old thing?"

"Fool!" snarled the Greek.

"Give me ear, my friends," said Mr. Maroudi quietly. "It is known to us that the scarab has a secret—the secret of the Eye of Osiris. That secret Kalizelos has read in an ancient papyrus, and it is known only to him. That secret he will now reveal."

"Never!" hissed the Greek.

Maroudi stood looking down at the bound man with a calm, grave face.

"These young English lords are my friends," he said. "In this land of Egypt my power is great enough to protect them; but soon they return to their own country, and my arm is not long enough to reach to an island in the North Sea. If you live, O Man of Evil Deeds, you will follow them to their own land. You must die, Konstantinos Kalizelos."

The Greek stared up at him. He uttered no word.

"Mr. Maroudi——" exclaimed Wharton.

The Egyptian raised his hand.

"Do not speak, my little friend," he said gravely. "It is written that men of evil deeds shall die for the wrong they have done. The life of this wicked man is in my hand, and only on one condition will I spare it."

He spoke in Arabic to Selim.

The man from Shellal took his scimitar in hand and approached the Greek, who stared at him with dilated eyes. The keen, bare blade flashed in the sunlight as it was raised.

"Listen to me, O Kalizelos!" said Hilmi Maroudi. "You who know the secret of the scarab utter that secret to the young English lord, who is the possessor of the Scarab of A-Menah. You who know what was written by the scribe of A-Menah, speak your knowledge." He struck a match and held it up, burning with a steady flame in the stillness of the desert. "If he has not spoken by the time this match has burned out, you, Selim, strike off his head."

"On my head be it!" said Selim.

There was a terrible pause. The juniors would have spoken, but they knew that it was useless. Maroudi was their friend and protector, but he was master there, and he was grimly, irrevocably resolved. Only by giving up the secret could the Greek be made harmless; and if he did not give it up, it was death! Sir Reginald Brooke opened his lips, and closed them again. It was for Maroudi to give orders, and opposition was futile. The Egyptian was grim, and in terrible earnest.

The still flame burned down.

The Greek panted, and great drops of sweat came on his brow. The secret was dear to him, but life was dearer.

The match burned out.

There was a flash of sweeping steel as Selim swept up the scimitar for the fatal blow. A scream broke from the Greek.

"Hold! I will speak!"

Maroudi signed to the man from Shellal. The scimitar remained poised in the air.

"Speak!" said Maroudi coldly.

"What I have read in the papyrus is this," said the Greek, in a hollow voice. "The great diamond, the Eye of Osiris, is hidden within the scarab. This was written by the scribe of A-Menah for the guidance of his son, Menarsis! The Golden Scarab is hollow, and the Eye of Osiris is within."

The Egyptian gave him a keen look.

"If this be true, you live!" he said.

"Oh gad!" said Lord Mauleverer. "Anybody got a pair of nut-crackers?"

The juniors laughed, relieved by the breaking of the tension.

Eager eyes were turned on the golden beetle.

The Greek's statement was simply amazing; such a thought had never crossed the minds of the juniors. To all appearance, the Scarab of A-Menah was made of solid gold. Yet they knew that Kalizelos must be speaking the truth; he had spoken it only to save his life.

The scarab passed from hand to hand; but the keenest eye could detect no sign of an opening. Maroudi's eyes turned doubtfully on the Greek; those of Kalizelos, in terror, on the gleaming scimitar poised above his head.

"Unwind the head of the beetle," said Kalizelos hoarsely. "Thus it is written in the papyrus—I know no more."

Watched breathlessly by all the juniors, Lord Mauleverer gripped the head of the beetle in finger and thumb and attempted to unwind it. For a full minute he failed—then there was a movement in the metal, and the golden head of the scarabeus unwound. It came off in Mauly's fingers, leaving the golden body of the beetle open.

From the opening came a dazzling flash, almost blinding in its brilliancy, from the hidden contents of the scarab. It was the flash of the great diamond that human eyes had not seen since the reign of Rameses the Second—the flash of the "Eye of Osiris."

Lord Mauleverer tipped it out into his palm.

It lay there, scintillating and blazing in the sun; a huge diamond, glowing with strange lights. The schoolboys stared at it breathlessly.

Kalizelos gave a groan. He was looking, at last, on the Eye of Osiris that he had so long and desperately sought; but he was looking his last on it. The great diamond, worth the ransom of many kings, was lost to him for ever.

"It is the Eye of Osiris!" said Hilmi Maroudi, in a hushed voice. "For three thousand years it has lain hidden —and now it is yours, my young friend."

Lord Mauleverer shook his head.

"Not mine!" he said quietly. "This diamond is the property of the Egyptian Government, and will be handed over to them."

"Oh, Mauly!" gasped Bob Cherry.

The Egyptian gave Mauleverer a very curious look.

"It is true," he said. "There is a law in Egypt concerning treasures that are found! Yet——"

"Fool!" muttered Kalizelos.

Lord Mauleverer glanced at the Greek with a smile.

"Take it, Mr. Maroudi," he said. "I can trust you to hand it over in the proper quarter! You approve, nunky?"

"My dear boy!" was all Sir Reginald could say.

"Take it, Mr. Maroudi! Hassan's got his eye on it already——"

"Oh, sar!" gasped the dragoman.

"I will take it and it shall be placed in the Museum at Cairo," said Mr. Maroudi gravely. "And there shall be an inscription that it was found and given to the people of Egypt by a noble English lord!"

"Like the scarab, Mr. Kalizelos?" asked Lord Mauleverer politely. "You can have it now, if you like—a parting present."

"Fool!"

Lord Mauleverer laughed, and slipped the hollow scarab into his pocket.

"I'll keep it as a jolly old souvenir," he said.

The Greek was released and allowed to take his camel. With a black and bitter brow, he rode away from the oasis and disappeared from the sight of the Greyfriars fellows—and they were glad to see the last of him.

• • • • • •

"I say, you fellows!"

"Hallo, hallo, hallo!"

"You've got back!" grunted Bunter, as the juniors came on board the dahabiyeh the following day with Mr. Maroudi and Sir Reginald, and the smiling dragoman. "Had a rough time, what? Did they give you anything to eat?"

"Ha, ha, ha!"

"I saved the scarab for you, anyhow, Mauly," said Billy Bunter. "I suppose old Brooke's told you. Foresight, you know, and presence of mind——"

"You fat villain!" said Lord Mauleverer. "I was goin' to kick you——"

"Oh, really, Mauly——"

"But it's all right! We've found the jolly old treasure."

"Oh crikey! Where is it?" gasped Bunter.

"In Mr. Maroudi's pocket."

"You silly ass! I don't believe in trusting these niggers! I say, Mauly, old man, I'll look after it for you."

"Mauly's handed it over to jolly old Egypt!" chuckled Bob Cherry. "It's going into the museum at Cairo."

"The silly idiot!" gasped Bunter.

"Ha, ha, ha!"

"You silly dummy—I mean, look here, old chap, get it away from that nigger and give it to a pal, and I say—yarrrroooop! Leave off kicking me, you beasts! I can call a nigger a nigger if I like, and I can jolly well say—yarooooh!"

• • • • •

Harry Wharton & Co. sailed back in the dahabiyeh to Assuan, where they took a kind and friendly farewell of Mr. Maroudi. From Assuan the train bore them to Alexandria, where they took the steamer for home. The holiday in Egypt was over—and they all agreed that it had been a great time! Still, they were glad that they were going to see Greyfriars again, and they looked forward cheerily to the new term at the old school.

THE END.

(That ends Harry Wharton & Co.'s holiday in Egypt. Next week they return to Greyfriars again, and are starred in the first grand story of a new and sensational series. The yarn is entitled: "THE WORST BOY IN THE FORM!" Tell all your pals about it.)

OUR THRILLING STORY OF HIGHWAYMAN ADVENTURE!

The Red Falcon!

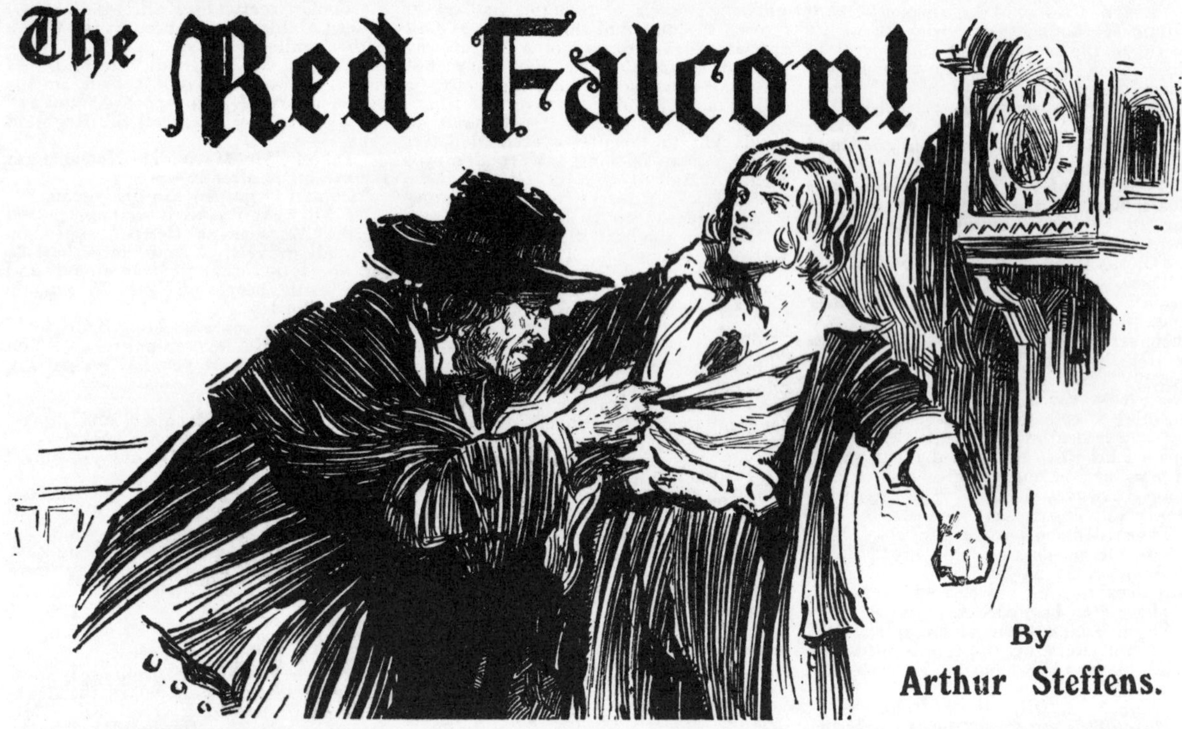

By

Arthur Steffens.

READ THIS FIRST.

Convicted of robbing the Earl of Huntford of a diamond star, Hal Lovett and Jerry McLean are conveyed to the convict hulk Ethalion, anchored at Woolwich—Hal to serve a sentence of seven years and McLean to await deportation. As the result of a prearranged plan, the convicts fire the ship, and Hal and Jerry escape in the blackness of the night, eventually reaching Blackheath, where they stay at an inn named the Swan With Two Necks. Hal and Jerry are returning from a trip to London when suddenly their coach is held up by a highwayman.

Held Up!

THE coachman's foot stepped on the brake and jammed it down on the iron-shod wheels. The postboy behind, searching for a weapon, was ordered fiercely to "Drop that and get down!"—an order he promptly obeyed. Then the horseman, whose eyes glittered like diamonds through the hole in the crude mask which hid his face, came up closer, with his second pistol levelled.

"Drop those reins!" he said to the driver, who was by this time shivering like a jelly.

The man obeyed.

"Now I'll trouble you gentlemen to drop your money in my hat!" said the highwayman sternly. "You may add your watches and your jewels, or anything of value you may carry! I'll advise you gentlemen inside who are searching for a pistol that I am fingering a hair trigger, and that my gun is liable to go off without warning! Ah! You are sitting up! That's better!"

The coach-robber urged his horse—a bony and sorry-looking steed, Hal was quick to notice—close up to the coach. Into the hat he held crown downwards the trembling passengers began to drop their money and their valuables.

Under the chin of one fat man inside the coach, who was more obstinate than the others, the highwayman jerked the cold steel barrel of his pistol.

"Come, come!" he roared. "You can't tell me a guinea is all you've got! Feel in your pockets, friend, and find some more, or my gun shall pop!"

With a savage oath, the passenger added a bag-purse to the rest of the loot, then subsided on the padded seat in a kind of faint.

Having ridden all round the coach, the highwayman came back to the front seat and covered McLean with his pistol extended at arm's length.

"Now, sirs, you look well-to-do!" he cried. "What about you?"

The coolness and daring of the robber thrilled Hal. But there was more about him and his horse which startled the boy. That bony steed, quite unsuited to the daring work of its master, was none other, Hal knew, than the wretched animal Jerry McLean had rescued from the shafts of the farmer's cart when he robbed the man of the clothes—the horse which had enabled him in safety to reach the Swan With Two Necks.

And not only was the horse familiar, but the rasping voice of the highwayman as well.

Hal gripped Jerry by the arm.

"You must know that voice, Jerry!" he whispered excitedly.

The highwayman was growing impatient. To rob a stage coach single-handed was perilous work. One had to be expeditious and stand no nonsense to get away with it.

"Come, gentlemen!" said the horseman, beginning to show anger. "Your money, IF YOU PLEASE!"

But Jerry did not hand out the little money he had left. Instead, he leant forward on his box seat and cried:

"Jack Pryse, don't you know me?"

If the driver of the coach heard, McLean did not care. Neither did Hal.

As for the highwayman—with a loud, bellowing laugh, he lowered his pistol-arm.

"Jerry, by all that's wonderful!" he cried. "And the kid, too! You may keep your money Jerry. Kid, I'll be seeing you later. Now, my bonnie mare, come up; we must away!"

Even as he swung his bony horse round there came a clattering of hoofs back along the way the coach had come. It was the echoing beat of horses ridden hard.

At that moment the moon swung out of a bank of cloud and silvered the highway. Looking back, Hal saw a posse of men coming along the road, leaving a cloud of dust behind them. He caught the glint of metal, and saw scabbards swinging as the horsemen rode along

Then the coachman began to yell.

"It's the Bow Street patrol! They'll catch the thief, by jiminy!"

Setting a leg up on the lower step, he reached out for a leather hold. As he did so, however, Hal leapt into the driver's seat, gathered up the reins, and began to pull the horses round. They obeyed in huddled, prancing confusion.

"Cut your stick, Jack!" shouted Jerry McLean.

Waiting for no further urging, Pryse rode his sorry horse into the night.

Hal had by this time got the leaders dancing up a grassy slope which bordered the road, and, yanking at the reins, he brought them round so violently that the coach reared up on its near-side wheels only.

The coachman, thrown into the dust as the coach moved, was scrambling to his feet, fuming wildly.

"Dang it!" he yelled. "You'll have the whole lot over!"

Which was exactly what Hal wanted to do—and did. One last mighty pull at the reins at the crucial moment, and over went the coach. It struck the ground with a rending crash, and the horses came down in a struggling heap with it.

Jerry and Hal were hurled from their box seat to the ground; passengers came tumbling from the top seats in a panic-stricken jumble; the men inside could

Printed and published every Saturday by the Proprietors, The Amalgamated Press, Ltd., The Fleetway House, Farringdon Street, London, E.C.4. Advertisement offices: The Fleetway House, Farringdon Street, London, E.C.4. Registered for transmission by Canadian Magazine Post. Subscription rates: Inland and Abroad, 11s. per annum; 5s. 6d. for six months. Sole Agents for Australia and New Zealand: Messrs. Gordon & Gotch, Ltd., and for South Africa: Central News Agency, Ltd.—Saturday, September 24th, 1932.

be heard shrieking and cursing as they struggled to get free.

Then up came the posse of Bow Street Runners, to find the whole road blocked and no way of getting through.

Jack Pryse, who had helped Hal and Jerry to escape from the convict hulk, had got a flying start.

As Hal picked himself up from the road and brushed the dust from his clothes he found himself staring into the cold, calculating eyes and grim, set face of Martin Cosgrave, the Bow Street Runner!

A Narrow Escape!

HAL LOVETT held his breath as he looked into the stern eyes of Cosgrave. The man's eyes seemed to bore right through him, to read his mind.

"I believe," said the Runner, bending in the saddle as he reached out for Hal's shoulder, "I've seen you before!"

Hal did not answer. He wanted to turn and run, but the way was barred by the overturned coach and the four struggling horses, who were plunging madly as they tried to regain their feet.

Hal believed that Martin Cosgrave had recognised him, and felt that he was lost.

"What madman overturned the coach?" Cosgrave demanded, drawing back the clutching hand and staring hard at Hal.

"Oh, it was the coachman!" answered Jerry McLean, who had sprung to safety when the coach crashed, and now loomed up beside Hal. "The fellow lost his head."

The coachman did not hear, for he was bent double trying to loosen straps and buckles and free the harnessed horses, the capes of his great coat floating over his ears.

"H'm!" grunted Martin Cosgrave, staring hard at McLean, and taking in appraisingly the faded finery which Jerry had that day bought at Isaac Sloman's, in London.

Hal Lovett bit nervously at his underlip. Had Cosgrave recognised Jerry, too, he wondered. He had been present at the trial at the Old Bailey. Often he had talked to Hal in the streets that abut on Covent Garden.

But the Bow Street Runner seemed suddenly to remember that the coach had been robbed. Swinging his fine horse round, he pointed in the direction Jack Pryse had gone.

"After him," he cried, "and take him dead or alive! Don't wait there, gaping like a lot of schoolboys! Get round that coach and ride him down!"

And he himself, since they were slow to move, pushed his horse among the others, gained the bank beside the road, and went slithering over it.

In a moment he was by, and the others made after him, finding a path in single file. Soon the last of the Redbreasts—as the Runners were popularly called—had scrambled past the barrier, the whole posse vanishing in a clatter of pounding hoof-beats and a cloud of flying dust.

And with their going the coachman gave tongue.

"Which of you overturned my coach?" he wanted to know. "Where's Jim? Hey, Jim! Come and help us get these horses up, and to right the coach!"

"Coach won't run no more to-night, Walter," answered the guard, as he came up holding his dented horn in gloved hands. "The rear axle's broke."

"Dang it! And darn it!" howled the driver, as he flung his hat down on the dusty road. "Did ye ever hear the like?"

And then the passengers joined in the chorus of lamentation, cursing the highwayman, blaming the driver, and wanting to know how they were going to reach Maidstone that night.

"Reckon some of you'll have to walk," said the coachman. "The Billings' coach won't have room for all of ye!" And then he caught sight of Hal, and strode up to him angrily. "Here's the one who toppled the coach over! Oh, he's a dark 'un, he is! He was workin' in wi' the highwayman!"

But Jerry McLean intervened.

"I'd advise you to keep your tongue quiet," he said. "The horses were scared. All my friend did was to try to quiet them."

Then Jerry drew Hal away.

"Let's get our luggage, lad," he said, "and we'll foot it to the inn."

And so they dragged their chests out of the bootikin, and shouldered them, and together they started upon their long walk to the Swan With Two Necks. The wooden chests were heavy, but they did not mind. And as soon as they were out of earshot and the overturned coach had been swallowed by a bend in the road, Jerry began to laugh.

"Fancy the highwayman being Jack Pryse, Hal, boy!" he said. "Jack's alive. I reckoned he must have got away from the burning hulk, but it's good to know he is safe."

"The Runners are splendidly mounted. I'm afraid they'll run him down," said Hal, as he swung the heavy chest from shoulder to shoulder without even changing stride.

"H'm! They have the pace of him. But Jack's cute. He can look after himself. I don't think they'll take him. And, thanks to your blocking the way with the overturned coach, he got a long start. That's not what is troubling me, boy."

"What then?" asked Harry.

"Cosgrave knew us. I saw the gleam of recognition in his eyes. Hal, he's the cleverest of all the Bow Street Runners. And since he did not apprehend us, I'm wondering what he is scheming in his mind."

They swung along with raking strides, two gentlemen of the town, to judge from their appearance, and each one weighted down by a heavy trunk.

"Hal," said McLean presently, "did you once tell me that Cosgrave liked you?"

"He seemed to. He used to talk to me whenever he passed my father's shop in Wych Street."

"And he saw that red falcon tattooed on your chest?"

"Yes."

"Did he ever refer to that?"

"Only once when he asked me how I came by it."

"Well, in my opinion, he gave us a chance to-night," said McLean, "because if he recognised us, he must know we both escaped from the convict hulk Ethalion. Then why did he give us the chance?"

But since Hal Lovett could not answer him, Jerry McLean lapsed into silence, and in this manner, trudging manfully on, they at last reached the Swan With Two Necks, and dumped the chests down within the hall, only too glad to ease the muscles of their aching arms.

In the hall they found mine host, Peter Davey, waiting for them, and holding in his palm a great silver turnip of a watch whose dial Peter eyed critically.

"Why, what's to do, gentlemen?" cried Peter. "Where's the coach? I've got a bowl of rum freshly brewed for the passengers. But not a sound of horn or rumble of wheel have we heard, though she's been overdue this hour past."

Jerry McLean told the story of the highway robbery, to which Peter Davey listened intently, whilst the sinister figure of Tom Kinch, the potman, hovered in the background.

A while later, over a bite of supper and a tankard of foaming ale, Jerry told Peter Davey more about the robbery, and told how he had recognised Jack Pryse, and how Jack had been responsible for his and Hal's escape from the convict hulk.

Peter nodded his grand old head approvingly.

"If your friend is one of the right kind, I'm glad he got away from that bloodhound Cosgrave," said he. "And if you think Cosgrave guessed who you were, I'd advise you to be on your guard, sir. Perhaps you would be wise to leave my inn."

"We'll stay another day, Peter," said Jerry, as with a yawn and a stretch, he prepared himself for bed.

The Runners Arrive!

IN the morning Hal and Jerry were up and about almost as soon as the bustle and clatter in the inn began. They ate a hearty breakfast in the coffee-room, during which they heard the lively chatter of travellers who passed in and out of the inn yard in a constant stream.

And with it all they gathered some news.

None of the passengers on the overturned Maidstone coach had gone on to their destination. The highwayman had got away with a rich haul. And, what was more, he had got the better of Cosgrave and his Bow Street Runners.

Jerry dropped a hand on Hal's across the table and winked.

"Did you hear that now?" he asked.

A little while afterwards they gathered from the ostler how the highwayman had hoodwinked the Runners.

"It seems he was a desperate cove, sir," said the ostler, as he chewed at a pipe of straw, "and a new 'un at the game, they say. Any rate, 'e's got nerve. He's the one who robbed the farmer out on Blackheath t'other night, for he was ridin' the stolen 'oss, a bag o' bones only fit for the knacker's yard. And 'ere's where 'is cleverness comes in. 'E 'ad a long start, but the Runners were finely mounted and on fresh 'osses. They rode him down. But one of them, an officer named Martin, eager to get his man, gained a long lead on t'others. And what does the 'ighwayman do?"

"What did he do?" asked Jerry lazily, his hands set deep in his pockets and his feet spread wide, whilst he grinned happily at Hal.

"Slips his 'oss in amongst the trees on Shooter's 'Ill, waits till the Runner rides up, then dashes out on him, ducks the bullet, and tips him outer the saddle on to his head as clean as a whussle. And then, the Runner being stunned, he pinches his fresh 'oss, and gets clean away on it!"

"Smart!" said Jerry.

"Ay," muttered the ostler, shaking his almost bald head, "I'll say it was smart. But a batch of reinforcements have galloped out of Lunnon town, and, what wi' highwayman abroad, and convicts at large, they're scouring every bush and copse and cottage and barn the county through. For Mr. Cosgrave, they say, is the last man to take it lying down."

Soon after lunch a coach arrived, and with it a messenger in charge of the saddles which Isaac Sloman had promised to send. Jerry tipped the messenger, unpacked the saddles, and had them carried out to the yard.

And there he told the ostler to saddle Galloper so that the horse should be ready for the road in case of emergency. Jerry had given measurements with accuracy, and the saddle was a perfect fit.

"Didn't know you wuz a military gent, sir," said the ostler, as he remarked upon the pistol holsters.

"I am not, Bob," answered Jerry, "but with highwaymen and escaped convicts around, I intend to go armed when I ride abroad."

Hal was not yet provided with a horse, but landlord Peter Davey lent him a smart grey, and this horse also was saddled. The holsters were filled. McLean and Hal packed black masks in their riding coats, and lists of inns and friendly landlords up and down the country which Peter Davey provided were pocketed as a further precaution.

The afternoon came and began to wane, and the only arrivals at the Swan With Two Necks were gossips from the villages, who came to talk over the coach robbery.

So evening came, and, feeling easier in their minds, Jerry and Hal sat down to dinner. Here Peter joined them.

"I tell you what it is, Tom Kinch," said Peter, angered by the long face of the man. "I shall have to give you marching orders. It's time I got another potman."

Kinch did not answer, but the look he shot at Peter and Jerry and Hal was full of venom.

Jerry had just helped Hal to a second serving of the prime, juicy rump steak which formed the basis of the meal when of a sudden there was a great hubbub and clatter in the yard. Hal put down his knife and fork, and drew back the curtain which screened the window.

Through the thick, small panes of glass he saw that the yard was full of horsemen. His keen eyes roamed over three-cornered hats and red waistcoats. His ears rang to the echo of clanking swords, ringing spurs, and voices raised almost to a shout. For a moment he sat as if frozen to his seat.

"Jerry," gasped Hal, as soon as he had recovered from the shock, "the Bow Street Runners!"

Peter Davey's chin drooped, his jovial, ruddy face lengthened. But in a moment he was himself again.

"Better not be trapped in your pew, gentlemen," he whispered.

Jerry McLean and Hal scuttled out of it, abandoning their meal.

"Come with me upstairs," whispered Peter, taking Hal by the arm. "The Swan is full of bolt holes."

But before they could get clear of the room there was a surge of men, who entered from the yard and from the front of the inn simultaneously, men in blue coats and scarlet waistcoats, who walked with ringing steps.

And in front of those who entered from the yard came Tom Kinch, who, pointing at Jerry and Hal, said, in a shrill, squeaking treble:

"There they are, Mr. Cosgrave! They're convicts escaped from the hulk Ethalion. Arrest 'em, and give me the reward!"

Jerry and Hal were surrounded in a moment by strapping, broad-shouldered men who eyed them fixedly. Some were jeering, some were smiling, others looked grim.

Martin Cosgrave alone betrayed no sign of emotion. His keen, sharp eyes looked into Hal's, into McLean's.

"H'm!" remarked the celebrated Bow Street Runner. "This man declares you are escaped convicts. What are your names?"

"My name is Palmer," said Jerry carelessly, and without hesitation. "This is my younger brother Ted. We live at Canterbury, and are riding there to-morrow."

Mr. Cosgrave's eyes wrinkled into a grim smile, his lips at the same time curving downward.

"Indeed!" he said. "And what would you say if I told you your name was Jerry McLean, and that your brother's name was Lovett, eh?"

His right hand sought his pocket and dived beneath the big flap. It came out again gripping a staff with a crown on top of it, and this he held up to view.

"Jerry McLean and Hal Lovett," he said briskly, "I arrest you in the King's name!"

(Hal and Jerry are in a tight corner now, through the treacherous Tom Kinch. Don't miss the thrilling developments in next Saturday's extra special number of the MAGNET. *And, remember, chums, the first SIX SUPER STAMPS will be presented FREE in this issue.)*